A HISTORY OF
ENDOCRINOLOGY

Victor Cornelius Medvei

CBE, MD, FRCP

Chevalier de l'Ordre National du Mérite de France

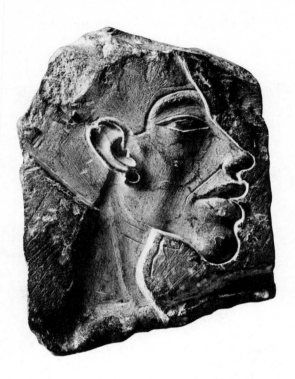

A HISTORY OF ENDOCRINOLOGY

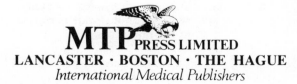

MTP PRESS LIMITED
LANCASTER · BOSTON · THE HAGUE
International Medical Publishers

Published in the UK and Europe by
MTP Press Limited
Falcon House
Lancaster, England

British Library Cataloguing in Publication Data

Medvei, Victor Cornelius
A history of endocrinology.
1. Endocrinology – History
I. Title
616.4   RC648

ISBN 0–85200–245–9

Published in the USA by
MTP Press
A division of Kluwer Boston Inc
190 Old Derby Street
Hingham, MA 02043, USA

Library of Congress Cataloging in Publication Data

Medvei, Victor Cornelius.
A history of endocrinology.

1. Endocrinology—History. I. Title.
QP187.M43   612.4   81–20782
ISBN 0–85200–245–9   AACR2

Text set in 11/12 pt Linotron 202 Bembo, printed and bound
in Great Britain at The Pitman Press, Bath

DEDICATED

to my wife; without her love, inspiration, continuous encouragement and active help, this work could not have been carried through;

to my teachers, especially to the memory of Professor Julius Bauer (1887–1979), my guide, mentor and friend during my formative years;

and to the memory of my true friend, Lt.-Commander Malcolm H. C. Young, BSc, RN (1903–1940), who was killed in action for his country and for the idea that others may live in freedom: *vir bonus, civis fortis, amicus fidelis*.

CONTENTS

PREFACE

No history of endocrinology can be written without reference to Sir Humphry Davy Rolleston, whose monumental study of the subject appeared in 1936 under the modest subtitle: *The Endocrine Organs in Health and Disease with an Historical Review*. It was based on the author's Fitzpatrick Lectures at the Royal College of Physicians of London in 1933 and 1934. The lectureship, which dates from 1901, is devoted to the History of Medicine.

Rolleston's work as regards scholarship and delivery cannot be surpassed and will remain the solid basis for any further study. It is of interest to note that Rolleston gave the Fitzpatrick Lectures when he was 71 years of age and had his book published when he was 74. By that time he had achieved most of his professional aims and all the honours a distinguished medical career can offer (see Section II). He perceived clearly that endocrinology was "an enormous subject in a most active stage of growth", which "recently has received most valuable help from organic chemists, who have devoted much time to the elucidation of the structure, isolation and synthesis of the hormones". He remarked that the knowledge of endocrinology was expanding with extreme rapidity, and it has been suggested that in this respect it would appear to be itself influenced by a growth hormone. He continued: "Before 1890 there were comparatively few publications dealing with the ductless glands, but in 1913, A. Biedl's book *Die Innere Sekretion* contained a bibliography of no less than 256 pages and references to about 8500 articles, and by 1925 there were more than 3000 articles published every year"; but even Rolleston could not foresee the present development of endocrinology which has proceeded at the rate of an atomic explosion. He did comment on the first special journals on the subject in the United States, in

Germany, in France and in Italy. The first International Endocrine Congress to be held in Marienbad, in the summer of 1934, was organized by Julius Bauer (see Section II), whose fame rested on the study of the constitutional aspects of disease and on the study of endocrine disorders. His efforts failed, because he had criticized the trend of medicine in Hitler's Germany. It took another 26 years before the 1st International Congress of Endocrinology took place in Copenhagen, in 1960.

The present writer was so impressed by Rolleston's book that he suggested to its publishers, the Oxford University Press, in March, 1949, that they should produce a second edition. I quote from their reply on 31 March:

> ... We are indeed gratified to have your appreciative comments on our publication of the late Sir Humphry Rolleston's *Endocrine Organs in Health and Disease*. Our own belief, and the opinion of impartial critics, make us endorse all you are good enough to say, yet it is a regrettable fact that this notable work did not enjoy a circulation fully commensurate with its merits. ... This fact makes us hesitant to embark upon a second edition, and we are further discouraged by the weight of our existing commitments. Nevertheless, if circumstances permit at any future time, we will gladly give due consideration to your suggestion; in any event we regard ourselves as privileged in having placed our imprint on a monograph which has been distinguished by the favourable notice of so many competent judges.

It was signed by the Medical Editor. It did not take into account that six years of war had had a damping effect on the pursuit of the study of endocrinology and, obviously, on the commercial aspect of scientific publishing. There has been no second edition to the present day.

In 1950, *CIBA Monographs* of CIBA Ltd. in Basle, produced a special number, devoted to 'Internal secretion', containing three essays by R. Abderhalden on 'The antecedents of endocrinology', 'From the history of endocrinology', and 'The development of clinical endocrinology', which the present writer rendered into English (published by CIBA Monographs in Bombay, July, 1951). Since that time, there has been a spate of papers on further developments in endocrinology. H. M. Bottcher (b. 1895) published (in German): *Hormone: Die Geschichte der Hormonforschung*, Cologne, 1963. Two books appeared on *The History of Diabetes Mellitus* by Nikos S. Papaspyros (2nd ed. Stuttgart, G, Thieme, 1964), and *The Story of Insulin: Forty Years Success Against Diabetes* by G. A. Wrenshall *et al.* (London, Bodley Head, 1962).

I have not been able to find another complete work in book form devoted to the history of endocrinology in the English language.

Various suggestions to several publishers to commission such an undertaking have been unsuccessful over the years, and I am pleased that the present publishers have shown the courage to support such a venture. I only hope that my endeavour will prove that there is a need for this book, and will not disappoint the public or the publishers.

In the second Hermon Ould Memorial Lecture on 'History as an Art', given by the late Bertrand Russell before the members of the P.E.N. Club in London on 4 May, 1954, which I attended, Russell presented his reasons for believing that the applications of scientific laws to the writing of history are not so important nor so discoverable as is often suggested. The most important modern inventors of general theories about human development and progress had been Hegel and his disciple Marx. They believed that the history of past events was subject to a logical schema which would enable its students to foretell the future. Neither could foresee the hydrogen bomb and the effect of that device. History could produce the best possible result in a non-historical reader only if it was made interesting not only to those who wished to know some set of historical facts for a special reason, but also to those who read it in the spirit in which one reads poetry or a good novel. It meant first and foremost that the historian should have feelings about the events he was telling about and the characters he was portraying. It was, obviously, imperative that he should not distort facts, but it was *not* imperative that he should not take sides in the conflicts depicted in the narrative. Russell disliked the tendency of some modern historians to tone down everything dramatic and pretend that heroes were not so heroic and villains not so villainous. There seemed to be a tendency in our time to pay too little attention to the individual and too much to the mass. We were so indoctrinated that we lived in the age of the common man, that men became common even when they might be otherwise. What was dangerously false was the suggestion that people regarded as heroes were merely representing social forces whose work could and would have been done by someone else if it had not been done by them. The worst of such a view was that, if it was held, it tended to become true. Heroic lives have always been inspired by heroic ambitions, and the young man who thought there was nothing important to be done, was pretty sure to do nothing important.

I was much impressed by Lord Russell's lucidly and brilliantly presented thesis. It will be seen – I hope – in the course of our progress through the history of endocrinology, that those views apply as much in this case as to the writing of political history.

In this book quotations from works in Latin, Italian, French and

German will be given in the original language, in most cases with an English translation. There are some exceptions where a translation is not offered. This is intentional, because it was felt that an unequivocal translation was difficult.

I am fully aware of the criticism that scientists in English-speaking countries – and especially in Great Britain – today believe that an English translation of a foreign text is sufficient. It will be seen in Chapter 13, p. 138, that H. H. Simmer felt that Thomas Willis and Richard Lower were wrongly credited with the suggestion of pituitary hormones. The key to such claims lies in the translation of one of Willis's sentences from the Latin, by Harvey Cushing. That translation is, however, faulty.

For the same reason, I was given to understand, (Sir) Charles Robert Harington, in his classic treatise on *The Thyroid Gland, its Chemistry and Physiology* (London, OUP, 1933), put his numerous citations from the Latin, French and German in the original, *without* an English translation, in order to avoid any misinterpretation. Sir (later Lord) Solly Zuckerman quoted an extensive passage from Lieutaud in French, with an English translation.

The present writer has come across quotations from Théophile de Bordeau, wrongly translated, but especially several translations from German sources which were incorrect. No excuse is offered, therefore, for the method employed in this book.

At this juncture I have to make another point. For those rigid adherents to the Imrad style of writing scientific papers, the presentation of the material in this book will be God's gift for critical reviews. From 1928 to 1981, however, I have been – as Sir Alan S. Parkes has put it (see p. 399), an eye-witness of the developments in the field of endocrinology, and at times these developments seemed to advance at an incredible pace. Personal experiences related by my teachers extended that span of time in retrospect by another thirty years (i.e. from 1898 onwards). Whenever possible, I have, therefore, attempted to relate the story of research and discoveries, as they occurred. In this endeavour I have occasionally been handicapped by three factors: One was ignorance, that is, when I did not know the true nature and sequence of events; secondly, by the needs of personal discretion, in cases when people, who were the dramatis personae, were still alive (David Marine, for example, was 97 when he died in 1977; Julius Bauer died in May, 1979 in his 92nd year; and so did Herrman Zondek; A. W. Spence is 80) or where their families and pupils would be embarrassed or distressed. Thirdly, because I could not inflict on my long-suffering publishers a further expansion of a book which originally – I hoped – would not exceed about 350 pages. On a number of occasions, I had to give what almost seems to amount to a list of the explosive progress of research; but this I did only if I thought that each discovery implied progress in the field. A strictly critical approach was used when it was felt that criticism was justified, for example in the case of the story of insulin. Otherwise, I have attempted to follow Descartes' method; when his critics declared that he should have presented his arguments in the strict form of mathematical and logical discipline instead of his informal and chatty style, he explained the two methods of exposition as follows:

> Analysis demonstrates the true way by which a thing was methodically discovered ... so that, if a reader cares to follow it and bestow sufficient attention to the (developing) argument, he will understand the matter no less perfectly and make it his own as if he had discovered it himself. ... On the contrary, the synthetic method uses an opposite procedure. It does demonstrate clearly its conclusions, employing a long series of definitions, postulates, axioms, theorems. ... The reader is compelled to give his consent, however hostile and obstinate his attitude may be; but this method is not so satisfactory as the first and does not make the keen learner equally contented, because it does not show the way in which the subject taught was (really) discovered.

J. N. Watkins, who compared Descartes' methodology with that of Isaac Newton, for example, comes down in favour of Descartes, in preference of "the dead-pan didactic" method of Newton. (Watkins, J. W. N.: Confession is good for ideas. In: *Experiment: A Series of Scientific Case Histories*. London, BBC, 1964.) He does not deny that Newton was a genius nor that he did not make fundamental discoveries, but he feels that Newton used his method mainly to silence – *a priori* – undesirable critics who are always ready to pounce on ideas different from the accepted ones, be they William Harvey, Descartes, Addison, or merely lesser fry. Does not the Imrad method do the same?

Finally, I was surprised, in the course of carrying out research for this book, in how many instances I was unable to find the date, place and cause of death of many well-known scientists in the field, born after 1850, or if they were dead at all! This applied to many people in the Americas; searches carried out most kindly by the Wellcome Institute for the History of Medicine and the Royal Society of Medicine in London and (in the USA) by the National Library of Medicine and the Endocrine Society yielded only a few dates. Many of the Institutions where the people concerned had worked, seemed to have lost track of them once they had left or retired.

This state of affairs may seem amazing, but it is a sad fact.

ACKNOWLEDGEMENTS

My grateful acknowledgements are due to The Wellcome Trust and to Messrs. Squibb and Sons Ltd., who so generously contributed towards the financial cost for preparing this book. I also acknowledge gratefully the great help I received from the Librarian of the Royal Society of Medicine in London and his staff; from Professor Erna Lesky and Universitäts-Professor Dr. Helmut Wyklicky of the University Institute for the History of Medicine in Vienna; the help of Mr. John L. Thornton, FLA, formerly Librarian of the Medical College of St. Bartholomew's Hospital, London; the kindness of Professor Hans H. Simmer of the University Institute for the History of Medicine, Erlangen; the help of Miss Merriley Borell, PhD, of the History of Medicine Unit, History Department of the University of Edinburgh and of Professor Peter M. Daniel of the University of London (Neuropathology), whose interest and encouragement proved invaluable. There are many others, whom I cannot name individually in the short space allotted, but to whom I am deeply grateful and much indebted. My grateful thanks are also due to Mrs. Joan Peake and Mrs. Sheila M. Rudge who so meticulously re-typed my first script. Last, but by no means least, I would like to acknowledge the help, patience and understanding of my publishers, especially of their Managing Director, Mr. D. G. T. Bloomer and the Editor, Mr. P. Johnstone, and their staff.

London, May, 1981   V.C.M.

THE HISTORY

INTRODUCTION

THE living organism is a very complex system. To stand up to the dangers of life, to feed, to digest, to procreate, to be born, to survive, to grow and to develop and – all the time – to remain in an equilibrium which is satisfactory, it needs the ability of quick decision and action. To be able to flee or fight, good internal communication is necessary. The higher the development of the living body, the more important such communication becomes. In the vertebrates, the mammals and the peak of creation, man, this sytem is most complex. The nervous system, comprising the brain, the spinal cord, the communicating motor and sensory nerves, supported by the sympathetic and parasympathetic nervous system, guarantee high-speed information and the ability to react. The transmission is by electric stimuli; the whole system is like a computerized telephone network.

Curiously, it has taken much longer to realize the existence of the somewhat slower, but equally important system of communication, the 'canal system' of the body. The circulation of the blood was first described correctly by William Harvey, an Englishman, at the beginning of the 17th century. It took another 250 years before it was realized that every organ of the body can send messages and messengers, using that system of circulation and its fluid, the blood, to other organs. At the target, those messengers link to receptors and deliver the message. For certain particularly important purposes, such as resistance to stresses, growth, procreation, pregnancy, child-birth and lactation, special organs have emerged, the main function of which is the production, storage and discharge of these compli-cated chemical messengers via the blood, by the 'humoral' method. The most important of these organs take on the shape of glandular

3

structures. Some of these glands, like the pancreas (or sweetbread) have a double function: They produce chemical substances which they 'excrete' or yield through special ducts, leading for example into the small intestine, to further digestion; at the same time, they have islands of groups of different cells, which produce special chemical messengers like insulin, which is discharged directly into the blood and regulates sugar-metabolism. Some glands produce only chemical messengers for blood transport: Such are the gonads or sex glands, the glands near the kidneys or suprarenal glands, the thyroid gland in the neck.

It soon became obvious that there is a complicated regulatory mechanism within this glandular system, and in the 1930s the concept was created of the 'endocrine orchestra', the glands which discharge their products into the blood directly being called 'endocrine' glands, as will be explained presently. The conductor of the orchestra was found to be the pituitary gland, below the brain.

In the last 50 years, however, it became clear that there is a close connection and co-operation between the communication network of the nervous system and of the humoral system; in fact, the release of hormones is controlled by the brain, the most important junction being the so-called hypothalamus part of the brain. Intensive research has been carried out in the last twenty years to unravel this connection; we are now going through a most exciting phase of these discoveries. It has been established that the 'master' endocrine gland is the brain itself, which produces, among others, its own painkilling hormone, the 'people's opiate', and links have been demonstrated with the working of the ancient Chinese procedure, acupuncture.

It is with the history and development of this field of natural sciences that this book is concerned.

A history of endocrinology must, at first glance, appear synonymous with the history of endocrine glands and with that of internal secretions. On second thoughts, the situation needs some clarification.

As Sir William Maddox Bayliss (see Section II) has put it in his *Principles of General Physiology*[1]:

> There are a large number of substances, acting powerfully in minute amount, which are of great importance in physiological processes.
>
> One class of these consists of the hormones, or chemical messengers, which are produced in a particular organ, pass into the blood current and produce effects in distant organs. They provide, therefore, for a chemical co-ordination of the activities of the organism, working side by side with that through the nervous system.
>
> The internal secretions, formed by ductless glands, as well as by other tissues, belong to the class of hormones.

> There are interrelations between certain of these internal secretions,
> but at present their nature is still very obscure.

This understanding of the role of the hormones is fairly recent. It
was Claude Bernard (see Section II), who first said in a lecture on 9
January, 1855, that the liver has an external secretion in the form of
bile and an internal one of sugar which passes directly into the
general circulation. The modern idea of internal secretion may,
therefore, be dated from the middle of the 19th century.

The anatomical knowledge of the organs in the body which are
now known as the 'ductless' or 'endocrine' glands, is from a much
earlier date. In recent years, the list of these organs has increased, as it
became known that some organs have exocrine and endocrine
capacity.

Evidence of abnormal endocrine function has, however, existed
since ancient times, and no history of the field of endocrinology can
omit that evidence. Moreover, it may give an insight into the social
and psychological response to such conditions in various communities and cultures.

There is also evidence that forms of treatment of diseases existed in
ancient times, in Chinese, Biblical, Greek, Roman and other cultural
antiquity, which nowadays would be regarded as attempts at hormone replacement.

A history of endocrinology must take these facts into account.

It must also take into consideration that endocrinology, as it has
developed in the 20th century, is a field, not a discipline, because it is
not unified by common techniques (like biochemistry or genetics)[2].
It has drawn on the labour of researchers from various disciplines
and – at varied periods – the field has been dominated by one or
more individual disciplines. During the past fifty years physiology,
biochemistry, immunology and molecular biology, especially, made
the greatest impact. "In all periods, however, practical clinical and
social concerns have prevented the total submersion of the field
within the dominant discipline."[2]

Accordingly, endocrinologists with a holistic outlook presented the
field in the manner of Sir Humphry Davy Rolleston. As a clinician
and student of the human body in health and disease, he defined
endocrinology as the study of all aspects of the ductless glands, from
the clinical to the biochemical.

In the same year that Rolleston's *The Endocrine Organs in Health and
Disease* was published (1936), the American endocrinologist Edward
A. Doisy (see Section II) delivered the Porter lectures on *Sex
Hormones*[3] at the University of Kansas School of Medicine. In his
historical approach he stressed "change rather than continuity in the

field". For him, endocrinology was just beginning, as the newly trained biochemical researchers laid the foundations for a reliable science of endocrinology. Doisy defines, therefore, 'four stages' of endocrinology:

(1) Recognition of the gland or organ as one producing internal secretion.

(2) Methods of detecting internal secretion.

(3) Preparation of extracts leading to a purified hormone.

(4) The isolation of the pure hormone, determination of its structure and its synthesis.

His presentation of the result of a hormone investigation is given in the following example:

Hormone	Preparation of active extracts	Isolation	Synthesis
Adrenaline	Oliver and Schafer 1894	Takamine 1901	Stolz 1904

A different approach appeared in Arthur F. W. Hughes' (see Section II) posthumously published paper, 'A history of endocrinology'[4]. His work on neuro-secretions influenced his outlook, especially when discussing the hypothalamo-pituitary axis and negative feedback. He also studied and analysed the statistics from the *Journal of Biological Abstracts*, which first appeared in 1926. Until well into the 1930s the annual level of laboratory studies in endocrinology was about 300. "Since 1946, however, the yearly number of papers has risen rapidly . . ." preceding a general increase in biological activity. Hughes' figures seem to indicate that the development of growth of biochemical endocrinology did not become apparent in the total growth of the endocrine field until over ten years after the publication of Doisy's chart, reaching a peak of nearly 1800 in 1951.

Long Hall and Glick[2] draw the important conclusion from this fact that ". . . one can see the complexity of development and conflicting historical interpretations that one would expect in a subject that is a field and not a discipline". Hughes concludes:

> The early history of the subject can appropriately be regarded as a sequence of clear-cut advances. Yet similar treatment of more recent phases inevitably involves wholesale arbitrary selection, thus obscuring the accompanying penumbra of contradictory and unconfirmed findings which necessarily form a prominent element of discussion in contemporary critical reviews. Only in this way can the history of science be related to its present course.

Before we begin, it will be appropriate to give a few derivations of some words, much used in the endocrine field, most of which date from the 19th and the present century.

In 1766 Albrecht von Haller (see Section II) grouped together the thymus, thyroid and spleen as *glands without ducts*, which pour a special substance into the veins and thus into the general circulation. He referred back to F. Ruysch (1638–1731), who had said that a peculiar fluid was made in such glands, which went into the veins.

As said before, Claude Bernard used first the term 'internal secretion' in 1855. 'Endocrine' and 'Endocrinology' came into use in the 20th century. ἔνδον (endon) is an adverb in classical Greek and means inside, within, in contrast to ἔξω (exo) which means outside, externally, hence exocrine glands = glands with external secretion. κρίνω (krino), a Greek verb, meaning to separate, sift. In 1905, Professor Ernest H. Starling (see Section II) used the word 'hormone' for the first time in his Croonian lectures at the Royal College of Physicians, 'On the Chemical Correlation of the Functions of the Body'. His actual words were: "... these chemical messengers, however, or hormones as we may call them". The reason for this was that Bayliss and Starling had felt – after their discovery of secretin in 1902 – that the term 'internal secretion' did not define the nature of a chemical substance produced in any tissue of the body, and not necessarily in a ductless gland, and carried by the blood to other parts, where it excites reactions which affect the organism as a whole. Considering the problem of correct terminology, eventually the word 'hormone' was suggested by Sir William B. Hardy of Gonville and Caius College, Cambridge, and his classical colleague W. T. Vesey. It is derived from ὁρμάω (hormao), a Greek verb, meaning to put into quick motion, to excite or arouse. Nearly 250 years before, John Smith (1630–1679), DM, FCP London, of Brasenose College, Oxford, had used the word 'hormetic' (ὁρμητικά meaning having the property of stimulating), in 1666, when writing of the "hormetick power and contraction of the muscles". Sir Edward Albert Schaefer (see Section II), while accepting the word 'hormone' for a messenger with stimulating effect, suggested the word 'chalones' (χαλάω = chalao = I relax) for chemical messengers with a depressing or inhibitory effect, in 1913. He also proposed, with Professor W. R. Wardle's help, the word 'autacoids' (αὐτός autos = self; ἄκος akos = a remedy) to cover both previous terms. Eugène Gley (see Section II), also at the International Congress of Medicine in London in 1913, suggested the word 'harmozones' (ἁρμόζω = harmozo, meaning I regulate) for the hormones of the interstitial cells of the testicles, the corpus luteum, the thyroid and the pituitary, which have influence on

7

growth and nutrition. For substances like CO_2, which are metabolic products, but modify activities in distant parts of the body, Gley suggested the term 'parhormones'. N. Pende (see Section II) used 'endocrinology' in 1909. Artur Biedl (see Section II) published his book *Innere Sekretion* in 1910[5], but Wilhelm Falta's (see Section II) book, published in 1913, bore the title *Die Erkrankungen der Blutdruesen*[6] (*The Diseases of the Bloodglands*), which became in the English translation in 1915: *Endocrine Diseases Including their Diagnosis and Treatment*.

The ductless glands were, in the first half of the 19th century, commonly spoken of as the vascular or blood glands, partly because it was thought that in some manner they modified the blood supply and partly because of their own rich blood supply. Falta argued that the "clinical definition of a number of those disease entities which we call today 'Diseases of the Bloodglands' is – to a certain extent – much older than the concept of internal secretion, obtained from experimental pathology". He pointed to the effect of human castration, known in antiquity, when eunuchs played an important role. Similarly, animal breeders had a good empirical knowledge of the effects of castration when attempting to fatten pigs, bullocks or capons, long before discussing the question in what manner the gonads influence the distribution of body fat. Falta concluded his introductory remarks as follows:

> One may define the sum total of all cell complexes, which are capable of internal secretion, as the hormopoetical system. There are, however, a number of organs (of the body), the specific function of which we have to regard as the production of especially important hormones, which possess powerful physiological characteristics. These organs have in common, that they yield their specific secretion directly into the blood circulation. They are, therefore, called 'Bloodglands', and their total expanse, the 'Bloodgland System'.

Both Biedl and Falta discussed the neuro-humoral influences of the 'bloodglands', but Biedl underlined the fact that an (empirical) knowledge of humoral organ-correlations existed *before* the knowledge of neuro-mechanisms. This is obvious from the existence of pre-historic organotherapy. Falta used the expression "hormopoietic" before W. S. Halsted, who did so in The Harvey Lectures (Philadelphia, 1913–1914).

In the United States, Charles Euchariste de Médici Sajous (1852–1929) was the first to publish, in 1903, a treatise on "The internal secretions and the principles of medicine"[7]. He allotted the control of the immunizing mechanisms of the body to the adrenal, pituitary and thyroid glands. He regarded the hormone of the adrenal medulla the dominant factor[7].

8

INTRODUCTION

The words 'dysfunction', 'dysthyroidism', and 'dyspituitarism' were originally used in two different senses, which is somewhat confusing. They meant (1) an abnormal secretion of a gland; and (2) irregular or overlapping syndromes, dyspituitarism meaning a combination of hyper- and hypo-pituitarism[8]. Similarly, toxic goitre with some features of myxoedema was also called dysthyroidism. This particular application seems today less popular. In the late 1920s the expressions 'Inkretion' and 'Inkretory glands' were used in Germany, but – happily – their use has faded away.

The idea of internal secretions was not readily accepted by some German universities; in 1914 a well-known professor called the theory a "Viennese humbug" ("Wiener Schmarren")[9].

REFERENCES

1. Bayliss, Sir William Maddox: Principles of General Physiology. 4th ed., p. 739. London, 1924.
2. Long Hall, Diana and Glick, Thomas F.: Endocrinology; a brief introduction. J. Hist. Biol. **9** (2), 229–233, 1976.
3. Doisy, Edward A.: Sex Hormones. Porter Lectures Delivered at the University of Kansas School of Medicine. Lawrence, University of Kansas, 1936.
4. Hughes, Arthur F. W.: A history of endocrinology, edited by Egar, Margaret Wells. J. Hist. Med. Allied Sci. xxxii (3), 292–313, 1977.
5. Biedel, Artur: Innere Sekretion. Berlin, Wien, Urban & Schwarzenberg, 1910.
6. Falta, Wilhelm: Die Erkrankungen der Blutdruesen. Berlin, Julius Springer, 1913.
7. Sajous, C. E. de M.: The Internal secretions and the Principles of Medicine. Philadelphia, F. A. Davis, 1903.
8. Cushing, H.: The Pituitary Body and its Disorders. Philadelphia, 1912.
9. Wiel, A.: The history of internal secretions. Medical Life, **32**, 73–97, New York, 1925.

CHAPTER ONE

PREHISTORIC TIMES

G ARRISON asserted the identity of all forms of ancient and primitive medicine. "One of the best accredited doctrines of recent times is that of the unity or solidarity of folk-ways."[1] This is true of all customs of primitive peoples which are concerned with the fundamental instincts of self-preservation and reproduction.

In prehistoric times, and even today among primitive races, the eating of heart, liver, brain, spleen and blood was not uncommon: raw, cooked or in the form of the ashes. Anthropophagi ate the organs of enemies killed in battle; this was ritual theophagy and religious in origin. Others worshipped a species of animal or vegetable (totemism) which was linked closely with the life of the individual member or of the whole of the tribe. The totem animal or vegetable was sacred and was not to be killed or eaten, otherwise the tribe or its member would be similarly afflicted[2]. The exception to this rule occurred at special religious festivities, when the totem was eaten as an act of communion, to increase the mental and physical power of the tribe and prevent moral degeneration. Later, when the origins of the cult had sunk into oblivion, some of the totem animals were used for medicinal purposes, as when – for example – vipers' flesh was used as an antidote to poison.

To eat the heart of an enemy killed in battle in order to obtain his bravery is called an act of cannibalism; it may, however, also be called organotherapy. To drink his blood or devour the extracts of the enemy's organs, Landouzy[3] called 'Opotherapy' in 1898 (ὀπός = juice; θεραπεία = treatment): a habit which still exists, for example, on the continent of Africa.

The question of fertility played an important role, if the tribe were to survive. A woman who failed to conceive and become pregnant

11

was a source of worry and shame. Fertility rites are well known in primitive communities from the earliest times. Probably the earliest known representation of the human figure is the 'Venus of Willendorf' (? 22 000 BC) which was found by Szombathy, in 1908. It is a limestone statuette of 4½ inches, which gives the impression of a female endocrine obesity, and is related to many other representations of a sedentary, overfed woman, vegetating in prehistoric caves,

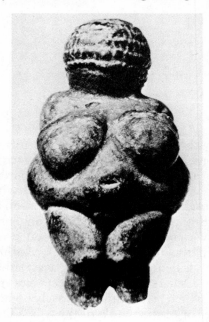

Figure 1 Venus of Willendorf (*ca.* ?22 000 BC) [Naturhistorisches Museum, Vienna]

but also resembles some of the Egyptian carvings or Babylonian bas-reliefs of women[4].

Effective contraceptive practices were rare among primitive people: the main substitutes for the control of conception were – on the few occasions when disease or starvation or natural disaster or defeat in war did not perform that task – abortion and infanticide. Some practices were - and are – coitus interruptus, coitus inter femora, or, in the case of others, the use of tampons of algae or seaweed (Eastern Islanders); the Achehnese women use a tampon with the very effective tannic acid. This applies, of course, only in the case of the primitives who realize that 'coitus makes babies'. Subincision is 'a status-giving ceremony', like circumcision, rather than a consciously employed method of contraception, and is, moreover, hardly effective[5].

The role of the male in the production of offspring was, at any rate, not always understood by some primitive people. Some believed that children were the result of some food the mother had eaten. The Euduna tribe insisted that the women bore half-caste children, because their native mothers had partaken of the white bread the white settlers had introduced, instead of eating the dark native bread. Some tribes share the belief that an invisible 'spirit-baby' enters the woman to produce the child[6]. Paternity is a social rather than a biological concept with most primitive societies.

REFERENCES

1. Garrison, Fielding H.: An Introduction to the History of Medicine. 4th Ed. p. 17. Philadelphia, W. B. Saunders, 1929.
2. Rolleston, H. D.: The Endocrine Organs in Health and Disease. p. 5. London, OUP, 1936.
3. Landouzy, L.: Les Seropathies. p. 9, Paris, 1898.
4. As 1: p. 49.
5. Himes, Norman E.: Medical History of Contraception. p. 54, New York, Gamut Press,1936 (reprinted 1970).
6. Johnston, Donald R.: The history of human infertility. Fertil. Steril. **14,** 262, 1963.

CHAPTER TWO

THE ANCIENT CHINESE

JOSEPH Needham and Lu Gwei-Djen mention that goitre was known in ancient China[1]. They seem to have used burnt sponge and seaweed for its treatment. It was to be taken twice in the spring and summer and three times in the autumn and winter[2], in the form of powder, pills or dissolved in wine (1600 BC).

The elder Polos took with them in 1271 AD, on their second journey to the East from Venice, young Marco Polo, when he was still less than 20 years of age. In his celebrated book *The Travels of Marco Polo*, the heading of Chapter 32 reads: "Of the Province of Karkan, the Inhabitants of which are Troubled with Swollen Legs and with Goitres". He says, "They are in general afflicted with swellings in the legs, and tumours in the throat, occasioned by the quality of the water they drink."[3] It has to be stressed, however, that the inhabitants, although subjects of the Grand Khan, were mainly "Mahometans, with some Nestorian Christians", and the province was not in China proper.

The *Pen Ts'ao ching* (*Great Herbal of the Chinese Pharmacopoeia*) dates back to Emperor Shen Nung (2737 BC) and the *Neiching* (*Canon of Medicine*) to the Emperor Huang-ti (2697 BC). The *Great Herbal* contained organic remedies, not only of vegetarian origin. There was toad's skin for dropsy, hen's gizzard for indigestion and gastric ulcers. Mice were particularly popular, but may have come from Egypt, where they had been used before. Of particular interest is the use of semen of young men for treatment of sexual weakness, a true organotherapy. Eunuchs played an important role at the Court of the emperors and in the civil service.

The effects of castration and infertility were well known and of great concern in Chinese society. Dwarfs acted in ancient China as

15

jesters from the earliest times[4]. Diabetes mellitus had already been studied by Chang Chung-ching, the Chinese Hippocrates (*ca.* 160– *ca.* 219 AD). It was still confused, however, with other ailments, as is shown by the enumeration of its symptoms: polyphagia, polydipsia, pollakisuria, glycosuria (sweet urine), clouding of the urine, frigidity and swelling of the lower limbs. The sweet nature of the urine was, however, not recognized until the 7th century AD[5]. The *Neiching* gives important measures of the bones and the alimentary tract; it is the beginning of physical anthropometry. Knowledge of anatomy was especially fostered by a remarkable work, the *Hsi Yüän Lu* (1241–43), produced during the Sun dynasty (906–1280). It consists of instructions to coroners, giving detailed guidance for the post-mortem examination – before or after burial – looking for the signs of wounds, strangulation, blows, poisoning, evidence of suicide, but also instructions for resuscitation and antidotes for poisoning[6]. Robert van Gulik's detective fiction, centred around Judge Dee Jen-djieh, rests on a sound basis of his extensive Chinese studies, although taking place during the Tang period (618–906 AD). During the Tang dynasty large medical encyclopaedias were published, covering the whole field of medicine. The extensive use of acupuncture with its charts and the intensive study of the pulse added to the general interest in the body. The Chinese took great interest in the philosophy of numbers, which also influenced their ideas on medicine and, within that field, on the difference between the sexual development of the male and female bodies. Female life is dominated by the number seven. Teeth grow at 7 months and 7 years. Puberty begins at 14 with the menarche, and the menopause at 49. For men, the dominant number is eight. Dentition occurs at 8 months and 8 years, puberty at 16 (!), and the male decline at 64. Ch'eng Ta-wei postulated in 1593 AD a mathematical formula for determining the sex of the foetus during intra-uterine life[7]!

The original text of the *Pen-ts'ao ching* was lost and is known only through an annotated edition by T'ao Hung-ching, the *Ming-i-pie-lu*. It contained some very old material, but was composed for the greater part under the early Han dynasty (206 BC–9 AD) by an unknown author. This work deals with 365 mineral, herbal or animal drugs, some of which were mentioned above[8]. (See also pp. 86, 93 and 189 on the use of seaweed for goitre.)

In 624 AD the study of medicine was reformed and put under the control of the T'ai-i-shu (Grand Medical Service), i.e. under state control. Important works, published under the same augury, dealt with a variety of subjects, including deficiency diseases (e.g. beriberi), rickets and goitre[9].

Early Japanese medicine was based largely on Chinese sources, brought over via Korea and partly directly by Chinese refugees.

If the use of male and female hormones from pregnant urine or the placenta appears very modern, it has to be remembered that some female animals eat their placenta, and chimpanzees have been observed to drink their own urine when in labour. Chinese women have been given dried placenta to improve their fertility, whereas Javanese women eat it for the same purpose. Strangely enough, in Kalotaszeg in Hungary a woman who does not want any more pregnancies burns her placenta and mixes the ashes in the drink of her husband[10].

Taoism, the rival of Buddhism, had complicated rules on sex life. The basis of these practices was coitus reservatus. The source of sperm was the brain (see also Aristotle); thus, the sperm which had descended from the brain to the bladder but had not been ejaculated returned to its source. This was called 'returning the essence' (*huan-tsing*). This form of deliberate contraception separated the sexual act for pleasure from that performed for procreation[11].

Confucius said: "There are three things which are unfilial, but the most unfilial of these is to have no sons". In China and Japan large families were regarded as essential, to provide ancestor worshippers and to serve as old age insurance. In the Tang period (618–906 AD) and much later, it was common to have three or four wives, at least in the well-to-do classes. "In fact . . . the rate of reproduction is so high, the arts of production so retarded . . ., and preventive medicine so ill-developed that a high death rate has generally prevailed". In view of this, contraception in ancient China was not seriously considered. Only fairly recently has Hagerty – on the instigation of Norman Himes – been able to obtain evidence that contraceptive prescriptions did exist, to be given mainly to women (usually of higher caste) who had experienced difficulty with childbearing and whose life or health was in jeopardy. In the *Thousand of Gold Prescriptions* by Sun Ssu-mo (who died in 695 AD), there were recipes based on mercury, which, no doubt, were effective, if not dangerous, and might have also acted as abortifacients. There is evidence that the ancient Chinese did practise abortion. "A pill made of oil and quicksilver fried and taken on an empty stomach will prevent one from becoming pregnant[12]."

REFERENCES

1.   Needham, J. and Lu Gwei-Djen: Proto-endocrinology in mediaeval China. Jpn. Stud. Hist. Sci. No. 5 (Tokyo) 1966.

2. Iason, Alfred, H.: The Thyroid Gland in Medical History. p. 14. New York, Froben Press, 1946.
3. Polo, Marco: The Travels. p. 95, London, J. M. Dent & Sons, 1908.
4. Tietze-Conrat, E.: Dwarfs and Jesters in Art. London, Phaidon, 1957.
5. Huard, Pierre and Ming Wong: Chinese Medicine. (Translation) p. 32, London, Weidenfeld & Nicolson, 1968.
6. Garrison, Fielding H.: An Introduction to the History of Medicine. p. 73. Philadelphia, W. B. Saunders, 1929.
7. As 5: pp. 64–65.
8. ibid.: pp. 12–30.
9. ibid.: p. 31.
10. Johnston, D. R.: The History of Human Infertility. Fertil. Steril. **14**, 261–272, 1963.
11. As 5: p. 56.
12. Himes, N. E.: The Medical History of Contraception, pp. 108–111. New York, The Gamut Press, 1936.

CHAPTER THREE

THE EGYPTIANS

WITH the deciphering of the Rosetta stone, the study of ancient Egypt expanded beyond expectation. The yield of information in every field has been enormous. The study of tombs – including the pyramids, of sarcophagi and temples, but especially the discovery of papyri, made it possible to obtain a detailed picture of life in ancient Egypt. In medicine, the Ebers papyrus (dating from *ca.* 1550 BC) from the tomb of El Assassif was one of the most important. Among other things, the diagnosis of pregnancy was discussed in it. It was also said that "women who had spots before their eyes were sterile"[1]. In the Brugsch (medical) papyrus (*ca.* 1350 BC), the following statement is made: "A watermelon pounded, is mixed with the milk of a woman, who has born a son, and is given the patient to drink: if she vomits, she is pregnant, if she has only flatulence, she will never bear again". This sounds like a modern pregnancy test, combined with one for infertility[2]!

It seems that there was a popular knowledge of ovaries in some parts of the Mediterranean world before Herophilus (see Chapter 6) and that the ancient Egyptians performed ovariotomy on human females for the (?) purpose of contraception[3].

Among the 640 cultural objects listed in Sudhoff's (see Section II) catalogue of the International Hygiene Exhibition in Dresden in 1911, there was a queen in labour in an obstetric chair, attended by four midwives (18th dynasty), a circumcision (4000 BC), and a plaque recording a suit for recovery of costs for a clitoridectomy (163 BC). Egypt was also regarded as the aboriginal home of prostitution[4].

The oldest papyri are the gynaecological and veterinary scripts of the Kahun papyri of the Petrie collection of the Middle Kingdom (2160–1788 BC). Gynaecology and obstetrics are represented particularly in the five principal texts by Felix Reinhard. The other important papyrus is the Edwin Smith one (dated *ca*. 1600 BC), which is mainly surgical; but there are five columns on the back with incantations, partly for the rejuvenation of old men; they may well belong to the New Kingdom (1580–1200 BC).

Although the ancient Egyptians were medically – as in many other respects – conservatives (Herodotus said, "they keep the ordinances of their fathers and add none others to them"), they had a surprising fund of medical knowledge. Whether the close connection of the priesthood with medicine was responsible for guaranteeing a high degree of intelligence and education in the case of the priest–doctor is difficult to say.

One of the chapters of the Ebers papyrus deals with anatomy and physiology. A pharmacopoeia provides prescriptions for acute and chronic illnesses: pound a cat's womb and add it to other ingredients; it will prevent hair from losing its pigment. For night blindness "in the eyes", take the roasted liver of an ox and crush it.

Many of the animal remedies used by man all over the world came from ancient Egypt. This applied especially to mice, which became very popular in China[5]. Yet mice were already suspected of disseminating disease (see the Bible, Isaiah, xvi, 17)

The Egyptians and the Babylonians were pioneers in organotherapy and became the teachers in medicine of other nations in the Middle East: "And Moses was learned in all the wisdom of the Egyptians" (Acts, vii, 22). Homer said of them, "[Egypt] teeming with drugs . . . the land where each is a physician, skilful beyond all men. . . ." (*Odyssey*, iv. 230–32). The 700-odd prescriptions mentioned above appear modern in the sense that they give weights and measures, but they are not as carefully chosen as those of Hippocrates.

Herodotus' view of them (in the 5th century BC) as doctors is interesting: "Medicine is practised among them on a plan of separation; each physician treats a single disease, and not more; thus the country abounds with physicians, some undertaking to cure the diseases of the eyes, others of the head, others again of the teeth, others of the intestine and some of those which are internal"[6]. They were, obviously, the forerunners of our modern specialists, the thyroidologists, the diabetologists, the neuro- and psycho-endocrinologists, the experts in conception and infertility and those in contraception. As to the thyroid, there is a relief from Dendera, representing Cleopatra, which shows a fullness of the neck, possibly due to goitre[7] (Figure 2).

Whether the Egyptian god Bes, usually depicted as a dwarf, is achondroplastic or myxoedematous has not been finally decided[8].

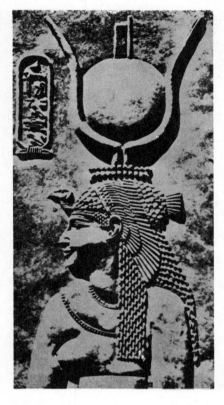

Figure 2 Egyptian carving showing goitre

Seligmann described a skull from Thebes of the 18th dynasty. It showed hypoplasia of bones laid down in cartilage, with signs of arrested growth in the floor of the posterior fossa. The forehead was prominent; the nasal bones and nasal processes of the superior maxillae showed arrested development. Seligmann thought that the formation of the nasal bones excluded achondroplasia and the skull was cretinous[9]. Keith[10] and Brothwell[11] are of an opposite opinion. This goes to illustrate how difficult it is to interpret such findings.

Aldred and Sandison studied in detail the monuments of the Pharaoh Akhenaten, and came to the conclusion that he had an acromegalic face and eunuchoid obesity, which may have been due to a pituitary adenoma, first with some α-cell activity, but later leading to pressure hypofunction of the pituitary gland[12].

According to Ghallioungui, the ancient Egyptians knew about polyuria and sugar-diabetes[13]. In the papyrus Kahun, there is a recipe: 'Treatment for a woman thirsty', which breaks off at this point[14]. Brothwell described a probably acromegalic skull from ancient Egypt in the Natural History part of the British Museum[11].

21

Ruffer concluded from his studies of tomb paintings, reliefs and statuettes, that dwarfs were probably not rare in ancient Egypt, many of them definitely achrondoplastic, e.g. Chnoum-hotep,

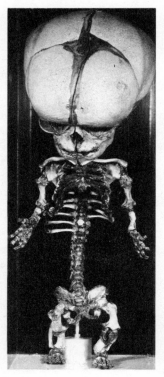

Figure 3 Achondroplastic dwarf, height 29 cm. Donated in 1842 by Robert Liston [By kind permission of the Royal College of Surgeons of England (London)]

whose statuette, found at Sakkara, showed typical disproportion between trunk and limbs and a large head[15].

The main importance of Egyptian medicine lies in its proximity to and in its lasting influence on Greek medicine, which existed before Homer's time and persisted into the Alexandrian and Graeco–Roman periods. Egyptian medicine proper had, however, become stationary and stale, especially from the time of Herodotus. In the Alexandrian period, it was the influence of Greek medicine which acted as a rejuvenator.

Elliott Smith, in a study of the Royal Mummies, found examples of slim, almost cachectic women, for example, the Queens Nofretari and Nedjmet and the Lady Rei. There were also very stout women like the Queens Henut-tawy and Inhapy. Stout – and bald – men were not uncommon in ancient Egypt, at any rate among the higher castes, e.g. the High Priest Masaherta, but the Pharaoh Tuthmosis

IV looked very emaciated[16]. There has been fairly recently a suggestion that the celebrated Tutankhamen was an intersex, because of the
gynaecoid features and proportions[17].

It is interesting to note that the ancient Egyptians used prolonged
lactation to reduce fertility. Primitive Egyptian women were not

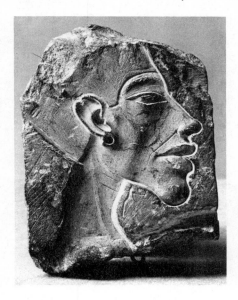

Figure 4 Acromegaly: limestone
portrait head of Akhenaten,
XVIIIth dynasty, *ca.* 1365 BC [By
kind permission of Staatliche
Museen zu Berlin, 102 Berlin 2/
Bodestrasse]

expected to bear children more frequently than once every three
years; accordingly they nursed their children for a corresponding
period[3]. The Ebers papyrus also contains the first reference to a
medicated lint tampon to prevent conception. The original prescrip-
tion contained tips of acacia; gum acacia is also generally used in the
production of modern contraceptive jellies as a vehicle[18]. All the
Egyptian prescriptions seem to have been made for the use of the
woman and not for the man; "this is in accordance with the best
modern theoretical thought on the subject"[3].

REFERENCES

1. Johnston, R. D.: The history of human infertility. Fertil. Steril. **14,** 261–272,
    1963.
2. ibid.: p. 262.
3. Himes, N. E.: A Medical History of Contraception. p. 67, New York, Gamut
    Press, 1936.
4. Garrison, F. H.: Introduction to the History of Medicine, 4th Ed., p. 53,
    Philadelphia, W. B. Saunders, 1929.

5. Iason, A. H.: The Thyroid Gland in Medical History, p. 10, New York, Froben Press, 1946.
6. Herodotus, II, 84.
7. Brothwell, D. and Sandison, A. T. ed.: Diseases in Antiquity. Chap. 43, pp. 521–531, Springfield, Thomas, 1967.
8. ibid.: p. 521.
9. Seligmann, C. G.: A cretinous skull of the 18th Dynasty. Man **12,** 17, 1912.
10. Keith, A.: Abnormal crania. Achondroplastic and acrocephalic. J. Anat. Physiol. **47,** 189, 1913.
11. Brothwell, D. R.: Digging up Bones. London, British Museum (Nat. Hist.), 1963.
12. Aldred, C. and Sandison, A. T.: The Pharaoh Akhenaten: A problem in Egyptology and pathology. Bull. Hist. Med. **36,** 293, 1963.
13. Ghallioungui, P.: Magic and Medical Science in Ancient Egypt. London, Hodder & Stoughton, 1963.
14. Griffith, F. Lt.: Hieratic Papyri from Kahun and Gurob. cit. after Brothwell and Sandison (see 7).
15. Ruffer, M. A.: On dwarfs and other deformed persons. Bull. Soc. Arch. Alex. **13,** 1, 1911.
16. Smith, G. Elliott: The Royal Mummies. Cairo, Musée de Caire, 1912.
17. Professor T. Chard, St. Bartholomew's Hospital, London. Personal communication.
18. As 3: pp. 63–64.

CHAPTER FOUR

THE HINDUS

THE main works which make up the body of Ayur Vedic medicine came from the oral tradition and were formed over a period of a thousand years, beginning 1400 BC. They were based on the theories of the breath, of the humours and of the constituent elements of the microcosm and the macrocosm. The most notable text is the *Susruta* (5th century AD), which is the great storehouse of Aryan surgery. This was, originally, a very different conception from the Chinese hypotheses, although later there was an exchange and interweaving of Chinese and Indian ideas. The golden age of Ayur-Veda medicine coincides with the rise of Buddhism (327 BC–750 AD) and the period of Indian expansion. Among Buddha's attendants there were two doctors, Kasparja and Jivaka. The latter became a patron of Tibetan medicine, to whom remarkable operations were ascribed: laparotomy, thoracotomy and cranial trepanation, under anaesthesia by Indian hemp (*Cannabis sativa*). The Chinese pharmacopoeia borrowed from India: Indian hemp, datura, caulmoogra, sandalwood, cardamum (from Malabar), Indian camphor, cinnamon (from Ceylon), long pepper and cane sugar[1]. The Suśruta mentions 760 medicinal plants. The soporific effect of hyascyamus and *Cannabis indica* were known and had been used in surgical anaesthesia since ancient times. In the Ayur Veda there is also reference to sweet urine with a syndrome of burning sensation in the hands and feet[2].

The Hindus knew that pregnancy lasted ten lunar months. They believed that some 'sealing spirits' were responsible for female sterility. They also thought that in the eighth month of pregnancy the vital force was drawn from the mother to the child and back again repeatedly; hence an eight months' child could not survive, whereas a seven months' baby had a better chance.

A hole in a rock was symbolic for a woman's birth passage and passing through such a narrow hole would give the Hindu woman improved fertility. (In Aberdeenshire women still squeeze through the 'Devil's Needle' and this is believed to bring them luck; but, originally, this was a fertility rite for barren women.) Similar customs exist in many other parts of the globe[3].

The Hindus were people with a balanced view of life: they were concerned with their religious duties, but interested in material welfare and also in a sophisticated love life which they elevated to poetical heights and a veritable *ars amandi*, witness for which is the *Kāma-Sūtra* (early 4th century AD) of Vatsyāyana Mallanāga, who was himself a physician. Accordingly, contraceptive techniques were of major interest. They were partly magical and ritualistic, such as the recommendation of swallowing three-year-old molasses, or of the roots of agni tree cooked in sour rice water; another group consisted of vaginal fumigations with the smoke of neem wood, or passiveness in coitus, or holding the breath. A third group might appear more rational, advising methods like coitus obstructus, or smearing the vagina with honey and ghee (butter converted into a kind of oil by boiling), or vaginal medication of rock salt dipped in oil, or the use of tampons of ground ajowan seed and rock salt with oil. Ordinary modern table salt is an effective spermicide[4].

For the cure of impotence and of obesity (!) the Ayur Veda recommended the administration of testicular tissue (organotherapy)[5].

Goitre (*Galaganda*) is caused by the

> deranged and aggravated vayu in combination with the deranged and augmented Kapham and fat of the locality affects the two tendons of the neck (Manya's) and gradually gives rise to a swelling about that part of the neck characterised by the specific symptoms of the deranged Doshas. . . . The swelling or tumour in the goitre is characterised by a pricking pain in its inside, marked by the appearance of blue or dark-coloured veins on its surface. It assumes a vermillion or tawny-brown hue. The goitre becomes united with the local fat in the course of time and gains in size, giving rise to a sense of burning in the throat, or is characterised by the absence of any pain at all. The swelling in the Kaphaja variety assumes a large shape and becomes hard, firm and cold. A case of goitre attended with difficult respiration, a softening of the whole body, weakness, a non-relish for food, loss of voice as well as the one which is more than a year's standing should be abandoned by the physician as incurable.[6]

Decomposing urine or cow's urine has been used in Southern India in many acute and chronic diseases. Essential diabetes mellitus was recognized as *madhumeha* or 'honey-urine', and the symptoms of thirst, foul breath, and languor were noted[7].

REFERENCES

1. Huard, Pierre and Ming Wong: Chinese Medicine. (Translation) p. 92, London, George Weidenfeld & Nicolson, 1968.
2. Brothwell, D. and Sandison, A. T.: Diseases in Antiquity. Chap. 43, p. 522. Springfield, Thomas, 1967.
3. Johnston, R. D.: The history of human infertility. Fertil. Steril. **14,** 261–272, 1963.
4. Himes, N. E.: Medical History of Contraception. p. 121. New York, Gamut Press, 1936 (reprinted 1970).
5. Iason, A. H. The Thyroid Gland in Medical History. p. 12, New York, Froben Press, 1946.
6. ibid.: p. 13.
7. Garrison, Fielding H.: An Introduction to the History of Medicine. 4th Ed. p. 71, Philadelphia, W. B. Saunders, 1929.

CHAPTER FIVE

THE JEWS AND THE BIBLE

T HE principal sources for Jewish medicine are the Bible and the Talmud. There were – of necessity – close connections with Egyptian, Sumerian and Babylonian medicine, as the Jews were in captivity for some 430 years in Egypt, in Assyrian captivity in 722 BC and in Babylonian captivity in 604 BC for another 70 years. Other important sources are, of course, the archaeological findings made in the Holy Land, which are still continuing.

According to the Old Testament, health is a gift of God, and disease the wrath of God. The latter can be prevented or removed only by submission, atonement, prayer, moral reform or sacrifice. The fundamental idea of visitation due to the wrath of God for sin, disobedience, moral turpitude, today still exists among orthodox Jews. The laws of hygiene were excellently designed and strictly observed. The priests were involved in hygienic measures to regulate everyday life and control disease (especially infectious), but did not otherwise act as physicians. The prophets did perform miracles – Elijah raised children from the dead (I Kings, xvii, 17–23) – and Elisha 'healed' the waters of Jordan (II Kings, ii, 21–22), but that was not identical with the practice of medicine. Apart from the priests, who acted as public health officers, and from the physicians, there were professional pharmacists: "Moreover the Lord spake unto Moses, saying . . . 'And thou shalt make it an oil of holy ointment, an ointment compound after the art of the apothecary'. . . ." (Exodus, xxx, 25), and in Nehemiah, iii, 8: "Next unto him repaired Hananiah, the son of one of the apothecaries. . . ."; there were also professional midwives, who played an important role (see the stories of Rachel and Thamar). There was a special reference to their use of the obstetric chair in labour, which was popular in the Orient:

29

> And the king of Egypt spake to the Hebrew midwives, of which the name of one was Shiprah, and the name of the other Puah[1]: And he said, 'When ye do the office of a midwife to the Hebrew women, and see them upon the stools; if it be a son, then ye shall kill him. . . .
>
> (Exodus, i, 15 and 16).

Shipra and Puah might have been the representatives of a number of (college) midwives, as it seems unlikely that a population of about a million people should have only two midwives.

Circumcision was first ordered by God to Abraham as a token of the covenant, in Genesis (xvii, 10–14). Abraham was on that occasion himself circumcised when aged 99 years (Genesis, xvii, 24). When they were in captivity in Egypt, the Jews stopped circumcision after the death of Joseph, except for the tribe of Levi. It seems that baby Moses, when found in his basket, was recognized by Pharaoh's daughter as one of the Hebrews, because he was circumcised, as he was of the tribe of Levi. Following the exodus from Egypt, Moses seems to have stopped circumcision, because of the exigencies of the wanderings in the wilderness. This applied to his own small sons. When he was taken dangerously ill, his Arab wife Zipporah feared that disease had struck because her son had not been circumcised. She carried out the circumcision with a sharp stone (Exodus, iv, 25–26), but on that occasion it was not to introduce a general hygienic measure, because she

> cut off the foreskin of her son, and cast it at his feet, and said, "Surely a bloody husband art thou to me". So he let him go: then she said, "A bloody husband thou art, because of the circumcision".

Only later (Joshua, v, 2) was Joshua commanded by God to make sharp knives and circumcise the children of Israel, born in the wilderness after the Exodus from Egypt. This is the only surgical procedure mentioned in the Bible, apart from the treatment of fractures and war wounds (Ezekiel, xxx, 22). We have already referred in Chapter 3 to the fact that "Moses was learned in all the wisdom of the Egyptians" (Acts, vii, 22), and to the idea prevailing that mice disseminate disease (Isaiah, xvi, 17).

Obstetrics were an important part of medical knowledge. "Be fruitful, and multiply, and replenish the earth" (Genesis, vi, 28) was God's blessing. Prolificacy was a reward for good life, barrenness a punishment for wickedness. ('Rachel said unto Jacob, "Give me children or else I die"'. Genesis, xxx, 1). But infertility was recognized to be due either to the man or to the woman: "Thou shall be blessed above all people: there shall not be male or female barren among you, or among your cattle". (Deuteronomy, vii, 14). The

30

only difference was that sterility of the man was no legal cause for divorce, in contrast to sterility of the woman[2].

When a woman's infertility presented itself in the form of disease, such as permanent uterine bleeding, there were miraculous cures, such as the case of the woman who had had an issue of blood for twelve years, "which had spent all her living upon physicians, neither could be healed of any"; she came behind Jesus and touched the border of his garment; "and immediately the issue of her blood was staunched". This was reported not only by St. Mark, v, 25–34, but also by St. Luke, ix, 43–48, who was himself a distinguished physician.

For all the reasons mentioned above, contraception for its own sake was not practised. When it became necessary for health reasons, there were definite methods in existence. 'Onanism' has most likely been misrepresented: it was more likely to have been coitus interruptus than masturbation, which would not have much sense if Onan would visit Tamar for the purpose of sleeping with her. Incidentally, his elder brother Er displeased God and was killed, because he also practised coitus interruptus in order to preserve the beauty of his wife Tamar and not to disfigure her by pregnancy[3]. If a woman was pregnant, and the pregnancy endangered her life, "the unborn child may be cut to pieces and removed, for her life takes precedence over the life of the unborn child"[4] (embryotomy).

Other methods of preventing conception were conceded when the woman was a minor (i.e. aged from eleven years and one day to twelve years and one day; the Orient, especially at that time, did not object to marriages with minors); when she was a pregnant woman with a normal pregnancy and when she was a nursing mother. The reasons given were, that a minor might become pregnant and die; that in a pregnant woman superfoetation might occur and result in the production of a foetus papyraceus; that a nursing mother might kill her child by losing her milk and being compelled prematurely to wean her child. In those conditions, the use of the sponge (spongy substances) was recommended, perhaps related to the lint used by the Egyptians; such knowledge of an occlusive agent might, indeed, have been passed on to the Hebrews during their long time in Egyptian captivity[5]. The sponge was put into the vagina to cover the os uteri before cohabitation. Prostitutes, or some women who had illegal intercourse, attempted sometimes to protect themselves by violent movements immediately after cohabitation. (Widows or divorced women were not allowed to remarry for three months in order to ascertain whether the paternity of the next child belonged to the first or second husband.) Removal of semen from the vagina after intercourse was another method of contraception (the violent movements had the same end in mind); this was advice given in the Talmud[6]. Finally, there were the many – mainly doubtful – potions, 'Beakers of Infertility' or 'Beakers of the Roots' given as contraceptives[7].

In the Bible there was a word for the human testicle (*eshek*) and for the testicle of an animal (*pachad*). The (later) Talmud seems to have used the same word for testicle and ovary (*bêçâ*)[8]. Any deformity, such as a testicle missing (undescended), will not only make a man unfit to approach the altar directly, but also exclude an animal from being used for sacrifice (Leviticus, xxii, 24). Men with hypospadias were not regarded fit for marriage (the Arabs, later, held the same view), because the ejaculate could not achieve conception.

Castration and castrates were well known in the Bible;

> And he lifted up his face to the window, and said, Who is on my side? Who? And there looked out to him two or three eunuchs
>
> (II Kings, ix, 32).

In the Book of Esther, i, 10, it is said that Ahasuerus "commanded Mehuman, Biztha, . . . the seven chamberlains (or eunuchs) that served in the presence. . . ." Potiphar, an officer of the Pharaoh, captain of the guard, an Egyptian (Genesis, xxxix, 1) was a married eunuch[9]. (In later times, the Aghawât (= eunuchs of the mosque) were also married.) The castrate was described as of soft hair, smooth skin, unable to urinate in an arc; his 'sperm' is watery, his voice soft and feminine. From the eunuchs, who had been castrated by man, were distinguished the eunuchoids, who were called 'sun-castrates'. This term, Preuss believes, is equivalent to the Egyptian 'castrated by Ra'; the sungod. For the sun-castrates there is hope for a (? miraculous) cure, for the 'man-castrates' there is none[5]. The sun-castrates may be people born without testicles or with ectopic testicles. The eunuchs (man-castrates) can be divided into those castrated by others and those who castrated themselves:

> [Jesus said] For there are some eunuchs which were so born from their mother's womb; and there are some eunuchs which were made eunuchs of men: and there be eunuchs which have made themselves eunuchs for the kingdom of heaven's sake. He that is able to receive it, let him receive it.
>
> (Matthew, xix, 12).

Many eunuchoids and some eunuchs possess some libido and can perform a type of intercourse; hence the existence of married eunuchs in Egypt and other countries. Self-castration for religious reasons is usually more radical and often involves removal of the penis as well. (See the Russian sect of the Skopzes which derived from the sect of the Valerians.) In our present age, we have the transvestites, some of whom have a complete removal of their genital organs performed. They seem to have managed to acquire the term 'transsexuals' which is, of course, genetically or morphologically not tenable.

Castration of animals used for breeding was illegal. Neither Buddha nor Confucius nor Mohammed commented against it, nor is there any relevant reference to it in the New Testament. Hebrew farmers sometimes bought castrated animals from the neighbouring non-Jewish tribes. Removal of the uterus was not regarded as castration.

For the treatment of (temporary or permanent) impotence, aphrodisiacs were used. The most popular were garlic (which is supposed to increase sperm), fish and even milk. Wine was also used, but regarded as dangerous. Salt, starvation, eczema, crying (emotional distress) diminish the amount of sperm; so do disease, venesection, and a tiring journey[10]. A plant, *dudaim* (? mandrake) was also used against infertility or as an aphrodisiac.

Women who had under- or undeveloped genitalia, lacked breast development, had a deep voice and suffered pain when attempting intercourse were called 'rams'. Female castration was, of course, unknown to the ancients, but Hebrew animal breeders knew that sows or cows could be fattened after hysterectomy, which prevented breeding. Hermaphrodites were known and described in the Talmud and caused legal and practical problems, because they could not be ascribed to either sex. He (?) had to be circumcised when eight days old, he could legally marry a woman, and divorce proceedings had to be carried out according to the law. Marriage to a man was, however, not permissible[11].

Woman during her menstrual periods was regarded as unclean, and intercourse during that time was not permissible. Yawning, rictus, lower abdominal pain, heaviness, vaginal discharge and irritability were regarded as signs of the impending period. During the period no religious functions could be carried out (the matrons of ancient Rome were not allowed to enter the temples while menstruating). Intercourse during menstruation was a *peccatum mortale* (morally speaking), while the Catholic Church regards it only as a *peccatum veniale*, for which – under certain circumstances – absolution can be given. Menarche was assumed to occur on the average at the age of 12. The intermenstrual period was usually 30 days. If it was less than 11 days, it was a sign of disease[12]. Women who had primary amenorrhoea should not marry and if they did, could be divorced. Breastfeeding was expected to last two years and more. Wetnurses were not common, although some were highly esteemed, such as Deborah, Rebekah's nurse (Genesis, xxxv, 8). In the case of twins, occasionally one was nursed by the mother, the other by a wetnurse.

Galactorrhoea in men (also mentioned by Aristotle, Hist. anim. III, chap. 20, para. 102) is also quoted in the Talmud, but regarded as an abnormality[13]. Much later, Albrecht von Haller (see Section II) collected quite a few cases[18].

The birth of uniovular twins is described in Genesis, xxxviii, 27–30, surrounded by drama. Tamar, wronged by her father-in-law Judah, succeeded in deceiving him and became pregnant by him. She was the widow of his sons Er and Onan, mentioned before. Judah promised her in marriage to his youngest son, but failed to keep his promise. She bore twin sons. There is comedy at the birth: Zarah put out his hand first; the midwife put a scarlet thread on it, saying, "This came out first". He withdrew his hand, however, and his brother, Pharez, was born first.

Also in the obstetric field, we find cardiac shock in precipitate labour, due to severe emotional upset. Phinehas' wife dies in childbirth, on receiving the news of her husband's and father-in-law's death in battle (I Samuel, iv, 19–20).

Whether Esau (the 'hairy one') (Genesis, xxv, 25) was simply a hirsute man or was suffering from adreno-genital syndrome is difficult to decide. His uniovular twin, Jacob, was apparently not hirsute, which could suggest a mild form of adreno-genital syndrome. 'Mild' because, like his brother, he lived to a biblical age of over 100 years.

Whether gigantism is racial as suggested of Arba "which Arba was a great man among the Anakim" (Joshua, xiv, 15) and his descendants, is also hard to say. They were living in the south of Canaan, in the city of Kirjath-arba, which became Hebron when it was given to Caleb, the son of Jephunneh, for an inheritance. There was also a reference to the Anakim in Deuteronomy, i, 28: "The people is [sic] greater and taller than we; the cities are great and walled up to heaven; and moreover we have seen the sons of the Anakims there". In Numbers, xiii, 32 and 33, they are spoken of as "all people that we saw in it are men of great stature. And there we saw the giants, the sons of Anak, which come of the giants: and we were in our own sight as grasshoppers, and so we were in their sight". They were divided into three families (? tribes), named Sheshai, Ahiman and Talmai. Although they struck fear into the hearts of the Israelites, Caleb drove them out of Hebron.

Giants were also mentioned in the story of Noah (Genesis, vi, 4) "There were giants in the earth in those days; and also after that when the sons of God came in unto the daughters of men, and they bare children to them, the same became mighty men which were of old, men of renown". Whether these were acromegalic, as A. H. Iason[14] maintains, is mere conjecture. Against such an assumption must be held the fact that acromegalics usually decline in energy and strength and in the progressive disease may suffer from severe headaches, encroached vision, hypogonadism with infertility and impotence, muscular weakness, osteoporosis, and occasionally also from diabetes mellitus and diabetes insipidus and cardiomegaly. They also have a high mortality rate, unless the disease becomes stationary.

One of the other famous giants in the Bible was Goliath of Gath. He was probably descended from the Rephaim (giants) of whom a remnant took refuge with the Philistines after being driven out by the Ammonites (Deuteronomy, ii, 20): "That also was accounted a land of giants: giants dwelt therein in old time; and the Ammonites call them Zanzummims; a people great, and many as tall as the Anakims;". In I Samuel, xvii, 4–7, Goliath of Gath is described as one " . . . whose height was six cubits and a span . . . and the weight of his coat [of mail] was five thousand shekels of brass . . . and the staff of his spear was like a weaver's beam; and his spear's head weighed six hundred shekels of iron". He held up the army of Israel for forty days. In the second book of Samuel (xxi, 15–22), in a later war of the Philistines against Israel, there were battles at Gob, in which four giants fought on the side of the Philistines, and all were slain. They were described "sons of the giant". One of them was the brother of Goliath the Gittite, the staff of whose spear

> was like a weaver's beam. And there was yet a battle in Gath, where was a man of great stature, that had on every hand six fingers, and on every foot six toes, four and twenty in number; and he also was born to the giant. And when he defied Israel, Jonathan the son of Shimeah the brother of David slew him . . . These four were born to the giant of Gath. . . .

Garrison suggests that the giant with the twenty-four fingers and toes was an acromegalic[15]. This seems unlikely for the reasons given above. Moreover, it is equally unlikely that he should have had a giant father and three brothers who were giants. We shall see later that tribes of giants were described in Nordic sagas. In most cases, however, there seems to be evidence that in many of these individuals there was pituitary dysfunction; if there are low gonadotropin values, the chances of procreation are considerably diminished. This remarkable occurrence of tribes and families of giants in Oriental and Nordic folklore must have a different explanation.

35

Dwarfs were regarded as misfits by the Hebrews[16] and had no access to the temple:

> Whosoever hath a blemish, he shall not approach to offer the bread to his God . . . or a man that is . . . crookbackt or a dwarf. . . .
>
> (Leviticus, xxi, 17 and 20).

> Only he shall not go into unto the vail, nor come nigh unto the altar, because he hath a blemish
>
> (Leviticus, xxi, 23);

but when Jesus entered Jericho,

> there was a man named Zacchaeus, which was the chief among the publicans and he was rich. . . . And he sought to see Jesus who he was; and could not for the press, because he was little of stature . . . and climbed up a sycamore tree to see him; for he was to pass that way. When Jesus saw him, he said: "Zacchaeus, make haste and come down; for today I must abide at thy house".
>
> (Luke, xix, 2–5).

Obesity, due to overeating, is described in Deuteronomy, xxxii, 15: "But Jeshurun waxed fat, and kicked; thou art waxen fat, thou art grown thick, thou art covered with fatness . . .", although the passage may have referred symbolically to Israel as a nation.

To sum up, there is no Jewish medicine in the sense of Egyptian or Greek medicine[17].

REFERENCES

1. Preuss, Julius: Biblish-talmudische Medizin. pp. 40–41, New York, KTAV Publishing House, 1971.
2. ibid.: p. 480.
3. ibid.: p. 534.
4. Himes, N. E.: Medical History of Contraception. p. 70, New York, Gamut Press, 1936 (reprinted 1970).
5. ibid.: pp. 72–75.
6. ibid.: p. 76.
7. As 1: pp. 439–440.
8. ibid.: p. 126.
9. ibid.: p. 257.
10. ibid.: pp. 538–539.
11. ibid.: p. 262.
12. ibid.: p. 141
13. ibid.: p. 476.
14. Iason, A. H.: The Thyroid Gland in Medical History, p. 22, New York, Froben Press, 1946.
15. Garrison, F. H.: Introduction to the History of Medicine. 4th ed., p. 66. Philadelphia, W. B. Saunders, 1929.

16.   As 1: p. 231.
17.   ibid.: pp. 254–260.
18.   Haller, A. von: Elem. physiol. tom. VII, lib. 28, Sect. I, para. 13, p. 18,
       Lausanne–Berne, 1757–66.

CHAPTER SIX

THE GREEKS

BEFORE HIPPOCRATES

THE Minoan culture corresponded, especially in its late period (1840–1400 BC), with the New Empire in Egypt. The Palaces at Knossos and Hagia Triada impress by their sanitary arrangements for ventilation, drainage, terracotta piping and latrines, which are almost modern in concept. The Mycenaean culture showed similar features. The Homeric period shows Minoan influence.

The Greeks were a mixture of peoples, some mountaineering and warlike, others athletic, fishermen and seafaring, but all restless and fiercely independent. Accordingly, they developed various types of medicine. They had many religious cults with local differences. Many of their chief gods could cause or prevent and cure disease; Artemis, Demeter, Hermes, Hera and Dionysus, to name just a few. There was also the medical magic, a darker ritualistic cult, of the chthonian deities of the earth and the nether world. Hades, Persephone, Hermes and Hekate were connected with this cult. Pre-Hippocratic medicine was mainly prophylactic and prognostic, based on atonement or catharsis by means of the sacrificial scapegoat (φαρμακός), and the drug (φάρμακον) was sacred and mystical. It was a sort of organotherapy, using the liver, spleen and heart in the form of 'homoeopathic magic', but by no means isotherapy in the sense of 'like cures like'[1].

Its practitioners became detached from the temples and priests and were magicians. The chief god of healing was Apollo Alexikakos, the averter of ills, who could produce epidemics or prevent and cure them. He was also the court physician to his fellow-gods, whom he cured with the peony root, hence his name 'Paean'; physicians were often called 'sons of Paean'. Artemis shared her brother's abilities. Both transmitted their knowledge of medicine to the centaur Chiron, the son of Saturn. He, in turn, brought up several heroes, including Herakles, but especially Aesculapios, a son of Apollo by the nymph Coronis. Aesculapios became so proficient in the art of healing that he reduced the number of shadows in Hades. After being destroyed by the thunderbolt of Zeus, he became the symbolic god of the healing arts. Temples were erected to him, which became sanitaria run by priest–physicians, the most famous being those at Cos, Cnidos, Epidauros and Pergamon. There the ritual of 'incubation' or temple sleep flourished. Medical education was also carried out at these health centres, and Hippocrates was born at Cos, of an Asclepiad family. Asclepiads were followers of Aesculapios, who had formed an organized guild of physicians; the temples dedicated to him were also called Asclepieia. Aesculapios' wife, Epione, and his daughters Hygieia and Panacaea participated in the cult and fed the sacred snakes. The snake was the companion of Aesculapios and held a similar position as in Crete, India and ancient Egypt, being entwined around the staff of the god.

Homer (? 1000 BC) has a record of 147 war wounds in the Iliad and is concerned mainly with field surgery[2]. Two of the leaders of the Greek fleet before Troy were Machaon and Podalirios, sons of Aesculapios, 'good physicians' or naval and military surgeons. Achilles, however, had also been brought up by the centaur Chiron, who had instructed him in medicine. The injuries inflicted in battle and reported by Homer show a remarkable knowledge of (local) anatomy, with a total mortality rate of 77%[2]. There is no observation of disease in Homer, but sanitation must have been fairly efficient, because during the 10-year siege there were only a few epidemics (see the opening canto of the Iliad); especially effective seems to have been the disposal of the dead by cremation.

Apart from the priests and the physicians, medicine was also practised and studied by the philosophers and the gymnasts. Greek philosophy at that period came from the East and Egypt via Ionia. Thales of Miletos (639–544 BC), who had been a student of the Egyptian priests, regarded water as the primary element from which all else is derived. One of his successors, Heraclitos of Ephesos (ca. 556–460 BC), thought that earth, air or fire are the primordial elements. Empedocles of Agrigentum in Sicily (504–443 BC), wandering philosopher, physician and poet, introduced the 'fourfold root of all things' into philosophy, namely earth, air, fire and water. The health of the human body depends on the balance of these elements, and disease stems from their imbalance.

Pythagoras of Samos (580–489 BC) had also studied in Egypt, and founded his school at Crotona. He was a philosopher, mathematician, physicist, numerologist and physician, and influenced the Hippocratic teaching of crisis and critical days in disease. Pythagoras was the first to regard the brain as the main organ of the higher activities (a view confirmed by Hippocrates and Galen, but opposed by Aristotle). He brought from Egypt the doctrine of transmigration of souls, and, above all, influenced the significance of the co-ordination of the four elements with the four qualities: dry, moist, hot and cold, producing the four humours of the body: blood, phlegm, yellow bile and black bile. These three sets of four would, by permutation and combination, explain the qualitative aspects of disease and the physiological action of drugs. Thus the doctrine of the four humours was – according to Garrison – "a vague foreshadowing of the endocrine and general biochemical aspects of human physiology"[3].

Democritos of Abdera (460–360 BC) first postulated the theory of atoms, i.e. that everything in nature is made up of atoms of different shapes and sizes, the movements of which are the cause of life.

The later division of Greek behaviour into two main streams, the military dour Spartans (Doric type) and the imaginative, brilliant Athenians (Ionians), also influenced the development of medicine. The Spartan lawgiver wanted to ensure the maintenance of a 'Herrenvolk' by strict rules for eugenic procreation. It is little known that Spartan women, whose husbands were away at the wars for years, not only looked after the domestic affairs and ran, efficiently, the family estates, but also could obtain permission from their husband to select a fit and eugenically suitable young man, who was not yet in the army, to become pregnant by him, and sons of such unions were acknowledged by the husbands and kept the family name going[4]. Crippled and deformed infants and newborn girls in excess numbers were exposed and thrown into the Eurotas. The Spartans held surgeons in high esteem: Lycurgos classed them as non-combatant officers.

The presentation of Artemis gives a good insight into the development of early obstetrics. She was, on the one hand, the virgin huntress, roaming the fields, woods, and mountains, loving dance and music and leading the life of an unmarried daughter of a feudal aristocratic family. On the other hand, there is the picture of the age-old nature goddess of Asia Minor, of Artemis of Ephesus. She was the goddess of all the wild beasts and especially of their suckling cubs, hence one of her statues in Naples depicts her having 16 well-formed breasts; but she also cared for (fresh-water) fish: there

41

was an image of her fish-shaped form from the waist down. When – at the age of three – she was asked by Zeus what presents she would like, she said, among other wishes, "Unfortunately, women in labour will often be invoking me, since my mother Leto carried and bore me without pains, and the Fates have therefore made me patroness of childbirth'[5]. The Greek word parthenos (πάρθενος), which is normally translated as 'maid' or 'virgin', has really no such meaning. Both Homer and Pindar use it as a reference to unmarried girls who are not virgins. The children of concubines in Sparta were called *partheniai*, indicating that their mother remained unmarried, 'parthenos' in name.

Zeus' wife Hera (did he really woo her for 300 years before he married her?) was the guardian goddess of marriage, and as such a helper for women in childbirth, except, of course, in the case of Zeus' girlfriends, such as Alcmene, the mother of Herakles' mother, when she prevented Eileithyia from mitigating the pangs of childbirth. Eileithyia, 'she who comes to aid in childbirth', had the moon as her symbol, as promoter of procreation and growth, and the cow as symbol of fertility. When Leto produced her twins, Artemis and Apollo, Eileithyia helped at their birth which was painless, as Artemis said in her previously mentioned discussion with Zeus. Actemia, on the other hand, horrified by her mother's suffering at her own birth, asked for and obtained from Zeus the gift of eternal virginity. Falling in love with young Endymion, she changed her mind and gave, eventually, birth to fifty daughters (obviously the forerunner of overfertilization after modern treatment of infertility!).

In Athens, nearer the age of Pericles, the medical profession became more specialized. General practitioners received fixed fees for their services. City and district public physicians were appointed at a comparatively high annual salary; some such posts had existed since Homeric times and were mentioned by Herodotus. In Thessaly, where horsebreeding was most important, they had a public veterinary surgeon (*hippiatros*). Anatomy was studied to a great extent during athletic contest or in the palaestra or, more painstakingly, in battle or during religious animal sacrifice. There existed a considerable knowledge of biology and medicine in Greek literature between the era of Homer and Hippocrates.

THE AGE OF HIPPOCRATES

Hippocrates (460–370 BC) lived during the best period of classic Greek and especially Athenian culture. Sophocles, Euripides, Aristophanes, Socrates and Plato, Herodotus, Thukydides and Phidias were contemporaries at the time when Pericles guided the fate of Athens. Born on the island of Cos, of an Asclepiad family, he was first a disciple of his father, then studied in Athens, travelled widely and practised in Thrace, Thessaly and Macedonia. He is supposed to have died in his ninth decade.

Hippocrates created medicine as an art, independent from religion or philosophy. He managed to collect and leave behind a concentrated body of medical scientific knowledge, based on close observation, intelligent conclusions and the use of long personal experience. He reinforced the already high status of physicians by giving them a high moral basis.

Hippocrates did not write much himself, but he became the great inspiration behind the schools of Cos and Cnidos, and the text written by his pupils and successors, such as Tzetzes and Soranus. He changed medicine from the mainly surgical experience of naval and military medicine into the general field, which opened up internal medicine, physiology, and pathology. He introduced clinical observation based on inspection and description, and his best descriptions of disease have never been surpassed. With great candour he admitted that of 42 clinical observations he described, 60% (25) ended fatally. His high ethical standard did not permit him to boast of his clever diagnoses or successful cures in the self-advertising manner of Galen. The style is an example of simplicity, lucidity and brevity. His book on ancient medicine is the first exercise on the history of medicine.

From the point of view of the present paper, the *Prognostics* and the *Aphorisms* (430–400 BC) are perhaps of the greatest importance. Hippocrates insisted on a careful, systematic and thorough examination of the patient, observing the general condition, the face (facies Hippocratica of the severely ill), the temperature, respiration, sputum, pulse, pains and tenderness, and movements of the body. The doctrine of the four humours was introduced, this humoral pathology being a forerunner of ideas of hormonal, although not necessarily endocrine, pathology. The pulse and Hippocratic theory persisted, remarkably, unchanged until William Harvey came on to the scene. The treatise on *Generation* (*ca.* 380 BC) deals with the incubation of hens' eggs for the study of embryology; it compares vegetable, animal and human embryology and discusses pangenesis, all the beginnings of biology before Aristotle. In the *Aphorisms*, it is mentioned that eunuchs do not suffer from gout or become bald[36], that gout in men does not occur before puberty[37] and that women develop gout only after the menopause[38]. In the section 'Diseases of Women', there is a connection noted between obesity and sterility.

Later, Soranus observed that amenorrhoea may occur in women of masculine appearance. Soranus of Ephesus also described clitoral enlargement in a manner expected in hyperadrenalism. Dorothy Thompson illustrated a terracotta figure of a woman from Boeotia, fourth century BC, which shows middle-age obesity or perhaps Cushing's disease[6] (Figure 5). Soranus also noted the

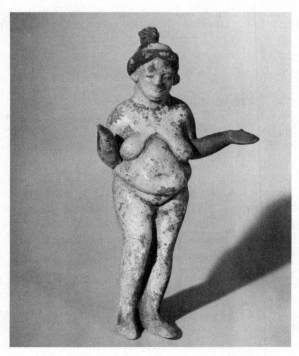

Figure 5 Pottery vase, Boeotia, 4th century BC. British Museum, height 19.2 cm. ?Middle-aged obesity ?Cushing's syndrome [Copyright British Museum, used by permission]

swelling of the neck after pregnancy, which he thought to be a form of bronchial tumour.

Herodotos, a contemporary of Hippocrates, described in his *History* (Book VII, 117) a man, Artachnaees of the Achmaenid family, who was 8 feet 2 inches tall (almost 5 royal cubits) and had the loudest voice in the world. In Book IX, 83, he mentions that among the Persian dead at Plataeae there was the skeleton of a man, $7\frac{1}{2}$ feet tall (5 cubits). Hippocrates says about the glands as follows (*De Glandulis*):

> The flesh of the glands is different from the rest of the body, being spongy and full of veins; they are found in the moist parts of the body,

where they receive humidity . . . and the brain is a gland as well as the mammae[7].

In order to cure a specific disease, it was necessary to restore the lost balance by the administration of the requisite 'humours' in its containing organ. The pituita, or nasal mucus, was the secretion of the brain that flowed through the lamina cribrosa of the ethmoid![7] Soranus later also noted the pigment changes in the face of pregnant women and the pigmentation of the areolae, which was also known to the Hindus.

In historical Greece, obstetrics became an important part of skilled medical practice and Hippocrates contributed towards its teachings, but – in fact – it was midwives who carried out a great deal of the actual practice of that discipline. One of their more pleasant tests for fertility was as follows: "If a woman do not conceive, and wishes to ascertain whether she can conceive, having wrapped her in blankets, fumigate below with oil of roses and if it appears that the same passes through her body to the nostrils and mouth, know that of herself she is not unfruitful"; is this Rubin's carbon dioxide insufflation test to determine tubal patency (1920 AD) anticipated by 2300 years?[5]

The Hippocratics failed to differentiate the thyroid from the cervical glands. Goitre was regarded purely as a deformity and was attributed to the drinking of snow-water. Hippocrates said (in *De Glandulis*): "Most diseases of the glands are not primary within themselves, and that when glands of the neck become diseased themselves, they become tuberculous and produce struma and the body is attacked with fever". The term 'struma' is still being used on the Continent (in Austria and Italy as a medical term for goitre)[7].

It is strange that the Hippocratics do not have a description of diabetes. Papaspyros[8] mentions Laennec's view ('Proposition sur la doctrine d'Hippocrate', Paris, 1804), that Hippocrates attached little or no importance to the exact names of diseases. "He cared far more for the signs of prognosis than those of diagnosis . . . the Father of Medicine, under the influence of Pythagoraean philosophy, did not make any attempt to cure an incurable disease. . . ." In the dialogue of Plato: Timaeus, one reads, "No attempt should be made to cure a thoroughly diseased system". Aretaeus was against this inhuman doctrine and in this point he surpassed Hippocrates.

ARISTOTLE

The greatest name in Greece after Hippocrates was Aristotle of Stagira (384–322 BC), another Asclepiad and the tutor of Alexander the Great. He himself had been a pupil of Plato. He was not a practising physician, but a philosopher and natural historian of the highest order. His work contained the systems of anatomy, comparative anatomy, botany, zoology, embryology and physiology. Anatomy was studied by the dissection of animals, by diagrams and by direct observation of nature; to all of this he applied the use of formal logic as an instrument of precision. He must be regarded as the founder of scientific biology. It was inevitable that there were many weaknesses in his final conclusions, but in logic, ethics, embryology and natural history he was very good.

For our present purpose, his *Generation of Animals* is of particular interest. Before his time, there was no single generally accepted theory of generation. There existed certain questions: "What is the nature of seed?" "What determines the sex of offspring?", "What of sex-linked characteristics?" The Pangenesis theory held that both male and female seeds come from all parts of the body, because they generate all parts. Hippocratic theories suggested that the brain and/or marrow are the source of seed; moreover, the four humours, phlegm, blood, bile and water, are blended in the seed. The testicles are either the source of seed or containers of seed drawn from elsewhere (the brain). It was also thought that the right testicle produced male offspring and the left, female; an alternative view was that with more heat (in the womb) males, and with less heat, females, were produced.

In Aristotle's *History of Animals* ovariotomy is described[9] in sows for increased growth and in camels for increased strength and endurance, and in both cases as a contraceptive device; yet the existence as an independent organ and the function of the ovaries was not known to Aristotle. It was Herophilos (3rd century BC) who is supposed to have described the ovaries. According to Strabo, however, the ancient Egyptians also performed ovariotomy on human females[10]. Aristotle regarded the brain as a gland which secreted cold humours to prevent overheating of the body by the fiery heart (via the lungs)[11]. Living things possessed a soul (*psyche*), vegetative in plants, sensitive in animals, rational in man. Inanimate things lacked a soul. He distinguished between species (*eidos*) as classes, having attributes common to all their members, and genus as a general similarity in size, shape or appearance. He also classified animals according to their reproductive status into viviparous, oviparous, gemmulous, and spontaneous generation. He studied the development of the chick embryo day by day and noted the possibility of superfecundation, and said that the semen is the formative, activating agent or 'soul', the female element being the passive soil to be fertilized or moulded as the potter's clay. He described reproduction in the dogfish and the Cephalopoda (verified by Johannes Mueller in 1842 and Racovitza in 1894).

One of the pre-Aristotelian theories suggested that only the male parent contributes to the genetic character of the offspring, the contribution of the mother being merely nutritional and formative externally[12]. This theory is used by Aeschylus[13] and by Euripides[14] in defending the matricide of Orestes. In Aeschylus, Apollo says:

> It is not the mother who begets the one called her child; she but nourishes the seed sown in her. The begetter is the man who fertilises her; she — a stranger — safeguards a foreign sprout, when the gods do not injure it.

Euripides makes Orestes say:

> My father begat me, your daughter bore me; she was a field which received the seed from another; without a father a child would never be.

Aristotle quoted Leophanes[15] who guessed that the testicles are the source of male genetic material, which also determined the sex of the child. The Hippocratics had even suggested that a good method to determine the sex would be to tie one testicle off![16]

Aristotle made it clear, however, that the correctness of Leophanes' assumption depended on a preformationist hypothesis, i.e. that the seed is like the adult, preformed as if it were on a minute scale with the male sexual parts from the right and the female from the left testicle.

Aristotle, based on his first-hand observations, presented an epigenetic theory: namely, that the actual differentiations unfold themselves in the course of the development of the embryo. In the case of parthenogenesis, it would be, obviously, the female who provides the seed. Aristotle believed, correctly, that some fish show parthenogenetic reproduction; he believed this also to be true of the bees, which assumption was wrong; but parthenogenesis was regarded the exception from the rule. The main stumbling point of the preformation theory was the explanation of resemblance of the child to the mother.

The earlier Empedocles (504–443 BC) had already suggested that both male and female seed, perhaps partly formed, blend together, after the two complete individuals in the seed are 'torn asunder', and the parts are then fitted – blended – together in the womb, anticipating modern ideas of genetics by more than 2400 years![17] As said before, the Hippocratic idea was pangenetic, i.e. the seed is secreted by the entire body, by the hard parts, by the soft parts and by all the fluid in the body, which would go a long way to ex-

plain the inheritance of acquired characteristics[18]. Aristotle's 'homo-
iomeries' or 'like-parts' are called 'seeds' (*spermata*) by Anaxagoras,
because they generate all things, just as in sexual generation.
Anaxagoras posed the famous question: "How can hair come from
not-hair, flesh from not-flesh?"[19] Anaxagoras was a representative of
the pangenesis theory, and committed also to the version of the
left/right theory. Democritos (460–360 BC), the atomist, had refined
the pangenetic theory. He held, according to Aristotle[20], that the
difference between male and female is the consequence of which seed
'prevails'.

> Sometimes the semen of the woman is stronger, sometimes it is
> weaker; the same for the man. In the man there is both female and male
> seed; same for the woman. . . . If the seed that comes from both is
> strong, a male is born; if weak, a female. Whichever prevails in
> quantity, that is what is born[21].

This theory can explain resemblance to parents in particular characteristics. In a modification, it can also explain the generation of
hermaphrodites.

One of the most important points of Aristotle's criticism of the
pangenesis theory was that it goes too far in postulating a large
variety of materials in the semen without stating the degree to which
nature may be present in a particular material. In Aristotle's theory,
the female provides the proximate matter for reproduction, the male
the source of matter and change. Conception is a paradigm in terms
of the four causes (matter, mover, form and end); the end is
continued existence of the species; the species is the form present
potentially in the matter from the female, and actively in the semen
from the male. When the semen and mense (or egg) come together,
an activity is begun which continues through the life of the new
individual; this activity is called the nutritive and generative soul.
The source of the seed is blood; the male seed is more 'concocted'
by the internal heat, and the menstrual fluid or fluid in the egg is less
concocted. The semen may be a 'foam' of 'pneuma', the active
principle, and water, the vehicle. Children resemble their parents
because the movements of the pneuma in the semen and mense are
formally the same as those which are present in the parents; the seeds
have 'powers' in them, and when they meet, one will gain mastery.
Pneuma (air) has a special psychic function in Greek thought about
life. If 'pneuma' is the material basis of soul, then it must be material
which carries the movement of the offspring[22].

Aristotle's application of the four-cause analysis and the theory of
power and activity to sexual generation was revolutionary. As we

shall see later, Galen criticized Aristotle's theory very intelligently and developed his own ideas, which were nearer to Hippocrates'.

Aristotle's *History of Animals* seems also to contain the first mention of a contraceptive in the medical writings of the Greeks. Conception is prevented "by anointing that part of the womb on which the seed falls, with oil of cedar, or with ointment of lead, or with frankincense, commingled with olive oil"[23]. Himes remarked on this in a footnote[24] that Dr. Marie Stopes states in a recent paper that "one of the most effective (contraceptive) things is simple olive oil"; in 2000 cases over two years using olive oil and a sponge her percentage failure rate was zero. Aristotle, however, did not understand the principle that olive oil reduces the motility of the spermatozoa and gums-up the external os; he regarded the 'smoothness' as the modus operandi.

In the section 'On the Nature of Woman' of the Hippocratic writings, written by his disciples, there is advice, such as the following: "If a woman does not wish to become pregnant, dissolve in water misy as large as a bean and give it to her to drink, and for a year she will not become pregnant"[25]. The same passage appears in the section 'On Diseases of Women'. The section 'On the Nature of Woman' also contains the passage: "After coitus, if a woman ought not to conceive, she makes it a custom for the semen to fall outside when she wishes this". The identification of 'misy' is difficult. Sulphur, sulphate of copper and iron sulphate have all been suggested[26]. Hippocrates seems to have understood clearly that both male and female elements had to unite to cause conception. Whether the fall of the semen outside should be achieved by coitus interruptus or by (violent) bodily movements, or by wiping out the vagina, is not clear. The last mentioned technique, followed by passing urine, is probably very old and persists to some extent even today[27].

Although Himes stresses[28] that the

> scanty evidence suggests that the contraceptive knowledge of antiquity was confined largely to the heads of medical encyclopaedists, to a few physicians and scholars. The average citizen was probably quite ignorant of the subject. . . . But this in no ways dims the torch of knowledge that a few gifted, independent minds of antiquity handed down to the modern world through Islam.

A. Preus wrote a very interesting and important paper on 'Biomedical techniques for influencing human reproduction in the fourth century BC'[29]. In it he stresses that Plato, Aristotle and other 4th-century thinkers were (theoretically) concerned about the problem of controlling the size of the human population in a well-ordered state. These social theorists developed their population policies based on the medical knowledge available from the Hippocratic treatises, especially the gynaecological ones. The medical technique to control male fertility was castration. Aristotle was well acquainted with the effects of this operation and its use in animal husbandry (see p. 194). He knew that it makes males infertile, although he believed that the testes are only weights, holding down the spermatic passages. To Aristotle the nature of the semen was similar to that of 'brain; its matter is watery, and the heat is an additional factor'. But he denied that semen and marrow are similar. Natural sterility was caused primarily by birth defects and secondarily by obesity and disease, because the semen was produced in less quantity, or became fluid and cold. "To test for fertility, put semen in water; if it sinks, it is fertile; if it floats, it is not"[30]. The Hippocratics knew that mumps can be followed by orchitis and sterility. This perhaps explains the idea that the seed somehow descends from the head; moreover, in the Hippocratic *Airs, Waters, Places*, a book used by Aristotle, there is a discussion on the infertility of the Scythians; among its causes is given the habit of some Scythians of 'cutting the vein behind the ear' to cure lameness and swelling due to continuous riding. The effect of this cure is to destroy sperm. In the contemporary gynaecological writers there is also a reference to hot baths discouraging conception[31].

In contrast to N. Himes, Preus does not believe that the Hippocratic gynaecological treatises suggest coitus interruptus as a contraceptive method. He also concludes that the Greek writers and Aristotle did not think that control of population would be effected by controlling male reproductive capacity.

The techniques for controlling female fertility were as follows:

(1) Climatic conditions: Cities exposed to the South and sheltered from the North have many barren women and frequent spontaneous abortions. Those facing North and sheltered from the South, have also barren women, because of the "hard indigestible cold water"[32]. Women in such places have scanty menses, difficult childbirth, but rarely abort spontaneously. Those facing West are even more unhealthy, but those facing East have women who conceive readily and have easy deliveries. Marshy water also affects fertility and childbirth adversely.

(2) Nutrition is the most important environmental factor: Aristotle notes that both underfeeding and overfeeding diminish women's capacity to conceive and bear to term. The Hippocratics knew that obesity may interfere with fertility. Similarly, underfed women, and especially nursing mothers, may not menstruate regularly. Of Scythian women it is said in *Airs,*

Waters, Places that they were so obese that "their womb could not absorb the seed; their periods are late and scanty, the womb is closed by fat; the slave girls in Scythia are in so much better condition that they conceive as soon as they have intercourse"[33]. There are many dietary recommendations to encourage conception.

(3) The menstrual cycle and the rhythm method: Remarkably, the Hippocratic writers and Aristotle knew that certain times of the cycle are propitious for conception and vice versa. This is made clear when a suggested treatment for achieving conception means a daily regime beginning on the first day of the period. Intercourse is set for the tenth day, which sounds a very modern arrangement.

(4) The surgical removal of the ovaries has already been mentioned, especially known in animal husbandry. Later, Soranus considered the removal of the uterus, at least in the case of a carcinoma of the cervix[34].

(5) The vaginal and cervical environment and its use for contraceptive measures advised by Aristotle has already been discussed. The Hippocratic writers knew also that displacement of the womb can be responsible for infertility. In the section 'Illnesses of Women' of the Hippocratic Corpus, digital redressment and the use of instruments made of wood or lead is recommended and prolapse of the womb is also discussed (II, 132). The wooden or leaden instruments were mainly probes, used for the treatment of eversions of the womb, but could easily cause injury and ulceration and endanger the life of the patient. If used on a pregnant woman they might cause abortion.

(6) The mysterious substance 'misy', taken in water, has already been discussed.

(7) Contraceptive movements: Like the ancient Chinese, Aristotle believes that a woman must feel pleasure in coitus in order to suck the semen up into the womb and conceive. If that is not the case, the semen cannot be sucked into the womb. Movements which prevent the deposition of the semen will have contraceptive effect.

The remaining two methods for controlling population were – according to Preus – abortion and infanticide, but these fall outside the consideration of our subject.

THE ALEXANDRIAN SCHOOL

In 331 BC Alexandria was founded and Greek science and culture flourished in the ancient civilization of Egypt. The Alexandrian School with its great university and library and its famous leaders became the conservator of Greek ideas and helped to spread them over the East. After Aristotle's death it took over the subjects of his studies, including sexual generation. Herophilos and Erasistratos (4th century BC) were the great Alexandrian anatomists who advanced the knowledge of the structure and functions of the human body. They were the originators of dissecting; Herophilos was the Father of Scientific Anatomy (Sudhoff), and Erasistratos was the first experimental physiologist. Both were accused by Celsus and Tertullian of carrying out human vivisection.

Herophilos of Chalcedon was a pupil of the dogmatist Praxagoras. He differentiated the cerebrum and cerebellum, described the meninges, the 4th ventricle, and, among many other organs, the ovary, which he called the 'female testicle', under which name it was still referred to by Vesalius in 1555 AD, in the second edition of his *De Humani corporis Fabrica*! Herophilos also described the cornua uteri, the seminal vesicles and the prostate. He counted the pulse with a water–clock and analysed its rate and rhythm. An aphorism of Herophilos was paraphrased by the poet Gay[35],

> Nor Love nor Honor, Wealth nor Power
> Can give the heart a cheerful hour,
> When Health is lost.

In the 3rd century BC, Alexandrian and thus Hippocratic medicine spread into Mesopotamia, embracing remnants of Assyro-Babylonian medicine, and eventually to Syria, which became the stepping-stone between Graeco-Alexandrian, Oriental, Graeco-Roman and Mediaeval medicine. Strangely enough, medical translations from the Greek texts were often made first into Syrian, then Arabic and Hebrew and, eventually, into Latin.

John Simon (1816–1904), in his prize-winning essay on the history of the thymus in 1845, suggested that this gland was probably known to the Alexandrian School since the time of Herophilos and Erasistratos[8].

REFERENCES

1. Garrison, F. M.: Introduction to the History of Medicine. 4th ed., p. 83. Philadelphia, W. B. Saunders, 1929.
2. Froehlich, H.: Die Militaermedizin Homers. pp. 58–60. Stuttgart, 1879.

3. As 1: p. 89.
4. Seltman, Ch: Women in Antiquity. London, Pan Books, Thames & Hudson, 1956.
5. Johnston, R. D.: The history of human infertility. Fertil. Steril. **14,** 261–272, 1963.
6. Thompson, Dorothy B.: Three centuries of Hellenistic terracottas. Hesperia **23,** 72, 1954.
7. Iason, A. H.: The Thyroid Gland in Medical History. p. 17. New York, Froben Press, 1946.
8. Simon J.: The Thymus Gland, a Physiological Essay, London, 1845.
9. Aristotle: History of Animals. **ix,** 50, 632, a21.
10. Strabo: xvii, 284.
11. As 1: p. 101.
12. Preus, A.: Galen's criticism of Aristotle's conception theory. J. Hist. Biol. **10,** 65–85, 1977.
13. Aeschylus: Eumenides. 657 ff.
14. Euripides: Orestes. 552.
15. Aristotle: Generation of Animals. iv, 1, 765a 24.
16. Littré, E.: Oeuvres complètes d'Hippocrate, viii, 501.
17. As 12: pp. 69–70.
18. Hippocrates: On Seed. 3, Littré vii, 474; also Hippocrates: On Intercourse and Pregnancy (translated by Ellinger, Tage U.H.) New York, 1952.
19. As 12: p. 72.
20. As 15: iv, 1, 764a 7.
21. As 12: p. 73.
22. As 12: p. 79.
23. As 9: iv, 583a.
24. Himes, N. E.: Medical History of Contraception. p. 80, footnote 4. New York, Gamut Press, 1936.
25. As 16: vii, 415, para. 98.
26. As 24: p. 81.
27. ibid.: p. 82.
28. ibid.: p. 100.
29. Preus, A.: Biomedical techniques for influencing human reproduction in the fourth century BC. Arethusa **8** (2), 237–263, 1975.
30. As 15: ii, 7, 746 b 12 ff.
31. As 29: p. 243.
32. ibid.: p. 244.
33. ibid.: p. 245.
34. ibid.: p. 246.
35. As 1: p. 103.
36. Hippocrates: Aphorisms, Section VI; No. 28. In: Hippocratic Writings, Edited by G. E. R. Lloyd. Translated by J. Chadwick, W. N. Mann *et al.* Pelican Classics, Penguin Books.
37. As 36: Section VI; No. 30.
38. ibid.: No. 29.

CHAPTER SEVEN

THE GRAECO-ROMAN PERIOD
(156 BC–576 AD)

THERE were two main periods of Roman medicine: the pre-Hellenic, mainly known from writings of Cato and Pliny the Elder, and from laws, inscriptions and allusions in Latin authors.

The second was the Graeco-Roman period proper, although the educated Roman at the time of Pliny was already greatly influenced by the Greek language (which he spoke as French was spoken by the educated English from the 18th century to the beginning of the First World War in 1914) by Greek literature, culture and science.

The early Romans were a mixture of central Italian tribes with the 'obese' Etruscans ("si urbanus esses aut Sabinus aut Tiburs aut pinguis Umber aut obesus Etruscus", = "If you were born a citizen of Rome, a Sabine or a Tiburtine a big-bellied Etruscan or an Umbrian pig", Catullus, XXXIX: 10–12, the celebrated poem in which he accuses one Egnatius of smiling endlessly and inanely to show off his white teeth; this, he alleges, is due to the fact that, as a native of Spain, he rubs his teeth and rosy gums every morning with what his bladder voids. "Those white teeth only show how much you've swallowed from your chamber-pot" = "ut, quo iste uester expolitior dens est, hoc te amplius bibisse praedicet loti"). The Etruscans were perhaps an Oriental race with a highly developed culture of their own[1]. Southern Italy and Sicily were inhabited by the Greek colonists of Magna Graecia from the 6th century BC almost throughout the Roman Empire, the cultural influences of which ended with the School of Salerno. Greek medicine migrated to Rome after the destruction of Corinth in 146 BC. Before that time, Pliny says, the Romans got on for 600 years without doctors. The itinerant Greek physician stood in bad odour as a quack, a possible conspirator and poisoner[1]. Greek surgeons like Archagathos (*ca.* 220 BC), the first to practise in Rome and nicknamed 'Carnifex' for his butchery[1], did not make them more popular, nor did the Greek physicians and confidantes of the empresses Livia and Messalina. In 293 BC the cult of Aesculapios was officially introduced into Rome in the form of a huge serpent from Epidauros, following which a great number of snakes were kept in private houses. This was a great step from the simple cabbage, which was the favourite household remedy of Cato the Elder. The Romans themselves excelled in their sanitary arrangements as regards sanitary engineering, public baths and public lavatories (Vespasian put a levy on their use; when his son Titus protested, he held a piece of money so obtained under the latter's nose and asked: "Olet?" ["does it smell?"] To the reply "Non olet" he remarked ". . . and yet it comes from urine" ["Atqui", inquit, "e lotio est".][2] The Romans were not successful in eradicating the malaria-infested island in the Tiber (where the monk Rahere had his vision of St. Bartholomew ordering him to found a hospital in London, when he had a severe attack of malaria in about 1120 AD).

The influx of Greek physicians was particularly from Asia Minor, from the medical schools of Pergamon, Ephesos, Tralles and Miletos. In the wake of the original Dogmatists and Empirics came, eventually, Asclepiades of Bithynia (124 BC), whose high ethical standards and outstanding knowledge made him highly respected. He, in fact, refuted the Hippocratic idea of Humoralism, i.e. diseases being due to disturbances of the balance of the body humours. He attributed disorder to the relaxed or constricted conditions of its solid particles, the strictum and the laxum, called solidism, derived from Democritos' atomic ideas and revived in more modern times as the Brunonian theory of sthenic and asthenic states, or Broussais' theory of irritation and counter-irritation[3]. Asclepiades' therapeutic method was that of systematic measures to counteract disease and not the *vix curatrix naturae* (the healing power of nature) of Hippocrates. Some of his pupils and followers replaced his theory of solidism by a system of medicine based on the vital air or *pneuma*, which we have discussed before (pneumatism).

Curiously enough, the best accounts of medicine in Rome at the time of the early Empire came from the pens of two Romans who were not professional physicians. Aurelius Cornelius Celsus (25 BC–50 AD) was a nobleman of the Gens Cornelia who had practical experience of medicine as the head of an important household; he also compiled extensive treatises on medicine, agriculture and other subjects, in the manner of gentlemen of leisure of all ages, like the gifted amateurs of the 18th century. He gave medical advice as a lord of the manor, without charge, and was regarded by his contemporaries (Pliny, for example) more as a gentleman of letters than a physician (an *auctor* and not a *medicus*). The contemporary professional physicians in Rome ignored him, but his work was rediscovered and printed in 1478 and reprinted in many editions. It was *De Re Medica* (30 AD, i.e. towards the end of the reign of Tiberius) – no doubt partly a translation from Greek sources. It was elegant in literary style and he was called the 'Cicero medicorum'. The work consists of eight books, opening with an interesting account of the evolution of medicine to his days. The first four books deal with diseases which should be treated by diet and a regulated mode of life; a disease characterized by polyuria and lack of pain, but weakness, must be diabetes, especially as it should be treated by a diet containing a minimum amount of food, although the observation that the fluid output is greater than the fluid intake is surprising[4]. The last four books describe diseases amenable to drugs and to the surgery of the Alexandrian school. The fifth book contains a classified list of drugs, with a chapter on weights and measures, pharmaceutical methods and prescriptions including nutritive enemas. Surgery and surgical instruments were highly developed in Rome at that time (over 250 different surgical instruments were found in the ruins of Pompeii). Celsus was among the first to make a distinction between various forms of the tumours of the neck. In Book VII (Chapters 6 and 13) he differentiated struma from other tumours, recommending treatment for it in Book V (Chapter 18)[5]. This enlargement of the neck Celsus defined as a bronchocoele, that is as a tumour "under the skin and the larynx which is fleshy only, or may contain a sort of honey-like substance [? colloid], sometimes even containing small bones and hairs mixed together." The connection with the thyroid was not known to him. He writes, however, in the chapter 'De Struma' (Book VIII, Chapter 13) that the use of the term merely refers to swollen lymph glands. Of goitre proper he writes in Book VII (Chapter 13), on 'De Cervicis Vitio'. He clearly describes cystic goitre; after discussing the use of caustics, he adds "sed scalpelli curatio brevoir est" (see also p. 191). A single incision should be made down to the cyst, which is then bluntly dissected and removed. If that is not possible, it should be destroyed with caustics[6]. Roman physicians at that time knew that a slave with bulging eyes was of poor market value because he was usually physically weak and of a nervous disposition.

It seems that the ancient Romans were in the habit of measuring the enlargement of the neck of young women with a thread in cases of alleged defloration or pregnancy, without, of course, connecting it with the thyroid. Catullus referred to it:

> Non illam nutrix orienti luce revisens
> Hesterno collum poterit circumdare filo.

> At dawn her nurse will not be able to wind
> The same thread round the bride's neck
> that was there last night. . . .[7]
> (Catulli, Carminia: LXIV Peleus et Thetis, lines 376–377).

Celsus also described a condition in which there was excessive excretion of urine (polyuria) and wasting (? diabetes mellitus).

The second non-medical informant is of general international fame: he was Pliny the Elder, or to give him his full name, Gaius Plinius Secundus (23–79 AD) (see Section II). He was another Roman of eminent family, and died when Vesuvius erupted. At the time he was in command of a small naval force in the Bay of Naples, and had orders to stand by and help people in distress caused by the natural disaster; but was so keen on observing the phenomenon that he ventured too near the site of the eruption and was killed. He was a naturalist by inclination, in the same sense as some of the 18th century and early 19th century amateur naturalists. His magnum opus was the *Natural History*[8], of which Books XX to XXXII dealt with medicine, although he briefly discussed the origin of the medical art in Book II, p. 224 and V, p. 370; the frauds of the medical art in Book V, p. 3; the practice of the medical art in Book V, pp. 156–158 and 376–381, and changes in the system of the medical art in Book V, p. 374.

Pliny was contemptuous of the Greeks for using human organ-preparations therapeutically. At the same time, he did recommend human bone marrow (from the femur) and the brain of young children for use against epilepsy. He also recommended animal organs as general remedies, and the healthy organs of animals as specific remedies, e.g. boiled brain of a crow or owl for headache; asses' liver for pain in the liver; for disease of the spleen, the use of raw spleen, removed from a dog which is still alive; against renal pain, the kidneys of a hare; against colic due to a stone in the bladder, eat a boar's bladder with its contents for men, for women the bladder of a wild sow. For impotence or improvement of sexual function in men, the testicles of male animals should be eaten; to achieve pregnancy, women should eat genitalia of a (female) hare[9]. From Pliny's writings (Book IX, Chapter 37), and also from Vitruvius' *De Architectura*, from Juvenal, "Quis tumidum gutter miratur in Alpibus" (Satire 13), it may be assumed that there must have been epidemics of goitre in the Alps in those days.

Goitre, according to Pliny, was caused by impurities in the water.

"Only men and swine are subject to swellings in the throat, which are mostly caused by the noxious quality of the water they drink"[10]. (See also the view of the Hippocratics on goitre, a deformity, being caused by drinking of snow-water, in Chapter 6).

Like Celsus, Pliny believed that the hot human blood of dying gladiators had a healing effect in cases of epilepsy. This seems to be a common belief among primitive people the world over. Arabs, before Mohammed, often drank their enemy's blood.

Pliny's Books XX to XXV are a great herbal, mainly derived from the work of Theophrastos of Ephesos (370–280 BC), the friend and pupil of Aristotle, to whom the latter bequeathed his library. He was not only a physician, but the 'proto-botanist', who did for the knowledge of plants what Hippocrates did for human medicine. His *De Historia Plantarum* contained careful descriptions of some 500 different plants. In the ninth chapter he summarized all that was known in his time of the medicinal properties of plants, "from the nepenthe and moly of Homer to the arrow poisons of African tribes"[11].

In Pliny's *Natural History*[8], aphrodisiacs are mentioned, including "hemlock applied to the testes at puberty" (hemlock was the poison which Socrates had to drink for his judicial execution). "Hempseed and condrion make men impotent" (Book XXII, Chapter 45). Sterilizing plants or animal products taken in drink or food are, among others, parsley and mint; the latter because it curdles milk and thus prevents "the seminal fluid from obtaining the requisite consistency" (Book XX, Chapter 53). Pliny gives a magic anti-aphrodisiac: "If a man makes water upon a dog's urine, he will become disinclined to copulation" (Book XXX, Chapter 49). When he repeats Aristotle, his advice seems better.

Curiously enough, both Pliny and Celsus had a precursor in their observations on human fertility and sterility and on the prevention of conception in the person of the great Latin poet and rationalist scientist Lucretius (99–55 BC). In his great work *De Natura Rerum*, he discusses the subject in Book IV (pp. 165ff). Sterility is caused by "too great thickness" or by "undue fluidity or thinness of the semen"[12]. "Some males impregnate some females more readily than others, and other females conceive and become pregnant more readily from other males. . . ." Diet and the "modes of intercourse" may be of importance.

Other leading surgeons and physicians, who were contemporaries or antedated Celsus, were Heliodorus and Archigenes of Apamea, who both used surgical ligatures, which at Galen's time could be bought at a special shop in the Via Sacra.

Of great importance was the work of Pedacius Dioscorides (54–68

AD), who was a Greek army surgeon in the service of Nero. He was the founder of Materia Medica, medical botany as an applied science. He described about 1600 plants or plant-principles, of which 149 were already known to Hippocrates, and ninety are still used today. "His classification was qualitative, as in a materia medica, rather than botanical . . ."[13]. His descriptions were followed 'word by word' for 16 centuries. *De Materia Medica* was published in more than seventy editions in all European languages except English. The original manuscript was discovered rather late in modern times by a Belgian in Constantinople and is now held in Vienna. The work consists of five books and discusses also animal products of medicinal value. It influenced Islamic physicians greatly and for a long time the knowledge contained in them was handed down from Arabic translations of fragments of the original. Prevention of conception is dealt with in four groups:

(1) Magic, e.g. wearing of amulets.

(2) Ineffective potions, e.g. finely ground willow leaves in water, iron rust (ferrum oxydatum) and the roots of fern, which – if taken by pregnant women – will cause miscarriage.

(3) Medicated pessaries, e.g. peppermint juice mixed with honey used as suppository before coitus (Book III, Chapter 36, p. 287), pepper, introduced as a pessary after coitus (Book II, Chapter 188, p. 238).

(4) Anointing the genitals with cedar-gum prior to coitus, applying alum in various forms to the uterus (? cervix) before coitus.

In addition, Dioscorides mentions certain substances causing sterility (in contrast to preventing conception), e.g. the bark of the white poplar taken with the kidney of the mule (Book I, Chapter 109, p. 101). This superstition persisted for centuries.

Fertility will be promoted by putting against the womb after menstruation a pessary made of the rennet of a hare, but hare rennet, when swallowed, can cause the death of an embryo, or – after menstruation – sterility. As mucopurulent discharge was the most frequent cause of sterility, rennet pessaries, which helped to digest and dissolve that type of discharge, were promoting fertility. If continually used, however, they might well cause contraception. If such pessaries were, therefore, controlled by the medical profession and their use, accordingly, limited[14], it is most likely that they were used mainly for the treatment of sterility. Young rundles of ivy leaves spread with honey, and introduced into the uterus, "provoke menstruation and evacuate the embryo", i.e. act as an abortefacient (Book II, Chapter 210, p. 255).

Aretaeos of Kappadokia, who lived under Dornitian (81–96 AD) or Hadrian (117–138 AD), came nearer than any other Greek of the Graeco-Roman period to the spirit and method of Hippocrates[15]. He gave classic descriptions of a number of major diseases, such as pneumonia, tetanus, diphtheria (ulcera Syriaca), the aura in epilepsy, but especially the first complete clinical description of diabetes mellitus, the first in Europe. He called it diabetes ($\delta\iota\alpha\beta\alpha\acute{\iota}\nu\omega$ = I pass through):

> Diabetes is a wonderful affection, not very frequent among men, being a melting down of the flesh and limbs into urine. The patients never stop making water, but the flow is incessant, as if the opening of aqueducts. Life is short, disgusting and painful; thirst unquenchable; excessive drinking, which, however, is disproportionate to the large quantity of urine, for more urine is passed; and one cannot stop them either from drinking or making water; Or, if for a time they abstain from drinking, their mouth becomes parched and their body dry; the viscera seems as if scorched up; they are affected with nausea, restlessness and burning thirst; and at no distant term they expire.[16]

Of other successors, Soranos of Ephesos (98–138 AD) is the most important and deserves special mention. After studying in Alexandria, he practised in Rome at the time of Trajan and Hadrian (91–117 AD). He was a follower of the Methodist School of Asclepiades. In his *Gynaecology* he wrote "the most brilliant and original account of contraceptive technique prior to the 19th century"[17]. Himes dedicated his *Medical History of Contraception* "To Soranos (98–138) most brilliant gynaecologist of antiquity, whose originality and distinguished career illumined a future path of medicine for nearly two thousand years". Soranos' original text was lost until 1838, and was known in the Middle Ages mainly through Moschion's treatise, *Gynaecia: De mulieribus passionibus*. Soranos was the author of 40 treatises, according to Emerius, a Dutch scholar[18]. In one or another of these he wrote on nearly all the subjects known to the healing art, though his main interest was in gynaecology, obstetrics and paediatrics. He described the anatomy of the female pelvic organs and the differences in girls, in pregnancy and in old women. He referred to the ovaries as *'didymi'* (paired organs),

> which are attached to the outside of the uterus, near its isthmus, one on each side. They are of loose texture, and like glands are covered by a particular membrane.[37]

He described the pigmentation of the face in pregnancy; he also noted that amenorrhoea tends to occur in women of masculine appearance. He described clitoral enlargement, perhaps in patients with adrenal cortical hyperfunction[19,20]. He used vaginal speculums, forgotten until the 19th century. "The most favourable time for conception", he thought "was shortly after the menstrual period". Remaining in bed after coitus might improve fertility. His discussion of contraceptive techniques is particularly rational. "On the Use of Abortefacients and of Measures to Prevent Conception" reads as follows:

> Atokion ... designates a remedy which prevents conception ... phthorion ... designates a remedy which kills the foetus ... ekbolion ... designates a violent convulsion of the body as for example in jumping.

Hippocrates, in his book *On the Nature of the Child*, had rejected abortefacients ("I shall never prescribe a phthorion") and advised a method to procure abortion by jumping, so that the buttocks are touched with the feet (the "Lacedaemonian Leap"[21]).

Soranos permitted the use of phthoria only in exceptional cases:

> when birth threatens to become dangerous ...; ... we think it surer to prevent conception than to kill the foetus. ... Abortion should not be resorted to in order to conceal the consequences of adultery, nor simply to maintain the chaste female form.

His main reliance was on an elaborate array of occlusive pessaries of various types, vaginal plugs, using wool as a base, and those were impregnated with gummy substances, such as sour oil, honey, cedar gum, opobalsam. Astringent solutions (e.g. alum and natron = native sodium carbonate) contract the os and thus make impregnation less likely. Soranos thought that the "damage done by drinking potions with the intention of preventing conception, can be very considerable", and he warned against it.

Oribasios, born at Pergamon *ca.* 325 AD, studied medicine (including the history of medicine) under Zenon of Chypre. He wrote an encyclopaedic *Medical Collection*, consisting of the 'Synopsis' and the 'Euphorists'. To prevent conception, he recommended (in Chapter 116)

> ... drink male or female fern root in sweet tasting wine, blossoms or leaves of the willow ..., but when one wants to prevent conception before copulation one anoints the virile part of the man with 'hedysome' (Fr.) juice. The application in a pessary after coitus of ground-up cabbage blossoms prevents the semen from congealing; before coitus, one injects a decoction of coronilla seed into the vagina.[22]

St. Jerome (Hieronymus), the Latin Church Father, a contemporary of Oribasios, strongly condemned methods used to prevent conception or to produce sterility.

Juvenal mentioned that Roman women had intercourse with eunuchs in order that they might enjoy themselves without becoming pregnant ("Sunt quas eunuchi imbelles ... tantum rapit Heliodorus"; Juvenal VI, 367).

Aetios was born in Amida, Mesopotamia, and lived at the time of Justinian I, 527–565. He was physician to the Byzantine court and the first doctor converted to Christianity. He wrote, in Greek, a medical encyclopaedia in sixteen books or discourses, in which he described goitrous enlargement of the neck and also gave a description of bestial insatiable appetite, that very much reminds us of diabetes[23]. In Book XVI he devoted two chapters to contraceptive technique, about which his ideas were similar to those of Soranos.

It is necessary to stress again Himes' repeated assertions, that in spite of such an interest among the leaders of the medical profession and some of the philosopher–scientists, "there was only a restricted diffusion of contraceptive knowledge in antiquity" and the broad masses of the population were ignorant of rational contraceptive techniques.

It is doubtful whether in Imperial Rome (or before) male or female protective sheaths were used, although Himes quotes a paper by C. E. Helbig on a religious legend indicating the use of a goat bladder[24].

It is interesting to note that the Romans, especially of the Empire, were very keen on having cretinous dwarfs. M. A. Ruffer tells the story that the poet Arisastus was reputedly so small that no one could see him (a similar anecdote circulated about the French actress Sarah Bernhardt, who was extremely thin)[25]. E. Tietze-Conrat quotes evidence from Plutarch, Martial and Suetonius for the existence of dwarfs in Ancient Rome, indicating a morbid taste for abnormalities[26].

The most important physician of the Graeco-Roman period, however, was Galen (130–200 AD), the greatest medical man of antiquity after Hippocrates (see Section II). Galen had an enormous influence on medicine throughout the Middle Ages and up to the 17th century, and became the founder of experimental physiology. He was a prolific writer and the most experienced and skilled practitioner of his time. He did not possess, however, the lofty ethical stature of Hippocrates, nor the lucidity and honesty of the latter's style. He had a tendency to self-advertisement, often omitting important facts in the description of his observations, but never a brilliant diagnosis nor a brilliant cure. Galen was a man of many talents, but perhaps not of genius like Hippocrates[27].

Galen's system of physiology and pathology was complicated and speculative. He worked out an answer to every possible problem, but often without the clinical observation and descriptive power of Hippocrates. His pathology was based on a combination of the humoral ideas of Hippocrates with the Pythagorean theory of the four elements, to which he added his own idea of an all-pervading spirit or *pneuma*. He presented this understructure of the great medical compendium he had created with complete assurance and dogmatic infallibility. Such a presentation, supported by monotheism and pious self-righteousness, appealed to the Moslems and to the mediaeval Christian Church, who were his inheritors in the field of medicine. It had the devastating effect of a rigid system which completely prevented the development of new ideas, virtually until the Renaissance.

His approach to treatment also differed from that of Hippocrates, who believed in assisting nature, fresh air, good diet, purgatives, bloodletting, barley water, honey and water (or vinegar), massage and hydrotherapy. Galen introduced a complicated system of polypharmacy, which survived in medicine until the 18th and even the 19th century. He produced nearly a hundred books on a variety of subjects, thirty on pharmacy alone. Three important books dealt with the temperaments and there were sixteen essays on the pulse.

His discoveries and achievements must not be overlooked nor belittled. He described aneurysms, the different forms of tuberculosis (phthisis), recognizing that it was transmitted, and separated pneumonia from pleurisy. His prescriptions were intelligently worked out and he understood the use of many drugs, which he collected during his continuous travels; especially of opium, hyoscyamus, hartshorn, turpentine, wine, honey, grape-juice and barley water, and cold compresses.

His analysis, knowledge and classification of the pulse was excellent and the *ars sphygmica* survived until the 19th century.

Galen introduced the theory of the four temperaments, which had a profound effect on his form of practice of medicine. He carried out many dissections on animals, on apes, oxen and swine, and also studied osteology. His contributions to the knowledge of anatomy were impressive, especially in the field of neurology and the anatomy of the brain. He also wrote the first manual on dissection (encheiresis), which remained valid until modern times. As an experimental physiologist he studied the result of experimental section of the spinal cord.

Concerning the endocrine glands, there is an allusion to the thyroid in a treatise on 'De voce', which has been attributed to Galen:

> The neck has two glands in which moisture is generated, as in the epiglottis a thick and viscid humor is secreted for the moistening of that organ. But from the true glands which are in the neck and from the substance of the epiglottis are no ducts through which the humor may

flow, as is the case in the two glands of the tongue. But those which are in the neck are of a spongy nature and from them the humor oozes out and trickles down [sic!] there being no necessity for ducts (which the others need) whereby the fluid may be carried.

The lack of a duct of the thyroid vexed the ancient anatomists. Galen looked upon these glands as filters through which the fluid portions of the blood are sieved. He thought that the 'secretion' of the thyroid lubricated the larynx and its cartilages (and so did Bartholin (1626–1690), Malpighi (1628–1694) and Morgagni (1682–1772)[10]. Galen produced aphonia by cutting the recurrent laryngeal nerve. He also studied experimentally the mechanism of respiration and showed that an excised heart will beat outside the body.

Galen mentions spongia usta made from fucus vesiculosus for treatment of goitre, as did the Hippocratics and Pliny before him[10]. It seems that the pituitary gland was known to Galen from his anatomical studies, but was first described as a separate entity by Vesalius.

G. W. Harris referred specifically to Galen in his Dale Lecture for 1971, delivered six months before his death (see also Section II). He called the lecture *Humours and Hormones*. 'Humours' because he began with the early views on the function of the pituitary gland. According to Galen the blood flows to and fro in the arteries, carrying *vital spirit* to the various parts of the body. *Animal spirit* was to be formed from 'vital spirit' in the brain, with the waste products of this chemical reaction flowing to the base of the brain, down the pituitary stalk and so to the pituitary gland. From this 'phlegmatic glandule' the waste products were supposed to be passed by ducts through the sphenoid and ethmoid bones to the nasopharynx, where they emerged as 'pituita' or nasal mucus. This view of the pituitary function was held for 1500 years, until Conrad Victor Schreiber (1614–1680) of Wittenberg[34,35] and Richard Lower (1631–1691) of Oxford[36] disproved the existence of a communication between the ventricles of the brain and the naso-pharynx, at least under normal circumstances (see also p. 138). Lower, whose theories were based on simple experiments and good clinical observations, formed the opinion that substances passed from the brain through the infundibulum and pituitary stalk to the gland, where they were distilled back into the blood. "It is interesting" remarked Harris, "to compare this early idea with our own views 300 years later, that neurosecretory material, formed in hypothalamic nuclei pass down the nerve fibres, through the infundibulum to the posterior pituitary where they 'distil' into the blood as the octapeptide hormones, oxytocin and vasopressin, and that hypothalamic nerve terminals liberate releasing factors into the portal vessels in the infundibulum and that these are carried down the stalk to the anterior pituitary, where they evoke 'distillation' of protein hormones into the blood." Galen, who worked at Alexandria *ca.* 155 AD, knew of the thymus, which he renamed ϑύμος, because it reminded him of a bunch of thyme flowers (ϑθμον). He thought the thymus was to protect the superior vena cava from pressure by the sternum and to stay and support the vessel and its branches. This view prevailed through the centuries. He also described a condition where a patient became emaciated because he could not eat – perhaps anorexia nervosa – but he did not specify the sex of the patients nor whether their periods stopped[28]. Soranos, however, wrote "more often anorexia strikes women who are suffering from amenorrhoea", implying that the disturbed function of the menstrual cycle caused the condition[28]. Galen did, however, criticize Aristotle's conception theory intelligently. In his treatise 'Peri Spermatos' ('On Seed')[29] and 'Kyomatos Diaplasmatos' ('On the Development of the Foetus')[30], he attempted to be faithful to the idea of reproduction of the Hippocratists, and did so by accepting many of their mistakes. He accepted the theory that the right testicle *and* the right side of the womb produce males and the left, females. This he did in spite of Aristotle's intelligent arguments against it. On the other hand, he learned and accepted from the Alexandrian anatomists the existence of the ovaries, which he also called 'female testicles'. This is, unfortunately, not evidence of an improved theory of sexual generation, because Galen believed, like Hippocrates, that the testicles are a storage depot for sperm, which has been collected from other parts of the body. Although Galen's view is an improvement on Aristotle's idea that the testicles are 'weights' to keep the seminal passage tight, Galen's theory cannot explain the fact that the 'female testicles' (i.e. the ovaries) are on dissection not storage containers, and are in fact, smaller than the (male) testicles. But Galen joins issue, correctly, with Aristotle in maintaining the Hippocratic point of view that there must be both male and female contributions to generation, and not – as Aristotle has claimed – only one (the male). By not ascribing any material role to the semen, however, Aristotle attempts to escape the difficulty in which Empedocles and Democritos found themselves, because they could not account for the way in which the material from the male seed mixed with that from the female. Moreover, Aristotle defends his theory of the soul as the form and active principle of the living being by ascribing active and formal principles to the male seed only. Galen, however, like the Stoics, believes in a complex material basis of the soul and wants this *pneuma* transferred to the foetus itself. Galen attacks the (Aristotelian) idea that the semen evaporates in the womb, with rather stringent arguments, as can be observed by dissection of recently impregnated animals; nor does pneuma escape via the female genitalia. Semen and menstrual blood mingle in the womb and it would not make sense for them to separate again. The semen, which has to remain long enough to do its work, cannot escape.

Galen thinks that there would be little time for the semen to escape, because his dissection studies seemed to confirm the Hippocratic assumption that there is an identifiable foetation six days after coitus, which is surrounded by a membrane which develops almost immediately after copulation[31]. Furthermore, Galen maintains that the male semen provides the material for the development of the nerves and of the walls of the arteries and the veins. Menstrual fluid is the source of blood, as semen could not be, because it does not have the characteristics of blood any more. Galen's theory is that female seed is expelled from the female testicles at the time of coitus, that both seeds meet in the womb, mix and form a membrane. The female seed serves as food for the semen in its development. The gonads are connected to all three systems of the body, a form of pangenesis against Aristotle's theory[30]. Galen does note that the female must provide not only matter, but also a source of movement if the offspring is to resemble the mother as much as the father; furthermore that excision of the ovaries practised in animals and by some people in women leads to an absence of libido and to sterility, which would indicate the existence of a female seed passing through and from the ovaries. By making the semen become a material part of the first foetation, Galen makes more plausible the transfer of form from male parent to offspring.

> . . . the theory is so fully developed that it has a schematic attractiveness, but also developed enough so that it is empirically testable – and consequently falsifiable. There are mistakes which it is a service to make; Galen's often are like that.[30]

In an interesting study, Professor Erna Lesky has added an important footnote to *Galen as Forerunner of Hormone Research*[32]. In 'Peri Spermatos' (= 'On Seed'), Galen asks: "What is, therefore, the cause, that castrates slow down in their whole vital capacity?" (IV, 574, K), after stating that castrated animals lose not only the power of procreation and libido, but also show changes as regards fat deposits, hair growth and distribution, voice, vascular tonus, etc. Galen stresses (IV, 628, K) that the sexual characteristics are expressed not only in the genital organs, but in the whole body: lion's mane, cox comb, boar's tusk, etc.; these he calls "ta hystera moria" = *Tá ὕστερα μόρια* = the later parts. In men, he talks about "maleness" (ἀρρενότης), and in women about "femaleness" (θηλύτης) (IV. 585,

K). Galen argues that in the same manner as a 'poison' or its effective 'antidote' act in a minute dose (ἐλάχιστον) on the whole body, the sperm (σπέρμα) can act in minute doses on the whole body to convey maleness or femaleness. In case of castration, the maleness or the femaleness are removed, and what is left is the basic structure, as it were. Thus, Lesky suggests, Galen has worked out by mere argument and analogy with the action of poisons and antidotes a scheme which comes very near our modern concept of hormone activity.

Galen described diabetes mellitus as a weakness of the kidneys; he did not refer to the sweet taste of the urine. He also called it "diarrhoea of the urine" (diarrhoea urinosa) and "dipsakos" (causing thirst)[33].

REFERENCES

1. Garrison, F. M.: Introduction to the History of Medicine. 4th ed., p. 105. Philadelphia, W. B. Saunders, 1929.
2. Suetonius: De Vita Caesarum. Vespasianus 23.
3. As 1: p. 106.
4. Celsus, A. C.: De Medicina. (With an English translation by Spencer, W. G. (3 Vols.) Book IV, Chap. 20:2, London, 1935–38.
5. Iason, A. H.: The Thyroid Gland in Medical History, p. 22. New York, Froben Press, 1946.
6. ibid.: p. 24.
7. The Poems of Catullus (translated by Michie, James). London, Panther Books, 1972.
8. Bostock, John and Riley, H. T. (translators): The Natural History of Pliny. London, Henry G. Bohn, 1857.
9. Biedl, A.: Innere Sekretion. Berlin, Urban & Schwarzenberg, 1910.
10. As 5: p. 26.
11. As 1: p. 102.
12. Himes, N. E.: Medical History of Contraception, p. 82. New York, Gamut Press, 1936.
13. As 1: p. 109.
14. As 12: p. 88.
15. As 1: p. 110.
16. Aretaeos the Kappadokian: The extant works. Edited and translated by Adams, F. London, 1856.
17. Lueneburg, H.: Die Gynaecologie des Soranos von Ephesuos. Geburtshilfe, Frauen-und Kinderkrankheiten, Diatetik der Neugeborenen. Uebersetzt von Dr. phil. H. Lueneburg, commentiert und mit Beilagen von Dr. J. Ch. Huber, Medizinalrath. Muenchen, Lehmann, 1894.
18. As 12: p. 89.
19. Brothwell, D. and Sandison, A. T.: Diseases in Antiquity. Springfield, Thomas, 1967.
20. Sandison, A. T. and Wells, C.: Endocrine Diseases. pp. 521–531. Springfield, Thomas, 1967.

21. Preus, A.: Biomedical Techniques for Influencing Human Reproduction in the Fourth Century BC. Arethusa Chap. 8.2. p. 250, 1975.

22. As 12: p. 93.

23. Aetios of Amida: ΒΙΒΛΙΩΝ ΙΑΤΡΙΚΩΝ, ΤΟΜΟΣ. A Venetiae, A. Manutii et A. Asulani, 1534.

24. As 12: p. 187.

25. Ruffer, M. A.: On dwarfs and other deformed persons. Bull. Soc. Arch. Alex. **13**, 1, 1911.

26. Tietze-Conrat, E.: Dwarfs and Jesters in Art. London, Phaidon, 1957.

27. As 1: p. 113.

28. Dunseith, Bridget L.: Personal view. Br. Med. J. **1**, 1694, 1978.

29. Preus, A.: Galen's criticism of Aristotle's conception theory. J. Hist. Biol. **10** (1), 65–85, 1977.

30. Ibid.: p. 84.

31. Hippocrates; On the Nature of the Child. Chap. 2.

32. Lesky, Erna: Galen als Vorlaeufer der Hormonforschung. Centaurus, I., pp. 156–162. 1950–51.

33. Papaspyros, N. S.: The History of Diabetes Mellitus. p. 6, London, 1952.

34. Schneider, Conrad V.: Dissertatio de osse cribriforme, et sensu ac organo odoratus. Wittebergae, Mevii, Mevii, 1655.

35. Schneider, C. V.: Liber primus de catarrhis. Wittebergae, T. Mevii and E. Schumacheri. 1660.

36. Lower R.: Dissertatio de origine catarrhi in qua ostenditur illum non provenire a cerebro. In Tractatus de corde. Londini, typ. J. Redmayne, pp. 221–239. 1670.

37. Temkin, O.: Soranus' Gynaecology. Johns Hopkins Press, Baltimore, 1956.

CHAPTER EIGHT

THE BYZANTINE PERIOD
(395–1453 AD)

As will be seen from the headings of the present and of the previous chapter, the Byzantine Period and the Graeco-Roman Period show a certain overlap. Little progress was made in medicine during the 1000 years of the Byzantine Empire, which itself eventually became fossilized. It was really surprising that it held out so long against the increasing pressure of the young and vigorous nations surrounding its frontiers. The civil administration of the Empire was run increasingly by eunuchs, who were actually efficient if hidebound. One of the ablest and most successful generals was Narses, the "elderly Armenian eunuch", who received his first command when he was in his mid-fifties and showed valour on the battlefield of Gualdo Tadino (552 AD), and afterwards as the first Exarch of Ravenna, "a good soldier and most prudent statesman"[1,2].

At best, some aspects of Greek medicine were maintained and Sir Clifford Allbutt summed it up correctly: "The chief monuments of learning were stored in Byzantium until Western Europe was fit to take care of them"[3].

Of the compilers during that long period, four names stand out:

The work of Oribasios (325–403), a friend and personal physician of Julian Apostata, was discussed in the previous chapter.

Aetios of Amida, Justinian I's personal physician, was also partly discussed previously. His collected writings, the *Tetrabiblion*, contained the teachings of Rufus of Ephesos, a contemporary of Soranos and a good surgeon who also wrote on gout, of Soranos, and of Philomenos.

Alexander of Tralles (525–605 AD) was a brother of the architect of the Hagia Sophia in Constantinople. After many years of a peripatetic existence, he eventually settled in Rome. His main work, the

71

Practica, although based on Galen, has some original observations and descriptions of disease and of remedies. He gives an especially good account of worms and their treatment, and seems to be the first to recommend colchicum for the treatment of gout, of which he gives an excellent description.

Paul of Aegina (625–690 AD), is the last of the four. His encyclopaedic work, the *Epitome of Medicine*, consisted of seven books, covering all the then existing medical knowledge without claiming any originality. It was really a case of "relata refero", although conscientiously executed. Goitre was still called "Bronchocele", the popular name being "Tumor gutturis" or "guttur tumidum"[4] (chronic swellings of the lymphglands were called "strumae". It is a Greek word for hogs, which are prolific and bear many offspring, since they have glandulous necks[4]. Paulus defined a "bronchocele" as a large round swelling, which was formed "in the neck from the inner parts, whence it obtains the name"; there are two varieties, the steatomatous and the aneurismatical.

> The aneurismatical we judge from the symptoms of an aneurysm, and abandon as hopeless, like all other aneurysms which it is dangerous to meddle with, as is the case most especially with those of the neck, owing to the size of the arteries. The steatomatous we operate on like steatomes in general, distinguishing and avoiding the vessels"[4].
>
> Concerning the tumour of the neck which is called a bronchocele. . . . There may be a large and round tumour in front of the neck, deriving its name from that interior part, which the Greeks call Bronchon. This tumour may be of two forms, in one the fat or soft parts swell; this kind belongs to the family of abscesses; which the Greeks call Steatomata, the other is derived from dilatation of these parts and this we must remember, and avoid it, for it might be an aneurysm.[5]

It is probable that Aetios (500 AD) and later, Ambroise Paré (1561 AD) regarded exophthalmic goitre, which was known to them, as a variety of aneurysm.

REFERENCES

1. Fisher, H. A. L.: A History of Europe. London, Fontana, 1960.
2. Medvei, V. C.: Senior appointments: age and health. Practitioner **199,** 322–324, 1967.
3. Allbutt, Sir Clifford: Science and Mediaeval Thought. C. J. Clay & Sons, London, 1901. (Harveian Oration, 1900.)
4. Iason, A. H.: The Thyroid Gland in Medical History, p. 28. New York, Froben Press, 1946.
5. Paul of Aegina. Epitome of Medicine, Book VI, chap. 38.

CHAPTER NINE

EVIDENCE OF ENDOCRINE DISORDERS IN OTHER PREHISTORIC AND ANCIENT COMMUNITIES

D URAN, in a paper entitled 'The Surgery of the Mayas' illustrated a statuette from Kaminal Juyu, which showed bilateral exophthalmos, which may have been connected with thyrotoxicosis. Wells found a similar condition presented in a head-shaped Peruvian pottery jug of the Mochica period[1] (Figure 6).

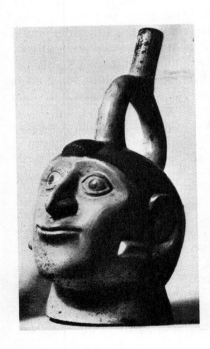

Figure 6 Pottery vase, Peru, Mochica period. Possibly intended to portray thyrotoxicosis [British Museum, London]

Tietze-Conrat found examples of hunchbacks from the Inca Empire. He also illustrated a Mayan 6th century AD pottery figure of a hunchback.

Giants, so popular in the Old Testament, also occurred in Greenland. Keith described in great detail a 12th century skull found in a cemetery of the cathedral in Gardar, at the Southern tip of Greenland. He diagnosed it as acromegalic "produced by normal . . . action" in primitive man. The skull must be one of a descendant of the first Norse settlers in Greenland[2]. Several of the Nordish sagas contain detailed references to people of immense stature and unusual appearance. The mere fact, however, that, in the same manner as in the Bible, there are whole genealogies through which the inheritance of these traits can be traced, seems to indicate that the diagnosis 'acromegaly' cannot be readily accepted. Although it is said that "this gigantism seems to have become endemic in the Fyrdafjord district of Sogn (Norway) and was commonly associated with personality changes", i.e. a "mental and physical precocity with a tendency to premature senility . . . associated with elements of pituitary hypofunction" and a parallel was found in Tanum (South Sweden), where rock-tracings indicated sea-raiders of immense size, the same caution has to be made as in the case of the families or tribes of giants in the Old Testament: Acromegalics are often sterile and suffer from muscular weakness, impaired field of vision (it was said on one occasion that Goliath had such visual defect and could not see David's action), thus they are hardly capable of the sustained physical effort which powerful warriors or seafaring people have to be able to maintain. It is just possible that giant tribes or families existed, certainly with a genetically increased growth-hormone production which, however, did not lead to acromegaly. The existence of such gigantism can still be observed today, although only sporadically. In fact, Larger has discussed the concept of 'racial gigantism' as a cause of extinction of fossil species[3]. The giant Saurians have been assumed to have been victims of this process, and Moore asks: "Did the tall Cro-Magnon people finally succumb to gigantism and are the Shillucks of today fated to follow them?"[4]. Mahoudeau rejected, however, Larger's hypothesis[5].

Todd examined the basis for the belief in the existence of palaeolithic giants and dwarfs. He thought that the concept of racial gigantism is related to that of pachyostosis in early animal groups. This idea has also been considered by Casati[6] in more recent times. It seems, however, that the whole question would have to be reconsidered and re-examined with the help of the tests and hormone-assays available at the present day.

It has been suggested that the characteristics of the Caucasian races are largely due to the influence of the pituitary gland: the colour, the large skeleton, and the long bones "point to an active anterior pituitary". The physical energy and the drive, so marked in the typical Caucasian . . . "is another characteristic for which the pituitary is responsible"[7]. Geikie-Cobb divided gigantism into three groups:

(1) Gigantism with infantilism.

(2) Gigantism with acromegaly.

(3) Gigantism with infantilism and acromegaly.

He thinks that all instances of real giants will fall into one of these classes. Some of the tall people are in fact eunochoids, as postulated in the classification by Tandler and Grosz[8].

At the other end of the scale, there are the Pygmies. The name is derived from the Greek word pygmé (πυγμή), meaning 'fist', and pygmaios (πυγμαῖος) = the length of a fist or thumb ('Tom Thumb'). It was used by Homer to describe a race of tiny men. Aristotle refers to a race of men of small stature, and Philostratos describes the "sleeping Hercules beset by swarms of Pygmies"[9].

Pliny refers to races of dwarfs both in Asia and Africa; and a Chinese author describes a tribe of dwarfs in the Philippine Islands. They would constitute the group of proportionate dwarfs, i.e. people of very small size as compared with average individuals of the same age and race (in contrast to the disproportionate group, such as the achondroplastic or rachitic dwarfs, or the forms of dwarfism due to disorders of various endocrine glands). Proportionate dwarfs are "normal human beings viewed through the wrong end of a telescope" (Meige): the condition is perhaps due to a genetically transmitted isolated growth hormone deficiency. Pliny was right: there are the African Pygmies, the Negrilloes, and the Asiatic Pygmies, the Negritoes. Both groups are dark-skinned, some tribes very black. Their average height is about 4½ feet, but sometimes considerably smaller. They have crisp, black, curly hair, flattened noses, long upper lips, prominent lower jaw, large mouths, short skulls, long arms, short legs, large feet, and relatively long toes. They are skilful tree climbers, using their long, subtle toes, and of nomadic habits in search of food. The anthropologists find it difficult to fit them into the usual order of classifiable groups. The eyes are often large and staring. They are daring and courageous hunters, very successful in shooting with tiny poisoned arrows, often from a blowpipe.

REFERENCES

1. Wells, C.: Bones, Bodies and Disease. London, Thames & Hudson, 1964.
2. Keith, A.: New Discoveries Relating to the Antiquity of Man. London, Williams & Norgate, 1931.
3. Larger, L.: L'acromègalie-gigantisme, cause naturelle de la dégénèrescence et, partant, de l'extinction des groupes animaux actuel et fossiles. Bull. Mém. Soc. Anthropol, Paris 6ᵉ, 3ᵉ sér. **7**, 22, 1916.
4. Moore, Sherwood: Hyperostosis Cranii. Springfield, Thomas, 1955.
5. Mahoudeau, A.: Comments on Larger (Q.V.) Bull. Mém. Soc. Anthropol., Paris. 6ᵉ sèr. **7**, 22, 1916.
6. Casati, A.: Le iperostosi intertabulari del cranio come fatto di variabilitá normale. Arch. Anthropol. Etnol., Firenze **89**, 127, 1959.
7. Geikie-Cobb, Ivo: The Glands of Destiny. London, Heinemann, 1947.
8. Tandler, J. and Grosz, S.: Die biologischen Grundlagen der sekundaeren Geschlechtscharaktere. Berlin, Springer, 1913.
9. As 7: p. 148.

CHAPTER TEN

L'ENVOY TO THE ANCIENTS

THE OLDEST KEY TO THE ENDOCRINE TREASURE TROVE: THE TESTICLES

As we have seen, it was the testicle that first drew the attention of man to the importance of a small organ. Damage to or loss of both testicles due to accidental or deliberate injury had dire consequences. Depending on the age when it occurred, it may mean loss of fertility, of sexual desire, of sexual capacity, or lack of development of secondary sexual characteristics and changes in bodily appearance[1]. The same applied in the case of diseased or undescended testicles, which had been damaged. It seemed as if nature had attempted to compensate for the vulnerability of this organ, in that it provided a double ration.

The importance of the testicles was well known to primitive man and during antiquity. The role of the seed and of the testicles in the theories of conception and the determination of the sex of the offspring have been discussed; and so have the ideas of the transmission of paternal and maternal characteristics.

Castration was practised on a large scale, not only on slaves and defeated enemies – to be used in service and in slavery – but also by the priesthood of various cults or in the case of male attendants in harems. The history of eunuchs is an important one in Eastern and Western cultures of antiquity. It has also been mentioned that there were various degrees of human castration; accordingly, there were married eunuchs, eunuchs in harems or in the society of Imperial Rome, who had love affairs of sorts and were even sought after by women, because there was no danger of pregnancy. Their role in the Civil Service of Imperial Rome and Byzanz and China was stressed. Some excelled even as generals.

Homosexuality in ancient Greece was not merely a psychological aberration. In the armies of Sparta it was a method of keeping the minds of the officers and soldiers off the temptations of foreign women during the long and dreary years of war service away from home; it was a means of ensuring training of future generations of military leaders by the generals of the present. Finally, it seemed that male lovers would excel in battle and wish to share the heroism, glory and death of the other partner. Similar sentiments were not uncommon among the other Greeks, between philosophers and their pupils and, later, between Alexander the Great and his close friends.

Impotence has always been regarded as disastrous, shameful or ridiculous. It might have been caused by defective testicular function, by castration, by injury to or disease of the testicles, by physical or sexual exhaustion or due to psychological reasons. The condition was represented in the ancient literature of most cultures, Chinese, Hindu, in the Bible and, of course, in ancient Greek and Roman literature. Ovid (Publius Ovidius Naso, a contemporary of Augustus and banished by him) was bewailing his (temporary) impotence in a celebrated poem so vividly, that the translator for Loeb's Classical Library, Professor Grant Showerman (Wisconsin), felt in 1921 and in 1947 unwilling to render it into English and printed the original Latin text as an Appendix[2]. He said that he did so because "a faithful rendering might offend the sensibilities of the reader, if not the literary taste". Yet Ovid's poetical ability was perhaps the most lyrical among the Latin poets of the Golden Age and in no way diminished on that occasion.

Primitive man and ancient man also had good knowledge of the effect of castration in animal husbandry. This knowledge was used to good account when turning some wild animals into domesticated ones and making them useful for the purposes of man. These facts must be borne firmly in mind. It will not be entirely surprising, therefore, that the first sound experimental knowledge of the working of the endocrine glands was derived, eventually, from Berthold's classic experiment; it is only surprising that it has taken so many centuries, until in 1849 AD, that the crucial experiment provided the key to the treasure trove.

REFERENCES

1. Tandler, J. and Grosz, S.: Die biologischen Grundlagen der sekundaeren Geschlechtscharaktere. Berlin, Springer, 1913.
2. Naso Ovidius P.: Amores, Book III, Song 7; (*not* in the Ars amandi). Loeb Classical Library. pp. 506–508. London, Heinemann, 1921 (reprinted 1947). (The volume is published as: Heroides and Amores.)

CHAPTER ELEVEN

THE MEDIAEVAL SCENE

LTHOUGH the Middle Ages appeared to be medically barren on the whole, there were a number of exceptions. In the first place, there was Arabic medicine, which had inherited the Greek tradition; it flourished and was enhanced by some Jewish physicians in Arab lands. Next, there were some interesting developments in the Far East, notably in China, which must be mentioned. Finally, there were some rays of light in the West, particularly where there were points of contact with the Arabs.

ARABIC AND JUDAEO–ARABIC MEDICINE (732–1096 AD)

The Arabs proved to be the main conservators of Greek medicine. The monotheistic tendencies of Aristotle and Galen had a strong appeal to Islam, once it had conquered a large empire; so did Galen's polypharmacy and tendency to dogma. Whereas the Arabs developed arithmetic and chemistry, also in the form of perfumes, they were averse to the handling of dead bodies (which they regarded as sinful) and hence also to anatomical dissection and to surgery and experimentation of that nature. They loved dialectic argumentation and, above all, authority. Although the authors of the Mohammedan era wrote in Arabic, many of them were, in fact, Persians, Spanish born or Jewish, and the basis of their medical knowledge was Greek. The two main sources of that body of knowledge were firstly, the Nestorian heretics, followers of the patriarch of Constantinople Nestorius (428 AD), who were exiled and took up the study of medicine. They founded a medical school in Edessa in Mesopotamia, but were driven out from there in 489. They fled to Persia, where they established a famous school at Gondisapor, which became one of the origins of Arabic medicine. The Caliphate in Baghdad was ruled by the Abbasides, whose outstanding members were Al-Mansur (754–775), Harun-al-Rashid, (786–802) and Al-Meiamun (813–833). During their reign, Greek texts were collected and translated, particularly those of Hippocrates, Galen, Rufus of Ephesus and Paul of Aegina. The principal translators (into Arabic) were Johannes Mesuë the Elder (777–837), also known as Janus Damascenus, and the Nestorian Honain ben Isaac or Johannitius (809–873). Mesuë the Elder was a Christian who became Director of the Hospital at Baghdad and physician to Harun-al-Rashid; he also translated Persian texts and wrote important medical aphorisms, later known in their Latin form as *Selecta Artis Medicinae*. He used testicular extracts as an aphrodisiac (a forerunner of Brown-Séquard) and other forms of organotherapy.

The greatest physicians of the Baghdad Caliphate (749–1258) were three Persians: Rhazes, Haly Abbas and Avicenna.

Al-Razi = Rhazes (860–932 AD)

Rhazes, whose full name was Abu Bakr Muhammed ibn Zakariya al-Razi, was born in Ray near Teheran, and later worked in Baghdad. He was an outstanding clinician and his descriptions of diseases are equal to those of Hippocrates or Sydenham. He made many contributions to various branches of medicine, gynaecology, and obstetrics and wrote classic descriptions of measles and smallpox. The most important encyclopaedic work he wrote was *Kitab-al-Hawi* or *Continens* in the Latin translation; it contains numerous original clinical histories, observations, experiments and a great number of extracts from many sources. Although theoretically a Galenist, he is really a Hippocratic by the rational simplicity of his practice. He described diabetes mellitus, but his method of treatment was not exceptionally impressive. In his other famous treatise: *Khulasai-al Tajarib* or *Quintessence of Experience*, he discusses in detail the sex organs, the various temperaments of the uterus, the diagnosis of pregnancy and its management, and 'The Means of Preventing Conception'. If there would be danger to a woman in pregnancy, there are several methods of preventing the semen from entering the womb, apart from coitus interruptus. One of them is the blockage of the uterine os by pessaries of cabbage, colocynth pulp, pitch, ox gall, whitewash and others. Expulsion of semen from the uterus would be achieved by violent physical bodily movements immediately after intercourse, or the application of certain drugs to the womb, such as sal ammoniae, sugar candy, potash, and others, which are supposed to bring on the period[1]. Finally, insertion of a stick or probe into the womb may bring on abortion, if left all night, without the use of force and without hurry. Dietary regulation, abdominal massage and hot baths are also recommended, in a similar manner as the 8th century Sanscrit suggestion.

Ali ibn Abbas, also a Persian, died in 994 AD

He wrote a treatise: *Kamil as-Sinaa* (*The Perfection of the Art*), or the *Royal Book* (*Liber Regius*). The work is divided into twenty discourses; some of the best are on materia medica, but he also dealt with the surgery of goitre (see the Bamberg Surgery, p. 91). The section on anatomy was the main source of knowledge for the next hundred years (to 1170) even at Salerno. It was not only systematic and concise, but more practical than Avicenna's *Canon*, which superseded it. He also gave a description of malignant anthrax ('Persian fire'). Contraceptive advice should only be given in cases where pregnancy was dangerous. Rocksalt introduced into the vagina before intercourse (or anointing the penis with it), will act as an effective contraceptive. Tar will act similarly, or cabbage seeds or the rennet of rabbits. His ethical precepts are noteworthy – that physicians should not pass information of such nature to prostitutes or to women with promiscuous habits. For the opposite purpose, the treatment of sterility, he prescribed pessaries containing arsenic[2].

Ibn Sina or Avicenna (980–1037 AD)

Ibn Sina (or Avicenna) was also called the 'Princeps doctorum', but his full name was Abu Ali al-Husain ibn Abdallah ibn Sina. He was the most famous scientist of Islam and one of the most famous of all races and times and his thoughts represent perhaps the climax of mediaeval philosophy. The work which interests us most is the *Qanum fit Tibb*, or *Canon*, better known under its Latin title *Canon Avicennae*. This enormous medical encyclopaedia contains about a million words and is a "codification of the whole of ancient and Muslim (medical) knowledge"[3]. Because of its formal perfection as well as its intrinsic value, the *Qanum* superseded Rhazes' *Hawi* (or *Continens*), Ali ibn Abbas' *Maliki* (or *The Royal Book*) and even the works of Galen; it remained supreme for six centuries. So great were Ibn Sina's encyclopaedic efforts in reporting facts in divers fields of learning and theorizing about them, that his very originality was dwarfed. So complete was the acceptance of the work that it stifled original investigation and sterilized intellectual life.

It may be said that Ibn Sina's authority approached that of Aristotle; he was at once oracle and magician. He was also eminently successful as court physician and vizier to different Caliphs, trod the primrose path at ease and died in the prime of life from the effect of its pleasures. He was physician-in-chief to the celebrated hospital in Baghdad and is said to have written over one hundred works on different subjects, only a few of which have been preserved. His wonderful description of the origin of mountains fully entitles him to be called the 'Father of Geology'.

Avicenna is said to have been the first to describe the preparation and properties of sulphuric acid and of alcohol. His *Canon*, which Haller styled a 'methodic inanity', is a huge, unwieldy storehouse of learning, in which the author attempts to codify the whole of medical knowledge of his time and to square its facts with the systems of Galen and Aristotle. Written in meticulous style (Arab mania for classification), this gigantic tome became the fountain-head of authority in the Middle Ages; for Avicenna's elaborated train of reasoning, a miracle of syllogism in its way, appealed particularly to the mediaeval mind and, indeed, set the pace for its movement in many directions.

Arnold of Villanova defined Avicenna as a professional scribbler, who had stupefied European physicians by his misinterpretation of Galen. In fairness to Avicenna, it is proper to say that his clinical records, which he intended as an appendix to the *Canon*, were irrecoverably lost, and only the Arabic text of the latter, published in Rome in 1593, and at Bulak in 1877, survives. That Avicenna must have been a clever practitioner, we should naturally infer from his great reputation.

Avicenna's recommendation of wine as the best dressing for wounds was very popular in mediaeval practice. He also described the guinea-worm[4], and described anthrax as "Persian Fire"[5]. He gave a good account of diabetes mellitus, describing the abnormal appetite and the collapse of sexual functions[6] and he noted the sweet taste of diabetic urine. He spoke of primary and secondary diabetes, just as Aretaeus did, and also described diabetic gangrene. As to his treatment of diabetics, repetition of his prescriptions in modern times have shown that his mixture of lupine, trigonella (fenugreek), and zedoary seed, produces a considerable reduction of the excretion of sugar[7]. The authority of the Latin texts of the *Canon* set back the progress of surgery, by preaching the doctrine – dear to the Arab mind – that the practice of surgery is an inferior and separate branch of the art of medicine, and by preferring the use of cautery to that of the knife. He regarded the prevention of conception indicated in case of a small woman for whom childbirth would be mechanically dangerous, or in cases of disease of the womb or weakness of the bladder.

Among the contraceptive techniques which he advocated were the following:

(1) Avoidance of intercourse at the time specially favourable for conception.

(2) Avoidance of simultaneous orgasm.

(3) Coitus interruptus.

(4) Violent jumps of the woman at the end of coition (7 to 9 times).

(5) Smearing tar into the vagina before and after intercourse, and/or anointing the penis with it, or with balm oil and white lead.

(6) Insert the flowers and seeds of cabbage into the vagina after the period and before and after coitus, preferably mixed with tar.

(7) Insertion of a pessary of colocynth, mandrake, sulphur, iron-dross and cabbage seed, mixed with tar.

(8) Smear the glans of the penis with sweet oil before intercourse[8].

Other physicians of the Eastern (Baghdad) Caliphate

Isaac Judaeus (855–955 AD), wrote a book on dietetics which became popular in Europe (De Dieta, Padua, 1487).

Jurjani (Zain al-din Abu-l-Fadail Ismail ibn al-Husain al Jurjani), was another Persian, who died ca. 1135. His Treasure of Medicine was written in Persian rather than Arabic and was completed ca. 1110 AD. It was among the earliest medical works to connect exophthalmos with goitre, something which did not happen again until the beginning of the 19th century[9]. He also described contraceptive methods similar to those of Avicenna. Finally, he gave the most complete account of the period for the examination of urine.

The Cordovan or Western Caliphate (655–1236 AD) prospered especially under the Ommiade Dynasty (755–1036). Their leading medical men were:

Albucasim, called Albucasis (1013–1106 AD)

Albucasim was born in Zahra, near Cordoba in Andalusia. He was mainly a surgeon, who used ligature and cautery to control haemorrhage during an operation. He was the author of a large medico-surgical treatise, the *Altasrif* or *Collection*, which contains illustrations of surgical and dental instruments. In it he mentions an operation for 'elephantiasis' of the throat (goitre). (See also pp. 81, 91 and 191.)

Avenzoar of Cordoba (died 1162 AD)

He was the greatest Muslim physician of the Western Caliphate. His *Teisir* or *Rectification of Health* is preserved in a Latin translation from the Hebrew (1280), published in Venice in 1490.

The Rabbi Moses ben Maimon called Moses Maimonides (1135–1204 AD)

Moses Maimonides became court-physician to Saladin. He wrote on personal hygiene (*Tractatus Regimine Sanitatis*) for Saladin's personal use; in the work dietetics as well as poisons are discussed.

Abu Mansur Muwaffak Bin Ali Harawi (ca. 970 AD)

He wrote the most important Persian work on pharmacology, mentioning 585 drugs, most of them of a vegetable nature. ("Liber fundamentorum pharmacologiae. . . ." Primus Latino donavit R. Seligmann, 2 pts. Vindobonae, Antonius Nob. de Schmid, 1830–1833.)

The Arabs derived their knowledge of Greek medicine from the Nestorian monks, many practical details from the Jews, and their astrologic lore from Egypt and the Far East. They upheld the Galenic pulselore and maintained to be able to determine the sex of a child before birth by inspection of the urine (uroscopy). They abstained from dissection because of religious conviction, left operative surgery and venesection to wandering specialists, and the care of women's diseases and obstetric patients to the midwives[10].

The Arabs founded a number of hospitals. In the one in Damascus (founded 1100 AD) treatment and drugs were given free for three centuries. The great Al-Mansur Hospital of Cairo had gynaecological wards, out-patients' clinics, was a teaching hospital with a large library, and also had diet kitchens. Male and female nurses were trained there. Sleeplessness was treated with soft music and story-tellers!

In Baghdad there were ophthalmic clinics and lunatic asylums, where the insane were treated with kindness – in contrast to the treatment employed in Europe.

Cordoba had a number of smaller hospitals and dispensaries. Medical teaching was carried out in all these centres, the Hall of Wisdom in Cairo being the most famous. Although anatomy and surgery were neglected, chemistry (alchemy) was of importance. Senna, sandalwood, camphor, cassia, tamarind, nutmeg, cloves, aconite and mercury were introduced as drugs. Hashish and Indian hemp were used to induce deep sleep and/or anaesthesia; syrups, juleps, alcohol and aldehydes were also Arab terms. Jewish physicians were prominent, especially in the Western Caliphate (or Cordoba), until their expulsion from Spain in 1492. Surprisingly, the schools of Salerno and of Montpellier used them as teachers until they had trained enough of their own. The policy of the popes vacillated and most European universities were closed to the Jews until the French Revolution.

THE CHINESE AGAIN

Marco Polo, who was mentioned in Chapter 2, really belonged to the Middle Ages.

Joseph Needham found evidence that the alchemy (chemistry) of the Arabs and Persians also had Chinese sources[11]. Moreover, Needham says, "Macrobiotics is a convenient term for the belief that it is possible to prepare, with the aid of botanical, zoological, mineralogical and above all chemical knowledge, drugs or elixirs which will prolong human life beyond old age, rejuvenating the body and its spiritual parts, so that the adept can endure through centuries of longevity, finally attaining the status of eternal life and arising with etherealised body as a true immortal"[12]. Truly, an anticipation of Brown-Séquard and Steinach!

> But there was another predisposing cause for alchemical ideas in China, the absence of any prejudice against the use of mineral drugs, analogous to that which existed so long under the Galenical domination in Europe; indeed, the Chinese went to the other extreme, compounding with remarkable persistence through the centuries all kinds of dangerous elixirs containing metallic and other elements (mercury, arsenic, lead, etc., as well as gold), which caused untold harm to those who resolutely took them.

The association of goitre with certain mountain regions, "was widespread in Chinese medicine from at least the 5th century AD onwards"[13]. There seems no doubt that the use of different kinds of seaweeds for the cure of goitre was known in China long before the knowledge in Europe. The great alchemist, Ko Hung, recommended an alcoholic extract (tincture) of seaweed for goitre in about 340 AD (see also p. 189). Later, at the end of the 5th century AD, there were written the *Goitre Prescriptions of the Abbot Shen*, who added nine more items, including the powdered shells of molluscs, as a source of calcium and iodine. In 1330 AD, the *Yin Shan Cheng Yao*, a book written by Hu Ssu-Hui, discloses great empirical knowledge of deficiency diseases caused by lack of vitamins, and repeats the fact that seaweed will cure goitre. According to Needham, their first use in Europe was at the end of the 12th century, at the time when the Europeans first knew of the magnetic compass, the windmill and papermaking, all techniques known to be "derived from the Chinese and Iranian culture-areas".

About 1475 AD Wang Hsi states in his *I Lin Chi Yao* that the thyroid gland lies in front of the larynx and looks like a lump of flesh about the size of a date (jujube = a Chinese date), "flattish and of a pink colour". He adds that for the treatment of goitre the glands of pigs, sheep and other animals should be desiccated over a tile and powdered, then taken with wine every night. He advocates air-drying of 50 pigs' thyroid glands, the powder of which should be drunk in cold wine by the goitrous patient. "Thyroid organotherapy was thus in China contemporary with Thomas Linacre".

The physician Tshui Chih-Thi, who lived about 85 AD, seems to have distinguished between solid (malignant) neck swellings which could not be cured, and movable (benign) ones which could. In about 650, the celebrated doctor Sun Ssu-Mo recommended the combined use of seaweed, powdered mollusc shells and thyroid gland (see also p. 189 of Chapter 14). Needham argues that the Chinese perception that 'hyperplasia' of the thyroid (goitre) was due to an 'incapacity', derived from their idea of thinking in terms of the organism as a whole; in goitre they saw an abnormality; normality,

> meant to them . . . . a correct balance between Yang and Yin (excitation and inhibition). The thung lei (identity of categories) principle therefore naturally suggested that tissues from the normal necks (of animals) should be employed to cure diseased necks (in man). . . . Thyroid organotherapy must clearly be counted a signal success of mediaeval Chinese medicine.

As mentioned in Chapter 2, the knowledge of some of the features of diabetes mellitus already existed in Ancient China, Hsiao Kho (dissolutive thirst)[14], but the sweetness of the urine was not recognized until later. In one of the earliest of the great medical classics, the *Huang Ti Nei Ching*, Su Wen, in Chapter 47, is the following passage:

> A patient suffering from this disease must have been in the habit of eating many sweet delicacies and fatty foods. Fatty foods make it difficult for the internal heat to disperse, while very sweet things give rise to obesity. Therefore the Chhi (pneuma) tends to overflow and thus causes Hsiao-Kho (dissolutive thirst)[14].

The pancreas was regarded as a very important organ, "neither fat nor flesh". It was also called the "gate of life" (ming men) and considered to be the fundamental organ (yuan) in the "three coctive regions". Li Shi-Chen said that the "pancreas is larger in obese people than it is in thin or normal subjects", and that it is "essential for the nourishment and management of life".

The first Chinese physician to mention the sweetness of the urine in sugar-diabetes was Chen Chhuan, who died in 643 AD. In his work, *Ku Chin Lu Yen Fano* (*Old and New Tried and Tested Prescriptions*), he distinguishes three forms of diabetes:

(1) Intense thirst, copious drinking and excretion of large amounts of urine, which is sweet to taste (Hsiao kho ping).

(2) The patient eats a great amount, has little thirst; the urine is less in quantity, though frequently passed, and has a fatty appearance (Hsiao chung ping).

(3) There is thirst, but the patient cannot drink much; there is oedema of the legs, wasting of the feet, impotence and frequency (Shen hsiao ping).

Needham thinks that the first form is diabetes mellitus, the second a polyphagic form of the disease with associated lipuria; the third refers perhaps to chronic nephritis[15].

Li Hsuan wrote a monograph: *Hsiao Kho Lun* on diabetes mellitus at the end of the 7th century AD. The author was perhaps identical with Director Li of the Bureau of Imperial Sacrifices (that Bureau was responsible for the medical qualifying examination). Director Li was perhaps the first to discuss at length the reason for the sweetness of the urine in that disease. He is quoted as saying that in Hsiao Kho illnesses (diabetes), three things must be renounced: wine, sex and eating salty cereal products. If this regimen is carried out, cure may be possible without drugs. One must also be on the look-out for the development of boils and carbuncles, because if such develop near joints, the prognosis is very bad. From the 8th century AD onwards other physicians emphasized the tendency of diabetic patients not only to obesity, but also to infective skin lesions, furuncles, rodent ulcers and troubles of the eyesight. Diabetic glycosuria was from then on mentioned by all medical writers and diagnosis consisted not only of the tasting of the urine, but also in the observation whether bees or ants would be attracted to it if a sample was placed near a hive or nest. Similarly, the tendency was realized to retinitis, night-blindness and cataracts.

The knowledge of sexual endocrinology began from the practical experience of castration. Eunuchs played a very important role at the Imperial Court, in business and other vocations. Animals were castrated since ancient times for medicinal purposes and for improvement of the meat used for food. There were also, in Chinese medical literature, early and frequent accounts of sex reversal, both in man and in animals.

Once the importance of the testes was recognized, they were used in pharmacology. In the *Pen Tshoo Kang Mu* there were numerous preparations made of desiccated or raw testicles from the pig, the dog or the sheep, which were given for male sexual debility, as treatment for spermatorrhoea, hypogonadism, impotence and other similar conditions. The first references occur in a book *Classified Fundamental Prescriptions of Universal Benefit*, printed in 1235 AD and ascribed to the eminent physician Hsu Shu-Wei of *ca.* 1132 AD[16].

Whereas testicular tissue was also mentioned in the materia medica of Dioscorides and in the Indian *Suśruta*, the use of preparations made from the human placenta was prominent in China. It was first mentioned in a pharmacopoeia of 725 AD, but rarely used until the 15th century AD, when Chu Chen-Heng encouraged its use for debility of all kinds. The placenta was carefully washed and drained, reduced to a small volume and combined with a number of vegetable drugs. Placentas of the horse and the cat were also used. "Barren women, those who only produce girls, those with dysmenorrhoea, those with miscarriages, difficult birth, if they take Ta Tsuo Wan pills, will get sons. . . ."

The most important development of Chinese medicine between the 11th and 17th centuries AD concerning the sex hormones, was "the veritable fractionations applied to urine". Pharmacists were engaged "almost on a manufacturing scale" to prepare active products from human urine by means of precipitation, re-solution, evaporation to dryness, sublimation and crystallization.

The origins of urinary therapy go as far back as ancient Taoism. The attitude of the Taoists to sex was not ascetic, but a magic–scientific one. In a history of the later Han Dynasty there is a passage which Needham quotes. There were three Taoist adepts at about 200 AD, who were

> all expert at following the techniques of Jung Cheng in commerce with women. They could also drink urine. . . . They were careful and sparing their seminal essence . . . and they did not boast with great words of their own powers. . . . All these people lived to between 100 and 200 years of age.

All people suffering from impotence, sexual debility, excess yang of burning feverish type which no medicine can benefit, will improve, according to Chu Chen-Heng (14th century AD), if urine is administered. The natural precipitate of the urine can also drive out the undue fire element affecting the liver and the bladder. As princes disliked taking it in the original state, the iatro-chemists began to purify the sediments. In these fractionations large quantities of human urine were used, up to 200 gallons. The whole amount was evaporated to dryness, including phosphates, urates and sulphates[17]. Another method was preliminary precipitation, using calcium sulphate, which would probably take down any protein that was present and, therefore, certainly also any steroid conjugates. In nearly all the methods, the process ends by sublimation. At first, this seemed difficult to understand, but – in fact – the urinary steroid sex-hormones do sublime unchanged in air between 180° and 300°, there being considerable differences in sublimation temperature between them. Indeed, this method is now used for their identification[18].

> There can be little doubt that between the 11th and 17th century AD, the Chinese iatro-chemists were producing preparations of androgens and oestrogens which were probably quite effective in the quasi-empirical therapy of the time. This must be considered an extraordinary achievement for any type of scientific medicine before the age of modern science.[19]

THE BARRENNESS OF MEDIAEVAL MEDICINE IN THE WEST

Feudalism and the Church dominated a scene which was based on obedience to authority. Intellectual independence and individual thought had no place in such a state of affairs. Of the ancient sources, the natural histories of the Elder Pliny and the Physics of Aristotle were accepted, but the biological works of Aristotle were not studied or understood. "Until the Renaissance there was neither induction nor experiment". As Allbut put it: "Logic . . . was for the Middle

Ages a means of discovery, nay, the very source of truth. . . . The dialectically irresistible was the true"[20].

"Through the Galenic dialectics . . . the medicine of the Middle Ages fell under the bondage of words, mistook the symbol for the thing, was decidedly backward in anatomy, physiology, pathology and internal medicine"[21]. The fundamental error of mediaeval medical science was in the divorce of medicine from surgery. Unlike Hippocrates, Avicenna and other mediaeval medical authorities regarded, like Galen, the surgeon as an inferior. This view was enforced by the Arabs and their followers, whose religion insisted that it was unclean to touch the human body with the hands. Surgery became, therefore, a domain of the barbers, bathkeepers and market operators. The Arab commentators of Galen, who regarded suppuration and "pus bonum et laudabile" as essential to wound healing, made operative surgery a dangerous form of treatment; in case of failure concerning an important person, the surgeon could be in danger of serious punishment. Not until the advent of Ambroise Paré and, later, of John Hunter, did surgery begin to emerge from the depth to which mediaeval thought and practice had banished it.

After the Dark Ages – following the downfall of Rome – Latin became the official language of Church and State in the West, and such science and learning as was permissible and still existed, was within the protection of the Christian Church. This initiated the period of Monastic Medicine from the 5th to the 10th century AD, in which the zeal for preserving the remains of ancient literature and the traditions of ancient and rational practice went hand in hand with the newly developed cult of the healing power of the Saints and Holy Relics. Supernatural powers were responsible for the great epidemics and heavenly aid was necessary to obtain relief from them. "Religious zeal and fanatical ascetiscism became the order of the day"[22].

The first account of a dissection of a human body in public is from about 1300 AD in Bologna. The first reference to a post-mortem examination is in 1288, that a physician in Cremona carried it out, to find the cause of death in a case of plague. As all diseases were regarded as divine visitations, most of them were mentioned in a religious connection. The Bishop of Emebert (7th century AD) put a curse on the wicked persons who despoiled the tomb of St. Gudula, that their offspring should be crippled and the women smitten with goitre[23]. Short accounts of endemic goitre are to be found in the Breviar (Lib. II, cap. 4) of Arnoldus Villanovanus (see also p. 812), for the province of Lucca and by Valescus de Taranta for the Comte de Foix (Philonium, Lib. VII, cap. 31). Algae were recommended as treatment, mixed with saltpetre or antimony.

In the Bamberg Surgery of the 12th century, in Chapter 33, which seems to have been copied from the *Royal Book* of Ali ibn Abbas (Haly Abbas, the Persian, see page 81), removal of goitre by surgery is advised:

> The skin is cut lengthwise and the tumour is withdrawn with all the material adherent to it. If you wish to be certain of this, you may cauterize with a large iron the whole interior of the cavity from which you have extracted the goitre. Care should be taken that the pulse of the nerves are not injured in surgery of this kind. If, however, such an accident occurs, you should suture or ligate each side of the wound. If you do not wish to cauterize when the tumour is removed, search diligently to make sure that nothing remains, for if anything remains, it will form again as before. When the region has been completely cleaned out, it is partly sutured and red powder is applied. A cloth is placed on the wound and treatment proceeds as stated already, but without a poultice[24].

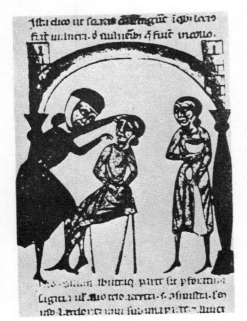

Figure 7 Operation goitre. Rolando's *La Chirurgia* (1264)

The aforementioned Arnold of Villanova (1235–1311) (see Section II) suggested burnt sponge and seaweed for the treatment of goitre, and so did Valescus de Taranta (1382–1417), but Guy de Chauliac (1300–?1370) (see Section II) recommends surgical removal of the diseased gland (see also pp. 81, 84, 109 and 191).

It was the School of Salerno in the 11th and 12th centuries which gave medicine in the West a new impetus after nearly 500 years of decay. Its creation amidst the clerical foundations around it is a mystery, as the School became a lay institution with free thought, in the best Hippocratic tradition, in a city which was the seat of a bishop and in about the year 1000, of an archbishop. The Benedictines had a house and a hospice there. However, the relations between the members of the medical school and the clergy were friendly. The anatomy was based on the study of swine, physiology and pathology were Galenic, but illnesses were studied by direct clinical observation, knowledge of the pulse and examination of the urine being of great use. Therapy was rational and included dietetics; surgery flourished; obstetrics and nursing were of a high standard. Greek was spoken, as it behoves a seat of Hellenistic culture; there was Arabic influence from Sicily and Jewish from some still existing centres in Rome, Genoa and Palermo (hence the four Founding Fathers of the school were supposed to have been a Greek, a Latin, a Jew and a Saracen). The High Salerno period of 1072–1224 (Sudhoff) began with Constantinus Africanus (*ca.* 1020–1087) (see Section II)[25]. The most important contribution of the School of Salerno to medicine was the *Tractatus de Aegritudinum Curatione*, the first example of an encyclopaedic textbook of medicine written by many authors. The celebrated *Regimen Sanitatis Salernitanum* (or *Flos Medicinae*), 1200–1300, was a poem (or poems) in double rhymed hexameters. It consists of sensible dietetic and hygienic rules and saw 240 editions in several European languages and in Hebrew. In several imprints it was dedicated to the King of England (Anglorum Regi scripsit schola tota Salerni). An English translation by the Elizabethan poet and courtier Sir John Haryngton was published in London in 1607 at the John Holme and John Press. A sample of both is given from a recent reprint (Rome, 1957) of the Ente Provinciale di Turismo-Salerno:

> Quatuor haec membra, cephe, cor, pes, hepar, vacuanda.
> Ver cor, hepar aestas, ordo sequens reliquas.
> Dat salvatelia tibi plurima dona minuta:
> Purgat hepar, splenem, pectus, praecordia, vocem,
> Innaturalem tollit de corde dolorem.

> The Heart and Liver, Spring and Summers bleeding,
> The Fall and Winter, hand and foot doth mend,
> One veine cut in the hand, doth help exceeding
> Unto spleene, voyce, brest, and intrailes lend,
> And swages griefes that in the heart are breeding.

Of the 'Ladies of Salerno'[25], Abella wrote "De natura seminis hominis" and Trotula (Madame Trotte de Salerno) "De passionibus mulierum", a treatise on gynaecology and cosmetics. Whether 'Trotula' was a collective name of all the midwives of Salerno, as

Sudhoff believed, or the name of a woman of the family of Ruggiero, seems irrelevant. (Karl Friedrich Jakob Sudhoff, 1853–1938, one of the greatest of medical historians, made a special study of the School of Salerno.)

From 1070 to 1170, Constantine's translation of the Almaleki of Haly (Ali ibn-) Abbas, was the sole source of anatomy, and the *Antidotarium* of Nicolaus Salernitanus (Praepositus, i.e. Praeses of the Faculty), the main pharmacopoeia, containing 139 prescriptions in alphabetical order. After its sacking by Henry VI in 1194, Salerno declined and with it the Medical School, which lost its influence after 1300, although it was not abolished until 1811 (by Napoleon).

Roger of Palermo (Ruggiero Frugardi), student and master at the school of Salerno, wrote a standard textbook *Practica* in 1170, in which he described cancer, and prescribed ashes of sponge and seaweed for the treatment of goitre. He also introduced suture of the intestines over a hollow tube, ligatures in haemorrhage; he recommended surgical removal of goitre, if necessary. A large goitre was transfixed with shoelaces and allowed to slough off.

Human dissecting, which had become permissible after the decree of Emperor Fredric II in 1240, improved the knowledge of anatomy. Mundinus of Bologna (Mondino de Luzzi, ? 1275–1326) completed his *Anathomia* in 1316; it was more a manual of dissection than a major textbook of anatomy. It went to 39 editions and translations and remained the most popular manual until 1530. Mundinus described the differences in the size of the uterus in virgins and multiparae. He also gave an anatomical description of the pancreas ($\pi\tilde{\alpha}\varsigma$ = all; $\kappa\varrho\acute{\epsilon}\alpha\varsigma$ = flesh) and mentioned its duct. The *Anathomia* (published first in Padua in 1487) was the first book devoted solely to anatomy and written for Mundinus' pupils.

Mediaeval English medicine did not differ fundamentally from that in the rest of Europe[26]. Sexual problems were known even in those days: if a man be too lustful "boil water agrimony in foreign ale, let him drink it at night fasting. However, if he should be too bashful in such matters, then he should boil the same plant in milk, for this gives him courage"[27]. Gilbertus Anglicus (see p. 98). (*ca.* 1180–1250) suggested that habitual sexual excess could weaken the joints, depriving them of their natural heat and moisture, thereby causing arthritis. John of Gaddesden (Johannes Anglicus, ? 1280–1361) wrote the *Rosa Anglica ca.* 1314 (*Rosa Anglica Practica Medicina a Capite ad Pedes*, the first printed medical book by an Englishman, Papie, 1492). In it he suggested that 'windy' foods, constipation and overeating at night, followed by intercourse may cause arthritis. He quotes Galen as saying that eunuchs never suffer from podagra[28].

The English attitude to contraception was succinctly expressed by

Geoffrey Chaucer (*ca.* 1340–1400). He said in *"The Persones (Parson's) Tale"* in *"The Canterbury Tales"*:

Eek whan man destourbeth concepcion of a child, and maketh a womman outher bareyne by drinkinge venemouse herbes, thurgh which she may nat conceyve, or sleeth a child by drinkes wilfully, or elles putteth certeine material thinges in hir secree places to slee the child;

or elles doth unkindely sinne, by which man or womman shedeth hir nature in manere or in place ther-as a child may nat be conceived; or elles, if a womman have conceyved and hurt hir-self, and sleeth the child, yet is it homicyde. (Verses 575–576.)

REFERENCES

1. Himes, M. E.: Medical History of Contraception. p. 137. New York, Gamut Press, 1936 (reprinted 1963).
2. Johnston, R. D.: The history of human infertility. Fertil. Steril. **14,** 266, 1963.
3. As 1: p. 141.
4. Avicenna: Libri V Canonis medicinae. Sect. iii, tract. II, cap. XXI. Romae, typ, Medicae, 1593.
5. Avicenna: Canon Avicennae. III, 118, ed. 1294. Bulak, 1877.
6. Papaspyros, N. B.: The History of Diabetes Mellitus. p. 8. London, 1952.
7. Abderhalden, R.: Internal Secretion. CIBA Monographs. No. 10, p. 339. Bombay, 1951.
8. As 1: p. 143.
9. Jurjani, Zain al-din Abu-l-Fadail Ismail ibn al-Husain al: Treasury of the King of Khwarazm (vi. 6). *ca* 1110.
10. Garrison, F. M.: Introduction to the History of Medicine. 4th ed., pp. 134–135. Philadelphia, W. B. Saunders, 1929.
11. Needham, J.: ΠΡΙΣΜΑΤΑ (Prismata). Festschrift für Willy Hartner. Wiesbaden, Franz Steiner, 1977.
12. Needham, J.: The elixir concept and chemical medicine in East and West. J. Chinese Univ. Hong Kong II (1), 244, 1974.
13. Needham, J. and Lu Gwei-Djen: Proto-endocrinology in Mediaeval China. Jpn Stud. Hist. Sci. Tokyo No. 5, 154, 1966.
14. ibid.: p. 159.
15. ibid.: p. 160.
16. ibid.: p. 166.
17. ibid.: p. 167.
18. ibid.: p. 168.
19. ibid.: p. 170.
20. Allbutt, Sir Thos. Clifford: Science and Mediaeval Thought. Harveian Oration 1900. London, 1901.
21. Garrison, F. H.: An Introduction to the History of Medicine. 4th ed., p. 143. Philadelphia, W. B. Saunders, 1929.
22. ibid.: p. 145.
23. Iason, A. H.: The Thyroid Gland in Medical History. p. 30. New York, Froben Press, 1946.
24. ibid.: p. 31.

25. Sudhoff, K. F. J.: Arch. Gesch. Med. VIII, 377, Leipzig, 1914–15; IX, p. 1, 1915–16.
26. As 2: p. 150.
27. Rubin, S.: Mediaeval English Medicine. pp. 124, 202. London, David & Charles, 1974.
28. ibid.: p. 206.

CHAPTER TWELVE

THE 16th CENTURY AND THE RENAISSANCE

A T the dawn of the 16th century, the supreme authority in the sciences and biology was still Aristotle, and in medicine, Galen. The study of the pulse and uroscopy (inspection of the urine) were still the most important actions of the learned physician, as can be seen on many contemporary miniatures. Notable advances had been made in the fields of eye diseases and optics, mainly by the Arabs and by the introduction of spectacles, which the Venetian glass workers began to manufacture as early as the end of the 13th century. On the other hand epidemics, especially waves of several forms of the plague, had decimated the population of Europe. Other epidemics, of such diseases as typhoid, paratyphoid, syphilis and tuberculosis, were caused by wars, povery, dirt and prostitution.

Albert von Bollstädt (1193–1280), better known as Albertus Magnus, the Dominican monk who later became Bishop of Ratisbon, taught at Paris and in Cologne, where he died. His main work was his book on animals (*De Animalibus*) which, although based on the work of Aristotle, contained many of his own observations. His versatility is expressed by the fact that he also wrote a popular book on cosmetics (*De Secretis Mullierum*), which was really compiled by a pupil. For us here, it is important that he recommended powdered testis of a hog in wine for men of poor sexual power and powdered womb of hare in wine to make women fertile[1].

Fertility played an important role: in 1532 Catherine of Medici, aged 14, was married to the Dauphin of France, aged 15, later to become Henry II. As king he took Diane de Poitiers as mistress; she was seventeen years older than he and had been his father's mistress. She almost persuaded him to divorce Catherine, because the latter had not become pregnant, and to marry her. Then – at long last –

Catherine did become pregnant and produced the future Francis II and during the next twelve years, had nine more children, including twins (in her last confinement). It was in 1569 that Dr. Wm. Chamberlen moved from France to Southampton, a member of a family who knew how to keep a medical secret!

The medical schools of Bologna, Padova and Montpellier had been founded. English medicine was represented by the *Compendium Medicinae* (London, 1510) of Gilbertus Anglicus (see p. 93). From monastic institutions came the physic gardens (herbulares). Collections of medical recipes were drawn up, such as the *Antidotarium Florentinum* (1498) and the *Pharmacorum Conficiendorum Ratio* (1546); the latter by Valerius Cordus (1515–1544) of Prussia. This was the first real pharmacopoeia and passed through 35 editions and eight translations; it was recognized as the official pharmacopoeia of Nüremberg[2].

François Rabelais (1490–1553), writer and physician, lectured at Montpellier and made one of the earliest Latin translations of Hippocrates.

It is Paracelsus, however, or to give his full name: Aureolus Theophrastus Bombastus von Hohenheim (1493–1541), who must be regarded as the most important medical thinker of the 16th century (see Section II). This Swiss, swashbuckling, but well educated physician, publicly burnt the works of Galen and Avicenna, but had a great respect for Hippocrates. He was a leader in chemistry, paving the way for chemical pharmacology, but regrettably, his novel ideas were usually embedded in a bombastic, fantastic and mystic language. He was well versed in the medical heritage of the Greeks, was an intrepid and often sound experimenter, and his pathology showed many good elements. His therapeutics were based on chemistry, but he discarded alchemy and attacked the belief in witchcraft, uromancy, and medicine practised by astrology only.

Paracelsus recognized miners' phthisis as an occupational hazard. He regarded gout and stone as diathetic diseases, i.e. 'tartaric' processes, due to precipitation of substances normally excreted from the body. He attributed goitre to mineral impurities in drinking water, especially sulphide of iron ('marchasita'), and also postulated a hereditary element in it. He was the first to realize the connection between cretinism, endemic goitre and congenital idiocy. "While goitre is not a characteristic of idiots, yet it is most commonly found among them." His references to cretinism are to be found in his *De Generatione Stultorum*[3]. His studies of endemic goitre were based on first hand observations in the Duchy of Salzburg. Paracelsus also made an unbiased study of diabetes mellitus, declaring it to be a severe generalized disease (in opposition to Galen). He explicitly recommended examination of diabetic urine[4], but did not refer to its sweet taste. However, when evaporating the urine, he noticed the formation of considerable amounts of a solid 'salt' (for which he must have mistaken the sugar). His intensive study of drugs made him say that everything is a poison, it is only the dose that matters: "Dosis sola facit venenum". He introduced laudanum (opium), sulphur, iron, arsenic, copper sulphate, mercury (especially in the treatment of syphilis), and potassium sulphate ('specificum purgans Paracelsi') into the pharmacopoeia, and made tinctures and alcoholic extracts popular. He also favoured mineral baths and mentioned several 'spas', such as Gastein in Austria and Plombières in France.

A remark should be made about contraceptive practices. The Catholic Church, the views of which were represented by the doctrines of St. Thomas Aquinas (1225–1274), was adamantly against any form of contraception. In spite of the dominance of the Church, however, there always existed some folkloric knowledge of contraceptive measures, but on the whole, the effective role of contraception in the Middle Ages was small. European folk beliefs and references in the lay literature after 1400 were mainly magical. The only occasional rational and more effective contraceptive methods were coitus interruptus, and the insertion into the vagina of a sponge saturated with lemon juice, e.g. in Constantinople[5].

The fall of Constantinople in 1453 brought many scholars from there to Italy. This meant a revival of Greek culture with the stress on Platonic and Hippocratic ideas in medicine, instead of the dialectics of Galen and Aristotle. Added to the neo-Platonists was the influence of the printers of the Renaissance.

Printed books took the place of handwritten texts and spread the newly developed thoughts and knowledge at a great speed; moreover, they were very much cheaper to produce and to buy. The Gutenberg Bible, printed in 1454, was followed by a veritable spate of books, and the craft of the printers became established all over Europe. William Caxton in England, the printers in Venice, Florence and Bologna, in Italy, followed suit and so did those in Paris, Basle, Antwerp and Leyden, and in many German towns such as Mainz, Bamberg and Strassburg.

Europe was in a fever of renewed spiritual activity, and in medicine the 'medical humanists' were the leaders of the new spirit. Niccoló Leoniceno (Leonicenus), 1428–1524, Professor of Medicine in Bologna and Padova, made a new translation into Latin of the Aphorisms of Hippocrates, but – even more important – he wrote a tract on the errors of the translators of Pliny and of the errors made by Pliny himself[6]. This was pioneer work which opened new vistas, in spite of attacks upon him by contemporaries. One of Leonicenus' friends was Thomas Linacre (1460–1524), the English physician who was an MD of Padova and DM of Oxford (see Section II). He was a student in Padova, when Venice became the most active centre of Greek and Latin printing in the world, and Padova was Venetian territory. Linacre published one of Leonicenus' translations in London much later, and also made translations from the Greek, which the famous Italian printer Aldus Manutius published in Venice in 1499, referring to Linacre as 'Thomas Anglicus'. Remarkably, he wrote two books on Latin grammar, one of which became very popular in France. Later he became physician to the Court, especially to Henry VIII and above all, became the Founder of the College of Physicians in London, which was legally a Royal foundation, as the King granted its Charter, granting what had been asked for in a petition signed by Linacre. On 23 September 1518, the King granted his Letters Patent under the Great Seal[7].

Printing brought about the publication of pharmacopoeias, i.e. collections of medical recipes. One of the most famous was the already mentioned *Antedotarium Florentinum* of 1498 (p. 98). The first pharmacopoeia to be approved by civil authority was the 'Pharmacorum omnium, quae quidem in usu sunt, conficiendorum ratio, vulgo vocant dispensatorium pharmacopolarum' (Nurimbergae, apud J. Petreium, 1546), written by Valerius Cordus (see p. 98). It was decreed by the City Authority of Nüremberg to be used by all dispensers under penalty of punishment. The word 'pharmacopoeia' was first used in 1560: "pharmacopoeia in compendium redacta", Anvers, by Johannes Brettschneider. This was followed by the "Pharmacopoeia medicamentorum, quae hodie ad publica medentium munia in officinis extant", Basil, 1561, by Ametius Foesius (1528–1595), who worked as a physician in Metz and who also wrote the important *Oeconomia Hippocratis* in 1588[8]. Much later, the College of Physicians in London produced the *Pharmacopoeia Londinensis*, of which there were ten editions between 1618 and 1851.

The earliest printed document on medicine, moreover in the vernacular, was the 'Laxierkalender' (purgation-calendar) of 1457, on a half sheet of paper. There was also an 'Aderlass-Kalender' (calendar for bloodletting), published in Mainz in 1462.

THE ANATOMISTS

Of equal importance was the revived interest in the study of anatomy. In this field the great artists of the Renaissance were just as much involved as the medical people and their great achievements

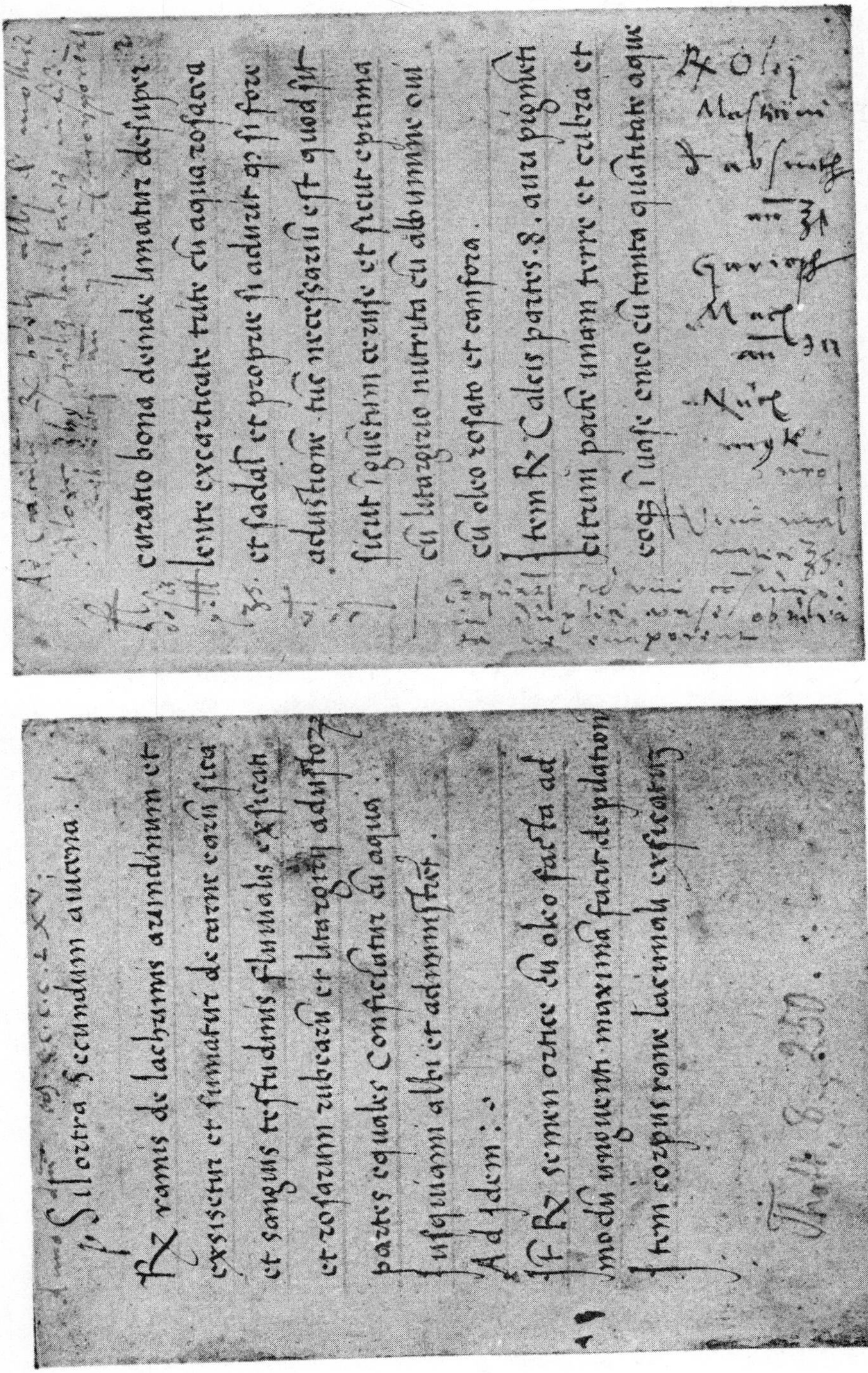

Figure 8 Table I of the Thottske Manuscript of a Florentine pharmacopoeia of 1465, discovered by Karl Sudhoff

were partly due to their ardent endeavour to gain first hand knowledge of the human body.

Leonardo da Vinci (1452–1519), who was also a scientist, declared that glands existed to close the gaps where muscles were missing, and that the thyroid gland separated the trachea from the clavicle.

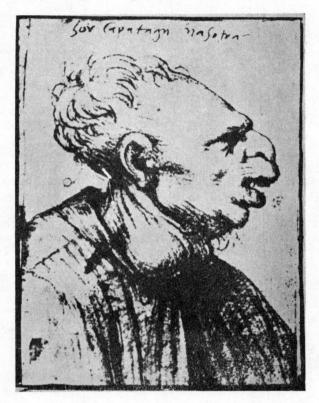

Figure 9 Leonardo da Vinci: *Goitreaux figure grotesque* (Man with goitre) [Rome: Bibliotheque Ambrosiana]

His chalk drawings of physiological anatomy (of *ca*. 1512) were buried and forgotten for 200 years or more, until they were noted by Wm. Hunter[9]. Hunter declared that their author was "the greatest anatomist of his epoch". The sketches were made at the dissecting table, because Leonardo believed that true knowledge of anatomy could be acquired only by dissection. He made over 750 of them, including those of muscles, heart and lungs, the blood vessels of the body, and cross sections of the brain at different planes. His studies of the valves, muscles and vessels of the heart are so outstanding that it seems surprising that he did not anticipate William Harvey in the discovery of the circulation, especially as he most likely injected blood vessels and investigated the hydrodynamics of the blood. He was the founder of cross-sectional anatomy, demonstrating important morphological relations of organs, vessels, nerves and bones. One of his drawings of the pregnant human uterus shows one of the ovaries, but, alas, also the cotyledonary placenta of a cow.

Michelangelo also carried out dissections, if not openly, at least stealthily. Iason[10] quotes Michelangelo's sonnet, written to a friend during the long-drawn-out work on painting the Sistine Chapel:

> I've grown a goitre by dwelling in this den
> As cats from stagnant streams in Lombardy
> Or in what other land they hap to be.

The Edinburgh anatomist Robert Knox (1791–1862) wrote an interesting book on *Great Artists and Great Anatomists*, containing among others, sketches of Leonardo da Vinci, Michelangelo Buonarotti and Rafael of Urbino[11]. His conclusions were as follows:

Learn anatomy by all means, but do not forget its object. . . . When you draw a dissected limb, be sure to sketch the living one beside it (like da Vinci did), that you may at once contrast them and note the differences. In drawing from the nude figure, contrast your sketch with the antique; you will find in it many defects. . . . The relation Anatomy holds to Art is to explain – first, how far the shapes and figures of the inward structures modify the external forms of man and woman; second, it informs the artist of the meaning of such forms; third, it explains to him the laws of deformation; . . . As an artist he must represent them, no doubt; but in doing so let him wisely follow Nature rather in her intentions than in her forthcomings. . . .

The great German painter Albrecht Dürer (1471–1528) may be added to this trio. He wrote a major treatise on human proportion[12] which was the first application of anthropometry to aesthetics. The superb woodcuts were also the first attempt to employ cross-hatching to represent shades and shadows.

The anatomy of the medical schools was still that of Galen, taught from the book, not by dissection and demonstration. The pioneer of modern anatomy became Andreas Vesalius (1514–1564) (see Section II). Trained in the Galenic tradition, his first writing dealt with a revision of Gunther's *Anatomical Institutions According to Galen*[10]. He soon, however, became a first-rate dissector, especially after five years' experience as public prosector in Padova, teaching to dissect and inspect the human organs *in situ*. The fruit of his labours was his crowning work *De Humani Corporis Fabrica Libri Septem*, Basileae,

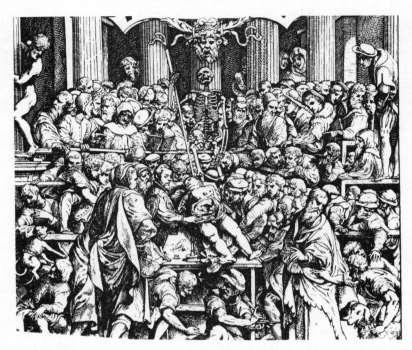

Figure 10 Title page of "De humani corporis fabrica librii septem" (Basileae, 1543) by Andreas Vesalius (1514–1564).

1543. This brilliant work, with all the new evidence gained from observation and experiment, was severely attacked by his old teacher Jacobus Sylvius, an inveterate Galenist, and also by some of his own opportunist pupils and, especially, by the established authority. His morale broke down, in a fit of despair he burned his manuscripts, left Padova and accepted a post as court physician to the Emperor Charles V in Madrid. He married and gave up anatomy completely for years. Meanwhile, his main pupil, Gabriele Falloppio (1523–1562), also known as Fallopius (see Section II), took up the torch and re-kindled the fire. The Fallopian *Observationes Anatomicae*, Venetiis, 1561, put Fallopius' name in the forefront of the critics of Galen.

Vesalius, still not old (47), but now a mere courtier, seemed almost forgotten. In 1563, he went on a pilgrimage to Jerusalem. On his way back, in 1564, he received an invitation to resume his Chair in Padova, but he died on the island of Zante, of a sudden acute disease, when aged only 50, a disappointed man. Vesalius described the thyroid as follows:

> This incision also shows two glands, one on each side of the root of the larynx, and these are large and somewhat fungus [sic!] and almost the

colour of flesh, but rather darker, with many prominent veins. . . .
This also do the glands which lie at the root of the larynx perform for
the trachea, since they moisten its orifice with a humor not indeed
fluid, but rather viscid and thick, for the glands themselves are thicker
and denser than the rest of the gland which secrete a humor.[10]

He called them: "Glandes laryngis radici adnatae"[13].

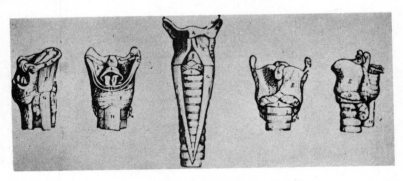

Figure 11   Drawings of the thyroid gland by Vesalius

The pituitary he named the "Glandula pituitam cerebri excipiens",
secreting the mucous discharge of the nose[13]. In the 1555 edition of
De . . . Fabrica, he described the ovaries as follows:

The testes of women contain, besides blood vesicles, some sinuses full
of a thin watery fluid which, if the testis has not been previously
damaged, but is squeezed and makes a noise like an inflated bladder,
will spurt out like a fountain to a great height during the dissection. As
this fluid is white and like a milky serum in healthy women, so I have
found it to be a wonderful saffron yellow colour and a little thicker in
two well-bred girls who were troubled before death with strangulation
of the womb; the testis of one of the girls, or at any rate one of the
sinuses in it, protruded like a rather large pea full of yellow fluid . . .

Surely, this is a description of the ovaries and perhaps of the corpus
luteum!

Interestingly, he also gave careful descriptions of the accessory
sinuses of the nose and of the ear. In his description of the brain he
was a pioneer of experimental and comparative anatomy, maintaining
that there was no fundamental difference in the cerebration of the
highest vertebrates from that of man. It is easily overlooked that he
was also a clinician of no mean skill, to be a physician to the court of
Spain, where he operated successfully on empyemas of the lung and
excised cancer of the breast[14].

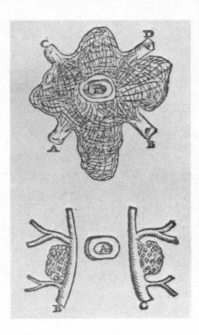

Figure 12 The pituitary body according to Galen and to Vesalius [From Ciba Monograph No. 10, by kindness of Ciba-Geigy Ltd.]

Fallopius, anatomist of Modena and Venice, was one of Vesalius' favourite pupils. He described the semi-circular canals, the trigeminal, auditory and glossopharyngeal nerves, but above all the corpus luteum (which was also noted by his pupil Volcherus Coiter (1534–1590), in 1573), thus controverting the idea that the ovaries contained semen. Coiter thought that the ovaries corresponded to the seminal vesicle rather than to the testes[15]. Already Vesalius had remarked in the second edition in 1555 of the *De Humani Corporis Fabrica* on the irregular surface of the 'testes muliebres', but the actual discovery of the ovarian follicles occurred only in the 17th century[16]. In 1561, Fallopius described the tubes named after him and the round ligaments.

That slender and narrow seminal passage arises from the horn of the uterus very white and sinewy but after it has passed outward a little way it becomes gradually broader and curls like the tendrils of a vine until it comes to the end when the tendril-like curls spread out, and it terminates in a very broad ending which appears membraneous and fleshy on account of its reddish colour. This ending is much shredded and worn as if it were the fringe of a worn piece of cloth and it has a broad opening which always lies closed by the coming together of those fringed ends. However, if they are opened carefully and spread apart, they form, as it were, the bell-like mouth of a bronze trumpet. Consequently since, whether the tendril-like curls be removed from this classical instrument or even added to, the seminal passage will extend from its head even to its uttermost ending and so it has been designated by me the trumpet (tuba) of the uterus. They are arranged in this way in all animals, not only in man, but also in fowls and cattle and in the corpses of all other animals which I have studied. . . .[17]

Nearly twenty years after Vesalius' *De Fabrica*, Realdus Columbus (1516–1559) (Matteo Realdo Colombo) observed for the first time that the thyroid gland in women appeared larger than in men. Columbus had succeeded Vesalius as lecturer in surgery and anatomy in the University of Padova in 1544 and in 1552 became lecturer in anatomy to the Papal University in Rome, where he practised surgery and where Michelangelo was one of his patients. He hoped to have his only work, a textbook of anatomy (*De re anatomica libri* XV. Venetiis, 1559), illustrated by Michelangelo, but was disappointed. The book contained a number of his discoveries and was written in a simple direct style: however, it was not completed and was published posthumously. The Royal College of Physicians in London have a copy in their Library. The frontispiece, the only illustration, shows Columbus dissecting and commenting, as was customary in Padova, whereas in London the lecturer employed a surgeon to do the dissecting, until after Harvey's time. Columbus was, however, in opposition to some of Vesalius' ideas.

In 1601, Giulio Casserio (Julius Casserius Placentinus), 1561?– 1616, described the thyroid as being a single organ in two parts and without an excretory duct. He was one of Harvey's teachers in Padova, whose 'Tabulae anatomicae' were as artistic as they were scientifically accurate[18].

Remarkably, another anatomist of outstanding merit, Bartolomeo Eustachi (Eustachius), 1520–1574, was among the opponents of Vesalius. Eustachius was professor at the Collegia della Sapienza in Rome and completed his *Tabulae Anatomicae* in 1552. They contained 147 superb plates, drawn by himself, but remained unprinted for more than one and a half centuries in the Papal Library, until Pope Clement XI gave them to the physician Lancisi, who published them with his own notes in 1714. They were the first anatomic plates on copper and more accurate in delineation than the earlier ones, including those of Vesalius. Although Eustachius did not oppose Galen, he was an outstanding discoverer in the field of anatomy. His discoveries included not only the Eustachian tube, the abducens

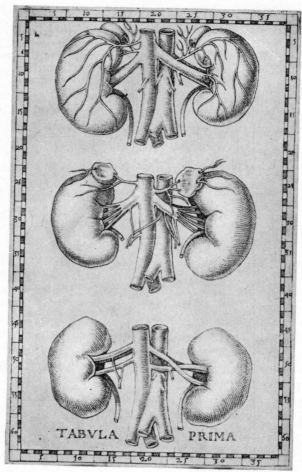

Figure 13 Eustachi (*ca.* 1501–74): Adrenal gland (1552), from "Opuscula Anatomica", Venice, 1563–4 [From Ciba Monograph No. 10, by kindness of Ciba-Geigy Ltd.]

nerve and the thoracic duct, but – of special interest for us – the suprarenal bodies, 'Glandulae renis incumbentes' in 1563, which were shown on the copper plates. In Chapter VI of his *Opuscula Anatomica* he stated that nobody had previously referred to the adrenals in any medical work:

> ... nihilominus ne aliquid in hac tractatione praetermissum esse quispiam mihi jure objiciat: consentaneum esse duxi de quibusdam Renum glandulis ab aliis Anatomicia negligenter praetermissis hoc loco scribere.[19]

He offered, however, no explanation of their function. The thyroid gland was called 'glandula laryngea' by Eustachius, who used the term 'isthmus' for the part connecting the two lobes. The theory that the thyroid is a lubricator for the wind pipe and the lungs was also supported by Bohelius, who wrote in 1585: "Lest constant respiration and the great difficulty of speaking and shouting should dry up too much of the trachea and the lungs, nature has provided those glands continually to prepare moisture for these."[20]

The existence of the suprarenal glands was also mentioned by Archangelus Piccolomineus (1562–1605), "Ferrariensis Civisque Romanus", in his *Anatomicae Praelectiones* in 1586[21] and by Caspar Bauhin (1550–1624), Professor of Anatomy, Botany, Medicine and Greek at Bâle, in 1588[22]. The aforementioned Giulio Casserio called them "Renes succenturiati". His pupil and successor Adrianus Spigelius (1578–1625) or Adriaan van den Spieghel, incorporated Casserio's fine plates in his posthumous work *De Humani Corporis Fabrica*, Venetiis, 1627, and talked of the "capsulae renales". To him, they merely served to occupy the space between the kidneys and the diaphragm[22]. Later, Nathaniel Highmore (1613–1685) agreed and added that they might serve to absorb humid exudates from the large vessels nearby[23].

After Paracelsus, there was an important study of goitre, being endemic in the Valais, Styria and the Pyrenees, by Muenster[24] and by Johann Lange (1485–1565) in 1554, for Salzburg, Styria and the Tyrol[25]. The Zürich chronicler Josias Simmler (1530–1576) also described cretins in the canton of Valais and another Swiss, Johannes Stumpf (1500–1558) recorded the incidence of goitre in the Grisons at Trimmis, Untervaz, Zizers and Igis. A Dutch physician, Pieter van Foreest (? – 1597) observed many cretins in the province of Vaitellina, on the Italian side of the Swiss border. In 1601, Johannes Jessenius, a physician in Prague, noted the occurrence of goitre in various parts of Bohemia and added that in some regions people regarded goitre as an adornment. In 18th century England endemic goitre in Derbyshire became known as 'Derbyshire neck' worn with a slight undertone of pride[26]. The surgeon Guy de Chauliac (1300–1370) (see also p. 91) wrote: "Botium aegritudo regionalis et hereditaria apud multos reputatur" (goitre = botium is frequently considered to be a local and hereditary disease)[26]. (See Marco Polo's observations on endemic goitre, p. 15.) Campbell reported it in the Rhine Valley above Lake Constance in 1524 (Beiträge z. medizinischen Topographie)[27]. On the border of the 17th century hovers Felix Platter (1536–1614). Having obtained his medical degree at Montpellier, he became professor of practical medicine in Bâle, his native city (see Section II). In his main work, published in 1602, the

Praxeos Medicinae, he gave a brief but precise description of the deaf and dumb, mentally defective (cretins), often seen in his native canton of Valais.

> Wherefore the disease is frequent in certain regions, in the beginning they write of Egypt, and in Valesia Canton Bremis, as indeed I have seen it myself, and in the Carinthia valley called Bintzgerthal many infants are wont to be afflicted: who besides their innate simple-mindedness, the head is now and then misformed, the tongue immense and tumid, dumb, a struma often at the throat, they show a deformed appearance: and seated in solemn stateliness, staring, and a stick resting between their hands, their bodies twisted variously, their eyes wide apart, they show immoderate laughter and wonder at unknown things.[28]

He also described death in an infant due to hypertrophy of the thymus, in 1614.

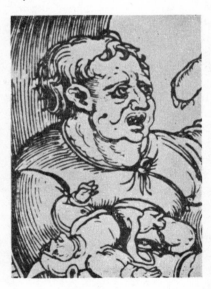

Figure 14 Ancient woodcut: goitre

Accounts of Roman authors of the prevalence of endemic goitre in the Alps: Juvenal (1st century AD) asked: "Quis tumidum guttur miratur in Alpibus?" ("who wonders at a swelling of the neck in the Alps?"). The Architect Vitriuvius (1st century BC) wrote: "Aequiculis in Italia et in Alpibus nationi Medullorum est genus aquae, quam qui bibunt afficiuntur turgidis gutturibus" (The Aequi in Italy and the Medulli in the Alps have a kind of water, from drinking which they get a swelling of the neck). Pliny the Elder (1st century AD) remarked: "Guttur homini tantum et suibus intumescit, aquarum qae potantur plerumque vitio" (Swelling of the throat occurs only in men and in swine, caused mostly by the water they drink). Ulpianus (2nd century AD) wrote: "Tumido gutture praecipue laborant Alpium incolae, propter aquarum qualitatem quibus utuntur" (The inhabitants of the Alps suffer from a big neck, caused by the quality of the water they drink). Caesar is credited with having noted the occurrence of a big neck among the Gauls as one of their peculiarities. In Hippocratic writings (4th century BC) there was the expression (gongrona) 'γογγρώνη', which Ambroise Paré thought to mean goitre (De gongrona ou bronchocoele). Littré (1840) also translated it as goitre. There was another Hippocratic expression which was also thought to mean goitre, namely (choiron) 'χοίρων'; it was used by Paulus of Aegina. Yet another term was 'botium' and Rogerius Salernitanus (12th century) wrote on 'De cura botii'. The word *struma* was apparently first used by Albrecht von Haller (1708–1777), who remarked: "Strumis longe plerumque thyroideam glandulam vitiari vulgo notum est". (It is generally known that goitre is mostly an affection of the thyroid gland.) Many more such expressions exist in various languages.

Reports of the existence of endemic goitre on the American continent before the arrival of the Europeans have been disputed, especially by I. Greenwald[29]. Yet our present knowledge of the causes of endemic goitre makes it seem unlikely that endemic goitre did not exist on such a vast continent before the 17th or 18th century AD. The exact meaning of the word 'coto' or 'ccotto' seems irrelevant.

Fallopius' pupil and successor was Hieronymus Fabricius ab Aquapendente (Girolamo Fabrizzi), 1537–1619. He built, at his own expense, the splendid anatomy theatre in Padova, which William Harvey attended as his pupil and which excites the admiration of the visitor even today. He wrote many important tractates on anatomy, some of which inspired Harvey in his research on the circulation. He also wrote on embryology ('De formato foetu', Venetiis, 1600) and later on 'De formatione ovi et pulli' (Patavii, 1621). He recorded in the first book the dissection of several embryos. In it he also gave one of the first illustrated accounts of the comparative anatomy of the female reproductive apparatus. In one drawing of the uterus and the ovaries of a pregnant sow, the corpora lutea are presented for the first time: "glandulae multae simuljunctae in utraque uteri parte". 'De formatione ovi et pulli' was left as a manuscript at his death and was published posthumously. It deals with the development of the chick in the egg. The illustrations show clearly the chick in the egg developing by epigenesis, whereas in the text he mysteriously and rigidly adheres to Galen's doctrine of preformation. A later printed copy of it is in the Library of the Royal College of Physicians in

London. These two writings were the basis for Harvey's studies on animal generation; yet Harvey did not hesitate to criticize some of Fabricius' ideas sternly. It has been claimed that the name 'ovarium' was introduced by Fabricius, "but according to Hyrtl, the name was first used by Niels Stensen (1648–1686)."[30]

R. V. Short summarized the events of the sixteenth century, concerning the ovaries, as follows: ". . . we may conclude that it was an era in which the ovaries received recognition as structures, even though their function was not appreciated."[38]

Vesalius' work had a direct effect on Renaissance surgery, one of the main representatives of which was the Frenchman Ambroise Paré (1510–1590) (see Section II). He wrote an epitome on De Fabrica in the vernacular, thus making it widely available to surgeons. Not only was he the greatest army surgeon of his time, but a surgeon in the class of Lister and John Hunter of later generations. Among his numerous discoveries, new methods of treatment, and writings, his outstanding merit was the refutal of the pseudo-Hippocratic doctrine "diseases (e.g. wounds caused in battle) not curable by iron, are curable by fire", which had caused many deaths by treating gunshot wounds with boiling oil. He was also the first to suggest syphilis as a cause of aneurysm. He did away "with the strolling surgeon's trick of castrating a patient in herniotomy"[31]. He also believed that cases of poly-orchidism existed and conferred supervirility "as in the case of the legendary man who was sexually active up to the age of 125 and lived to reach that of 169 years"[32]. This, of course, means exclusion of the cases where there present multiple cysts of the epidydimis, or the subdivision of the body of one testicle due to an irregularity in its embryonic development. Although now proved to be extremely rare, cases of true polyorchidism do seem to occur, as described, for example, by R. Hodgson Boggon in 1933[33]. In 1550, Paré described varicocele as "a compact pack of vessels quite filled with melancholic blood"[34]; whether he already attributed it to inadequate sexual relief, often due to late marriage, as thought of later, is not known. Nor is it known if he connected the existence of a varicocele with subfertility in the patients afflicted; it is known now that the reported incidence among men attending subfertility clinics is between 19 and 39 per cent. The pooling of blood around the testicles increased the scrotal temperature and makes ineffective the function of the scrotum as a box for cool storage, depressing the sperm count with poor motility and an increased number of abnormal forms[35].

Ambroise Paré seems to have regarded cases of exophthalmic goitre, erroneously, as examples of aneurysm – as did Aetius before him (500 AD)[36]. (See p. 63.)

In the English translation of 1649 of Paré's *Of Man's Body*, he says in Chapter XVI,

Of the Glandules in general, and of the Pancreas, or sweet-bread. . . . Besides this, we have spoken of glandules in general, we must know that the Pancreas is a glandulous and fleshlike body, as that which hath every where the shape and resemblance of flesh. It is situate at the flat end of the liver, under the Duodenum, with which it hath great connexion, and under the gatevein, to serve as a Bulwark both to it and the divisions thereof, whilst it fills up the empty spaces between the vessels themselves, and so hinders, that they be not pluck'd asunder, nor hurt by any violent motion as a fall or the like.

The second, enlarged edition of his anatomy, in the original French, was published in Paris in 1561, under the title *Anatomie Universelle du Corps Humain* (etc.). He obviously assigned to the pancreas a similar function as others did to the thyroid and to the suprarenals, dictated by the fear of the vacuum of his times[37].

REFERENCES

1. Rolleston, Sir Humphrey: The Endocrine Organs in Health and Disease. p. 7. London, Oxford University Press, 1936.
2. Cordus, Valerius: Pharmacorum omnium, quae quidem in usu sunt, conficiendorum ratio, vulgo vocant dispensatorium pharmacopolarum. Norimbergae, 1546.
3. Bombastus ab Hohenheim, A. P. T. (Paracelsus): De Generatione Stultorum. Opera II, pp. 174–182. Strassburg, 1603.
4. Paracelsus: De Urina, Chap. IV. Opera, 1603.
5. Himes, N. E.: Medical History of Contraception. p. 82. New York, Gamut Press, 1936.
6. Leoniceno, N.: De Plinii et Plurium Aliorum in Medicina Erroribus. Ferrara, 1492.
7. Clark, Sir George: A History of the Royal College of Physicians of London. Vol. I, p. 41. Oxford, Clarendon Press, 1964.
8. Garrison, F. H.: An Introduction to the History of Medicine. 4th ed, p. 197. Philadelphia, W. B. Saunders, 1929.
9. ibid.: pp. 215–216.
10. Iason, A. H.: The Thyroid Gland in Medical History. p. 37. New York, Froben Press, 1946.
11. Knox, R.: Great Artists and Great Anatomists. H. Renshaw, London, 1852.
12. Dürer, A.: Vier Bücher von menschlicher Proportion. J. Formschneyder, Nürnberg, 1528.
13. Abderhalden, R.: Internal secretion. CIBA Monographs. pp. 308–310. Bombay, 1951.
14. As 8: p. 220.
15. As 1: p. 399.
16. As 13: p. 307.
17. Falloppio, G.: Observationes Anatomicae (translated by Wilson, L. G.). pp. 196–197. Venice, 1561.

18. Casserio, G.: Tabulae Anatomicae. lxxiix. Venetiis, 1627.
19. Eustachi, Bartolomeo: Opuscula Anatomica. Chap. VI. Venice, 1563–64.
20. As 10: p. 40.
21. Piccolomineus, Archangelus: Anatomicae Praelectiones. p. 145. Rome, 1586.
22. Bauhin, C.: De Humani Corporis Partibus Externis. Bale, 1588.
23. Highmore, N.: Corporis Humani Disquisitio Anatomica. Bk. I Pt. 3, Chap. 4, pp. 82–84. Hagae, 1651.
24. Muenster: Cosmographia. University of Basle, 1550.
25. Lange, Johann: Medicinalium Epistolarum Miscellanea. Basileae, 1554.
26. Endemic Goitre. pp. 12–13. World Health Organization, Geneva, 1960.
27. As 10: p. 41.
28. Platter, F.: Praxeos seu de cognoscendis, praedicendis, praecavendis, curandisque affectibus homini incommodantibus. Basileae, 1602–03.
29. Greenwald, I.: The early history of goiter in the Americas, in New Zealand and in England. Bull. Hist. Med. **17,** 229, 1945.
30. As 1: p. 399.
31. As 8: p. 225.
32. As 1: p. 389.
33. Hodgson Boggon, R.: Polyorchidism. Br. J. Surg. **1,** 630–639, 1933.
34. Annotation: Varicocele and subfertility. Br. Med. J. **1,** 1304, 1978.
35. ibid.: p. 1305.
36. As 10: p. 29.
37. See Chapter 13.
38. Short, R. V.: The Discovery of the Ovaries. In: The Ovary, 2nd edn., Vol. 1. New York, San Francisco, London, Academic Press, 1977.

CHAPTER THIRTEEN

THE 17th CENTURY AND THE MICROSCOPISTS

ROM ancient times until the Renaissance and beyond, the term 'glands' was applied to many organs of soft consistency. The brain, the liver, and the spleen were all called glands at one time or another. The thyroid, the thymus, the salivary glands and the lympathic glands were known, but had not been studied much. Moreover, the structure of the glands could not be studied before the advent of the microscope.

It was known that some glands had excretory ducts as an outlet for their secretions, but others gave rise to speculations and futile theories: the pituitary – as we have seen – was assumed to discharge its phlegm (pituita) through the lamina cribrosa into the nasal cavities, according to Galen. This method of passing fluid from one place to another was a common idea; even Vesalius accepted Galen's favourite theory that in the heart the blood was moved from the right to the left ventricle by numerous foramina in the interventricular septum, invisible to the naked eye. The study of the finer structure of the organs was made possible only by the invention of a new technique, the anatomic injection. It became especially important for Harvey's study of the circulation of the blood. Stephanus had filled the blood vessels with air, Eustachius with coloured fluids, Malpighi and Glisson with ink, and Willis discovered the circulus arteriosus in the brain, named after him, by injecting the blood vessels of the brain with 'aqua crocata'[1]. Swammerdam, de Graaf and Ruysch used the method of alcoholic injection. These three belonged to the group of the 'microscopists', about whom we must now say a little more.

THE MICROSCOPISTS

In 1609 Galileo Galilei made available two instruments which were very important to the development of modern science. They were the telescope and the microscope. Although these early compound microscopes failed to give a clear picture, after 1650 a way was found of mounting simple lenses of a high power[2]. Many of the important microscopical discoveries of the 17th century were made with a simple lens. Robert Hooke (1635–1703), a pupil of Robert Boyle, was a mechanical genius who built one of the earliest compound microscopes. The results of the observations made with it, he published in London in 1665 in his "Micrographia, or some physiological descriptions of minute bodies made by magnifying glasses; with observations and inquiries thereupon". It illustrates vegetable histology and contains the first reference to the "little boxes or cells distinct from one another"[3].

It is believed that the first microscopist to use the instrument for the investigation of disease was Athanasius Kircher of Fulda (1602–1680), a Jesuit scholar. He was an Orientalist, musician, physicist, mathematician, optician and a medical man.

The short-lived Jan Swammerdam (1637–1680) of Amsterdam rose to greater fame as an expert in microscopic dissection and experimental physiology; he described the red blood-corpuscles and the lymphatic valves. He invented a method of injecting blood vessels with wax, which was later claimed by Ruysch.

Of even greater importance was Antonj van Leeuwenhoek (1632–1723) (see Section II) of Delft. He was a draper and had no medical or scientific training and was secretive about his manner of working. He always used a simple microscope with lenses of short focal length. He had, during the course of his long life, some 247 microscopes with 419 lenses, most of them ground by himself. He became a Fellow of the Royal Society of London, to which he donated 26 microscopes and sent 375 scientific papers. Among his many great discoveries, the one of the utmost importance here, is his description of the spermatozoa, "originally pointed out to him by the student Hannen in 1674"[4].

Leeuwenhoek's[5] first report on the "little animals of the sperm" dates back to November, 1677[6]. These observations concerned fresh seminal fluid, "immediately after ejaculation, before six beats of the pulse had intervened" and showed that it swarmed with a multitude of "animalcules" that could propel themselves about with serpentine movements[7]. He made one mistake by giving the size as smaller than that of a red blood-corpuscle (*ca.* 7.2 μm in diameter) as compared

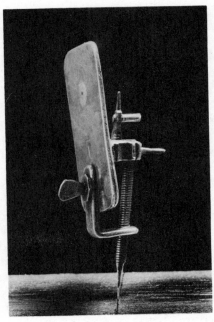

Figure 15   Leeuwenhoek's microscope [Copyright Museum Boerhaave]

with the true size of *ca.* 58 μm, but otherwise his description has remained valid.

> Their bodies which were round, were blunt in front and ran to a point. They were furnished with a thin tail, about five or six times as long as the body, and very transparent and with the thickness of about one twentyfifth of the body[8].

Castellani rightly stresses that "Leeuwenhoek's position was that of an observer who, completely free from preconceptions, strives to describe whatever occurs under his own eyes as faithfully as possible". He confined himself to drawing on his observations (exactly as Bonnet would recommend that naturalists should do, a hundred years later), only "les consèquences les plus immèdiates" – that is, "unfiltered through the screen of theory"[9]. (Charles Bonnet, 1720–1793, believed in the preformation theory, that the organism is already preformed in the ovum or spermatozoon.) Leeuwenhoek's very 'innocence' enabled him to classify the spermatozoa as 'animalcules'. From his point of view . . . "they were born, they grew, they moved by their own means through the seminal fluid, they died"[10]. In 1683 and 1684, Leeuwenhoek found out by experiment that in dogs' seminal fluid kept in a glass tube, spermatozoa began to die as time passed and that after seven days very few of them were still alive and swimming about "as if they had just come from the dog"[11].

In his next experiments, on a bitch and on female rabbits, killed at various times soon after mating, he found spermatozoa in the first part of the uterus or (later) in the Fallopian tubes, swarming under the microscope, briskly moving about. In the rabbits killed six hours after mating he found one cornu uteri teeming with live spermatozoa. Keeping the other cornu in a box with moist paper for 16 hours, there were, on examination, only a few living animalcules to 25 or more dead ones. After another five hours they were all dead[12].

The greatest figure among the microscopists was, however, Marcello Malphighi (1628–1694) (see Section II). He was professor of anatomy in Bologna, Pisa and Messina. He studied the embryology of the chick and the histology and physiology of the 'glands' in 1665. He maintained that the acini (grana glandulosa), i.e. little round bags in the substance of the glands continuous with the excretory duct, are identical with the simple follicles and muciparous crypts. His studies of the embryology of the chick, 'De formatione pulli in ovo' (= On the formation of the chicken in the ovum) (1673) and 'De ovo incubato' (= On the incubated ovum), are the foundation of descriptive embryology, with an accurate notation of the aortic arches, the neutral grove, the cerebral and optic vesicles. He correctly assumed that the (Graafian) follicle was a protection for the real ovum that was within it. He also coined the name 'corpus luteum', which, in cows observed by him, is yellow, but not in cats, sheep, sows, mares or human females. He did not, however, realize that it was formed from the lining of the ruptured follicle. According to Spallanzani (see pp. 187–188), he also attempted experimental artificial insemination, but was unsuccessful.

The 'corpus luteum', which – as we have seen – was first described by Fallopius (see p. 106) and noted by his pupil Coiter, was given a detailed account of by Regner de Graaf (1641–1673) (see Section II). He did this in his treatise "De mulierum organis generationi inservientibus" (= On the organs of women which serve the purpose of procreation) (Leiden, 1672), and it seems fully justified that the follicles of the ovaries were named the 'Graafian follicles' (vesiculae Graafianae) at Albrecht von Haller's suggestion. In that work there occurs the famous quotation: ". . . secundum illud Proverb. cap. 30 'Tria sunt insaturabilia . . . infernus, et os vulvae, et terra.' . . .", ". . . (according to the quotation from Proverbs, Chap. 30, . . . 'there are three things which are insatiable: . . . hell, and the os vulvae, and earth' . . . ") so tamely translated in the authorized version of the Bible. The most important part is

118

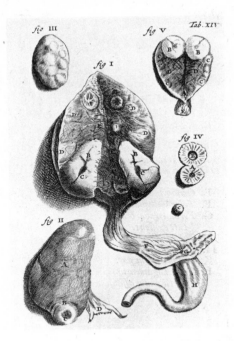

Figure 16 One of the earliest illustrations of the ovaries (cow's), from Regnier de Graaf's "De mulierum organis generationi inservientibus", Leyden, 1672 [From Ciba Monograph No. 10, by kindness of Ciba-Geigy Ltd.]

Chapter 12: 'De Testibus Muliebribus Sive Ovariis' (= On the Female Testicles or Ovaries) and Chapter 13: 'De Semine Muliebri' (= On the Female Sperm). He says: "Ova in omni animalium genere reperiri confidenter asserimus". (We may assert confidently that eggs are found in all kinds of animals, since they may be observed not only in birds, in fishes, both oviparous and viviparous, but very clearly also in quadrupeds and even in man himself. Dr. George W. Corner's translation.) "Communis itaque foemellarum Testiculorum usus est, Ova generare, fovere, et ad maturitatem promovere, sic, ut in mulieribus eodem, quo volucrum ovaria, munere fungantur; hinc potius Mulierum Ovaria, quam Testes, appellanda veniunt; siquidem nullam similitudem tum forma tum contento cum virilibus Testibus proprio dictis obtinent . . ."[13]. (Thus the general function of the female testicles is to generate the ova, to nourish them, and to bring them to maturity, so that they serve the same purpose in women as the ovaries of the birds. Hence, they should rather be called ovaries than testes because they show no similarity, either in form or contents, with the male testes properly so called

REGNERI DE GRAAF

DE

MULIERUM
ORGANIS

GENERATIONI INSER-
VIENTIBUS

TRACTATUS NOVUS,

DEMONSTRANS

Tam Homines & Animalia cætera omnia,
quæ Vivipara dicuntur, haud minus quàm
Ovipara; ab Ovo originem ducere.

AD

COSMUM III.

MAGNUM ETRURIÆ DUCEM.

De Mulierum Organis, &c.   303

nere fungantur; hinc potiùs Mulierum Ovaria, quàm Testes, appellanda veniunt: siquidem nullam similitudinem tum formâ
tum contento cum virilibus Testibus pro-
prie dictis obtinent: quapropter ut inutilia
quædam corpora à multis habiti fuerunt; at
minùs rectè, quandoquidem illi ad genera-
tionem summopere necessarii exsistant; quod
probat mira vasorum Præparantium circa il-
los contortio, atque confirmat ipsa fœmel-
larum castratio, quam sterilitas infallibiliter
concomitatur: licet *Varro* scribat, vaccas
exsectis Testibus, si statim cöeant, conci-
pere ; quod quidem de masculis verum,
quatenus vesiculæ feminales adhuc femine
turgeant; non autem de fœmellis, quæ
vesiculas illas non habent: adeòut *Hofman-
ni* assertio veritati minùs congrua appareat,
quod pluribus ostenderemus, nisi dà *Whar-
tono* factum foret. Quomodo autem Ova illa
fœcundentur, & ad Uterum perveniant,
sequentibus capitibus elucidabitur.

TABULA DECIMA-QUARTA

Vaccæ & Ovis Ovarium exhibet, ut ea, quæ
post coitum in illis eveniunt, conspi-
ciantur.

Figura I. Exhibet Testiculum Vaccæ.
A.   *Testiculus secundùm longitudinem apertus.*
BB. Glan-

304   REGNERUS DE GRAAF

BB. *Glandulosa substantia, quæ post Ovi expulsionem in
Testibus reperitur, per medium divisa.*
CC. *Cavitas, in quâ Ovum contentum fuit, sere abolita.*
DD. *Ova diversæ magnitudinis in Ovario contenta.*
EE. *Vasa sanguinea ad Ova excurrentia.*
F. *Tuba Fallopiana membranosa expansio complicata.*
G. *Foramen in extremitate Tubarum exsistens.*
H. *Tuba Fallopiana pars abscissa.*

Fig. II. Exhibet Testiculum necdum apertum.
A. *Testiculus.*
B. *Glandulosa substantia extra Testiculum protuberans.*
C. *Foramen in ejus medio exsistens.*
D. *Tuba Fallopiana membranosæ expansionis portio.*

Fig. III. Exhibet Testiculum Ovillum cum transpa-
rentibus Ovis necdum masculino semine irroratis.

Fig. IV. Exhibet glandulosam globulorum substantiam
ex Ovis Testiculo exemptam prout Ovum adhuc
continebat.
A. *Glandulosa globuli substantia adaperta.*
B. *Locus ex quo Ovum exemptum est.*
C. *Ovum ex eo exemptum.*

Fig. V. Exhibet Testiculum Ovis, ex quo Ovum ab
aliquot diebus expullum fuit.
A. *Testiculum per medium divisus.*
B. *Glandulosa globulorum substantia cum cavitate suâ
propemodum abolitâ.*
CC. *Ova diversæ magnitudinis in Testium superficie la-
tentia.*
DD. *Vasa sanguinea ad Ova excurrentia.*
E. *Ligamenti Testiculorum portio.*

TABU-

Figure 17   Tabula XIV and title page of de Graaf "De mulierum organis generationi inservientibus"

120

. . . .) "On this account, many have considered these bodies useless, but this is incorrect, because they are indispensable for reproduction. . . . This is . . . confirmed by the castration of females, which is invariably accompanied by sterility."[14] It was Malpighi, however, who called the "substance glanduleux faisant hernie hors du testicule femelle" of de Graaf the "Corpus luteum" in 1687, but suggested that it gave rise to the formation of the ovarian follicle and ovum (i.e. regarded it – wrongly – as an early stage of the follicle).

In a searching study of de Graaf's contributions, B. P. Setchell has made a number of important observations[15]. As will be seen (pp. 125–127), William Harvey had published his book on reproduction in 1651, 21 years ahead of de Graaf's (companion) volume on reproduction in the female. Harvey was

> misled because he could find no trace of the male semen in the uterus after coitus and because he could detect no changes in the ovaries (or female testes as they were then called) of deer during and after mating. He therefore concluded that the ovaries played no part in reproduction[15].

We now know that stags start to rut a full month before the hinds begin to ovulate[90]. Harvey's work was known to de Graaf. He himself said: "The bodies which are always found naturally in the membranous substance of the 'testicles' just described are the vesicles full of liquid. . . ." ("De Mulierum etc. . . .", p. 176). These fluid-filled vesicles, as de Graaf was careful to point out, had been seen by others long before; "Vesal, Fallopio, Volcher Coiter, De Laurens, De Castro, Riolan, Bartholin, Wharton, Dom. de Marchetti and others have described these vesicles under various names." ("De Mulierum . . .", p. 179). In 1667, Stensen (who had been his fellow student at Leiden) had suggested that the female testes of viviparous animals also contained ova and should therefore be called 'Ovaries', and the vesicles had been called "ova" by Van Horne in 1668 ("De Mulierum . . .", p. 180). "De Graaf described and illustrated the ovarian vesicles in several species and fitted the ova into a reasonable scheme, which is substantially what we believe today . . ."[15]. He also made the important observation, from a carefully-timed series of dissections of rabbits after mating, that the vesicles changed into something quite different which he called "globules", but which we now call 'corpora lutea'. De Graff used the terms vesicles (vesicula) or egg (ovum) for what we now call the follicle. "He did use the term follicle (folliculus) but in quite a different sense, meaning the structure which surrounded the egg and which was left behind when the egg left the ovary. . . ." It is therefore unfortunate that we now use the term 'Graafian follicle' for what de Graaf called eggs or vesicles, especially as de Graaf, as he pointed out himself, was certainly not the first to describe these structures. . . . "The term Graafian follicle as a synonym for Graafian vesicle appears to have first been used by Bischoff (1842), presumably to avoid confusion with 'germinal vesicle', a term introduced about 1830 for what we now know to be the nucleus of the ovum"[15]. The real and great contribution of de Graaf was to realize the essential importance of these vesicles or eggs to reproduction in the female. (See "Communis itaque . . .", p. 184.) De Graaf assumed correctly that the eggs travel from the ovary to the uterus through the Fallopian tubes and cites several cases of tubal pregnancy as proof of this. The 'egg' to de Graaf included the follicular fluid and an outer membrane – the fluid being analogous to the white of the hen's egg, which analogy is a good one. He actually said: ". . . if they [the ova of women] are boiled, . . . the liquor contained [in them] acquires upon cooking the same colour, the same taste and consistency as the albumen contained in the eggs of birds". "It must have required some courage", R. V. Short remarks, "even in those days, to eat the boiled ovaries of a rotting human cadaver, in order to see what they tasted like."[90] Von Baer referred to what he had discovered, which "we now call the ovum, as the foetal ovum or ovule, and it would have saved a lot of confusion if this latter term had been retained"[15].

Hans H. Simmer, in his outstanding study[16] "Ludwig Fraenkel versus Vilhelm Magnus", mentions Ludwig Fraenkel's last scientific contribution, received in 1951, five days after his death, which has a direct link to de Graaf's observation in 1672 that in the rabbit the number of corpora lutea equalled that of embryos[17]. Similarly, Ludwig Fraenkel (see also p. 510) examined the corpus luteum of *Dasypus hybridus*, an armadillo. He found it to be lobulated and recognized an equal number of corpus luteum segments and of embryos[18].

De Graaf was also perhaps the first in the field to study the pancreas and its function. In his 'Disputatio medica de natura et usu succi pancreatici"[19] (= Medical discourse on the nature and the use of the pancreatic juice) he reported on his experiments of collecting the pancreatic juice of dogs by artificial pancreatic fistulae. He remarked on the small amount secreted, except during his fifth experiment when he managed to collect a large amount within five hours, but – unfortunately – "intermixed with bile", bitter to taste and yellowish in colour, "by reason the Intestine was not first cleansed"[20]. The reaction of the juice in the various experiments – acid or alkaline – was also equivocal (although he thought it more

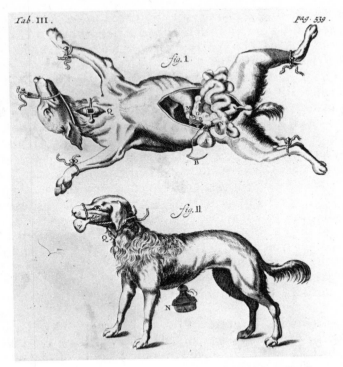

Figure 18   de Graaf's dog with pancreatic fistula

likely to be acid). de Graaf regarded the pancreas a glandula conglomerata (he was a pupil of Sylvius);

> . . . has vero appellamus illas quae ex pluribus glandulis minoribus simul junctis conflantur, quales sunt Pancreas, Salivales et plures alias in Faucibus, Naribus, oculis, imo ipsum Thymum constituunt. . . ."[21]
> In contrast to the 'Glandulae conglobatae', they are not only ". . . substantiae suae connexionis ratione differunt, . . . sed etiam vasis peculiaribus. Conglobatae enim vasis lymphaticis donatae sunt, conglomeratae autem liquorem suum in peculiares cavitates deponuntur. . . .

> . . . those we truly call conglomerate glands, which are made up from several smaller glands joined together, such as the pancreas, the salivary glands and several others in the pharynx, nostrils and eyes; they even constitute the thymus gland. . . . In contrast to the 'Glandulae Conglobatae', they are not only . . . different by reason of the connection of their substance . . . but also because of the peculiarity of their ducts. The conglobate glands empty into the lymphducts (vessels), the conglomerate ones deposit their fluid into specific cavities.

The pancreatic duct was found by J. George Wirsung in 1631. He was the Bavarian prosector of J. Vesling (1598–1649), professor of anatomy at Padua. Wirsung was murdered in 1632 by a Dalmatian colleague and did not publish his observation, which was announced by Vesling in 1641[22]. The pancreatic duct had been described by Wirsung twenty-two years before its successful chronic cannulation by de Graaf. It took de Graaf six attempts before he succeeded, and it is not always realized that animal experiments in those days before anaesthesia were often extremely cruel. This emerges clearly from de Graaf's description of the technique. We do not think it necessary to give all the gruesome details, but would like to mention that the larynx of the dog was first operatively damaged, thus "his troublesome cry to the standers-by being removed" yet "a respiration be procured" ("Disputatio medica de natura et usu succi pancreatici"; see also Fig. 17). Moreover, in order to disprove the theory that the pancreas was the excretory organ of the spleen in analogy of the gall bladder to the liver, he splenectomized a dog and then collected pancreatic juice two months later. The fact that this remarkable experimental achievement did not yield more positive results was due to the state of knowledge of chemistry in his day. It was not until the 19th century that Claude Bernard again took up the quest.

It is sometimes forgotten that the short-lived de Graaf, who crammed so many achievements into barely fifteen working years, also studied the testis and gave a minute account of the structure of its substance and of the course of the seminiferous tubes in his 'Tractatus de virorum organis generationi inservientibus' in 1668, four years before his observations on women[23]. He also, incidentally, practised ligation of the vas deferens.

"Probably the most significant original observation de Graaf made was, that the testis consists largely of tubules (which de Graaf called vascula seminalia) and was not glandular, porridge-like or marrow-like as had been believed until then"[15]. As he says:

> Not everybody will get the opportunity to try this laborious and sordid experiment, and so I shall describe another experiment by which without labour or unpleasantness, the tubules of the testicles can be perceived far better than in the previous experiment. Take the testicles of an edible dormouse and you will see clearly through the tunica albuginea the tubules of the testicles white with semen. If the tunica albuginea is removed and the tubules thrown into a basin of water and shaken about a little, you will behold a delightful and surprising sight; the tubules will separate from one another in such a way that without any help from instruments it can be seen with absolute clarity that the substance of the testicles consists wholly of tubules.
>
> (De Virorum . . . p. 56).

In fact, this discovery was first made by Claude Aubery (Claudius

Aubrius Lotharingus), who published 'Testis Examinatus' (1658) in Florence, under an (anagrammatic) pseudonym 'Vauclius Dathirius Bonglarus'. It was republished in the *Philosophical Transactions of the Royal Society of London* in 1668[24], a little later than a review of de Graaf's treatise, "but it is unlikely that de Graaf was aware of Aubery's work and even contemporaries agreed that de Graaf's description of the tubules went much further than Aubery's"[15] (p. 3). Setchell concludes his paper:

> There is one other thing for which modern science should remember de Graaf. At the end of a letter in Latin dated 28th April 1673 to the Royal Society of London accompanying his reply to Swannerdam (Partium Genitalium Defensio), he says, 'I would like to tell you briefly that a certain most ingenious man named Leeuwenhoek has devised microscopes, which surpass by far those which we have seen until now made by Eustachius Divinus and others . . .' and he appends a letter in Dutch from Van Leeuwenhoek which the Royal Society had translated and published in their Philosophical Transactions. This letter contained Van Leeuwenhoek's first published observations with his microscopes and thus de Graaf should be accorded some credit for bringing this humble draper with the knack of making such good lenses to the attention of the scientific community. De Graaf himself died soon after writing this letter, just after this thirty-second birthday[15] (p. 12).

In these studies de Graaf was preceded by the Frenchman Jean Riolan the Younger (1580–1657)[25], the contemporary and pedantic opponent of William Harvey's circulation (Huxley called him "a tympanitic Philistine, who would have been none the worse for a few sharp incisions"[26]). In 1926 Riolan described the seminiferous tubules. It was also he, incidentally, who introduced the term 'capsulae suprarenales' for the adrenal glands in 1628.

De Graaf was also preceded by the English physician Nathaniel Highmore (1613–1685), who in 1651 described the seminal ducts in his *Corporis humani disquisitio anatomica*[27].

In this chapter we cannot omit the name of William Harvey (1578–1657), best known as the discoverer of the circulation of the blood (see Section II). He was, of course, also one of the leading anatomists and experimental physiologists of his time, a physician to St. Bartholomew's Hospital in London, a clinician with a large and smart private practice, a courtier and friend of King Charles I, a traveller, accompanying major Royal embassies and ambassadors. His other major treatise *Exercitationes de generatione animalium*[28] established him not only as one of the pioneers of embryology and endocrinology, but also as one of the first English writers on obstetrics. Johnston remarks that Harvey, interested as he was in

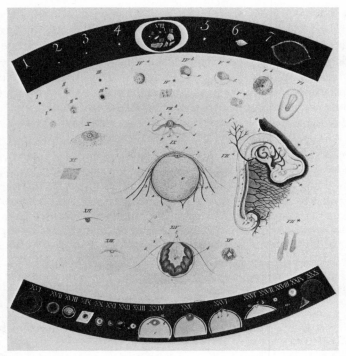

Figure 19   Testicle and epidydimis. Engraving from "Corporis humani disquisition anatomica" by Nathaniel Highmore, The Hague, 1651

obstetrics and in the problems of fertilization, did not seem interested in fertility, and he himself – to his regret – did not have any children[29]. In that treatise, he refuted the doctrine of the preformation of the embryo, but suggested the gradual building up of the organism from the ovum.

> In the dog, rabbit, and several other animals (and in the deer), I have found nothing in the uterus for several days after intercourse. I therefore regard it as demonstrated that after fertile intercourse among viviparous as well as oviparous animals, there are no remains in the uterus either of the semen of the male or female emitted in the act, nothing produced by any mixture of these two fluids, as medical writers maintain, nothing of the menstrual blood present as 'matter' in the way Aristotle will have it; in a word, that there is not necessarily even a trace of the conception to be seen immediately after fruitful union of the sexes. It is not true, consequently, that in a prolific connexion there must be any prepared matter in the uterus which the semen masculinum, acting as a coagulating agent, should congeal, concoct, and fashion, or bring into a positive generative act, or by drying its outer surface, include in membranes. Nothing certainly is to

be seen within the uterus of the doe for a great number of days, namely from the middle of September up to the 12th November . . . (the rutting season being now ended, and the females having separated themselves from the males)[30].

The remarkable feature of Harvey's great work on both the circulation and embryology, is that he had no access to the microscope, although he was a contemporary of the 'microscopists'. As Keynes has pointed out[31] at a meeting of the History Section of the Royal Society of Medicine in 1914, a painting of Harvey with a compound microscope beside him on a table was shown, but this was obviously a recent forgery. Whoever is finally credited with the invention of the microscope (was it Zacharias Janssen of Middelburg, as Pierre Borel (1620–1689) tried to prove in his 'De vero telescopii inventore' (Hagae-Comitum, 1655) ?), one such instrument, $2\frac{1}{2}$ feet long and made of gilded brass was brought to England by Cornelius Drebbel of Alkomaar, mathematician to James I, in 1619. Harvey could, therefore, have known this instrument, "but perhaps he was too unfamiliar with the science of optics to be able to seize upon the advantages he might have had by its use". After all, Nathaniel Highmore published a small book, *The History of Generation*, in the same year as Harvey, in which he repeatedly refers to the use of a microscope in examining the development of the embryo in a hen's egg[31]. Highmore was known to Harvey for many years and Highmore dedicated his book *Corporis humani disquisitio anatomica*[32] to Harvey.

If Harvey made use of the artificial incubation of eggs in his studies, he never mentioned it. This method, which the Egyptians had used for many centuries, was well known to Harvey's friend John Greaves at Merton College, who wrote a description of it, although it was not published until twenty years after Harvey's death. In spite of not being able to demonstrate the capillary connection between arteries and veins, his demonstration of the circulation was amazingly correct and never surpassed. In his 'De generatione', the inability to study the development of the embryo microscopically, he got the account of the fertilization of the ovum wrong (see pp. 66 and 205). In spite of this, Harvey's second great line was of fundamental influence on the further development of the study of embryology. The term 'Ovary' was – in its Latin form 'Ovarium' – coined either by Fabricius ab Aquapendente in 1621, or perhaps by Niels Stensen (1648–1686), as Hyrtl maintained. Stensen (or Steno) of Copenhagen was incidentally the discoverer of the parotid duct, named after him. In 1667, Steno described in his book "Elementorum Myologiae Specimen . . ." the dissection of the

127

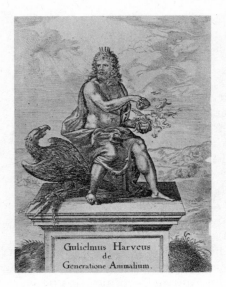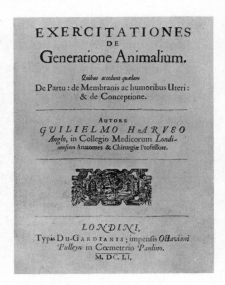

Figure 20 Wm. Harvey "De generatione animalium"

dogfish; there he put forward for the first time the view that the female testes of mammals contained eggs and were analogous to the ovaries of oviparous species:

> Inde vero, cum veridum, viviparorum testes ova in se continere . . . quin mulierum testes ovario analogi sint.[91]

In 1675, Steno described in his book on "Ova Viviparorum . . .", discussing specifically ovaries (called by him female "testicles") the ovaries of two mules. He concluded that a mule might become pregnant and produce offspring on those rare occasions when the ovaries did contain some eggs, the absence of which must be the cause of her well-known infertility, a view which still seems to hold good (see also Chapter 23, p. 678)[92].

In 1668, Ysbrand van Diemerbroeck (1609–1674) maintained in a letter to Werner Rolfink (1599–1673) that it was J. C. van Horne (1621–1670) of Leyden who discovered the ovarian follicles, which he called 'ova'. Be this as it may, the accurate description of the ovarian follicles by de Graaf in 1672 must grant him an honoured position in the subject, although he himself did not claim any priority, but referred to the observation of the celebrated van Horne[33]. The true significance of the ovary was recognized much later (see p. 366). The nature of woman was linked to the womb: "Propter solum uterum mulier est quod est", was a saying of the Dutch physician Johan Baptist van Helmont (1577–1644). He was a Belgian mystic, one time Capuchin friar, and one of the founders of biochemistry. He invented the word 'gas'; he was also the first to observe and describe the lipaemia of diabetes mellitus[34]. It was only in the 19th century that the French physician and medical poet Achille Chéreau (1817–1885) paraphrased Helmont's saying: "Propter ovarium solum mulier est quod est".

The best account of "The Discovery of the Ovaries" has been written by R. V. Short[90], both as regards historical research with critical scientific evaluation and literary merit. Lack of space prevents me from reproducing it in greater detail, but the concluding sentences deserve quotation:

> "This brief account of the history of our knowledge of the ovaries outlines the value of a broad comparative approach to the subject. By our increasing tendency to specialize we have lost the breadth of interest which our predecessors had. Many of their observations were close to what we now believe to be the truth, but they could not be developed in the prevailing scientific climate. A similar problem exists to-day, for with the enormous volume of research findings now being published, a new concept is only 'on top of the pile' for a short time. A concept may remain unrecognised or be swamped by newer material, and it may actually need to be rediscovered at the 'right' time to be influential in scientific thinking.
>
> Although much is known, much still remains to be discovered; and much of what has already been discovered needs to be uncovered."[90]

To sum up, at the end of the seventeenth century, Harvey and some of his followers still believed, as had Aristotle, that the ovaries were of no importance for reproduction. Wharton, Descartes and others thought that the female 'testicles' produced their own 'semen' (the follicular fluid). It had to mix with the male sperm to become an embryo. Stensen, de Graaf, Bartholinus and others represented the 'ovists'. They thought that the whole follicle was an egg and that fertilization occurred in the ovary itself. Leeuwenhoek's discovery of the spermatozoon gave rise to the emergence of an "Animalculist" school. C. Drelincourt's suggestion in 1685 that the real ovum was within the Graafian follicle, remained a cry in the wilderness[90].

The scientific, mathematical and philosophical discoveries could not but exert a strong influence on medicine. As so many scholars embraced a great number of disciplines, from mathematics, botany, chemistry, optics to philosophy, mysticism, anatomy and experimental physiology, this is not surprising. René Descartes (1596–1650) (see Section II), wrote – perhaps inadvertently – the first textbook of physiology: *De homine figuris et latinitate donatus a Florentio Schuyl*[35]. He regarded the human body a material machine, controlled by a rational soul, which was seated in the pineal body.

The treatise covered the whole field of 'animal physiology' and was meant to be an appendix to the celebrated *Discourse on method* (1637). Its first edition was published in French (not in Latin) in 1644, hence "latinitate donatus".

Descartes was also one of the first to consider the brain as an organ integrating the functions of mind and body.

> For the parts of the blood which penetrate even into the brain do not serve merely to nourish and maintain its substance but instead chiefly to produce a certain very subtle breath or rather a very lively and very pure flame which they call the animal spirits . . .[36].

> In proportion as the animal spirits enter the cavities of the brain, they pass hence into the pores of its substance, and from these pores into the nerves . . .[37].

"whence they proceed through the hollow nerves to the rest of the body"; but when the spirits in the ventricles were uncertain about their proper destination, the pineal directed them "by leaning to one side or other of the middle line"[38].

His forerunners in antiquity were Anaxagoras (500–428 BC) and Herophilus of Chalcedon (4th century BC, the observer of the 'female testicle'), who suggested that the soul was situated in the cerebral ventricles[39].

Descartes, incidentally, described a form of compound microscope in 'Dioptrique', a treatise appended to his *Discours de la méthode*[40]. He belonged with Giovanni Borelli (1608–1679) and Sanctorius (Santorio Santorio of Padova, 1561–1636) to the iatro-mathematical school, according to which physiology was governed by the laws of mechanics and physics. Sanctorius used a clinical thermometer and a 'pulsilogium' (pulse-clock) and weighing. He carried out the first classic experiment to prove the 'insensible perspiration of the body' ("Ars de statica medicina", Venetiis, 1614 and "Commentaria in primam seu primi libri canonis Avicennae", Venetiis, 1625). Rolleston[41] wrote that "Modern theosophists believe that in the later perfection of the human race the pineal will accommodate the seventh sense, the power of divine insight; the sixth sense, that of comprehending unvoiced thought or of psychic receptivity, is placed in the pituitary"!

The word 'gland', which had been used somewhat indiscriminately in the past (see the beginning of this chapter), gained a more accurate definition after Thomas Wharton's (1614–1673) studies (see Section II). His *Adenographia: sive glandularum totius corporis descriptio*[42] (there was a London edition in 1656, according to Garrison and Morton[43]) was remarkably compact. Under glands he included the lymphatic glands, the pancreas, the thymus, the salivary glands, the thyroid, pineal and pituitary glands, the capsulae renales, which he called 'glandulae ad plexum', the testicles, vesiculae seminales, the prostate, the ovaries and the mammae. He did not clearly separate the thyroid gland from the submaxillary glands, but gave it its modern name, based on a wrong deduction. He chose θυρεός (thyreos) = an oblong shield, because "it contributes much to the rotundity and the beauty of the neck, filling up the vacant spaces round the larynx [another example of the horror vacui of his times; V.C.M.] and making its protuberant parts almost to subside, and become smooth, particularly in females, to whom for this reason a larger gland has been assigned, which renders their necks more even and beautiful"[42]. He observes that the thyroid is more full of blood than any other gland. Therefore, he suggests three other functions of the thyroid, apart from that quoted above: (1) to take up, like a sponge, superfluous moistures from the recurrent nerve (see also p. 155); (2) to "cherish" the cartilages; (3) to lubricate the larynx and make the voice sweeter. He postulated on the basis of his discovery of Wharton's duct of the submaxillary gland, presented in the same work, that all 'glands' must have a secretory function. Of the pituitary he wrote: The "Glandula pituitaria σφητοειδής vel cunealis, that the use of the gland is, according to Bauhin to drain off the moisture of the brain." This theory goes back to Galen and Vesalius ("Glandula pituitaria cerebri excipiens", 1543, in *De Fabrica* . . .), that the waste material excreted by the brain (a 'glandular' organ) passes through the infundibulum into the pituitary and from there to the nasopharynx[44]. On this theory were based pills and sneezing powders "to purge the brain".

. . . glandulae vero non ta sanguini qua nervi famulantur.

the glands serve not so much the blood as the nerves.

. . . aliae succum nutritium nervis ministrant, aliae secrementa eorum excipiunt, et per lympaeductus in venas reducunt; aliae excrementa eorum foras exportant, adeoque omnes nervorum ministerio incumbunt.

. . . some procure the nutritional juice for the nerves, others take over their secretions and bring them back to the veins viâ the lymphatics; yet others remove their excreta outside: thus all administer to the nervous system.

The suprarenal glands, called by Wharton 'Glandulae ad plexum', "certo possumus statuere, non esse materiam plane excrementitiam, sed utilem, quia in venas perpetuo recipitur" ("we can state with certainty, secrete not only stuff which is excreted, but also useful ones, because continually taken up by the veins"). Like Francis Glisson (1597–1677), Wharton regards the adrenals as 'glandulae redutrices'. In his 'Anatomia hepatis . . .'[45] Glisson discusses the glands and their functions: "De actione et usu Lymphae ductuum sive canalium aquosorum". He attempted a classification of the various types of gland, based on their various functions, as far as they are connected with the needs of the nervous system[46]:

. . . a variis glandium officiis, quatenus ad nervos referuntur. . . . Earum enim aliae excretioni, aliae reductioni, aliae vero nutritioni famulantur: hinc, adeo divido illas in excretrices, reductrices, et nutritias. Prima illarum, est verum excrementum, altera, quaerundum partium respectu, est excrementum, aliarum vero, est liquor desiderabilis, ac propterea reducundus, tertia autem est succus vere nutritius.

The first is solely a product for excretion, the second type (of secretion) is partly for excretion, but partly a desirable fluid and will, therefore, be returned (to the veins). The third type is a true juice of nutrition[47].

To the first type of gland, the 'glandulae excretrices' belong, for example, the testes; to the second group, the 'glandulae reductrices' the suprarenal capsules; to the third group, the 'glandulae nutriciae', belongs – among others – the thymus.

Because (the thymus) is fairly big in comparison with the other glands of the whole body in the embryo and the newly born, who grow most at that period of life and need, therefore, nourishment most; in old age, however, when little nourishment is needed, the thymus is hardly discernible and is recognized only rarely. Moreover, the gland has no excretory duct, nor a cavity in the manner of the larger reducing glands. One has to group it (the thymus), accordingly, into the class of the 'glandulae nutritiae'[48].

(All translations by V.C.M.)

Caspar Bauhin (Bauhinus) (1560–1624), Professor of Anatomy, Botany, Medicine and Greek at Basel, wrote the *Theatrum anatomicum*[49] and *Anatomica corporis virilis et muliebris historia*[50], which contain important historical data.

Wharton referred to the adrenal glands as "glandulae renales" or as "glandulae ad plexum nerveum sitae", he described them with a cavity. He put forward the interesting theory that some humor imbibed from the spleen by the nerves common to both organs was deposited in the adrenal cavity, and "being not purely excrementitious (though perhaps unprofitable to the nerves), is restored to the veins, as being of some use to the venal blood"[51]: shades of 'Blutdruesen' of Johannes Mueller and of Wilhelm Falta several centuries later? Wharton says

Glandulae renales, vel ad nerveum plexum abdominis sitae, earumque usus[52]. Bartholinus de his haec habet. Prima inventio horum corpusculorum Bartholomeo Eustachio debetur, qui earum sub glandularum nomine meminit; et post eum Archangelus et Bauhinus, Casserius renes succenturiatos vocat. Nos ab usum, quam iis tribuimus capsulas atabrilarias . . . vocabimus. Alia quoque nomina his forte coaptari possunt; mihi videtur maximiis quidrare, nimirum, ut dicantur glandulae ad plexum sive glandulae ad plexum nervosum sitae[53].

Renal glands, sited at the nerveplexus of the abdomen, and their function . . . Bartholinus says this about them. The first discovery of these little bodies was due to Bartholomeus Eustachius, who mentioned them under the name of glands; and after him, Archangelus and Bauhin and Casserius called them 'renes succenturiatos'. We call them 'capsules atabilarias', because of the function we allot to them. Other names can also be given to them; to me it seems that certainly, they should be called glands at the plexus or glands sited at the nervous plexus.

These were the names given to the suprarenal glands by various authors:

Casserius: Renes succenturiati; C. Bartholinus: Capsulae atrabilariae; Thos. Wharton: Glandulae ad plexum; Spigelius: Capsulae renales; van Diemerbroeck: Glandulae renales; Morgagni: Glandulae majores ad renes; Winslow: Glandulae suprarenales; Riolan the Younger: Capsulae suprarenales.

The Elder Riolan (1538–1605) thought the suprarenal glands supported a group of nerves above the kidney[54], but Antonio Molinetti refuted this[55].

Caspar Bartholinus (1585–1629) of Copenhagen was the first to believe that there was a humour, which he called 'atrabilia' and which was contained in a cavity of the adrenals and passed by communicating channels to the kidneys and so to the urine[56]. His son, Thomas Bartholinus (1616–1680), described a cavity in the centre of the thymus in 1673 and had noted fluid (see also p. 175) in it. He thought it to be a diverticulum from the lymph[57], which view was supported later (in 1732) by G. I. Pozzi.

The aforementioned Jean Riolan the Younger (1580–1657) (see p. 152) noticed that the adrenals in the foetus were much larger than in post-natal life; hence he concluded that they were active in foetal life only[58]. One of his fellow countrymen, Pierre Dionis (?–1718), who was professor of operative surgery in Paris, said in 1707 that the "capsulae atrabilariae functioned as kidneys during foetal life by means of a duct opening into the emulgent [renal] vein, there being a valve between the cavity of the adrenal and the duct;" at birth they begin to atrophy, because their useful activity has ceased. (See also p. 152.) This theory found followers as late as the mid-19th century! Two people who took it up were Antonio Mollinetti and G. I. Pozzi (1697–1752) (Giuseppe Ippolito Pozzi of Bologna, who became Archiater Extraordinarius to Pope Benedict XIV; see also

Chapter 14, p. 176). Pozzi eulogized Molinetti's thesis of 1732, that the adrenals acted as diverticulae of the blood, diverting most of the arterial blood away from the kidneys and thereby preventing the secretion of the urine in the foetus, since this would be disastrous[59]. This idea was later modified by Théophile de Bordeu (1722–1776), whose important contribution to endocrinology will be discussed in greater detail in the next chapter.

Samuel Collins (see also p. 176) suggested in 1685 that ". . . a further use . . . may be to impart a Fermentative Liquor, flowing out of the Termination of the Nerves, by some secret passages (not yet discovered) into the body of the glands belonging to the kidney, to dispose the Blood in order to the Secretion of the serous and saline parts, from the Vital Liquor . . . and watry particles conveyed into the Roots of the Urinary Ducts . . ."[60].

Wharton also gave a good description of the pineal gland and referred to Riolan, according to whom its function was that of a valve between the third and fourth ventricles.

> De Glandulis Capitis et primo de Pineali (p. 135); . . . est substantiae durioris cerebro, coloris pallidi et membrana tenui obducitur (p. 136).
>
> . . . vasa habet trium generum; arteriam, venam et nervos . . . Sylvius nerveos funiculos appellat (p. 137). Ne esse sedem intellectus . . . (p. 140).
>
> . . . it has three types of vessels; an artery, a vein and nerves . . . Sylvius calls the nerves canals. . . . It cannot be the seat of the intellect.
>
> . . . Assero itaque, quo defaecatior haec pars cerebri servetur, glandulas duas, pinealem et pituitariam, eidem appositas esse . . . (p. 141).

Wharton noticed the similar structure of the pancreas and of the salivary glands (see also p. 175). He thought that the pancreas removed a supposed excrement from the 'plexus of the vagus'.

> De pancreate (p. 64). . . . substantia ejus, si modo membranas et vasa excipias, tota glandulosa est. Ex multis quasi globulis, frustulis vel nodulis communi membrana inclusis, et partim membranarum, partim vasorum connexione junctis, compacta videtur . . ..
>
> On the pancreas . . . its substance, if one excepts the membranes and the vessels, is entirely glandular. It seems to consist of many lobes, crumbs and little nodules, enclosed in a common membrane and partly by vessels, partly by membranes connected, it appears a compact mass . . ..

Before de Bordeu there was no real concept of 'internal secretion', in spite of the view occasionally expressed that some organs may influence or change the composition of the blood[61]. Such an opinion was presented by Franciscus Sylvius (Frans de la Boe), 1614–1672, Professor at Leyden, supporter of Harvey, and physiological chemist; also by Thomas Willis and Frederick Ruysch (1638–1731). However, most researchers continued to look for ducts in the ductless glands, and often claimed to have found them. Three such researchers were: Marco Aurelio Severino (1580–1656), a pioneer of surgical pathology, who published one of the earliest works on comparative anatomy (*Zootomia Democritaea*, Noribergae, 1645) with microscopical studies; he was followed by Ambrosius Rhode (1605–1696) in 1661, and by Antonio Maria Valsalva (1666–1723), a pupil of Malpighi and best known for Valsalva's manoeuvre, in 1719, in reporting an excretory duct in the adrenals. Rhode and Valsalva claimed that this connected the adrenals with the gonads (Valsalva from the adrenals to the epididymis and to the ovary). Valsalva, therefore, assumed that the adrenals must be grouped (see p. 237) with the sex organs or adjuvant to them. It was left to John Ranby (1703–1773), of London, known for his services for setting up a company of surgeons, in 1725, and to Johann Duvernoy (1691–1759), professor of anatomy in Tuebingen, in 1756, to show that the alleged duct of the suprarenal gland was an artery, often found and passing from the renal artery to the gonads. Similarly, a duct of the thyroid was supposed to exist in the opinion of Theophile de Bordeu, among others (see next chapter). In 1659, Walter Charleton (1619–1707) presented the view, generally held in the 17th century, about the glands which had no obvious ducts (in *The Natural History of Nutrition*). He divided glands into (1) those with ducts; and (2) those

> inservient to the secretion of a humor, and the reduction of it into the veins afterward, to which belong the glandulae renales or deputy kidneys (i.e. the adrenals), those adjacent to the oesophagus, the parotides, axillary, inguinal etc. glandules. They all receive from the nervs a certain humor more rough and acrimonious (and approaching the nature of the blood) than is agreeable with the succus nutritius: and therefore the nervs, by the help of these glandules, discharge themselves of it, and retain only the more sweet, mild and profitable juice. . . . The humor, thus rejected by the nervs . . . is not excluded out of the body as an absolute excrement, but is inbibed by the glandules adjacent to the veins, and by them imported into the veins.

> (3) (Inservient to the preparation of the true succus nutritius): the glandules of the mesentery, the thymus[62].

As Rolleston put it: "The second category might, as with some later statements, such as those of Richard Lower and de Bordeu, be thought to show a glimmering of the conception of internal secretions"[63].

William Cowper (1666–1709), in his *Anatomy of Human Bodies*[64] (in which, to a great extent, he plagiarized Bidloo's *Anatomia* of 1685), published at Oxford in 1698, regarded the thymus as a "lymphatic gland" which varies "its magnitude according to the quantity of the lympha that is necessarily transmitted through it from the superior part" (of the body). He thought that the thyroid had "the same office" as the thymus[65] (see also his views on the pineal body, p. 140). Govert Bidloo (1649–1713) was later physician to William of Orange (William III) in England (see p. 176).

Richard Wiseman (1622–1676), surgeon to Charles II, referred in 1676 to Andreas Laurentius (Du Laurens) (1558–1609), physician to Henry IV of France, who had written in his treatise 'De mirabili strumas sanandi', Paris, 1609, that goitre was contagious. Wiseman thought, therefore, that bronchocele was a species of "the King's evil"[66]. The word 'bronchocele' was a concoction of the Greek

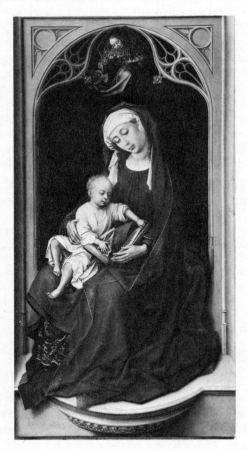

Figure 21   *Virgin* (with goitre) *and Child* – Roger van der Weyden (1399–1464) [Derechos reservados © Museo del Prado – Madrid]

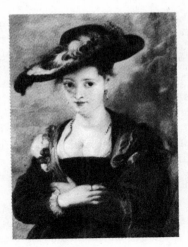

Figure 22 Rubens: *Chapeau de poil* (his sister-in-law Suzanne Fourment with goitre)

'windpipe' with tumour and was a synonym for goitre (see p. 111) when the thyroid enlargement was thought to be due to a herniation containing air from the windpipe. The first reference to 'bronchocele' in English is in 'A Medicinal Dispensatory containing the whole body of Pharmacy . . . Anglicized and revised by R. Tomlinson, Apothecary, London, 1657'.

Shakespeare mentioned goitre in *The Tempest*: Act III, Scene 3:

Gonzalo: (an honest old counsellor of Naples):
          Faith, sir, you need not fear. When we were boys,
          Who would believe that there were mountaineers
          Dew-lappéd like bulls, whose throats had hanging at them
          Wallets of flesh; or that there were such men
          Whose heads stood in their breasts? which now we find
          Each putter-out of five for one will bring us good warrant
          of.

Many pictures of old masters show goitre (Figures 21 and 22).

H. M. Brown quoted Baccius (?–1600) as saying "the people are strumous, but the women more than the men, because of the evil of the water (as they think) that they drink"[67].

Two of the most important figures on the English 17th century canvas were Thomas Willis (1621–1675) and his pupil and friend Richard Lower (1631–1691), of Oxford (see Section II). Willis, who later moved to London, was Sedleian Professor of Natural Philosophy. He was a man of many talents: an acute clinical observer and teacher, interested in chemistry (fermentation), and materia medica.

His main work, however, was in the field of neurology and of the anatomy and the function of the brain, witness of which was the publication of 'Cerebri anatome; cui accessit nervorum descriptio et usus' (London, 1664), in which he had been assisted by Richard Lower. The illustrations were by his friend and pupil, Sir Christopher Wren. Willis was the man of ideas and theories while Lower was more the experimenter.

Galen's idea that the 'pituita' of the pituitary is discharged into the nasal cavities had already been refuted by the careful studies of Conrad Victor Schneider (1614–1680) of Wittenberg, who first published an account of 'Schneider's membrane', the pituitary membrane, in 1655 ('Dissertatio de osse cribriforme, et sensu ac organo odoratus', Wittebergae), followed five years later, in his 'Liber primus de catarrhis' (Wittebergae, 1660), by the proof that only the macerated ethmoid bone displays pores. In the living person, those 'pores' are completely filled with vessels. The pituitary did not contain a cavity or any liquid. He also compared the relative weights of the brain and of the pituitary gland and found this quotient very low in man in comparison with that of certain other animals. Richard Lower, in his 'Dissertatio de origine catarrhi in qua ostenditur illum non provenire a cerebro'[68], confirmed Schneider's views experimentally. As already mentioned (p. 65), G. W. Harris would regard this idea as modern in its endocrine conception.

Willis voiced the same idea when writing: "The blood pours out something – through the spermatic arteries to the genitals, so also it receives as a recompense a certain ferment from these parts – to wit certain particles imbued with a seminal tincture are carried back to the bloody mass, which make it vigorous and inspire into it a new and lively virtue". Willis, in fact, freely and frankly acknowledged his indebtedness to Lower, whom he – in his turn – helped in his private practice in London.

Hans H. Simmer made an interesting contribution: *The Beginnings of Endocrinology*[69]. He felt that Willis and Lower were wrongly credited with the suggestion of pituitary hormones. The key to such claims lies in the translation of one of Willis' sentences from the Latin: "sanguis . . . seri superflui partem aliquam glandulae pituitariae demandet, partemque aliam in furculos venosis, versus cor reducendam instillet"[70]. Harvey Cushing translated the first part of this sentence as "The blood . . . takes some part of the superfluous serum *of* the pituitary gland . . ." S. Pordage (who translated into English in 1681 *The Remaining Medical Works of that Famous and Renowned Physician Dr. Thomas Willis*, London, 1681; Facsimile published in Vol. II of Feindel, ed. Willis), used the word *to* instead of *of*: . . . the blood of the arterial circle 'might carry away some part of the superfluous Serum *to* the pituitary Glandula . . .[71]. This, in Simmer's opinion, is the correct translation as

> Willis spoke indeed of uptake by the gland and not of discharge. . . .
> An experiment convinced Willis of a receptive function of the pituit-ary. When he injected ink into a carotid artery, part of the ink appeared in the pituitary tissue.

"The foregoing analysis", Simmer continues, "removes the temp-tation to read into Lower's or Willis' statements the germ of the conception of an internal secretion".

Willis' concept of Gonadal Ferment was different. His concept of gonadal function was a modification of that of Galen (see p. 67 ff), and was also based on clinical observations. Willis did not need an analogy for the way of propagation; he had the knowledge of blood circulation at his disposal. For the action of the testes, however, he still required an analogy; instead of Galen's analogy of poison, he used that of ferments. In 1659, Willis' two treatises 'De fermenta-tione' and 'De febribus' were published as *Diatribae duae medico-philosophicae*. In the first, he described the influence of the glands. "In the uterus are active principles which are necessary to form the embryo"; also, "as it were with a living ferment, they inspire (inspirant) through all the body, the whole mass of blood." Thereby, femininity is achieved.

> . . . When 'fermentation' from the womb (womb = uterus plus ovaries) is lacking, women became pale, short-winded and unfit for any motion. In man, . . . the ferment (fermentum) of the testes causes 'abundance of heat, great strength, a sounding voice and a manly eruption of Beard and Hair'.

The result of testicular defect is the eunuch, vividly described by Willis. It is of interest that Willis did not discuss hermaphrodites, although Thomas Bartholin had described such patients in 1654, and Jacobus Buerlinus wrote his medical thesis on 'De foeminis ex suppressione mensium barbatis' (Nuernberg, 1664). ". . . in pro-posing the release by the testes of a substance into the blood and assigning a specific action to this material, Willis apparently was the first to forecast internal secretion correctly in all regards"[69].

Ysbrand van Diemerbroeck (1609–1674) of Utrecht, the medical chronicler of the plague, put forward in 1672 the view that the pituitary,

> separated from the arteries of the rete mirabile (which prevented too impetuous an access of blood to the brain [see next chapter, p. 155], similar to the idea of the rôle of the thyroid as an organ of vascular shunt), (produces) a part of the phlegmatic serum and transmits it through the infundibulum to the middle ventricle through the funnel

139

that lives above it, as so ascending to the superior ventricles it may flow through the papillary processes to the nostrils and to the roof of the mouth[72].

This complicated speculation could not stand up to Lower's elegant experimental results. Another speculation was put forward by Thomas Gibson (1647–1722), an M.D. Cambridge and Leyden and a Fellow of the College of Physicians in London. His unusual career was topped by his appointment as physician-general of the army at the age of 71. His only book *Anatomy of Humane Bodies Epitomised* (London, 1682) was really a new edition of Alexander Reid's (*ca.* 1586–1641) *Manuall of the Anatomy or Dissection of the Body* (London 1634). In the preface to the 4th edition (1694), Gibson states that the "ornaments" in it were obtained from the works of thirty-four anatomists! In the summary of his theory on the structure and function of the pituitary, he indicates that it is perhaps concerned with the secretion of the cerebro-spinal fluid, as believed also by Sylvius and Raymond Vieussens (1641–1715) of Montpellier in his 'Nevrographia universalis' (Lugduni, 1684), perhaps the best-illustrated work of the 17th century on the configuration and structure of the brain, spinal cord, and nervous system (see also p. 171).

Willis also dealt with the pineal body in his *Cerebri anatome*[73]. The pineal was known to the Greeks and to Galen as the 'little pine' (ϰῶνος = pine-cone; ϰωνάριον = the pineal body) because of its shape. It also had a Latin name: 'turbo' (whorl) and the 'glandula turbinata'. Willis merely latinised 'konarion' into 'pineal body'. In 1682, Thomas Gibson, in his *Anatomy of Humane Bodies Epitomised* (p. 316), referred to it as "The glandula pinealis", "or penis, because it represents the pine-nut of a man's yard". It has also been called the 'penis cerebri', 'virga cerebri', and – much later – the 'epiphysis cerebri' (in contrast to the 'hypophysis'), and the 'glandula superior'. This was the name given by Bishop Niels Stensen (Nicolaus Steno), 1638–1686, of Copenhagen (and Paris, Padova, Pisa and Florence) in his 'Discours sur l'anatomie du cerveau', Paris 1669), in order to correspond with the 'glandula inferior'; (i.e. the pituitary). We have already mentioned Wharton's and Riolan's ideas as to its alleged function. This differed from Galen's teaching, that it was a secreting gland, or from the later view, that – because of its position – it controlled the flow of cerebrospinal fluid. Willis, in 1664, suggested that it was collecting the cerebro-spinal fluid as it was "to receive and retain within it the serous humors deposited from the arterious blood"[73]. Humphrey Ridley (1653–1708), in his *Anatomy of the Brain* (London, 1695, p. 83), put forward a theory which William Cowper also accepted. He had drawn the illustrations for Ridley's work, that "the glandula pinealis which we take to be a lymphatic gland, receiving lympha from the lymphducts which pass the third ventricle of the brain to the infundibulum and glandula pituitaria"[64]. This view prevailed throughout the next two centuries (Magendie), up to the beginning of the 20th century! Rolleston's quotation of the views of modern theosophists has been mentioned on p. 130.

In contrast to Descartes, Borelli and Sanctorius, Willis belonged to the iatro-chemical school, whose founder was Jean-Baptiste van Helmont (1577–1644) (see p. 128): as some other representatives may be regarded Franciscus de le Boë (Sylvius) (1614–1672), de Graaf and Bishop Stensen (Steno). They all regarded the vital phenomena as chemical in essence[74].

Willis contributed to another discipline of the endocrine field: in his 'Pharmaceutice rationalis sive diatriba de medicamentorum operationibus in humano corpore" (2 vols., Oxford, London 1674–1675) he said that the urine of diabetics tasted sweet. He also differentiated between the polyuria with sweet urine and without it (? diabetes insipidus). Rolleston, however, pointed out that Willis said that this sweet taste occurred in all cases; "he therefore cannot be said to have thus separated diabetes mellitus from other forms of polyuria, though he paved the way for this"[75]. Willis said, ". . . that the urine of diabetics tasted sweet and that this was characteristic of their condition", which he considered to be a disease of the blood.

Quod autem plerique Autores potum aut parum aut nihil immutatum reddi asserunt, a vero longissime distat: quoniam urina in omnibus (quos umquam me novisse contigit, et credo ita in universis habere) tum a potu ingesto, tum a quovis humore in corpore nostro gigni solito plurimum differens, quasi melle aut saccharo imbuta mire dolcescebat. (Pharmaceuticae rationalis, Section IV, caput III, p. 64).

What, however, most authors assert, is far from being the truth, namely, that too little is returned of what is drunk (or nothing unchanged), because the urine in all of those I ever knew (and I believe that this is so in all of them), is much different from the usual, because it is strangely sweet, partly from the drink imbibed, partly from the fluid created anywhere in our body.

Accordingly, Willis concluded that the sweetness of the urine, which is observed in the 'pissing evil' must be preceded by the appearance of sweetness in the blood[76]. Willis seems also to have been the first to use under-nourishment and lime-water in the treatment of sugar-diabetes[76]. He also observed that "sadness and long grief, also convulsion affection" may cause the malady. Before him, the Venetian Vittore Trincavella (1496–1568) mentioned grief and persecution among the causes that may bring on diabetes[77]. Incidentally, furunculosis of the skin and tuberculosis had been noted as complications of diabetes as early as the 5th century AD. Amatus and Zacutus Lusitanus, Portuguese doctors in the early 16th century, believed excess of food, alcohol and sex to be contributory causes of diabetes. Lusitanus regarded diabetes to be an affection of the stomach, a view also expressed a century later by Thomas Sydenham (1624–1689)[78]. One of Molière's (1622–1673) early adaptations and improvisations of Italian comedies was Le mèdecin volant (1650), which already contains the figure of Sganarel (Sganarelle), whom we later meet again in Sganarelle (1660) and in Le mèdecin malgré lui (1666). In it, Sganarelle, the valet, pretending to be a doctor, tastes the urine and notes that it is sweet.

Johann Conrad à Brunner (1653–1727) of Diessenhofen, Switzerland, who discovered Brunner's glands in the duodenum of dogs and man (1672), surgically removed the spleen and pancreas in the dog[79]. He kept the dogs alive and noted extreme thirst and polyuria. Thus he carried out the pioneer experiment concerning the internal secretion of the pancreas and almost discovered the cause of diabetes mellitus. It seems likely, however, that Brunner's dogs survived because he had not removed the whole pancreas[80]. Wharton had already used the microscope in some of his studies of structure, but – obviously – his instruments were not powerful enough to enable such fine distinctions of cellular architecture as was possible for Langerhans, two-hundred years later.

Herman Boerhave (1668–1738) was a vitalist, who (see p. 154) regarded experiments as rather crude and dangerous procedures. Having said that, Boerhave speculated remarkably intelligently on the pancreatic juice. In 1745, he wrote:

> Hence the Uses of the Pancreatic Juice, when mixed and incorporated with the Chyle, the Faeces, the Bile and the Mucus, are to dilate the thick parts of the fluids, to produce a due Mixture of them, to render the Chyle capable of mixing with the Blood, to fit it for its passage through the Lacteals, to correlate the acrimonious parts of the Fluids, to correct the Vicidity and bitterness, . . . and lastly, to go and return, and consequently answer all these ends, with the utmost Expedition[80].

Robert Boyle (1627–1691) was another of the great scientists of the age. He was given the title D.M. at Oxford in 1665, although he was never a practising physician. He did, however, prove that air was necessary for life as well as for combustion. His most important medical work was 'Memoirs for the natural history of humane blood, especially the spirit of that liquor' (London, 1683). He defined chemical 'elements' and discovered Boyle's Law. He was a friend of Sydenham's. He also left behind 'Medical experiments or a collection of choice and safe Remedies', which – on 9 November, 1691 – were officially approved by Robert Southwell (1635–1702), the ninth President of the Royal Society[81]. It contained many remedies for urinary calculi, from which Boyle himself suffered. A later addition, not from Boyle's hand, contained a number of doubtful animal preparations, such as powdered crabs' eyes and other organic remedies. Organotherapy of the worst sort was rife in the 17th century; snails' shells, frogs' spawn and all the contents of the witches' cauldron in Shakespeare's Macbeth:

Eye of newt and toe of frog – Wool of bat and tongue of dog – Adder's fork and blind-worm's sting – Lizard's leg and howlet's wing – For a charm of powerful trouble – Like a hell-broth boil and bubble.

The official London Pharmacopoeias of the London College of Physicians did not always appear to be very much different! (see p. 100). One of the standard textbooks, published in Madrid in 1613, was devoted entirely to the use of animals in pharmacy. It was Velez de Arciniega's 'Historia de los animales mas recebidos en el uso de Medicina: donde se trata para lo que cada uno entero, o parte del aprouecha, y de la manera de su preparacion'[82]. One of the best-known European pharmacopoeias was in 1697, the 'Dictionnaire Universelle des Drogues Simples' by Nicolas Lémery (1645–1715), who discovered iron in the blood. This contained a summary of the parts of the human body which are put to medicinal use. Human fat was one of the most important ones, used especially for embrocations against rheumatism. The public executioner in Paris had a nice little sideline and income from selling it. 'Goddard's drops', which Charles II bought from Dr. Goddard for a large amount of money, contained dried human bones distilled. Goddard's drops were used for preparing the famous sal volatile oleosum.

We have already mentioned the contribution of Thomas Willis, the 'Pharmaceutice rationalis'. The London Dispensatory of 1694, "with medicines both Galenical and Chymical" gives an attempt at (?glandular) therapy as follows: 'Oyl of Foxes', in Latin, 'Oleum Vulpinum'. A complicated decoctum of it is good "for payns of the joynts, sciatica and aches and for convulsions and palsies". The standard French dictionary of drugs of the eighteenth century contains the following advice: "Fresh urine, two or three glasses drunk in the morning, fasting, is good against gout, hysterical vapours and obstructions"[83]. (See also p. 55, Catullus, and pp. 88–89, urinary therapy in China.)

What about contraception? The knowledge of contraceptive techniques did not seem to have made great advances in the 17th century. It is here, perhaps, that the beginning of the use of the sheath or condom should be mentioned. It is known that many primitive people and the early Egyptians used various forms of penis protectors, though mainly as protection against tropical and other diseases[84]. Whether the sheath (in form of the bladder of a goat) was known and used in antiquity, as Antoninus Liberalis claims in his *Metamorphoses* (No. 41, 'The Fox'), is difficult to decide. Fallopio (1523–1562) was one of the early writers on 'De Morbo Gallico', i.e. syphilis, in 1563. He advocated a linen sheath, cut to shape for the glans, as protection against syphilis[84]. In the 17th century, it was mentioned in the letters of Mme. de Sévigné (1626–1696) in 1671, to her daughter, the Countess of Grignan. She mentions a sheath made of gold-beaters skin as "armour against enjoyment, and a spider web against danger".

Whether a slaughterhouse worker hit by chance upon the idea of using one of the thin animal membranes as protection against syphilis, is open to conjecture. Whether the term 'condom' stems from a Dr. Condom or Conton, a physician at the court of Charles II, is also not definitely proved. Others thought that the 'inventor' was not a physician, but a courtier of the King, but the existence of either person has not been established. It seems certain, however, that the sheath – of whatever material – was first used as protection against venereal disease, long before its use as a contraceptive. It also appears certain that the two outstanding diarists of the epoch, Samuel Pepys and John Evelyn, never mention a Dr. Condom or Conton, nor the contraception being used. It was Joseph Hyrtl, the 19th century anatomist of Vienna, who suggested it should be called Gondom, after a courtier of Charles II (*Handbuch der Topographischen Anatomie*, Wien, 1847).

Daniel Turner (1667–1742), the founder of British dermatology, uses the word 'Condun' in a treatise on syphilis in 1717, but, in fact, all the various theories as to the origin of the name have remained conjectural. Himes remarks[85] with interest, if not with 'Schadenfreude' (he is American),

> how each of two nations refuse to accept the 'honor' of association with it. The French call the condom "la capote anglaise", or the English cape; the English have returned the compliment: to them it is the "French letter".

Nathaniel Highmore of the antrum Highmori fame, also gave a good account of the seminal ducts and the epididymis in 1651[86]. We have already mentioned Highmore's book on *The History of Generation* (p. 127) published in the same year as Harvey's, but with the addition of microscopical studies. The tunica albuginea below the tunica vaginalis extends at the posterior border for about 8 mm as a triangular area of condensed fibrous tissue, the 'corpus Highmorianum'.

Regnier de Graaf had also given a description of the testicle in 1668 (as mentioned on p. 124), which he described as made up of small tubes forming lobules.

Pregnancy and childbirth are certainly conditions greatly controlled by hormones. Both conditions were, however, often handled by midwives rather than physicians. The earliest printed textbook for midwives dates really back to the 16th century. There was in about 1500 an early German popular little handbook for lying-in women by Ortollf of Bavaria, the *Frauenbuechlein*[87], which was followed in 1513 by the important *Der swangeren frawen und hebammen roszgarten* by Eucharius Roeslin, which was the earliest printed textbook for midwives (and pregnant women), published in Worms. There was an early English translation (*The byrth of mankynde*, London, 1540) and translations into Latin. It went some 40 editions, and there are several copies in the Library of the Royal College of Obstetricians and Gynaecologists in London. It was based mainly on Soranus' of Ephesos teaching as transmitted by Moschion (Muscio), who worked *ca.* 500 AD, and whose treatise was arranged in catechism form. It was re-edited by Caspar Wolff (in *Gynaeciorum*, Basel, 1566) and F. O. Dewez in Vienna in 1793, and contained drawings of the female genitalia and of the foetus *in utero*. An improved version of Roeslin was published by Jacob Rueff (1500–1558), *De conceptu et generatione hominis* (Tiguri, 1554) translated into German by Froschauer in the same year under the title *Trostbuechle* (little book of comfort).

Ambroise Paré had written in 1549 on the handling of problems of actual childbirth. There was also the very interesting book by Louise Bourgeois (1563–1636), who was accoucheuse to the French Court and a pioneer of scientific midwifery. She attended Maria de Medici through her six labours. Her 'Observations diverses sur la stérilité, perte de fruict, foecondité, accouchements, et maladies des femmes, et enfants nouveaux naiz' (Paris, 1609), cover a much larger field than the usual textbooks of midwifery. Similarly comprehensive was Francois Mauriceau's (1637–1709) of Paris book: 'Traité des maladies des femmes grosses et accouchées' (Paris, 1668) covering diseases of pregnancy and puerperium, with reference to tubal pregnancy. He had also met Hugh Chamberlen (see p. 98) of the family which kept the invention of the forceps a secret for 200 years. Mauriceau referred a rachitic dwarf woman for delivery, but Chamberlen did not succeed on that occasion[88]. Mauriceau's book was illustrated with exquisite copper plates. It must not be forgotten that

William Harvey's work *Exercitationes de generatione animalium* (London, 1651) contained an important chapter on labour (De partu), which is the first original work on obstetrics by an English author. Harvey was, in fact, a highly skilled obstetrician, or – perhaps more correctly – in that chapter acting as an adviser on obstetrics[89]. There were, of course, a number of important books on operative gynaecology and obstetrics, which appear beyond the scope of the present subject under discussion.

REFERENCES

1. Garrison, F. H.: An Introduction to the History of Medicine. 4th ed., pp. 251–252. Philadelphia, W. B. Saunders, 1929.
2. Singer, Chas.: A Short History of Medicine. pp. 105, 115–122. Oxford, Clarendon Press, 1928.
3. As 1: p. 253.
4. As 1: p. 254.
5. Castellani, Carlo: Spermatozoan biology from Leeuwenhoek to Spallanzani. J. Hist. Biol. **6**, 37–68, 1973.
6. van Leeuwenhoek, Anthonj: Collected Letters. Vol. II. Letter No. 35 to the Royal Society of London in November 1677. Amsterdam, 1941; published as 'Observations de natis e semine genitali animalculis'. Philos. Trans. R. Soc. **12,** 1040, 1679.
7. Ibid.: Collected Letters, Vol. II, p. 285.
8. Ibid.: p. 287.
9. As 5: p. 41.
10. As 5: p. 42.
11. As 6: Collected Letters, Vol. V. A'dam, pp. 143–145, 1957.
12. As 11: p. 195.
13. de Graaf, R.: De Mulierum Organis Generationi Inservientibus. Chap. XII, p. 302. Lugduni Batavorum, 1668.
14. Fulton, John F.: Selected Readings in the History of Physiology. Completed by Wilson, L.G. 2nd ed., p. 387. Springfield, Thomas, 1966.
15. Setchell, B. P.: The contributions of Regnier de Graaf to reproductive biology. Eur. J. Obstet. Gynecol. **4,** 1–13, 1974.
16. Simmer, Hans H.: The First Experiments to Demonstrate an Endocrine Function of the Corpus Luteum, Part II: Ludwig Fraenkel versus Vilhelm Magnus (Sudhoffs Archiv. **56,** Heft 1, 76–99, 1972).
17. de Graaf, R.: De Mulierum Generationi Inservientibus Tractatus Novus, p. 178. Leyden, Hackiana, 1672.
18. Fraenkel, L.: Arch. Gynaek. **181,** 217, 1952.
19. de Graaf, R.: Disputatio Medica de Natura et Usu Succi Pancreatici. pp. 545, 551, 553, 565. Lugdunum Batavorum 1664 and Fulton, J. F. (as 14) p. 167.
20. As 14: p. 168.
21. As 19: p. 541.
22. Rolleston, Sir Humphrey: The Endocrine Organs in Health and Disease. p. 419. London, Oxford University Press, 1936.
23. de Graaf, R.: Tractatus de Virorum Organis Generationi Inservientibus, de Clysteribus et de Usu Siphonis in Anatomia. Lugduni Batavorum, 1672.

24. Aubery, C.: Testis examinations. Philos. Trans. R. Soc., Lond. **3**, 834–844, 1668.
25. Abderhalden, R.: The Antecedents of Endocrinology. CIBA Monographs, No. 10, p. 306. Bombay, 1951.
26. As 1: p. 248, footnote 1.
27. Highmore, Nathaniel: Corporis Humani Disquisitio Anatomica. The Hague, 1651.
28. Harvey, William. Exercitationes de Generatione Animalium. London, 1651 (English translation, 1653).
29. Johnston, R. D.: The history of human infertility. Fertil. Steril. **14**, 266, 1963.
30. As 14: pp. 384–386 (in: X Sexual Generation. Wm. Harvey).
31. Keynes, Sir Geoffrey: The Life of William Harvey. p. 341. Oxford, Clarendon Press, 1966.
32. Highmore, Nathaniel: Corporis Humani Disquisito Anatomica. The Hague, 1651.
33. As 22: p. 339.
34. As 1: p. 261.
35. Descartes, René: De Homine Figuris et Latinitate Donatus a Florentio Schyl. Lugduni Batavorum, 1662.
36. Descartes, René: Des Passions de l'Ame. Amsterdam, 1649.
37. As 14: p. 264.
38. As 22: p. 452.
39. As 22: p. 454.
40. As 31: p. 340.
41. As 22: p. 454.
42. Wharton, Thomas: Adenographia sive glandularum totius corporis descriptio. p. 139. Coll. Lond. Socii. Amstelaedami, 1659.
43. Garrison, F. H. and Moreton: A Medical Bibliography, 3rd ed., No. 1116, p. 141. London, Andre Deutsch, 1976.
44. As 42: p 169.
45. Glisson, F.: Anatomia hepatis . . . subjiciuntur nonnulla de lymphae – ductibus nuper repertis, Chap. 45, p. 401. Londini, typ. Du-Guardianis, 1654.
46. Ibid.: p. 438.
47. Ibid.: p. 439.
48. Ibid.: p. 443.
49. Bauhin, C.: Theatrum Anatomicum. Basle 1590.
50. Bauhin, C.: Anatomica corporis virilis et muliebris historia. Leyden, 1597.
51. Shumacker, H. B.: The Early History of the Adrenal Glands. Bull. Inst. Hist. Med. **4**, 39–56, 1936.
52. As 42: Chap. XIII, p. 77.
53. As 42: Chap. XIII, p. 78.
54. Riolan, Jean the Elder: Opera cum physica tum medica . . . Francofurti, 1611.
55. Molinetti, A.: Dissertationes anatomico-pathologicae. Bk. 6, Chap. 7, pp. 302–303. Venetiis, 1675.
56. Bartholinus, C.: Anatomicae Institutiones Corporis Humani. Wittenberg, 1611.
57. As 22: p. 435.
58. As 22: p. 317.
59. As 22: p. 317 (also Pozzi, G. I.; Orationes Duae, Bononiae, 1732).
60. As 51: pp. 42–43.
61. As 25: p. 316.
62. As 22: pp. 15–16.
63. As 22: p. 16.

64. Cowper, William: Cowper's Table X, in his The Anatomy of Human Bodies, Oxford, 1698.
65. As 22: p. 142.
66. Iason, A. H.: The Thyroid Gland in Medical History. p. 52. New York, Froben Press, 1946.
67. Brown, H. M.: Wisconsin Med. J. xiv, 240, 1917.
68. Lower, R.:Tractatus de Corde, pp. 221–239. London, 1670.
69. Simmer, H. H.: The Beginnings of Endocrinology, in Medicine in Seventeenth Century England. Symposium held at UCLA in honour of C. D. O'Malley, 30 March–1 April 1971, Chap. 9, pp. 215–236. University of California Press, Berkeley, CA, 1974.
70. Willis, T.: Cerebri Anatome, p. 56. Amsterdam, 1664.
71. Pordage, S.: translation of 70, p. 86.
72. Diemerbroeck, Isbrand van: Anatome Corporis Humani, Geneva, 1672.
73. As 70: p. 169.
74. As 1: p. 257.
75. As 22: p. 430.
76. Papaspyros, N. S.: The History of Diabetes Mellitus. p. 11. London, 1952.
77. Ibid.: p. 12.
78. Ibid.: p. 13.
79. Brunner, Johann Conrad à: Experiments Nova Circa Pancreas, Amsterdam (Amstelaedami), 1682.
80. Henderson, J. C.: Personal communication.
81. As 22: p. 11.
82. As 66: p. 53.
83. As 66: p. 55.
84. Himes, N. E.: Medical History of Contraception. Reprinted 1963. pp. 188–190. New York, Gamut Press, 1936.
85. Ibid.: p. 194.
86. As 27: p. 90.
87. As 1: p. 198.
88. As 1: p. 277, footnote 2.
89. As 31: p. 358.
90. Short, R. V.: The Discovery of the Ovaries. In: "The Ovary". 2nd edn, Vol. 1. New York, San Francisco, London, Academic Press, 1977.
91. Stensen, N.: Elementorum Myologiae Specimen. Seu Musculi Descriptio Geometrica. Cui Accedunt Canis Carchariae Dissectum Caput, et Dissectus Piscis ex Canum Genere. Florence, 1667.
92. Stensen, N: Ova Viviparorum spectantes observationes. In: Thomae Bartholini, Acta Medica et Philosophica Hafniensa. Vol. II, pp. 219–232, Hafniae, 1675.

CHAPTER FOURTEEN

THE 18th CENTURY AND THE BEGINNING OF THE 19th CENTURY

THERE were many people during the 18th century who had a great impact on the development of endocrinology. Let us start with two of the most important ones: Théophile de Bordeu (1722–1776) and Albrecht von Haller (1708–1777) (see Section II).

THÉOPHILE DE BORDEU

De Bordeu wrote in the 'Analyse mèdicinale du sang', which formed the sixth part of his verbose[1] *Recherches sur les maladies chroniques*, published in 1775, that each organ of the body gives off 'emanations', which are necessary and useful to the whole body. This concept of emanations from all organs of the body is, therefore, much wider than that formed 70 years ago, when the idea was restricted mainly to the endocrine glands. de Bordeu's concept approached the present day view, that we have kidney hormones, gut hormones, hypothalamic hormones, and that neuro-secretion and negative feedback have become an essential part of studies in the endocrine field. More recently, molecular biology and immunology have also taken their share in such studies. de Bordeu had expressed, however, his concern with this theme much earlier. What he said in the above treatise was:

> What I believe with certainty is, that every organ occupying its own nook . . . and living its own life . . . diffuses about itself, into its environment and its particular system, exhalations, or certain emanations, which have taken on its characteristics, are integral parts of itself. I do not regard these emanations as useless, or of purely physical

149

necessity. I believe them useful and necessary to the existence of the organism as a whole. I conclude that the blood bears within itself extracts of all organic parts, each of which components, I repeat again, are necessary to the well-being of the whole, possessing specific qualities and properties beyond the reach of the chemist's experiments . . . each (of the organs) serves also as a factory and laboratory for a specific humor, which it returns to the blood after having prepared it within itself and imparted to it its own specific character.

(J'en conclus que le sang roule toujours dans son sein des extraits des toutes les parties organiques . . .).

I postulate as many specific cachexias, as many principal mixtures of the humours as there are distinct organs and different humors. The mucus tissue in particular seems to me the seat of most of these cachectic revolutions. . . . Moreover, there is no gland which does not draw from the cellular tissue around it a large amount of serosities . . . these serosities commingle with the specific humour formed and secreted within the gland. . . . Now these serosities, not being always supplied as they are needed, come to a congestion, a cachexia which flows back into the humours and inundates the whole region. . . . It remains for physicians to follow up and to classify the various reflexes consequent upon the defective functioning of each particular organ[2].

de Bordeu placed great importance on the tonic effect of testicular and ovarian secretions: "The semen imparts, as is well known, masculine tone to all parts . . . considered"[2].

Twenty-three years before, in 1752, de Bordeu's book *Recherches Anatomiques sur la Position de Glandes et sur leur Action* was published[3]. In it, he attacked Herman Boerhave's (1668–1738) mechanistic chemical doctrines and thus became one of the founders of the vitalistic school of Montpellier, together with Paul-Joseph Barthez (1734–1806), his successor at Montpellier. Although a zealous adherent of Hippocrates, Bordeu had this to say in the treatise on the glands, concerning the pituitary[3]:

On l'a toujours traité de corps glanduleux, & Galien lui faisoit l'honneur de l'appeller Glande simplement, comme par excellence, cependant il n'en a ni la forme, ni même les usages, si ce que les anciens & les modernes en ont dit se trouve vrai. Les Anciens croioient qu'il étoit fait, en premier lieu, pour retenir les esprits animaux; il sert, disoient-ils, de 'bouchon' à l'entonnoir, & sans lui tous les esprits, contenus dans les ventricules, se dissiperoient bien aisement. 2°. Il pompoit les humidités superflues du cerveau; elles alloient toutes aboutir à l'entonnoir, & la Glande pituitaire les recevoit, & les dégorgoit dans la cavité des narines; . . . Les Récens . . . ont cru que cette Glande étoit réellement faite pour repomper quelques liqueurs superflues. . . . Il n'ya rien de démontré sur cette question; il n'est pas aisé de sçavoir si la Glande pituitaire n'a pas quelque conduit excrétoire;

on trouve souvent à la portion moienne de sa selle sphenoidale, un trou plus ou moins apparent; scavoir si ce trou n'est pas fait pour donner passage à quelque conduit particulier, ou à un vaisseau sanguin, qui établiroit entre la Glande pituitaire et la cavité des narines, un commerce de sang don't l'usage est inconnu?

One has always dealt with the glandular body, and Galen honoured it by simply calling it 'the Gland' above all; nevertheless neither the form nor its function have proved correct, in the manner both, the Ancients and the Moderns said of it. The Ancients believed that it existed for the retention of the animal spirits; it served, they said, as a plug to the funnel, and without it, all the spirits contained in the ventricles would easily disperse. 2. It sucks up the superfluous moisture(s) from the brain; they all go to end in the funnel, and the pituitary gland receives them and discharges them into the cavity of the nostrils. . . . The moderns believe that this gland really exists to re-absorb some superfluous humours. . . . There is nothing proved concerning this question; it is not easy to find out whether the pituitary gland has an excretory duct or not; one often finds in the middle part of the sella (of the sphenoid) a hole, which is fairly conspicuous; whether this hole exists to be a passage for a special duct or for a bloodvessel, which connects the pituitary gland with the nostrils, for the purpose of an unknown function of the blood, is not known.

He was also thought to have detected very fine canals leading from the thyroid gland into the trachea, at least in the body of a man who had died a violent death, thus making the thyroid a true gland with excretory ducts. Through these fine ducts the thyroid secretion drizzled into the larynx "like tender dew" (. . . les liqueurs destinées à humecter la Trachée, doivent tomber, non point à grosses goutes . . . mais former comme une pluie ou une rosée douce et imperceptible . . .)[4]. Another of his observations on the thyroid was happier[5]:

Aiant été à même d'observer le long de la partie occidentale de Pyrenées des Goiietres qu'on y trouve communement dans quelques cantons, et qui sont presque tous formés par le gonflement de la Thiroide, nous avons vu bien des cas particuliers, parmi lesquels nous en choisirons deux, qui ont quelque rapport avec les questions qu'on examine dans ce traité. . . . 1°. Les femmes sont plus sujettes que les hommes à avoir des Goiietres; elles ont même naturellement la Glande Thiroide plus grosse à proportion; la plupart de celles qui ont des Goiietres, ont la voix fort rauque; bien des gens disent qu'ils ne sont pas étonněs de ce Phénomène . . .

Having been able to observe along the Western part of the Pyrenées goitres which one finds there generally in some cantons, and which are nearly all formed by the swelling of the thyroid, we have truly seen special cases from whom we selected two, who have some relevance to the questions examined in this treatise. – 1. Women are more liable to have goitres than men; they have somewhat larger thyroid glands; the majority of those who have goitres have a very hoarse voice; truly, people say that they are not surprised at this phenomenon. . . .

151

De Bordeu also notes that the adrenals are especially large in the foetus, compared with their small size in adults[6] (see also p. 133 in Chapter 13). They may have two uses in the foetus: (1) to separate from the blood a humour as in adults; (2) to take the place of the kidneys or to prevent the excretion of urine – not only by receiving a certain amount of the blood, which should otherwise go to the kidneys, but by removing bodies which might damage the foetus: "On pourroit avancer encore, . . . que les humeurs du fétus ne deviennent urineuses, ou excrémentitielles et nuisibles".

Further considerations as to how the secretions of the various glands occur led de Bordeu to assume that the two essential predispositions were the presence of the blood in the blood-vessels and the action of the nerves surrounding them. The difference of the secretions is due to the specific taste of the gland and its orifice which will reject any secretions alien to it. There is also present – in various degrees – a tension of glands in some cases, leading to an erection, spasms, rubbing movements and convulsive ejection, most marked in the case of the male (and female) seminal ejection and of milk secretion. Not knowing anything about ovarian function, de Bordeu mistook female orgasm for evidence of secretion of the female sperm, akin to that of the male. The idea of the specific "taste" of the gland, giving rise to the specific secretion, is not too far from the idea of the production of specific hormones:

> . . . les parties propres à exciter telle sensation passeront et les autres sont rejettées; chaque Glande, chaque orifice aura, pour ainsi dire, son gout particulier; tout ce qu'il aura d'étranger sera rejetté pour l'ordinaire. . . . Ne pourroit on pas dire qu'une humeur retenue dans le sang le gâte, et dérange par tous les organes?

> . . . The specific parts to excite such a sensation will be passed on and the others are rejected; each gland, each orifice will have, as it were, its own style; everything which is foreign, will be rejected as a rule. Can one not say that one humour (moisture) retained in the blood will cause damage and unsettle all organs?

and, finally,

> Nous avons supposé jusqu'ici que les humeurs étoient contenues *formellement* dans le sang; cette opinion semble plus vraisemblable que celle des Auteurs qui assurent le contraire; . . .[7]

> We have so far assumed that the humours are strictly contained in the blood; this opinion appears more likely correct than that of (other) authors who assert the contrary. . . .

He discusses the difference between excretion and secretion in terms which also sound modern:

> Ces deux fonctions sont bien differentes dans les Glandes passives qui

ont des réservoirs, la secrétion se fait peu à peu dans ces organes, et l'excrétion a ensuite son temps; au lieu que les Glandes actives rejettent autant d'humeur qu'elles en reçoivent; elles ne sçauroient en conserver une certaine quantité; cette réflexion ne laisse pas que d'avoir ses usages, ne fût-ce que pour distinguer les Glandes, les unes des autres. (p. 421.) "On peut faire l'application de cette remarque à tous les autres organes: chacun d'eux domine dans les tempĕramens qu'il régit. Ce régime est sans doute dû à la sensibilité organique, radicale et nerveuse; mais cette vie elle-même est entretenue et conservée par l'humeur propre et innée qui entre dans la constitution de chaque organe. Chacun d'eux a un département marqué sur les solides, sur les vaissaux, le tissu cellulaire et les nerfs: chacun aussi sert de foyer et de laboratoire à une humeur particulière qu'il renvoie dans le sang après l'avoir préparée et fécondée dans son sein, après lui avoir donné son caractère radicale . . . d'ailleurs il n'est point de glandes qui ne retire du tissue cellulaire qui l'environne, une grande quantité de sérosités, en les pompant . . . Ces sérosités se mêlent à l'humeur spécialement formée et séparée dans la glande[2].

These two functions are quite different in the passive glands, which are reservoirs, the secretion occurring gradually in these organs, and the excretion after that time; in contrast, the active glands return (throw back) as much of the fluid as they have received; they are not able to conserve a certain quantity (of it); such a reflexion has, nevertheless, its uses (usefulness), if (no other) but to distinguish between the glands. . . . One can apply this remark to all the other organs: each of them holds sway within the constitution it governs. This régime is, without doubt, due to the organic sensitiveness, both radical and nervous; but the life itself is maintained and conserved by the proper inborn tissue fluid which enters into the constitution of every organ. Each of these has a subdivision mapped out upon the solid parts of the body, on the vessels, the cellular tissue and on the nerves; each one also serves as a centre and a laboratory for a specific liquid which returns into the blood, after having prepared and fertilized it (in its bosom), and after having passed on to it his main (root) characteristic . . . moreover, there is no part of the glands which do not return to the surrounding tissue a great quantity of serous fluid, while they move it on (pump it) . . . these serous fluids mix with the humour specially formed and separated (secreted) in the gland.

Max Neuburger (1868–1955), the medical historian of Vienna, who had rediscovered de Bordeu, said in an address to the 74th Meeting of 'Deutscher Naturforscher und Aerzte' in Karlsbad in 1902, that he (de Bordeu) was "der wahre Urheber oder mindestens Vorlaeufer der Lehre von der inneren Sekretion". (The originator or – at least – forerunner of the theory of internal secretion)[8]. This view was also supported by Arthur Biedl in his *Lehrbuch der Inneren Sekretion*[9], but opposed by Eugène Gley (1857–1930) in his textbook of internal secretion, because – according to his interpretation – de Bordeu did not make his statements so definite as Neuburger and Biedl had maintained. Be this as it may, de Bordeu came nearest to the modern theory of internal secretion and certainly influenced later workers in the 19th century, although his contemporaries did not seem to have paid much attention to him. In 1818 Richerand wrote[10]:

> Les physiologistes modernes n'ont rien ajouté de satisfaisant à ce que renferment sur le mécanisme des sécrétions les Recherches anatomiques sur les glandes, que l'on doit regarder comme un des plus beaux monuments élevés à la science de l'homme.

> The modern physiologists have added nothing satisfactory concerning the mechanism of secretions and the anatomic researches on the glands, which one should regard as one of the most beautiful monuments erected towards the science of man.

Why was de Bordeu not more accepted by his contemporaries, one may wonder? Mainly, it seems, because as one of the leading 'vitalists', he did not perform many experiments but believed that he could build up an argument starting from fundamental truths. Alas, he did not have, like Thomas Willis, a Richard Lower to test and support or refute his ideas. To vitalists, experiments were rather crude and dangerous procedures;[11] dangerous, because they so easily upset what was known to be true on *a priori* grounds.

ALBRECHT VON HALLER

The other giant of the medical stage of the 18th century was Albrecht von Haller (1708–1777) of Bern, the greatest physiologist of his generation and as such the forerunner of Claude Bernard and Johannes Müller. Haller is the eminent representative of the 'systematists'. Some other members of the group were Bernardino Ramazzini (1633–1714), the founder of occupational medicine, Peter Süssmilch (1707–1777), the pioneer of medical statistics, and Johann Peter Frank (1745–1821), who not only became one of the founders of preventive medicine and public hygiene, but also defined diabetes insipidus (see p. 174).

The thyroid

Before de Bordeu there had been several authors like Frederick Ruysch (1638–1731), the Leyden anatomist, who – according to von Haller – adopted the "only remaining possible opinion concerning the thyroid, that a peculiar fluid was elaborated in that gland and poured into the veins"[12]. In 1776, von Haller grouped together the thyroid, the thymus and the spleen as ductless glands, pouring their special fluid into the general circulation. The German surgeon

Lorenz Heister (1683–1758), whom de Bordeu had attacked, believed (in 1747), like Haller, that "The thyroide glandule . . . is full of serous, yellowish and somewhat viscid humour, but whether it emits the same into the windpipe or gula, is not yet determined (Heister thought it did). "At least there are no ducts certainly known to open into either of them . . . yet that the use of this gland is very considerable, may appear from the largeness of the arteries which it receives from the carotids (1754)"[13]. This was underlined later by Christopher Wm. Hufeland (1762–1836), court physician at Weimar, who wrote in 1797 in his book *Die Kunst das menschliche Leben zu verlaengern* (Jena, 1797): "The organs of generation have the power of secreting the finest and most spiritual parts of our nourishment; but at the same time they are so organised that these perfected and ennobled juices can again return and be received into the blood". Others, who were equally impressed by the lavish blood supply of the thyroid gland, thought that it was an organ of a vascular shunt, which should prevent a sudden onrush of blood into the brain, an idea which was still occasionally supported in the 19th century[14]. (See also Chapter 13, pp. 131 and 139.) So was the opinion that the thyroid was part of the vocal apparatus:

> The act of uttering a tone or speaking, stops the return of blood from that organ (the thyroid), distends it and renders it tense and from the nature of its attachment round the top of the trachea and in the free side of the alae of the larynx, renders them fixed and tense also. . . . The importance of the thyroid body must be admitted when it is shown to be necessary for the perfection of the voice and hence of speech. (Martyn, 1857)[14].

Haller's description of 1776 no doubt influenced Johannes Müeller in 1830, and even 20th century authors like Wilhelm Falta, to adopt the name of 'vascular' or 'blood'-glands for the ductless glands. Haller also made a contribution to knowledge of the function of the ovary. He showed that the corpus luteum was formed from a thickening of the wall of the Graafian follicle after it had ruptured[15], but he turned down Boerhave's (his teacher's) idea that the ovum must escape from the ovary, leaving a scar (corpus luteum) behind (Praelectiones Academicae . . ., Vol. V, 1744).

Precocious puberty

Haller mentioned eighteen patients with precocious puberty. He himself had described the case of Anna Mummenthaler, born at Trachselwald, Canton Berne, in 1715. Her menstruation had started

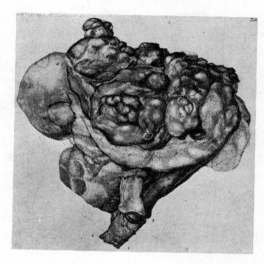

Figure 23 Preparation obtained at necropsy of a case of precocious puberty, described by Carl Emil Gedike, 1825. Right ovary much enlarged [From Ciba Monograph No. 10, by kindness of Ciba-Giegy Ltd.]

at the age of two. At the age of eight she became pregnant by her uncle and nine months later she was delivered of a stillborn child. Although von Haller did not understand the pathology of the condition, he thought that it needed scientific debate and should not be regarded merely as a freak condition due to supernatural influence[15]. It was Johann Friedrich Meckel the Younger (1781–1833) (see also pp. 172 and 237), the greatest comparative anatomist before Johannes Müeller, in the first systematic work on human abnormalities[16], and Étienne Geoffroy Saint-Hilaire (1772–1844)[17], who made a close study of precocious puberty.

The thyroid (continued)

The aforementioned Lorenz Heister, 1683–1758 was the founder of scientific surgery in Germany. His book *Chirugie*[18] was an up-to-date exposé of the state of surgery, with excellent illustrations. The thyroid, he agreed with Haller, had no definite ducts known. He wrote:

> If a tumour arises in the anterior part of the neck from the resisting Flatus or air, some humour or other violence, as straining in labour, lifting of weights, etc., the disorder is then usually called a Bronchocele. In my opinion it should rather be termed a Tracheocele. It is remarkable that some nations are quite free from this disorder, while

156

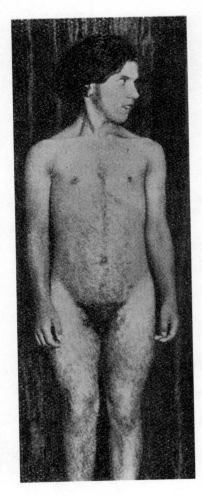

Figure 24 Girl of 9 with precocious puberty due to adrenocortical hyperplasia (Bauer and Medvei; see p. 240)

others are grievously afflicted therewith. Among which latter we may recognise the inhabitants of Spain, Germany, Sweedland, Bavaria, France, Helvetia and especially the inhabitants of the Tirole, who have these tumours (but flaccid) sometimes to such a degree that they can extend to the navel even down to their knees.[18]

To begin with, Heister advocates the use of ointments, but if the condition is chronic and disturbing, surgical removal is advisable. He obviously carried out the operation on several occasions. Fortunately, he never had haemorrhage as a complication, and did not have to use red-hot iron.

In exstirpating these strumae or scrophulae, there is no small danger of wounding some of the large arteries, veins or nerves of the neck by the

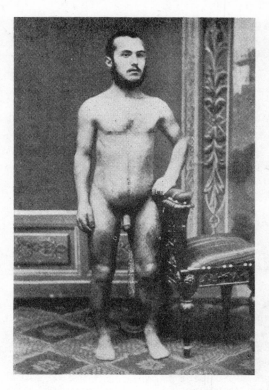

Figure 25 9-year-old boy with precocious puberty and gigantism (pedomacrosomia) (Ercole Sacchi. 1895) [From Ciba Monograph No. 10, by kindness of Ciba–Geigy Ltd.]

scalpel, which would occasion death or some very bad symptom. . . . As these tumours are usually without pain, it is not at all surprising that they should be neglected by the generality of people, who are both poor, careless and fearful of the surgeon's hand; and that more especially if they think the tumour an ornament, like the inhabitants of Tirole. If a patient should be desirous of being freed from the disorder without the knife, it may be done with caustics. But you must be careful not to undertake this method of cure in any but soft and mild kind of strumae, seated not near any large vessel nor too deep in the neck; otherwise the tumour may be converted from a strumous to a cancerous disposition, or at least malignant symptoms brought on, which would endanger the patient's life by injuring the large veins, arteries, nerves or trachea seated in these parts[18].

Heister had in 1715 already refuted J. Vercelloni of Asti's (b. 1676) suggestion[19] that the thyroid was a receptacle of worms, the ova of which mixed with the chile and passed by ducts into the oesophagus. Giovanni Battista Morgagni (1682–1771) of Forli (see Section II) was a pupil of Valsalva, and later a professor at Padova. He became the founder of modern pathological anatomy by his great work *De sedibus et causis morborum per anatomen indagatis*[20]. It was completed when he was 78 years old and consists of 700 reports of necropsies, correlated with the clinical case history, told in 70 most readable letters. It was the first attempt to localize the seat of disease in a scientific manner. He believed that

> the neck has two glands, in which a moisture is generated. But from the two glands which are in the neck, there come forth no vessels by which moisture may flow out, as those do from glands of the tongue[20].

He states in a later paper that the two lobes of the thyroid are connected by an isthmus[21]. He is not definite on the existence of a thyroid excretory duct (or ducts), but it could be that there was one opening into the trachea artery, the pharynx or on to the foramen caecum of the tongue[21].

P. Lalouette (1711–1792), before him, discussed the pyramidal lobe and the minute structure of the thyroid and observed that the vesicles seem to communicate with one another.

Giuseppe Flajani (1741–1808) reported "Sopra un tumor freddo nell' anterior parte del collo detto broncocele"[22]. He observed, in fact, two cases with thyroid enlargement, in the first case with pressure (see p. 259) symptoms, in both with palpitations and exophthalmos, without realizing the connection of the triad; nor did Antonio Testa (1756–1814) in a report on a similar patient in 1800[23]; or Charles de Saint-Yves (see p. 262) (1667–1733) in his *Nouveau traité des maladies des yeux* (Paris, 1722).

The credit for the first and classical description of exophthalmic goitre goes, without doubt, to Caleb Hillier Parry (1755–1822), of Bath (see Section II). In 1786, he observed a patient with goitre, palpitations and protrusion of the eyes, but his collection of eight cases of *Enlargement of the Thyroid Gland in connexion with Enlargement or Palpitation of the Heart* was published only posthumously, in 1825. In it, he remarked: "My attendance on the three last patients having occurred at the same time (in 1813), first suggested to me the notion of some connexion between the malady of the heart and the bronchocele". In patients three and eight: "the thyroid had been previously enlarged for a long time". But in an earlier publication, 'Elements of Pathology and Therapeutics' in the *Medical-Chirurgical Journal and Review*, 1815, 'one of the editors' referred to two patients under his care, with enlargement of the thyroid and cardiac disease (without mentioning exophthalmos)[24].

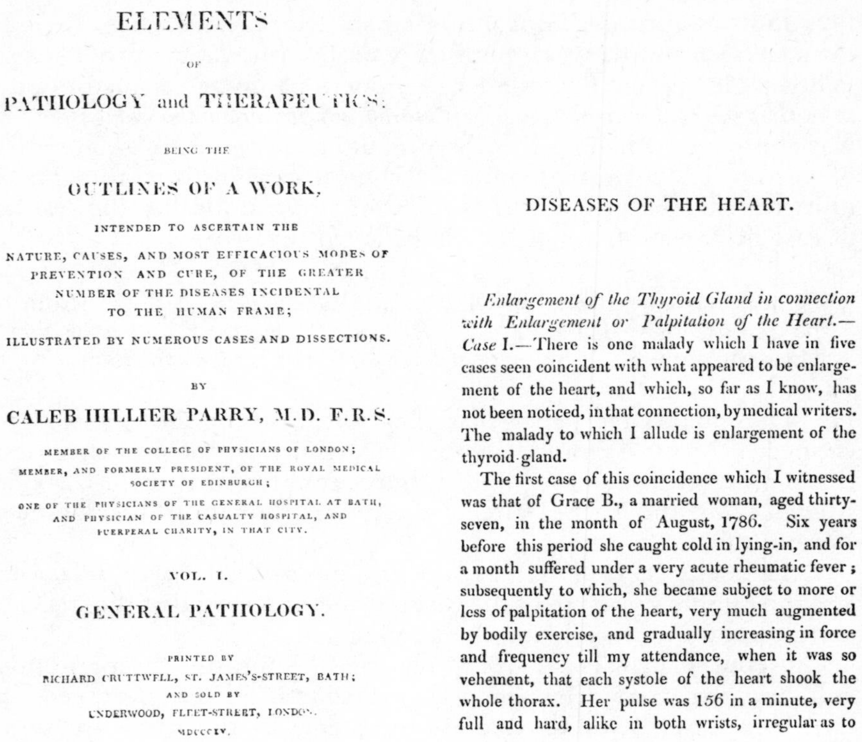

ELEMENTS

OF

PATHOLOGY and THERAPEUTICS:

BEING THE

OUTLINES OF A WORK,

INTENDED TO ASCERTAIN THE

NATURE, CAUSES, AND MOST EFFICACIOUS MODES OF
PREVENTION AND CURE, OF THE GREATER
NUMBER OF THE DISEASES INCIDENTAL
TO THE HUMAN FRAME;

ILLUSTRATED BY NUMEROUS CASES AND DISSECTIONS.

BY

CALEB HILLIER PARRY, M.D. F.R.S.

MEMBER OF THE COLLEGE OF PHYSICIANS OF LONDON;
MEMBER, AND FORMERLY PRESIDENT, OF THE ROYAL MEDICAL
SOCIETY OF EDINBURGH;
ONE OF THE PHYSICIANS OF THE GENERAL HOSPITAL AT BATH,
AND PHYSICIAN OF THE CASUALTY HOSPITAL, AND
PUERPERAL CHARITY, IN THAT CITY.

VOL. I.

GENERAL PATHOLOGY.

PRINTED BY
RICHARD CRUTTWELL, ST. JAMES'S-STREET, BATH;
AND SOLD BY
UNDERWOOD, FLEET-STREET, LONDON.
MDCCCXV.

DISEASES OF THE HEART.

Enlargement of the Thyroid Gland in connection with Enlargement or Palpitation of the Heart.—
Case I.—There is one malady which I have in five cases seen coincident with what appeared to be enlargement of the heart, and which, so far as I know, has not been noticed, in that connection, by medical writers. The malady to which I allude is enlargement of the thyroid gland.

The first case of this coincidence which I witnessed was that of Grace B., a married woman, aged thirty-seven, in the month of August, 1786. Six years before this period she caught cold in lying-in, and for a month suffered under a very acute rheumatic fever ; subsequently to which, she became subject to more or less of palpitation of the heart, very much augmented by bodily exercise, and gradually increasing in force and frequency till my attendance, when it was so vehement, that each systole of the heart shook the whole thorax. Her pulse was 156 in a minute, very full and hard, alike in both wrists, irregular as to

Figure 26 Caleb Hillier Parry: Frontispiece of his description of a patient with goitre, palpitations and exophthalmos

JOSEPH LIEUTAUD

Joseph Lieutaud (1703–1780) described in 1759 a girl who, after a fright due to a clap of thunder, developed a goitre and lost her periods[25]. Lieutaud was professor of medicine in the University of Aix-en-Provence. His work as anatomist was highly regarded by his contemporaries and he was elected a foreign member of the Royal Society of London in 1739, the same year as his eminent fellow-countryman, the Comte de Buffon, and Albrecht von Haller. Louis XIV made him a Conseiller du Roi.

Lieutaud's observations on the endocrine glands were recently reconsidered by Lord (then Sir Solly) Zuckerman in his 'Seventh Addison Memorial Lecture', delivered at Guy's Hospital, London, on 16 December 1953[26], on 'The Secretions of the Brain; Relation of Hypothalamus to Pituitary Gland'. He said:

His observations about the pituita are no more than a historical curiosity; but those he made about what we now know as the hypothalamo-hypophysial connection are extremely interesting. For it so happens that in the course of his studies he stumbled on what is called today the pituitary–portal system of veins.

The record of this discovery is in a volume that was published in 1742 under the title *Essais Anatomiques*[27], essentially a general textbook of anatomy. Its fifth section deals with the central and peripheral nervous systems, and in his description of the third ventricle of the brain, Lieutaud drew attention to a deep fossa anteriorly, the aperture of which gradually narrows as it approaches the base of the pituitary stalk. According to Lieutaud, the stalk, contrary to usual belief, is not canalized, but instead is a kind of cylinder 'two or three lines' thick, formed of a grey substance, and covered by pia mater. On the other hand, running along it are very small longitudinal vessels which communicate with those of the pituitary gland below.

> La tige, qui s'éleve de la glande pituitaire, répond véritablement à la partie la plus profonde de cette fosse; mais elle n'a point de cavité, comme on le prétend; c'est une espèce de cilindre de deux ou trois lignes de hauteur, formé par la substance cendrée, et recouvert de la pie-mère. On remarque de très-petits vaisseaux qui marchent dans son axe, communicant avec ceux de la glande qui reçoit cette colomne ou qui la soutient. J'ai donné à cette partie le nom de "tige pituitaire", parce que j'ai crû que celui d'entonnoir ne sauroit lui convenir. Il n'est point difficile de montrer la solidité de la tige pituitaire, j'en donnerai la manière dans l'administration.

> The stalk, which arises from the pituitary gland, corresponds exactly with the deepest part of that pit, but it has no cavity as has been assumed. It is a kind of cylinder, two or three lines high, formed of grey matter and covered by the pia mater. One perceives very small vessels, which pass along its axis, communicating with those of the gland, which receives this column or which sustains it. I have given the name 'pituitary stalk' to this part because I believe that the term funnel would not be suitable for it. It is not difficult to demonstrate the solidity of the pituitary stalk and I shall describe the method for doing so.

Nine years later de Bordeu attacked Lieutaud's views:[28]

> D'aileurs cette circulation singulière de l'humeur des ventricules qui se rend à la Glande par l'entonnoir, & qui rentre ensuite dans la masse du sang, pourroit-elle se faire, si que M. Lieutaud dit de la solidité de la colomne pituitaire, se trouvoit vrai? (p. 145).

> Moreover, this remarkable circulation of the fluid in the ventricles, which makes its way to the (pituitary) gland through the funnel and which re-enters afterwards into the mass of the blood, could it develop if what M. Lieutaud said (about the solidity of the pituitary column) be found true?

161

De Bordeu pointed out that the (three) functions which Lieutaud attributed to the brain as a glandular organ could just as well have been applied to almost any organ or tissue of the body. De Bordeu was equally unimpressed with Lieutaud's view that the solidity of the pituitary stalk can be easily demonstrated by cutting it in successive sessions. The stalk, he found, is too delicate, and is only crushed by such treatment. He admits, however, the existence of axial vessels along the stalk, and in doing so, leaves the impression that in describing them, Lieutaud had implied that they were a channel for the humours of the brain to the pituitary. He was unconvinced, too, by Lieutaud's assumption that the axial-stalk vessels communicate with those of the pituitary gland[26].

As we now know, Lieutaud and de Bordeu were both right and wrong. de Bordeu was wrong and Lieutaud right in suggesting that the axial-stalk vessels communicate with those of the pituitary below; while de Bordeu was well justified in attacking Lieutaud's conception of the structure and function of the brain, and in doubting that a vital fluid flows from the base of the brain to the pituitary.

Portal circulations

This is a 'History'. Occasionally, it may seem justified to look far ahead. What does what Lieutaud described in 1742 look like now, in 1982? The *Quarterly Journal of Experimental Physiology* has recently published a paper by J. R. Henderson and P. M. Daniel on 'Portal circulations and their relations to countercurrent systems'[29]. They have reviewed the distribution of portal circulations throughout the animal body:

they are commoner than is generally supposed. Most portal circulations consist of two serial capillary beds connected by one or more larger vessels. We have called these 'convergent' portal circulations; examples are hepatic portal, placental, hypophysial, renal, ovarian, and testicular circulations, as are parts of the lymphatic circulation. A second type of portal circulation, which is less common, consists of two serial capillary beds that are not connected by larger vessels. These we have called 'continuous' portal circulations: adrenal and pancreatic circulations are examples of this type. When a countercurrent concentrating mechanism exists in the body it is always part of the primary or secondary bed of a convergent portal circulation, though some convergent portal circulations are not associated with countercurrent mechanisms. . . . What characterises portal circulations is that they possess two serial capillary beds (supplying different cell types) that are not separated by the heart. We will refer to the two capillary beds as 'primary' and 'secondary' respectively (p. 355)[29].

About the "Circulation of the pituitary" Henderson and Daniel say the following:

> Popa and Fielding (1930) first realised that the vessels running along the pituitary stalk connected two capillary beds, and formed a portal system analogous to the portal vein of the liver. These workers actually mistook the primary for the secondary bed, thinking that the blood passed up the stalk. We know now that blood flows down the stalk in the long portal vessels, carrying neurohormones from hypothalamic nerve cells to the epithelial cells of the adenohypophysis. . . . It seems, however, that the original idea about the direction of the blood flow in the pituitary stalk was not entirely wrong, for Page, Munger and Bergland (1976) have described portal vessels in the stalk in which blood could flow from the neurohypophysis up to the median eminence. Oliver, Mical and Porter (1977) have shown experimentally that neurohypophysial hormones do in fact pass up the stalk to influence the release of hormones from the median eminence (p. 359)[29]. These authors make the suggestion that there is a counter-current exchange of hormone(s) between the ascending and descending portal vessels; . . .
> Such is the course of history: Soothsayers were the first serious students of the liver, and thought of the entry of the great vessels into the liver as the gate of the organ – the porta hepatis. Rufus of Ephesos, a Roman surgeon, described this arrangement in about 100 AD . . . and some time after the discovery of capillaries in 1660 by Malpighi, it became evident that the portal vein was at least unusual in having capillaries at both ends (p. 355)[29].

Long before Popa and Fielding[30], Lieutaud suggested that the axial-stalk vessels communicate with those of the pituitary below; and he was also responsible for the term "tige pituitaire"; la tige, from the Latin tibia, meaning stem, stalk, trunk.

Another surgeon, Pierre-Joseph Desault (1744–1795), was one of the first professors of the "École pratique de Chirurgie" in Paris and Bichat's teacher. He wrote the 'Observation sur l'exatirpation d'une partie considerable de la glande thyroide' in the *Journal de Chirurgie* (Paris, 1792). He dissected and ligated the superior and inferior thyroid arteries before cutting them. He seems to have been the first to dissect the firmly adherent gland from the windpipe (see p. 191). All the other surgeons, right up to 1874, found it necessary to carry out a ligature of the tumour en masse, when it was firmly attached to the windpipe[31].

Guillaume Dupuytren (1777–1835) was one of the most brilliant surgeons-in-chief at the Hôtel Dieu in Paris. He was the first to describe the flattening of the windpipe, caused by prolonged pressure of a goitre[31].

THE THYROID

Astley Cooper

Sir Astley Paston Cooper, Bart. (1768–1841) of Norfolk, and of St. Thomas's and later, Guy's Hospital in London, was a pupil of John Hunter. He was a pioneer in vascular and experimental surgery. In lectures given in 1798–1799, he said – according to notes taken by Mr. Earl, surgeon of Cromer: ". . . as the thyroid gland has no duct, it is possible the absorbents perform that office and that they convey the fluid into the thoracic duct"[32]. He collaborated with a younger colleague at Guy's, Mr. Thomas Wilkinson King (1809–1847) (see Section II), adding "Notes on the same subject" to King's most remarkable paper "Observations on the Thyroid Gland" in Guy's Hospital Reports (Vol. I, pp. 429–446; 1836), which earned King the name of 'Father of Endocrinology'.

Thomas Wilkinson King

King described the colloid of the thyroid gland, based mainly on his own experiments and observations, and showed that it passed into the lymphatics and from there into the great veins. He said (p. 437):

> The most important novel fact concerning the thyroid gland is doubtless this, that its absorbent vessels carry its peculiar secretion to the great veins of the body, (this had been, indirectly, surmised by Morgagni and others), and the most simple and satisfactory method of demonstrating this fact is, to expel the contents of the healthy gland by repeated and gentle compressions, into the lymphatics of the surface and then to coagulate the fluid in these vessels.

In healthy adults, such compressions are achieved by the muscles, by the movements of the larynx and the oesophagus. He concludes, prophetically (p. 441):

> Whilst the nourishment of a part is indispensable to its existence, the influence which it exerts upon the circulating fluids, may be more or less needful for the healthful subsistence of the entire animal.

In a table (p. 442), he presents his findings as follows:

Organs	Receive	And yield
Bones, muscles, appendages; coats of vessels; spleen; thyroid and thymus glands, and capsulae renales.	Blood 'arterial'	Blood 'venous' and lymph (in 'lymphatics')

(429)

OBSERVATIONS

ON

THE THYROID GLAND,

BY MR. T. W. KING.

WITH NOTES ON THE SAME SUBJECT,

BY SIR ASTLEY COOPER, BART.

PART I.—LOBES—CELLS.

THE present contribution is chiefly intended to supply a succinct view of the peculiar structure and adaptations of the thyroid gland; so that the more generally established anatomical relations of the organ need only be introduced as they may appear essential to these points*.

For a general history of the thyroid gland, it will be sufficient to refer the student to the volumes of descriptive anatomy. The account given by Cloquet will be found tolerably concise; but that of Meckel is the more complete.

Many recent anatomists seem to have observed that the thyroid gland contains a fluid; a few have adverted to its lobular structure; and others to an opinion that its more minute organization is granular.

The circumstances to be expatiated on in these observations relate principally to the form and arrangement of the lobules of the gland; to the nature of its cells and secretion; to its varying states of mechanical compression and sanguineous injection; and also to the transmission of its peculiar fluid, by the lymphatics, to the venous system. For the knowledge of these particulars, the author has depended solely on his own investigations and experiments, excepting where it will appear otherwise stated. It may also be advanced, in corroboration of the

* It is well also to state here, that there are many circumstances in the anatomical history of the class Mammalia which materially affect the subject; but without entering upon a detail of these, the Author has availed himself of his researches in comparative anatomy just so far as they seemed directly illustrative of particular facts within the scope of the present inquiry. These references will be made chiefly in the form of notes.

Figure 27 First page of Thomas Wilkinson King's paper

. . . yet it is difficult to set aside the inference, that something analogous to a reservoir function obtains in this part. (p. 443) . . . The dissection of a very great number and variety of glands has led me to infer that the quantity of the secretion must naturally be variable.

In his appended 'Notes', Sir Astley Cooper described his experimental thyroidectomies. The first were performed in England *ca.* 1827, the puppies recovering after malaise and stupidity.

Astley Cooper (continued)

Sir Astley Cooper published in 1832 *The Anatomy of the Thymus Gland*. He described the "reservoir" of the thymus as lined by smooth mucous membrane running spirally through the gland. His surgical experiments in dogs led to great progress in vascular surgery and we have already mentioned his report on the experimental removal of the thyroid gland in two puppies, in 1824.

DISEASES OF THE TESTES

In 1830 Astley Cooper's major treatise *Observations on the Structure and Diseases of the Testis*[33] was published. It is of interest to note that in the Preface he was constrained to say:

> I feel great regret at the price of this work; but it arises from the number of Plates. He who understands the expence of printing, drawings, of engravings, and of colouring, will at once discover that my object in publishing is not pecuniary advantage. . . .

Such sentiments still apply 150 years later! The work was based on his 40 years of experience of macroscopic examination of the testis. He described the corpus Highmorianum (see p. 127) as the mediastinum testis "from its situation".

As in the breast, he talked of "hydatid or encysted disease", not necessarily implying a cyst of parasitic origin. Malignant tumours he discussed as follows[33]:

> The testis is often the subject of a malignant disease, which I shall call 'fungoid', but which has been described by different authors under the terms of 'pulpy, medullary, soft cancer', and 'fungus haematodes' . . . but as a multitude of names for the same thing serve only to confuse, and as simplicity is the very soul of surgery, I shall confine its appellation to 'fungous' or 'fungoid'. The term fungus is most applicable to it; because, when it ulcerates, it forms a large fungoid projection, which is full of blood, and which bleeds freely from the slightest laceration, as well as often spontaneously (p. 116).

He discussed "scirrhus" as being a different condition from the 'excessively hard (Scirrhous) swelling of the breast'. This confusing nomenclature persisted until the middle of the century.

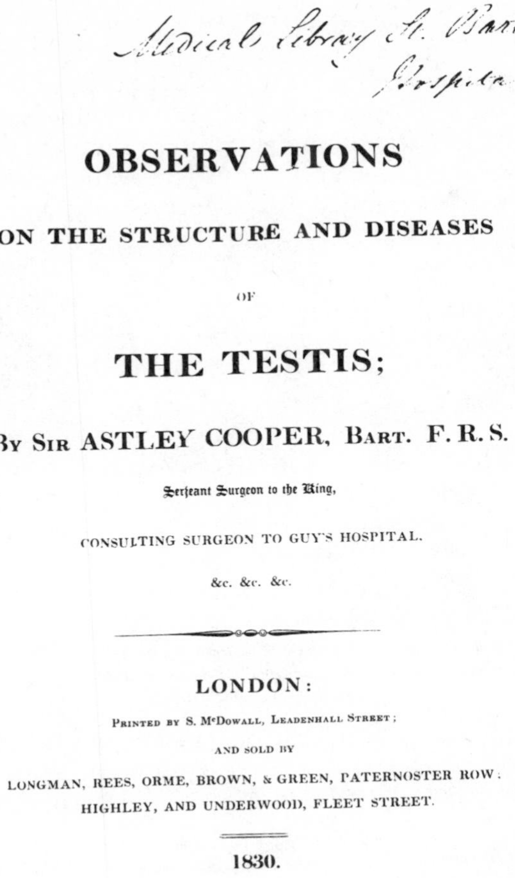

Medical Library St. Bartholomew's Hospital

OBSERVATIONS

ON THE STRUCTURE AND DISEASES

OF

THE TESTIS;

By Sir ASTLEY COOPER, Bart. F. R. S.

Serjeant Surgeon to the King,

CONSULTING SURGEON TO GUY'S HOSPITAL.

&c. &c. &c.

LONDON:

PRINTED BY S. McDOWALL, LEADENHALL STREET;

AND SOLD BY

LONGMAN, REES, ORME, BROWN, & GREEN, PATERNOSTER ROW.

HIGHLEY, AND UNDERWOOD, FLEET STREET.

1830.

Figure 28   Title page of "Observations on the structure and diseases of the testis" by Sir Astley Cooper [Print copyright Department of Medical Illustration, St Bartholomew's Hospital, London EC1]

DISEASES OF THE BREAST

A year earlier, in 1829, there had appeared Sir Astley Cooper's *Illustrations of the Diseases of the Breast* (London), which contained the first description of 'hydatid disease', which was his term for hyperplastic cystic disease of the breast.

ENDEMIC GOITRE AND CRETINISM

The question of endemic goitre cropped up again and again. We have already seen that Felix Platter referred to cretinism in his native

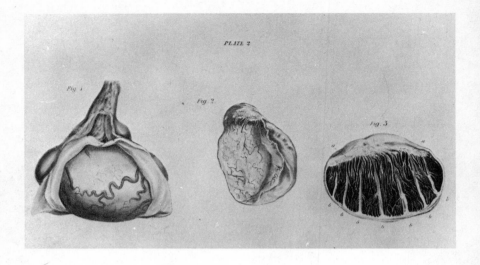

PLATE II.—PART I.

Fig. 1 shews the external portion of the tunica albuginea cut
open, and turned aside, to shew the internal vascular layer,
with the spermatic artery taking its tortuous course upon
it. With care, this layer may be entirely dissected from
the thicker tendinous coat.

Fig. 2.—The internal layer of the tunica albuginea injected, and
the tubuli removed, to exhibit this vascular membrane.

Fig. 3.—The tunica albuginea cut perpendicularly through its
centre :—

a a, its process, which I have called the mediastinum.

bbbbbbb, the ligaments which connect the sides of the
tunica albuginea, and which form strong bands of union
between them, to prevent the injurious effects of violence.
Between these pillars are seen ligaments, which are shorter
and more delicate, some of which proceed from the mediastinum, and a few from the opposite edge of the testis, from
which membranes are extended, to envelope the lobes of
the tubuli.

Figure 29 Mediastinum testis (as Figure 28)

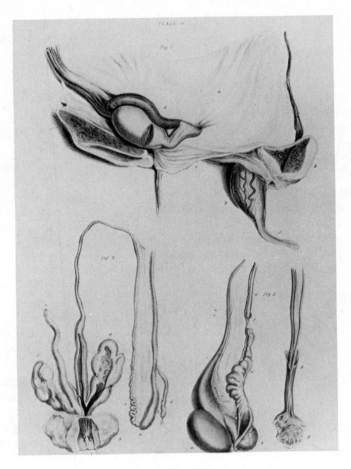

PLATE X.—PART I.

Exhibits an undescended testis in the adult, and a wasted testicle. It also contains the result of an experiment upon a
dog, of dividing the spermatic artery and vein upon one
side, and the vas deferens upon the other.

Fig. 1.—*a*, peritoneum lining the abdominal muscles.
    b, pubes.
    c, ilium.
    d, testis and epididymis.
    e, gubernaculum at the inner ring.
    f, gubernaculum passing through the external ring.
    g, pouch of peritoneum protruding through the external
      ring, which precedes the descent of the testis.—From
      the Collection at Guy's Hospital.

Fig. 2.—A wasted testis in the adult :—
    a, testis.
    b, epididymis.
    c, vas deferens.
    d, vesicula seminalis.
    e, right vas deferens.
    f, right vesicula.
    g, prostate gland.
    h, veru montanum with its two openings—two bristles in
      the one, and one in the other.

Figure 30 Undescended testis (as Figure 28)

169

Valais (see p. 109), but Paracelsus (see p. 99), Muenster, Lange, Stumpf and Campbell (see pp. 109–110) had also referred to it. After Platter there was the (only) book by Wolfgang Hoefer (1614–1681): *Hercules medicus sive locorum communium liber* (Vienna, 1657), which discussed the cause of goitre by air, water and food.

H. B. de Saussure (1740–1799), in 1786 (*Voyages dans les Alpes*, Neuchâtel), and Francois Emmanuel Fodéré (1764–1835), both thought that goitrous cretinism was due to the concentrated air in the deep valleys rather than to water. In his *Essai sur le goitre et le crétinage* (Turin, 1792), Fodéré also described the skeletal changes and especially the changes at the base of the skull (see also Chapter 15, pp. 250–251). De Saussure satisfied himself that drinking melted snow or ice, or alcoholism, coarse food or debauchery, were *not* the cause of endemic goitre, which he never encountered in villages over 3800 feet above sea level, nor in open plains. He found it only in confined narrow valleys, which were under 3000 feet above sea level and where – he thought – the air became stagnant and overheated[34].

The first book in which endemic goitre was discussed was published in 1789 by Michaele Vincenzo Giacinto Malacarne (1744–1816): *Sui gozzi e sulla stupidità . . . etc. dei cretini* (Turin). It was based mainly on his studies in the Aosta valley. Malacarne also described the results of his examinations of the bodies of three cretins in 1780. In the Valais of Switzerland, 'crétin' has been the word used for centuries, to denote goitrous, dwarfed, deaf and dumb unfortunates, who occurred there more often than in other places. In the valley of the Aosta (Piedmont), such human beings were lumped together with the insane, all being called 'Pazzi'. In the report of a Royal Commission on cretinism in the Kingdom of Sardinia in 1848, the incidence of cretinism in the Aosta valley was put as high as 28%. Three groups were described: crétins, semi-crétins and crétineux[35]. In the Pyrenées, such cretins were called 'Cagots' or 'Capots', in Navarre: 'Canos'. Whether the word 'Crétin' is derived from the 'Cretira', or from the Latin 'Creta' (= chalk, because of the white complexion of the sufferers) is open to conjecture[36].

Jean Etienne Dominique Esquirol (1772–1840) was the successor of Philippe Pinel (1745–1826) at the Salpetrière in Paris, and became the first Lecturer in Psychiatry there. In his major work: *Des maladies mentales* (Paris, 1838) he advanced yet another theory on the derivation of 'crétin':

Might not the denomination crétin come from the obsolete word 'crétine' which has the same meaning as alluvium? Has not this name been transferred to individuals who have become infirm in consequence of having dwelt upon an alluvial soil? In fact, is not

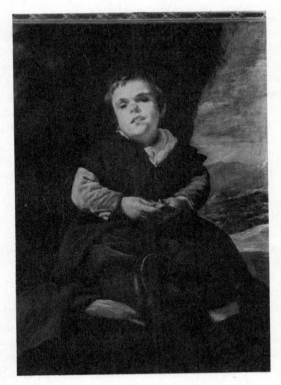

Figure 31   Velazquez *El Nino de Vallecas* [Museo del Prado, Madrid]

cretinism endemic in such mountain gorges as are very swampy and exposed to damp air?

The brothers Joseph (1768–1808) and Carl (1769–1827) Wenzel published a treatise in 1802: *Ueber den Cretinismus* (Wien), in which they attempted a classification:

(1) complete cretins, incapable of speech and reproduction;
(2) demi-cretins, capable of only the elements of speech, but able to create offspring;
(3) simple cretins or imbeciles, somewhat more intelligent than those in groups (1) and (2). There was no precise distinction of cretins from (mentally retarded) idiots[35].

THE PITUITARY GLAND

The *pituitary*, last discussed in the previous chapter, seemed to attract less interest until the end of the 18th and the beginning of the 19th

171

century. Franz Joseph Gall (1758–1828), of phrenology fame, thought that the gland was a large ganglion[37]. Samuel Thomas von Soemmering (1755–1830) introduced the less committal name of 'Hypophysis cerebri' in 1778 (*Dissertatio de basi encephali et originibus nervorum cranio egredientium libri quinque*, Goettingen). This term has persisted especially in the German speaking countries and in Italy. Pierre-Francois–Olive Rayer (1793–1867) of Calvados, renamed it in 1823, 'l'appendice sus-sphénoidal', a term soon forgotten. The above-mentioned Joseph Wenzel suggested in a paper 'Observations on the hypophysis cerebri of epileptic persons' (Beobachtungen ueber den Hirnanhang fallsuechtiger Personen, Mainz, 1810) that epilepsy was caused by a disease of the pituitary gland. This was later refuted by Joseph Engel (1816–1899), a pupil of Carl von Rokitansky, in his MD thesis: 'On the hypophysis cerebri and the infundibulum' (Ueber den Hirnanhang und den Trichter, Vienna, 1839). From his physiological and pathological studies he concluded that the hypophysis was a replica of the cerebellum, "the smallest brain, as it were, in the cranial cavity", and was of major importance for the body movements and the maintenance of balance. Engel pointed out that drunkards often have diseases of the pituitary, anticipating the most recent observation of Cushingoid symptoms in alcoholics by nearly 140 years! The sense of balance was also impaired in the inebriated state. This was due to the fact that the cerebellum was governing the forward movements of the body and the pituitary the backward ones. Moreover, he allotted to the gland an important function in "creative intellectual activity", especially in arousing emotions of pleasure and distaste. Although Engel hoped that "greater experience" might confirm or contradict his work, it was only after his death that more knowledge was forthcoming on the function of the pituitary.

Johann Friedrich Meckel the Younger of Halle, (see p. 156), the 'German Cuvier'[38], believed that the pituitary produced fluid which nourishes the brain.

Carl Gustav Carus (1789–1869), a friend of Goethe, thought on similar lines as Gall, saying that the pituitary was the head end of the nervus sympathicus. Ernst Burdach (1801–1876), also in the 19th century, regarded the pituitary body as the upper end of the spinal cord, the anterior and posterior lobes being a faithful replica of the anterior and posterior tracts of the spinal cord[39].

Morbid anatomical changes had been known in the pituitary body for a long time. Théophile Bonet (1620–1689), in his book: *Sepulchretum, sive anatomia practica ex cadaveribus morbo denatis* (Geneva, 1679) – the first collection of systematized morbid anatomy of nearly 3000 cases from Antiquity to the date of publication – referred to an

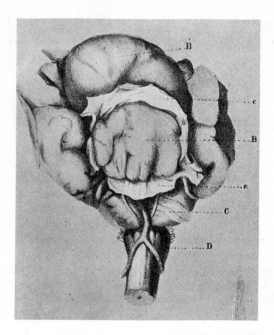

Figure 32 Greatly enlarged and lobulated pituitary (B) constricted by dura mater (C) (Joseph Engel, Vienna, 1839) [From Ciba Monograph No. 10, by kindness of Ciba-Geigy Ltd.]

enlargement of the pituitary. Raymond Vieussens (1641–1715) (see also p. 100) also referred to this enlargement in his *Novum Vasorum Corporis Humani Systema*[40] and Matthew Baillie (1761–1823) in *The Morbid Anatomy of some of the Most Important Parts of the Human Body*[41]. Baillie, from Lanarkshire, was a nephew of William Hunter and physician to George III. He was the last to inherit the 'Gold-headed Cane' of John Radcliffe (1650–1714) and others. In spite of these curiosities of morbid anatomy, Matthew Baillie remarked in 1797 on the pituitary that "this gland is very little liable to be affected by disease" and that the only change he had ever experienced was "one of enlargement to twice the normal size of fibrous tissue" (without any clinical details being given).

The pressure symptoms affecting the surrounding tissue in case of enlargement of the pituitary, especially blindness, were well known before the clinical disease entities were described. In 1718, Jean Louis Petit (1674–1750), the first director of the Académie de Chirurgie in Paris, who had been the first to open the mastoid process, remarked that in most cases of hydrocephalus the pituitary was "squirrheuse"[42]. Vieussens and, in 1833, T. H. Hedlund (1791–1847) reported on patients with blindness[40,43]. Joseph Wenzel connected the diseased pituitary with epileptic fits.

DIABETES

Diabetes insipidus

Johann Peter Frank (1745–1821) of Rotalleen (Palatinate) (see also p. 733) first defined diabetes insipidus and separated it from diabetes verus or mellitus[44]. He was the founder of modern public hygiene with his four volumes of *Complete system of Medical Police* ('System einer vollstaendigen medizinischen Polizey'), Mannheim, 1777–1788). Frank called diabetes insipidus, or spurius, a diabetes without glycosuria.

Michael Ernst Ettmueller in 1683 and John Latham (1761–1843) in 1811 analysed diabetes and examined the clinical aspects of diabetes insipidus[45,46]. John Latham, father of Peter More Latham, was appointed physician to St. Bartholomew's Hospital in London in 1792 and lectured on medicine.

Diabetes mellitus

Francis Home (1719–1813) in 1780 and Johann Peter Frank in 1791 proposed the yeast test for the detection of sugar in the urine[47,48]. Frank also repeated the observation of William Cheselden in his *Anatomy of the Human Body* (London, 1713) that diabetics often suffer from boils and carbuncles. Aretaeus the Cappadocian first used the word "diabetes" and his views have already been discussed, as have the views and method of treatment of Willis. William Cullen (1712–1790), of Edinburgh and Glasgow, reported on patients with non-sugar diabetes in 1787[49]. More important were, however, Matthew Dobson (1713–1784) of Liverpool's *Experiments and observations on the urine in diabetes*[50]. By evaporating urine, Dobson proved that its sweet taste was caused by sugar, and he showed that the residue underwent vinous and acetic fermentation. He also found the sweet taste of the blood in diabetics. As Sir Archibald Garrod said in his Lettsomian Lectures on Glycosuria in 1912: ". . . if Willis discovered or rediscovered glycosuria, to Matthew Dobson must be assigned the credit of having discovered hyperglycaemia"[51] (see also p. 724). Michel Eugène Chevreul (1786–1889) of Paris proved in 1815 that the sugar in diabetic urine is glucose[52]. In 1788, Thomas Cawley published a 'singular case of diabetes, consisting entirely in the quality of the urine; with an inquiry into the different theories of that disease'[53]. The pancreas of that patient was full of calculi, and Cawley suggested a connection between the diabetes and the condition of the pancreas, noting that the disease may follow injury to that organ; he was the first observer to do so. Similar cases of patients were reported later by Friedrich von Recklinghausen (1833–1910) in 1864[54] (calculi), Étienne Lancereaux (1829–1910) in 1877 (two cases with calculi)[55], and Lancereaux was definite in connecting the two conditions causally. Patients with other pathological changes in the pancreas were described by Richard Bright (1789–1858) of nephritis fame, in his *Reports on Medical Cases Selected with a View of Illustrating the Symptoms and Cure of Diseases by a Reference to Morbid Anatomy*[56] and by Apollinaire Bouchardat (1806–1886), in 1851[57]. Bouchardat was, incidentally, the first to use chemical and polariscopic methods for the detection of diabetes, and to attempt a rational dietetic treatment[58]. He invented gluten bread and suggested the use of green vegetables and the avoidance of alcohol.

Friedrich Theodor von Frerichs (1819–1885), famous experimental pathologist in Goettingen, Breslau and Berlin, and pioneer of liver pathology, found that in his experience, 20% of diabetic patients showed gross pathological changes in the pancreas! He also discovered leucine and tyrosine in the urine of acute yellow atrophy of the liver, in 1855[59].

William Prout (1785–1850), an English chemist, first recognized diabetic coma[60]; he also claimed to have recommended the treatment of goitre with iodine a year before Coindet (see p. 191). John Rollo (?–1809), a Surgeon-General in the Army, published in 1797 an account of two diabetic patients successfully treated with a restricted meat diet[61].

THE THYMUS

A complete history of the *thymus gland* up to the early 19th century was given in 1831 by F. C. Haugsted (1804–1866)[62], and in 1845 by John Simon (1816–1904) in his *The Thymus Gland, a Physiological Essay* (London), which won the first Astley Cooper Prize. Thomas Bartholinus' (1616–1680) observation of a cavity and fluid in the centre of the thymus (and a cavity in the adrenals) has already been mentioned (see p. 133). Wharton had already pointed out the resemblance of thymus tissue to that of the pancreas (see also p. 134)[63]. Later the thymus was classed among the glandulae conglobatae because of its structure and the absence of a duct[64]. Eventually, Johannes Mueller (1801–1858) put them into the group of 'blood glands'.

Govert Bidloo (1649–1713) was the Dutch physician and anatomist who accompanied William of Orange as his personal physician to England. He assumed that during foetal life an enlarged thymus held the space in the chest which the lungs would fill after birth when expanded by air, thus preventing the occurrence of the 'vacuum horrendum' of some physical philosophers[65]. Joseph Lieutaud accepted that view in his *Essais anatomiques* (Paris) in 1742 and so did several others: Jean Baptiste Senac (1693–1770)[66], Michaele V. G. Malacarne (1744–1816)[67] and J. H. Kopp (1777–1858) in 1830, who also wrote on 'asthma thymicum' and 'thymus-death'[68].

This mechanical theory was, however, refuted by Sir Astley Cooper, in *The Anatomy of the Thymus Gland* in 1832[69].

G. I. Pozzi (1697–1752), 'the Italian poet and physician', thought in 1732 that the thymus was capable of contraction (due to muscle fibres) and acted as a central pump for the lymphatic system (see also pp. 133–134); accordingly, he also described a communicating duct between the thymus and the thoracic duct[70]. William Cowper (1666–1709), in his *Anatomy of the Human Body* (Oxford, 1698), wrote: "It is a lymphatic gland and varies its magnitude according to the quantity of the lympha that is necessarily transmitted thro' it from the superior parts (of the body)".

William Hewson (1739–1774), a pupil of the Hunters, who studied the lymphatic system, regarded the thymus as an appendix to the lymphatic glands and a factory for the manufacture of the colourless corpuscles, which pass through the thoracic duct to the spleen where they are transformed into red blood-corpuscles[71]. Sir Astley Cooper denied that the thymus was a lymphatic gland at all. Long before them, J. T. Schenk (1619–1671), of Jena, suggested in 1664, that the chyle passed through the thymus and was changed in transit[72]. Samuel Collins (1618–1710), president of the College of Physicians of London in 1695, said in 1685 "the most noble use of the animal liquor, dropping out of the terminations of the nerves into the substance of the thymus, is to contribute its mite to the gentle fermentations of the blood"[73].

Francis Glisson (1597–1677) (see also p. 115), in his *Anatomia hepatis*[74] described the thymus as a "glandula nutritia" for the foetus, a view which was also accepted by Walter Charleton (1619–1707) in 1659[75]. by Pierre Dionis (? – 1718) in 1716[76] (see also p. 133) and by F. Bellinger in 1717[77]. F. Caldani[78] decided that the food brought by the umbilical vein was conveyed by the lymphatics of the liver to the thymus, and that after birth the thymus atrophied as its function

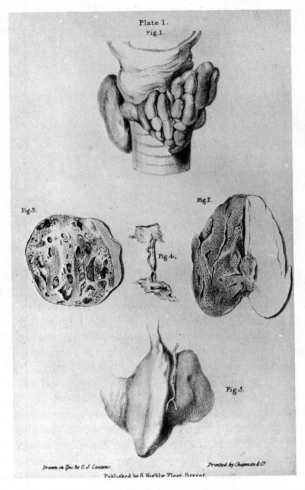

Figure 33 Frontispiece of Sir Astley Cooper's monograph on the thymus

was taken over by the mesenteric glands. In his treatise of 1832[69], Sir Astley Cooper confirmed Glisson's view that the thymus prepared a fluid for foetal nourishment and growth. He said (p. 44):

As the Thymus secretes all the parts of the blood, viz. albumen, fibrin and particles, is it not possible that the Gland is designed to prepare a fluid well fitted for the foetal growth and nourishment from the blood of the mother before the birth of the foetus, and consequently before chyle is formed from food, and this process continues for a short time

177

after birth, the quantity of fluid secreted from the Thymus gradually declining as that of chylification becomes perfectly established?

He also described a girl of 19, who died of a "Diseased growth of the Thymus and of Bronchocele or an unnatural growth of the Thyroid Gland" (p. 47)[69].

We have already seen that Thomas Wilkinson King listed the thymus in his table among the Organs, together with the spleen, the thyroid and the capsulae renales.

A digressing view on the rôle of the thymus was that it was a fat or hibernating gland; this was introduced by G. Velsch (1618–1690) in 1670 and accepted by John Simon in 1845 in his prizewinning essay.

THE ADRENALS

The *adrenals* were other glands where speculation was rife as to whether they had a central cavity and whether they had a special rôle in foetal life only. The views of Antonio Mollinetti and of Pozzi of Bologna have already been discussed. Joseph Lieutaud stressed that the blood supply of the foetal adrenal was much larger than of the foetal kidney, "d'où on pourrait tirer diverses rèmarques physiologiques, relative à la secretion de l'urine"[79]. ". . . from which one could draw various conclusions (physiological remarks) concerning the secretion of urine".) Sir Charles Bell (1775–1842) revived Mollinetti's theory[80], so did John Redman Coxe, Professor of Materia Medica at the University of Pennsylvania in 1828[81]. The views of the aforementioned Samuel Collins, PCP of London, which were given in 1685 in his *System of Anatomy*[82] have already been quoted and so have those of Wharton, Caspar and of Bartholinus. Glisson held a similar view to Wharton concerning the function of the adrenals (see p. 132)[83]. Three years before Thomas Addison, John Goodsir (1814–1867) of Edinburgh, considered "The suprarenal capsules, the thymus and the thyroid, as organs essentially similar in structure, as developments of the remains of the blastoderma, being formed of a continuous portion of that part." As all three are situated along each side of the spine and neighbouring major bloodvessels, he speculated that the three organs perform functions, "whatever these may be, analogous to those of the blastoderma", with a difference: "the three organs in question only elaborate the matter which has already been absorbed by the other parts, and is now circulating in the vessels of the more perfect individual"[84]. Is that another forerunner of the idea of internal secretion?

178

As progress toward discovering the real function of the adrenals was slight during the 18th and early 19th century, there was no real interest in the subject. So in 1716, the Académie des Sciences in Bordeaux offered a prize on the theme: "Quel est l'usage des glandes surrénales?" Although many essays were submitted, none of them was considered of sufficient merit to warrant a prize. This decision was publicly conveyed in 1718, in the most elegant manner by the Secretary of the Académie, the celebrated Charles de Montesquieu (1689–1755), then only twenty-nine years of age: he closed his discourse with the words: "Le hasard fera peut-être quelque jour ce que tous ces soins n'ont pu faire" (Perhaps chance will one day bring about what all these labours failed to do).

However, as Shumacker said so correctly: "The real impetus to modern investigation and the first great contribution to modern knowledge of adrenal physiology, after three centuries of unproductive speculations, came with Thomas Addison." His accurate observations and clear insight are directly responsible not only for his own very lucid description of adrenal insufficiency in man, but also for the experimental and clinical efforts of recent workers[85].

THE SPERMATOZOA

Two important achievements occurred towards the end of the 18th century. The first of these was the advancement of knowledge about the spermatozoa and fertilization.

Lazzaro Spallanzani

Lazzaro Spallanzani (1729–1799) (see Section II), Abbé (Abate), lawyer, professor of Greek studies, microscopist, medical scientist, traveller and travel writer, professor in Modena and later in Pavia, was one of the most versatile minds of his time. Among his varied scientific discoveries, there is one of particular importance to our theme. In 1785, he produced evidence that in lower animals, such as frogs, the silkworm, and others, fertilization of the ova occurred by the live spermatozoa, and that the spermatozoon was essential to fertilization (see p. 186). He also demonstrated the shape of the spermatozoon. His *Nouvelles Recherches sur les Découvertes Microscopiques et la Génération des Corps Organisées* was unfortunately available to me only in the French translation of 1769: "Traduit de l'Italien de M. l'Abbé Spallanzani, Professeur de Philosophie à Modène . . . par

179

M. l'Abbé Regley. . . . A Londres et à Paris, 1769''. On page xxiii, it is said:

On a accordé à la femelle du merlus une prodigieuse quantité d'oeufs. De compte fait, on en a trouvé dans une Jusque' à neuf millions trois cens trente quatre mille, et comme il faut à Leeuwenhoek, dix mille animaux dans le mâle pour chaque oeuf de la femelle, et il va se trouver qu'un merlus mâle contiendra seul un bien plus grand nombre de merlus vivans qu'il n'y a d'hommes existans sur toute la surface de la terre.

One has accorded to the female of the hake a prodigious quantity of ova. Having attempted to count them, one found in one [such female], nearly nine million three hundred and thirty four thousand; according to Leeuwenhoek, there are 10 000 'animals' (spermatozoa) in the male hake for each ovum of the female, and one will find that one male hake alone will contain a much greater number of living hakes (=spermatozoa) than there are human beings on the surface of the earth.

With a slightly critical eye, he says of Harvey (p. xxiv):

Harvey a jette un coup d'oeil bien different sur l'ouvrage de la génération . . . Harvey, fier de sa découverte, crut pouvoir renverser le système oeufs et des animalcules microscopiques. Il imagina que ce punctum saliens étoit le premier principe de l'organisation animale, et que les autres parties du corps venoient s'y adapter et s'y unir par *juxtaposition*, de la manière que les visceres se formorent toujours avant les organes du dehors.

Harvey took a a look of a quite different nature in his work on procreation . . . proud of his discovery, he thought that he could reverse the system of ova and the microscopic 'animalculi' (=spermatozoa). He imagined that the punctum saliens was the prime principle of the animal organization and that the other parts of the body would adapt themselves and thus unite by juxtaposition, in the manner in which the viscera always formed themselves before the organs outside did.

Il y a, suivant M. de Needham, deux espèces d'êtres simples; l'un est un être mouvant, l'autre un être résistant; c'est de leur union, et de la variété infinie de leurs combinaisons dans toutes les proportions possibles, que nait la collection générale des êtres, depuis la masse la plus brute jusqu' à la matière la plus exaltée, . . . et comme ces êtres font matériels, quoique simples, il est en droit d'appeller leur union un composé matériel (p. xlvii).

There are, according to M. de Needham, two kinds of simple beings; one is a moving (mobile) being, the other a resistant one; it is through their union and their infinite variety of the combinations in all possible proportions that is created (born) the general collection of beings, from the most primitive mass to the most exalted material . . . and as these beings create material, although of a simple structure, it is right to call their union a compound material.

After Leeuwenhoek[86] (see p. 117) there were no systematic microscopical observations of the biological characteristics of the spermatozoa until the mid-18th century, when the naturalist Comte George Louis Leclerc Buffon (1707–1788) published his great *Histoire naturelle*[87] in 44 volumes (1749–1804), in the first modern attempt to cover all scientific knowledge in one work. In co-operation with the Englishman John Turberville Needham (1713–1781), he decided on a systematic research programme on the problem of generation. Needham was a Catholic priest, living on the Continent, whose experiments had led him to the conclusion that there existed spontaneous generation. Buffon, who shared this view, had already outlined his theory about the 'molécules organiques' and the 'moules intérieurs'. When Needham arrived in Paris in 1747, their biological views were, therefore, already very close. The molécules organiques Buffon described as very small organic particles, incorruptible and indestructible and unmodifiable, which nature keeps using again and again to form new organisms, "grouping them into organs and tissues with the help of a sort of mold (moule intérieur), which is an integral part of the organism itself". If Buffon was the theorist, Needham was an accomplished microscopist[88–90].

Buffon and Needham denied the 'animality' of spermatozoa, which they considered as mere aggregations of organic matter with the task of initiating the formation of a new being. Seminal fluid appeared to Buffon to consist of a number of large filaments which would undergo a longitudinal separation in a few hours' time. A string of globular formations (corpuscles) along each of these filaments made it look like a rosary. The true nature of these 'filaments' cannot be determined. Five to six hours after obtaining the sperm, it had become completely liquid, and a certain number of the corpuscles lost their tail, and some seemed to change size and shape. After a further hour, all corpuscles had lost their tails and their movements were particularly brisk. "I have seen some of them divide and break up, one oval or globular becoming two", Buffon added[91]. 24 hours after the beginning of the experiment, only very few corpuscles were still motile under Buffon's eyeview through the microscope. In human sperm, the corpuscles were all tail-less:

> I observed that many of these globules changed shape; they stretched out considerably and became long, like little cylinders. Afterward, the two ends of the cylinder puffed up and they divided into two other globules, both in motion[92].

In fact, Buffon gave one of the first correct descriptions of the infusoria and of how certain species multiplied by division. His unfamiliarity with these organisms and his keenness to prove the non-specificity of the supposed animalcules of the sperm caused his lack of insight to recognise his mistake[93]. "Is it not natural", he asks, "to regard them as living organised parts of the animal or vegetable, parts which must . . . unite to produce moving and living beings and to form the animals and vegetables?"[94]

Spallanzani was engaged in research on infusoria from 1761 to 1765, as a result of which he felt compelled to attack Buffon and Needham's 'organic molecules' theory and the correlated 'generation system'[95]. Needham's defence of the system[96] induced Spallanzani to undertake a study of the spermatozoa, in which he was strongly urged on by Charles Bonnet (1720–1793)[97]. In a letter which Spallanzani wrote to Bonnet only a few months afterwards, he already gave him an account of his observations, almost as complete as they were in his monograph of 1776[98,99].

Spallanzani went about his task with great care and according to a careful plan. His investigations of the sperm covered – as already mentioned – a large variety of animals: man, bull, horse, dog, ram, fish; his methodical experiments were only limited by the optical equipment available at that time[100] and were, in many ways, similar to Leeuwenhoek's (he also made the same mistake as regards the actual size of the spermatozoa). He did remark that the 'corpicciuli' vary in size and are not globular but oval. He was also able, by a lucky coincidence, to give a good description of the 'tail' which he found *ca*. six times the size of the body and getting broader towards it. There seemed no major difference between the corpicciuli of several species, except in the fishes, which showed some movements characteristic of the infusoria.

Spallanzani also made use of the clock and thermometer to design almost classical experimental conditions. A short extract from a table will illustrate this:

Temperature			Period of motility (sperm of various animals)
2°	Réaumur	(1.6°C)	Less than 45 min
5.5°	R	(6°C)	120 min
12.5°	R	(10°C)	3 h 45 min
22°	R	(17.6°C)	8 h

Each sperm sample was divided into three test tubes which he exposed to different temperatures. He proved that sperm exposed to air would die (possibly due to evaporation of the seminal fluid). In a vacuum produced in an air pump, spermatozoa kept their motility for 2–3 hours after those exposed to air had lost their motility. Sperm enclosed in sealed capillary tubes remained motile for up to 3 days, whereas those exposed to air became motionless after 7–8 hours[101]. Like Leeuwenhoek he called them 'animals'[102]. By his experiments he also invalidated some views of Carl von Linnaeus (1702–1799) (Linné, C.)[103]. "Yet the most significant section in Spallanzani's *Osservazioni* is no doubt the one in which Needham's and Buffon's observations are critically dismissed"[86].

In a particularly brilliant experiment on male salamanders Spallanzani showed the existence of spermatozoa *in vivo*, concluding: "that the little worms of the sperm of man and animals exist in the semen before any alteration or decomposition in it caused by the air . . . even when it is restricted in the genital organs of man as of animals"[104]. He also proved that, contrary to Buffon's views, the spermatozoa did not change their shape ('losing their tails') neither in life nor in death[105]. He further demonstrated, by adopting rigorous experimental conditions, that Buffon's motile formations, which seemed to reproduce by division, were simply ordinary infusoria, which had contaminated the seminal fluid Buffon had used. Spallanzani showed that at a higher temperature, infusoria would appear in a sample after 14 hours![106] Accordingly, the main points in Buffon's arguments that spermatozoa were not animals were disproved, as his observations really referred to contaminating infusoria.

Iris Sandler pointed out in a careful study re-examining Spallanzani's interpretation of the rôle of the spermatic animalcules in fertilization[107], that in 1784 Spallanzani obtained two fractions from filtered frog's semen: a liquid portion (denuded of its fertilizing power) and a thick residue, containing the 'spermatic animalcules', left behind on the filter paper, which upon suspension in water were capable of fertilizing frogs' eggs. In spite of these clear results of his experiment, Spallanzani believed that the fertilizing capacity of the semen was in the fluid portion! This was not due to the usual assumption that Spallanzani was one of the 'preformationist-ovists' who believed that the embryo was already preformed in the ovum, getting from the semen only the stimulus to activate its growth.

We have seen Buffon's ideas (pp. 181–182), maintaining that there were no eggs in viviparous animals, "rather, he thought, the female possessed a semen like the male, which was the definite contribution of the female to fertilization"[107]. Moreover, there was doubt as to the occurrence of external fertilization; Linnaeus stated categorically: "Never, in any living body, does fecundation or impregnation of egges take place outside the body of the mother"[107].

Since Aristotle (see Chapter 6), the idea was prevalent that the sperm had a material portion and the pneuma, the 'aura seminalis' which was supposed to be the fertile portion carried by the liquid vehicle to the menstrual material of the female. This view was still held by Fabricius ab Aquapendente (see Chapter 12, pp. 111–112), in *De Formatione Ovi et Pulli*[108], as he could find no trace of semen in the ovum or uterus after copulation, a finding confirmed by William Harvey in 1651 (see Chapter 13, pp. 125–127):

> It is to the uterus that the business of conception is chiefly intrusted; without this structure and its functions conception would be looked for in vain. But since it is certain that the semen of the male does not so much as reach the cavity of the uterus, much less continue long there, and that it carries with it a fecundating power by a kind of contagious property, (not because it is there and then in actual contact, or operates, but because it previously has been in contact); the woman, after contact with the spermatic fluid in coitu, seems to receive influence, and to become fecundated without the co-operation of any sensible corporeal agent, in the same way as iron touched by the magnet is endowed with its powers and can attract other iron to itself. When this virtue is once received the woman exercises a plastic power of generation, and produces a being after her own image; . . .[109]

Fabricius also encouraged the view that the male semen was able to act at a distance, to produce fertilization. The term "aura" seminalis was introduced by Swammerdam (see also p. 116)[107]. De Graaf also accepted that view and extended it to the mammals (1672). He stated that the most subtle part of the (male) semen, called the aura seminalis, traversed the oviducts in order to reach the ovaries where it would fertilize the eggs. So did Charles Bonnet (1720–1793), who was one of the pen friends of Spallanzani a hundred years later, in 1779[110]. Bonnet mentioned that Haller also shared the view "that the power to animate the heart of the germ resides in the vaporous part of the sperm"[107]. In Buffon's theory of the 'organic molecule' (1749), the 'seminal animalcules' were rejected, in favour of an "infinity of living organic particles" from which all living beings were composed. These 'organic molecules', of which there were a definite number, could not be destroyed, only separated, so that the death of one organism freed them to be used again as bricks for the building of another living organization (i.e. plant, animal or human being). The shape of the new 'organization' was determined by an existing mould, the "moule intérieur". In the reproductive organs, the superfluous organic molecules assembled, forming the seminal liquor. It was Spallanzani's intention to prove that Buffon's organic molecules were, in fact, a class of (microscopic) animals but he realized the difficulty in proving this: "Ils son trop éloignées de nous, et des animaux les plus connus, pour prouver sans réplique qu'ils sont dans la même categorie" (=they are too far removed from us and from animals best known, to prove beyond question that they are in the same category). Spallanzani's experiments were designed to prove that these animalcules were true animals with division and propagation, subject to damage by poisonous fumes[107]. Using the fact that the vas deferens of fasting salamanders becomes transparent, he was able to observe and to conclude that "The spermatic animals of men and animals exist in the semen prior to any alteration or decomposition caused by the air"[107]. These results from the fresh semen of humans, horses, dogs, sheep, birds and fish were in agreement with Leeuwenhoek's observations.

The only thing Spallanzani could not establish was the manner in which the spermatic animals propagate themselves. He did, however, manage to demonstrate clear cut evidence of external fertilization in frogs, and a definite negation of the belief that the aura seminalis was responsible for the fertilization of eggs[111]. Swammerdam had before him mentioned his observations (in the *Biblia Natura*, 1752) on the fertilization of the red frog, where the female released the eggs, which were then covered by the release of seminal fluid from the male companion. The German naturalist Roesel gave a similar account of the fertilization in the green frog in 1758, in his *Historia Naturalis Ranarum*. But it was Spallanzani who proved by an ingenious experiment that fertilization in frogs was really external. Females discharged their eggs, when coupling with males, into a vessel filled with water. Normal development of embryos resulted. He next dissected eggs from the ovary, oviduct and uterus of the same females and put them into a vessel filled with water. These eggs did not develop. Although copulation normally occurred in water, Spallanzani found that it also occurred in an empty vessel, into which male and female frogs had been placed, and it could be observed that the males released semen onto the eggs simultaneously with their release by the females. If these eggs were placed in water, normal development of tadpoles took place. Finally, when the males were put into tight fitting taffeta pants before mounting the females, the released female eggs were not fertilized. If the droplets of semen were removed from the inside of those tight fitting pants and mixed with the released eggs, normal development resulted again: Quod erat demonstrandum![107] (Beatrix Potter was, obviously, not conversant with this experiment of Spallanzani when she wrote *The Tale of Mr. Jeremy Fisher*.) The last experiment was, in addition, the first in the line of demonstrating the possibility of successful 'artificial fecundation'. They were of importance because they served to prove "that fecundation in the foetid toad is not the effect of the aura seminalis, but of the sensible part of the seed"[112].

Iris Sandler makes out a very good case that the puzzling inter-

185

pretation by Spallanzani of some of his subsequent artificial fecundation experiments was not due to his being a dyed in the wool
preformation-ovist, as his critics maintained (for example, C. D.
Darlington[113].) These critics argue (1) that Spallanzani asked the
proper question: In what part of the semen does the fertilizing power
lie?; (2) that he devised and carried out the appropriate experiments
by separating the liquid from the sperm and testing each for its
fertilizing capacity; (3) that he obtained the correct results, that the
sperm containing portion had all the fertilizing ability; and that –
after all that, he came to the conclusion that the liquid was the active
principle! Sandler, however, makes two important points. Firstly,
that the experiments were, originally, designed to answer the
question of the 'aura seminalis', and this they did. Secondly, that
Spallanzani did not bend the results of his experiments to fit in with
the ovist theory. For some reason, it is possible that what he firmly
believed to be the seminal fluid, "upon two occasions . . . totally
destitute of such inhabitants (i.e. the enormous numbers of spermatic
worms)", and yet able to fertilize ova, was not, in fact, free from
spermatozoa; in which case, "the conclusions drawn by Spallanzani
as to the functions of the spermatic animals in fertilization were
logical inferences drawn from his experiments, and not a misinterpretation of facts generated by his belief in the theory of
preformation"[107]. Moreover, from his previous work, Spallanzani
was convinced that the 'spermatic animals' were – like the infusoria
he had studied – real animals, which happened to require for their
existence this rather specialized environment, and as such he did not
necessarily associate them with the generative process of the host
animal (the toad).

Finally, although Spallanzani tried to achieve development of the
ova by using electricity, blood, and visceral juices from organs other
than the testicles or seminal vesicles, instead of semen he did not
succeed; but it is known that artificial parthogenesis can occur in the
natural life cycle of some insects (e.g. aphidae), and Charles Bonnet
(in a letter of 15 August, 1778) drew Spallanzani's attention to an
experiment by Achard of hatching chickens in an incubator. Sandler
refers to the successful experiment of Bataillon who, in 1910,
reported on parthenogenesis in the frog, if the ovum is pricked by a
glass needle or micropipette[107]. Spallanzani was known to use a
needle ("his usual method of application") when applying sperm-
free semen to eggs. He recorded: "At this time I could take up with
the point of a needle, at the edge of the liquor, many drops that were
entirely destitute of worms. . . . My long experience in the world of
microscopical animals, whether belonging to man or animals, will, I
hope, vouch for me that I was not deceived in this delicate

investigation"[114]. Thus, Sandler feels justified in concluding with a quotation from the *Dissertations* . . . (part II, iii)[114]:

> It is said by many that fecundation is among the mysteries of nature: and like many of her operations, an object of admiration rather than enquiry . . . but, since the appearance of Haller and Bonnet, this gloom has been rendered much less thick. I am very far from thinking that I would have dissipated it entirely, yet I would fain hope that by my efforts, it has been somewhat cleared and that a light less feeble and uncertain, now shines through it.

It is little known that Spallanzani continued to study the problem of 'artificial fecundation' and carried out the first known successful experiments in various amphibia, an insect and in the dog, although he gave the priority in this matter to Malpighi; the latter's experiments, however, were unsuccessful[88]. I was fortunate enough to see and read the extremely rare short paper on the subject by Spallanzani, which was part of a preliminary volume of a projected Italian encyclopaedia, which, however, never seemed to have come off the ground, perhaps because the editor, Abbé Alessandro Zorzi, died suddenly. In that paper[115] Spallanzani discussed the problem in plants and animals, remarked that he was carrying out a number of experiments and promised a further detailed report when he had assembled sufficient new facts. In his experiments he used both the discharged semen and the expressed juice of the testis. He hoped that artificial fecundation would in future make it possible to carry out experimental cross-fertilization of species, e.g. frog and toad, perhaps even frogs and fishes, or mammals, for which latter a lead already existed in the breeding of mules. He referred to the subject again in the second volume of his now rare and important work: *Dissertazioni di Fisica Animale, e Vegetabile dell' Abate Spallanzani*[111]; further, in *Risposta al sig. Pietro Rossi* (Pisa, 1782); and in *Lettera al Marchese Lucchesini* (Milano, 1783); finally, in *Nuove esperienze sulla fecondazione di una cagna* (=bitch) (Padova, 1794).

It was another 42 years before Rudolph Albert von Koelliker (1817–1905) demonstrated the true cellular origin of the spermatozoa[116].

The ovum

It was also in 1827 that Carl Ernst von Baer (1792–1876) published his discovery of the mammalian ovum: *De ovi mammalium et hominis genesi*[117] (see also pp. 270 and 271). He was Professor in Dorpat, Koenigsberg and St. Petersburg, and one of the pioneers of comparative embryology and of the theory of germ-layers, histogenesis and

129

FECONDAZIONE ARTIFICIALE

ARTICOLO *del Sig. Abate Lazaro Spallanzani, pubblico Profeſſore di Storia Naturale nella Reale Univerſità di Pavia.*

FECONDAZIONE ARTIFICIALE. Vuolſi intendere quell' attitudine al naſcere, che dall' arte viene comunicata alle ſemenze delle Piante col mezzo della polvere degli ſtami, e all' uova degli Animali col mezzo del liquore ſpermatico. Riſchiariamo l' idea con eſempj tolti dai due Regni, Vegetabile, ed Animale.

I. Sembra omai che più non dubitino i Naturaliſti dell' eſiſtenza dei due ſeſſi nelle Piante. Si ſa che ſecondo queſta Teoria gli ſtami fanno l' ufizio del maſchio, e i piſtilli queſtò della femmina (Vedi STAME, e PISTILLO). La polvere dei primi entrando nella cavità dei ſecondi s' innoltra fino all' ovaja, dove ſuccede la fecondazione delle ſemenze.

La neceſſità di queſti due generi d' organi per la fruttificazione viene abbaſtanza provata dalla privazione o dall' alteramento dei medeſimi: conciosſiache ſe recidanſi gli ſtami o i piſtilli, ovveramente tralignino gli uni o gli altri ſubito che apronſi i fiori, ella è coſa certa che tali Piante o non danno ſemi, o li danno ſoltanto infecondi.

Che poi concorrano alla fruttificazione, in quanto che gli ſtami ſono gli organi maſchiii, e i piſtilli gli organi femminili, pare che lo provino ſenza replica quelle Piante che hanno due fatte d' individui, altri cioè provveduti ſoltanto di piſtilli, ed altri di ſtami. Imperocchè ſe le Piante a piſtilli non ſieno in vicinanza delle Piante a ſtami, ſi rimangono ſterili. E queſta è ſtata la cagione che ha indotto gli uomini a procurare queſte fecondazioni o maritaggi, dirò così, artificiali non poco vantaggioſi alla ſocietà in alcuni paeſi; obbligazione che abbiamo a' Ruſtici ſteſſi, da' quali ſi può dire che abbiano appreſo i Fiſici l' eſiſtenza dei due ſeſſi nei Vegetabili. Le Palme dattilifere (Vedi PALMA) ſono nel novero di quegli Alberi, che hanno gl' individui a ſtami oſſia maſchj, e gl' individui a piſtilli oſſia femmine. E la neceſſità di tenere in compagnia queſta doppia fatta d' individui per averne la fruttificazione era conoſciuta dai coltivatori di queſta Pianta fino ai tempi di Aleſſandro. Erodoto pure ci atteſta, e il fatto viene confermato dal celebre Botanico Tournefort, eſſere antica uſanza de' ruſtici abitatori dell' Oriente, dove faſſi un uſo sì grande di datteri, il maritare le Palme coll' attaccare i rami degl' individui maſchj a quelli degl' individui femmine. E un ſimil coſtume, per quanto ne riferiſce il Geoffroy, ſi pratica in Sicilia per rapporto ai Piſtacchi (Vedi PISTACCHIO). Intorno alle quali ultime Piante ſappiamo altresì dal Duhamel, che una di eſſe che trovavaſi in Parigi, e che era femmina, non produſſe mai frutta feconde, ſe non ſe quando le fu dato a compagno un Piſtacchio maſchio, dal quale eſſendo ſtata priva in ſeguito, tornò la medeſima alla primiera infecondità.

Ma di queſta fecondazione artificiale nelle Palme abbiamo fatti più luminoſi e più deciſivi in quella ſpezie che dal Boerave ſi appella *Palma dactylifera major, ſpinoſa, femina, folio flabelliformi*, e *Chamairops* dal Linneo. Una di queſte

R Pal-

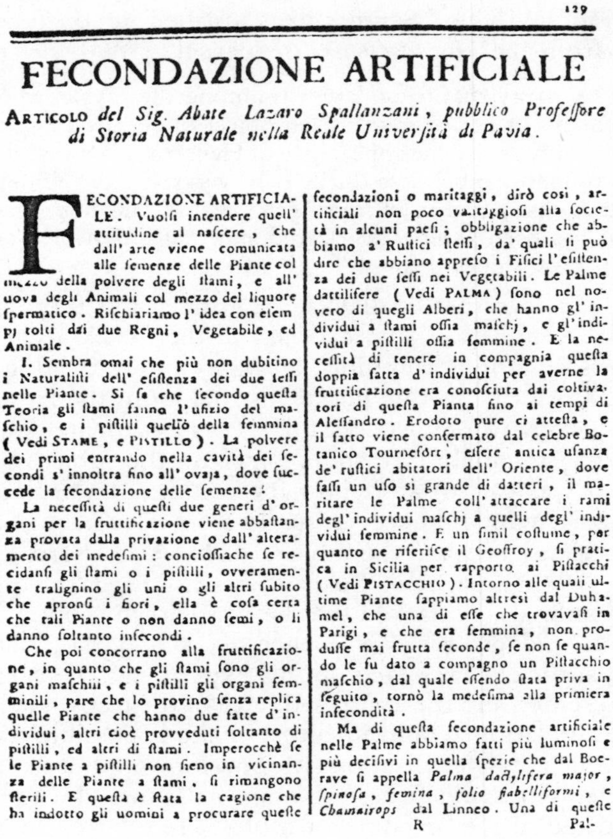

Figure 34 Front page of Spallanzani's paper on artificial insemination in the proposed Italian Encyclopaedia, Siena, 1779

morphogenesis (see Section II). With Frédéric Cuvier (1773–1838), he was the founder of modern morphology. His main work in this direction was *Ueber Entwicklungsgeschichte der Tiere*[118]. In 1797, J. Haighton published his observations on his experiments on rabbits which made him the first to describe induced ovulation. He concluded ". . . that the ovaries can be affected by the stimulus of impregnation, without the contact either of palpable semen, or of the *aura seminalis.*"[182]

Giovanni Battista Morgagni (1682–1771) (see p. 159) described in 1761[119] the 'hydatid', renamed by L. Gosselin (1815–1887) in 1848, the 'appendix' of the testicles[120], which is present in 90% of the bodies. It is the remains of the blind end of the Wolffian duct and resembles the fimbriated end of the Fallopian tube. It corresponds with the hydatid of Morgagni in the female, is near the globus major of the epididymis and is composed of fibrous tissue and blood vessels.

THE DISCOVERY OF IODINE

The other outstanding event at that period was the discovery of iodine. In 1811, Bernard Courtois (1777–1838), a self-taught chemist and dealer in chemicals and manufacturer of saltpetre in Paris, was washing the ashes of seaweed – used as a source of potash – and was using vitriol, when he noted violet fumes. With the help of two other chemists, Clément and Desormes, the violet gas was condensed into crystals (Substance X). This "Substance X" was soon identified as one of the halogen elements by Sir Humphry Davy (1778–1829), who happened to be in Paris at that time[121], and by Louis Gay-Lussac (1778–1850)[122]. Courtois, Clément and Desormes published a paper on the discovery in the *Annals of Chemistry*[123]. From the Greek *ιοειδής* = 'ioeides' = violet coloured, the new element was named 'iode' in French, 'iodine' in English, 'iodum' in Latin, 'Jod' in German. As mentioned before (p. 93), Roger of Salerno had used seaweed in the treatment of goitre in 1170 AD. It was also recommended by Ko-Hung in China in *ca*. 340 AD and, later, by Sun Ssu-Mo, *ca*. 650 AD, and in the *Pen Tsao*, the herbal of the Chinese pharmacopoeia (1596 AD), based on Emperor Shen Nung's prescriptions, twenty seven centuries BC.

Arnold of Villanova (1235–1311), consultant to Peter III of Aragon (see p. 99), doctor of theology, law, philosophy and medicine, alchemist, translator of Avicenna, mentioned burnt sponge and seaweed in his writings (*Parabolae*, dedicated to Philip the Fair, 1300). He was followed by Valescus de Taranta (1418) and Carlo Musitano (1635–1714), the latter using mainly burnt sponge[124]. In England, the first use of burnt sponge was the secret 'Coventry treatment' for goitre. Bradford Wilmer, a surgeon in Coventry, said that a physician named Bate administered it successfully to his daughter. The daughter's husband, a general practitioner called Keeling, then used it in his practice and so did his successors. It was mainly calcined sponge[125]. Thomas Prosser, in 1769, used calcined sponge in powder form for two weeks[126]. Jean François Coindet (1774–1834) of Geneva, is usually regarded as the first to have given iodine in the treatment of goitre[127,128]. Coindet also wrote an English version of his 'Observations on the Use of Iodine as a Remedy for

Bronchocele'[129], which was originally read to the Helvetian Physical Society on July 25, 1820. He begins:

> About a year since, when looking for a formula in the work of Cadet de Gassicourt, I found that Russell recommended the varec (fucus vesiculosus) as a remedy for bronchocele, under the name of 'aethiops vegetalis'. Not knowing what relations there might exist between this plant and sponge, I suspected, from analogy, that iodine might be the active principle common to those two substances. I tried the iodine; and the astonishing success I obtained from it, encouraged me to pursue my enquiries.

He continued to say:

> Two different causes have appeared to me to be productive of bronchocele in Geneva: the first is the use of hard waters, or the pump-water of the low streets of this city; they produce bronchocele in a very short space of time. Thus the soldiers of the garrison, principally composed of young men, strangers to the canton, on drinking those waters, become affected with it in a manner as remarkable as it is sudden. This form of the malady, rarely severe, promptly disappears of itself on the drink being changed.

The burned sponge, which had been used since the time of Arnold of Villeneuve in form of wines, lozenges, powders, etc. almost always combined with tonic medicines, "to remedy its bad effects on the stomach" will give rise,

> whatever correction be employed . . . to spasms or cramps of that organ, which often remain for a long time after the use of the medicine has been discontinued, and which in some cases become a chronic disease very difficult to cure. . . . What is the substance in the sponge that acts in a specific manner against bronchocele? It appears to me probable that it is iodine. I was confirmed in this view when I learned that Mr. Fife, of Edinburgh, had found iodine in sponge towards the end of the year 1819; when I had for six months witnessed its surprising effects in this disease.

Coindet preferred the use of 'hydriodate of potash' (KJ).

> I have used that of soda with equal success. The hydriodate of potash is a deliquescent salt, forty-eight grains of which in an ounce of distilled water represent about thirty-six grains of iodine. It is this preparation, in this dose, which I have most frequently used.

In his "tincture of iodine" he used forty-eight grains of iodine to one ounce of spirit of wine of 35°. He prescribed for adults ten drops of the tincture, in half a tumbler of 'syrup of capillaire' and water, three times a day, the dose being increased after a few weeks to 15 or even 20 drops. "In a great number of cases, [the bronchocele] subsides and is destroyed in the space of from six to ten weeks, so as to leave no trace of its existence".

Dr. Coindet thought that bronchocele is especially connected with a certain(?) state of the genital organs, from the influence of which it originates. Iodine will "in able hands, become one of the most powerful remedies, with which modern chemistry has enriched the materia medica".

William Prout (1785–1850) (see also p. 175) claimed, however, that – after taking it himself, to see if it was safe – he gave it to a patient with goitre[130] and recommended it to John Elliston (1791–1868), who used it in 1819 in St. Thomas's Hospital. Alexander Manson (1774–1840) of Nottingham read Coindet's report and used iodine in 1821 for a number of conditions, and was especially successful with goitre patients[131]. J. Inglis of Ripon recommended in 1838 a culinary salt, containing one two-thousandth part of iodine[132].

Jean Guillaume August Lugol (1786–1851), in his 'Mémoire sur l'emploi de l'iode dans les maladies scrofuleuses' (Paris, 1829), recommended Lugol's solution – an aqueous solution of iodine to which he later added iodide of potassium instead of tincture of iodine. In 1831 he received a prize of 6000 francs from the Institute de France for his book on behalf of the tuberculous.

Toxic effects of iodine

With the spread of the use of iodine, toxic effects soon appeared and Frédéric Rilliet (1814–1861) of Geneva described in his paper "Constitutional iodism"[133] (see p. 255) the danger of even small doses in the case of some people.

Surgical treatment of goitre

The surgical treatment of goitre had been mentioned by Celsus (25 BC – 50 AD) in his writings: '. . . sed scalpelli curatio brevior est'. Albucasis (1013–1106) is said to have operated for 'elephantiasis of the throat (goitre)'[134]. Pierre Joseph Desault (1744–1795), Bichat's teacher and one of the founders of vascular surgery, dissected in 1791 an adherent thyroid from the trachea[135]. Johann A. W. Hedenus (1760–1836) reported on six cases of successful excision of a goitre for impending suffocation. He published his report in 1822 (Tractatus de Glandula thyreoidea, Lipsiae), but the first of these operations was performed on 8 October, 1800. In London, Joseph Henry Green

(1791–1863) (see p. 248) removed the right lobe of the thyroid gland at St. Thomas's Hospital, the patient dying from sepsis 15 days later[136].

Luigi Porta (1800–1875), Scarpa's successor in Pavia, "initiated the enucleation of adenomas in 1849"[137], but in three patients he attempted ischaemic atrophy of the thyroid by ligating the thyroid arteries. He succeeded only in the third case by ligating both superior arteries, but the benefit was only temporary. He concluded that both the inferior and the superior thyroid artery on the same side should be ligated. Ligature of the superior thyroid arteries was also attempted before 1811, by William Blizzard (1743–1835), but the patient died from hospital gangrene[138]. H. Coates was more successful in performing the same operation in 1819[139]. He was followed by Henry Earle (1789–1823) in 1823[140] and Charles Aston Key (1793–1849)[141] on patients whom Halsted thought to have been suffering from Graves' disease.

JOHN AND WILLIAM HUNTER

The present chapter cannot be concluded without mentioning the brothers William and John Hunter and William Cumberland Cruikshank. William Hunter (1718–1783) dissected about 400 pregnant uteri, on which he based his superbly illustrated folio *An Anatomical Description of the Human Gravid Uterus Exhibited in Figures*, published in Birmingham in 1774. The text to it was published posthumously in London in 1794 as *An Anatomical Description of the Human Gravid Uterus and its Contents*. He commented in it on the corpus luteum:

> When there is only one child, there is only one corpus luteum, and two in the case of twins. . . . in some of these cases there were two distinct corpora lutea in one ovarium.

John Hunter (1728–1793) (see Section II) was, in fact, one of the most versatile medical geniuses: anatomist, experimental physiologist, ardent and successful collector for his museum of comparative anatomy, biologist, army surgeon and general surgeon, dental physiologist and dental surgeon, interested in hospital administration and many more things. There are many biographies in the form of papers, books, and, indeed, of a novel, which try to do justice to the monumental work of this restless genius; one of the fairly recent, excellent ones, is by Miss Jessie Dobson, for many years Curator of the Hunterian Museum at the Royal College of Surgeons in London[142]. John Hunter was attracted by problems which were posed by puzzles of nature. It is perhaps not surprising, therefore, that some of those problems were in the field of endocrinology.

John Hunter and Berthold's transplant experiments

The Danish writer C. Barker Jørgensen published an important paper in 1971: 'John Hunter, A. A. Berthold and the origins of endocrinology'[143]. It deals with some of John Hunter's and A. A. Berthold's transplantation experiments and some other puzzles, such as 'Pigeon's milk', the 'Free-martin', 'Effect of gonads on sexual behaviour', etc. Jørgensen says in his 'Introduction':

> The techniques of extirpating and transplanting organs became important tools early in experimental endocrinology. . . . If symptoms produced by extirpation of an organ could be prevented by transplanting the organ to a site remote from its original place in the body, this was considered strongly to indicate that the organ exerts its function by means of an internal secretion, a hormone, given off to the blood. Quite naturally, therefore, students of the history of endocrinology have been interested in early experiments on transplantation of endocrine organs. Two men came into focus, John Hunter (1728–1793) and Arnold Adolf Berthold (1803–1861): Hunter because he performed the first successful transplantation of testis, and Berthold because he interpreted the results of such transplantations which, in his view, suggested that the testes maintain the male secondary sex characters through their action on the blood.
>
> Despite the central position of Hunter's and Berthold's transplantation experiments in the history of endocrinology, their work and its background are still incompletely understood. The present paper aims at elucidating the place of Hunter and Berthold in the history of endocrinology by considering their work in relation to contemporary knowledge and concepts of the integrative mechanisms of the body. That the organism and its parts function as a harmonious whole, which attempts to maintain its integrity in a changing environment, such a holistic view has been in existence with varied intensity since antiquity. At the time of Hunter, these functional correlations were usually called 'consensus' or 'sympathy'. Hunter talked of 'universal sympathy', where the whole organism sympathizes with some action of a part. By 'partial sympathy', he meant, when distinct parts sympathized with some local action or sensation[144].

Hunter subdivided 'partial sympathy' into three kinds:

the remote, the contiguous and the continuous. The remote sympathy is, where there is no visible connection of parts that can account for such effects, e.g. pain in the shoulder as a result of inflammation of the liver.

the contiguous sympathy is that which appears to have no other connection that arises from the contact of separate parts,

e.g. stomach and intestines sympathize with the integument of the abdomen.

The continuous sympathy is where there is no interruption of parts, and the sympathy runs or is continued along from the irritating point as from a centre . . .: an example of it we have in the spreading of inflammation.[143]

The sympathies of special interest are those between the gonads and secondary sex characters. These were already known to Aristotle, when he reported on the effects of castration and spaying in man and animals (see p. 50) (in De Generatione Animalium and Historia Animalium). Hunter remarked that sex characters "depend upon the effects that the ovaria and testicles have upon the constitution". The sympathies between the gonads and their target organs belong to the 'remote sympathies'. Jørgensen says: "Today we distinguish only between two types of mechanisms of sympathy between remote parts of the body, the nervous and the humoral mechanism"[143]. Especially the sympathy between the testes and secondary sex characteristics of the male became some of the best examples of interaction between the parts of the organism (remote sympathy). It must be particularly noted that the re-absorption of sperm from the testicle was held important for maintaining the male secondary sex characteristics[145–147]. In Hunter's days, however, there were fundamental differences in the concepts of the above-mentioned mechanisms. Nerves were still regarded as pipes, carrying fluids into the organs they innervated; they were, therefore, not entirely distinguished from the blood-vessels in their method of function (see also Wharton's Adenographia, where he entertains a similar notion; see p. 131). Nor was there a sharp dividing line between the nerves and the humoral mechanism. There were also the newly-studied physical forces which also 'flow', especially electricity and magnetism. In addition to all that, there was the all important vital force, living principle or spirits, which were also supposed to be capable of acting directly through and on the body tissues. John Hunter's main experiments in this field concerned the transplantation of the testes of cocks to the belly of hens[148]. Hunter made, however, experiments on other subjects, which were later to appear as important contributions to endocrinology.

Experiments with endocrine results

In his paper on 'vesiculae seminales', Hunter concluded that "It is reasonable to infer that the use of the vesiculae in the animal oeconomy must, in common with many other parts, be dependent on the testicles"[149]. This was proved by the effects of castration, especially in young individuals. Removal of only one testis showed that both vesiculae seminales remained of normal size in man and animals. Hunter also noticed that castration prevented the re-growth of antlers in stags. This later became a subject of study by Berthold. Strangely enough, these and the following experiments by Hunter seem to have escaped the attention of F. G. Young in his important contribution 'Ideas about animal hormones' to *The Chemistry of Life*, edited by Joseph Needham (1970).

Burrows referred to Hunter's experiments on transplantation of spurs in fowl as "the earliest recorded experiments in endocrinology"[150]. They showed that the spur of a hen would grow to the size of a cock spur, if transplanted to a cock; the small spur of a young cock, on the other hand, would not grow if transplanted to a hen.

The effect of removing one ovary

In a further paper in *The Observations on Certain Parts of the Animal Oeconomy*[149], Hunter discussed 'The effect of extirpating one ovarium upon the number of the young produced'[151]. He carried out the experiment in pigs as being the most easily managed, and producing several at a litter and breeding perfectly well under the confinement necessary for experiments.

He selected two females of the same size and one male, all litter mates. The result was that the spayed animal produced 76 young in eight farrows, and then it stopped breeding. The normal sister produced 87 young in the first eight farrows; however, it continued breeding and had another five farrows, producing altogether 162 young. Hunter's conclusion was:

> That the constitution at large has no power of giving the one ovarium the power of propagating equal to both. . . . But that the constitution has so far a power of influencing one ovarium as to make it produce its number in a less time than would probably have been the case if both ovaria had been preserved . . .

Hunter also found that unilateral oophorectomy in the sow did not prevent twinning.

Jørgensen comments (p. 12): "What this 'power of the constitution' stands for is today a central problem in endocrinology and continues to be a matter of discussion". (See Refs. 152, 153.)

Anne McLaren remarked:

When one ovary of a mouse is removed, the number of eggs shed by the female does not diminish, since the ovulation rate of the remaining ovary doubles. The increased stimulus to the single ovary might come (1) from compensatory growth of the organ, enabling it to take up more follicle-stimulating hormone (FSH) from the blood in a given time, or (2) from a compensatory increase in FSH output from the pituitary, or (3) from consumption by the remaining ovary of an increased proportion of the circulating FSH. The experiments described below support the third of these alternatives. A twofold increase in ovulation rate by the remaining ovary was already apparent 3 days after removal of its partner[153].

Three years later, however (in 1969), Benson, Sorrentino and Evans wrote:

It has been suggested that increased gonadotrophin secretion follows unilateral ovarian removal and leads, *a priori*, to the compensatory hypertrophy of the remaining ovary. Recent studies have failed to substantiate this increase, possibly because the techniques employed were insufficiently sensitive to determine the subtle alterations in gonadotrophin levels. . . . It is postulated that the increase in serum FSH following unilateral ovariectomy results from a decrease in circulating ovarian hormones which partially releases the hypothalamico-hypophyseal system from feedback inhibition. As the remaining ovary hypertrophies and is stimulated to secrete these hormones, the level of inhibition is restored and serum FSH returns to preoperative levels. Our hypothesis is that an increase in FSH secretion is an important component in the mechanism of compensatory hypertrophy. . . .[152]

It should be made clear at this point that Hunter's transplant experiments of the spurs in fowl and of the testes in cocks (to follow), were intended to study the 'vital principle', assumed to be responsible for the union of the graft with the host, and for the survival and growth of the graft. This 'vital principle' was supposed to work independently of the nervous system and humoral mechanisms acting as integrating factors in the body. These experiments were, therefore, not carried out with any underlying endocrine speculations, the knowledge of which did not exist in a clear-cut manner; they happened to fit – subconsciously, as it were – into the endocrine framework of a later era. Nor did Hunter's contemporaries understand or appreciate the great importance of his experiments.

Other observations, such as compensatory hypertrophy of testicular tissue in incompletely castrated young cocks (published long after his death, in 1861)[154] and the masculinization of old female birds[149], were not followed up.

'Pigeon's milk' (and prolactin)

Similarly, Hunter's discovery that 'pigeon's milk', i.e. a substance secreted by the parents, female *and* male, to feed the young pigeon, is secreted by the crop, and the crop behaves like "The udder of females of the class Mammalia in the term of uterine gestation". He called the substance "curd, . . . as resembling that more than anything I know"[155]. It was not until 1933 that Oscar Riddle identified the pituitary hormone controlling the secretion of 'pigeon's milk' as prolactin, which also controls milk secretion in mammals[156]; pigeon's milk has also played an important role in establishing a bio-assay for prolactin[157]. Incidentally, in 1786 John Hunter knew of the atrophy of the prostate in man, after castration.

An eye-witness account of Hunter's experiments

The *Lancet* of February 18, 1928 published a letter of Dr. W. Irvine in London to Professor Thomas Hamilton, University of Glasgow, of June 17, 1771. The publication was entitled: 'John Hunter's Experiments: Evidence of an Eye-Witness'[158]. At that time, John Hunter was in his forty-fourth year and had been surgeon to St. George's Hospital for three years. Dr. Irvine and Professor Thomas Hamilton had both been students of Dr. William Hunter. In his letter, Dr. Irvine writes:

> The cutting of spurs from the heel of a cock and making them grow in his head, J. Hunter has often performed and has such cocks at present. Nay more, he has many hens just now into whose abdomen, when young, he has put the testis of a cock just separated from his body and this testis has got blood vessels and nerves from the part of the abdomen or viscera to which it is applied; has increased in size, yields a white liquor when it is cut into, but has not, as he had imagined, impregnated their ova nor altered their natural disposition.

In a footnote to the letter, it is said: the sole record of these experiments is a brief paragraph in John Hunter's lecture (Vol. i, p. 391, Palmer's *Life of Hunter*, 1837). This passage runs: "Here is the testicle of a cock, separated from that animal and put through a wound made for that purpose, into the belly of a hen, which mode of turning hens into cocks is much such an improvement for its utility as that of Dean Swift when he proposed to obtain a breed of sheep without wool". Did Hunter ultimately find that the disposition of these engrafted hens did become changed? The extract from his lectures (1792) seems to suggest he did. Berthold of Goettingen (1849) is usually supposed to have been the first to transplant with success the genital glands of fowls.

Another passage from Dr. Irvine's letter reads:

> Not to bore you I will mention one other thing out of a great number – Viz. male animals of the more imperfect kind have small testes in the winter and a very large in Breeding time. Mr. Hunter has preserved six male sparrows, killed betwixt December and the middle of April. The one killed in December has testes not bigger than a small pin's head, the rest are gradually larger, the testes of the last, killed in April, are as large each as the top of your little finger. Same in frogs; remarkable in the skate which in winter is not half-an-ounce and in summer near half-a-pound . . . He (Hunter) begs leave to add to your stock of facts some which he has found by his own experiments. A cow, free of her milk, after being in case, kept from the bull, has a show of blood every month after that, and frequently external. He has observed the same in deer, bitches, monkeys, etc . . ." . . .

These observations on the influence of warmth and light on the development of the growth of gonads of sparrows, frogs and the skate are well ahead of his time. Jørgensen points out that W. Rowan, in his pioneer studies 'on photoperiodism, reproductive periodicity, and the annual migrations of birds and certain fishes, in 1926'[154] "refers to R. Owen (1866) concerning the observation that, in birds, testicular development precedes migration and breeding; he was in fact referring to Hunter's findings on the English sparrow 150 years previously; Owen (1866) cited Owen (1836)[159,160] who reproduced Hunter's pictures of five pairs of sparrow testes taken at intervals from January to the middle of April". The testes of six male sparrows, killed by Hunter between December and the middle of April to demonstrate the gradual increase in size, are still in the Museum of the Royal College of Surgeons in London. Hunter's opinion on the effect of gonads on sexual behaviour is expressed in a posthumous essay[161]:

> Let us take a testicle from a cock and put it into the belly of a gander. If it was possible that the ducts could unite so as to carry the seed that was secreted in that testicle to the female, the produce would be the same as if a cock had trod the goose; so that the powers of the testicle would remain the same as if they had never been transplanted, and would continue to secrete the same kind of semen. The inclinations would not be towards the hen but towards the goose; for, although the testicles are the cause of inclinations, yet they do not direct these inclinations: the inclinations become an operation of the mind, after the mind is once stimulated by the testicle.

The freemartin

Hunter was extremely interested in the problem of the bovine freemartin. In 1786 he wrote an 'Account of the free-martin': "It is a fact known and I believe almost universally understood, that when a cow brings forth two calves, and one of them a bull-calf, and the other to appearance a cow, that the cow-calf is unfit for propagation; but the bull-calf becomes a very proper bull". He "eagerly fought for the opportunity to see and examine a free-martin", but his anatomical studies of three such cases did not get him nearer to a solution[149]. The word 'freemartin' is probably a corruption of the words 'ferry', i.e. a cow that is not in milk, and 'martin', being a spayed

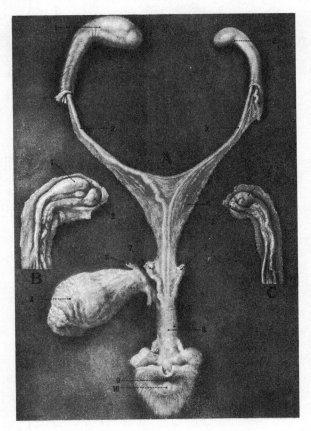

Figure 35 Lillie's classical drawing of the reproductive tract of a freemartin cow: (A) 1 and 2: scrotal testes; 3: vas deferens; 4: broad ligament; 5: ureter; 6: bladder; 7: seminal vesicle; 8: vagina; 9: vulva; 10: clitoris. (B and C) 1: testis; 2: epididymis

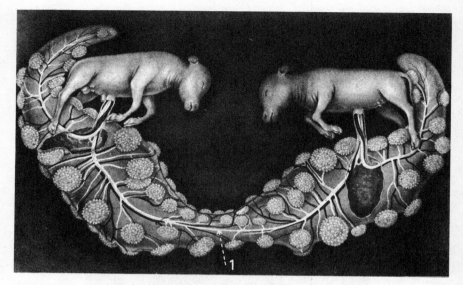

Figure 36 Lillie's drawing of the anastomosing blood vessels connecting the placental circulation of a male and a female bovine foetus

or barren animal killed for food at Martinmas[162,163]. Freemartins are always sterile; they have female external genitalia with little or no evidence of masculinization but, internally, the gonads are hypoplastic and usually contain testicular tissue. "The Fallopian tubes and uterus are poorly developed or even absent, and seminal vesicles, vasa deferentia, and epididymides are usually present"[162]. It occurs in about 90% of opposite-sexed twins in cattle, but only rarely in sheep, goats and pigs. The Viennese anatomists Julius Tandler and K. Keller were, in 1911, the first to appreciate that the condition only occurred when opposite-sexed twins shared a common placental circulation[164]; placental vascular anastomoses are rare in sheep, goats and pigs. In horse, twin pregnancy is rare and usually ends in the death and resorption of one or both of the embryos[165].

Frank Rattray Lillie (1870–1947) in 1916[166] and 1917[167] came to the conclusion that the cow-foetus must have been masculinized by the sex hormones produced by the testes of the bull-twin. Although many people still accept Lillie's explanation, including apparently Jørgensen, it all depends on "what is meant by 'sex hormones'", as R. V. Short points out[168]. He also stresses that the administration of androgens to the female foetus has no effect on the normal course of development of her ovaries. "It seems unlikely, therefore, that the male twin's androgens are responsible for the freemartin's ovarian hypoplasia." As germ cell sex is uniquely a phenomenon occurring in mammals, perhaps to protect the sexuality of the foetus *in utero* from interference by maternal sex hormones, but also from placental ones of possible neighbouring foetuses, Short suggests that "some factor must pass from the male to the female foetus to cause the development of medullary cords in the ovary, and there is also a suggestion that something may pass from female to male, since a number of bulls born co-twin to freemartins become relatively infertile or completely sterile in later life"[169]. Ohno *et al.* first proposed in 1962 that germ cells might be exchanged between the conjoined twins, and recently there has been more indirect evidence to support this view[169]. Short maintains, however, that even if XX-germ cells can successfully migrate into the testis, there has been no evidence of such XX-cells completing meiosis there[170]. Studies of the progeny even of like-sexed twins have failed to prove any evidence of germ cell exchange.

The gonads of the freemartin itself often contain medullary cords[170,171], which may be populated by germ cells during foetal life, but the germ cells all disappear from the medulla by the time of birth. This seems yet another example of the failure of XX-germ cells to survive in an environment of compatible genotype but incompatible phenotype, since the freemartin gonad secretes testosterone[170]: this seems further confirmation of the fact that an XX-testis can produce androgens in the absence of a Y-chromosome.

In a special paper, 'The bovine freemartin: a new look at an old problem', R. V. Short discusses John Hunter's original study[172]. Characteristically, Short's paper was published in the *Philosophical Transactions of the Royal Society of London* (Series Biology), in 1970, the same as Hunter's 191 years before! In it, Short reproduced a drawing by William Bell from John Hunter's dissection of a certain Mr. Wright's 'freemartin', the specimen of which can still be seen in the Hunterian Museum of the Royal College of Surgeons, Lincolns Inn Fields, London, in an excellent state of preservation. As the gonads were clearly testicular in appearance and "more than twenty times larger than the ovaria of the cow, and nearly as large as the testicles of the bull" (Hunter), Short concludes that the animal cannot have been a freemartin, as "the gonads of true freemartins . . . are always small and atrophic, even though they may take on the morphological appearance of testes"[173]. Moreover, there was no history of this particular animal having been born co-twin to a bull. The large intra-abdominal testes of Mr. Wright's animal were examined histologically by Berry Hart in 1910 and, more recently, by J. J. S. Stewart; there were almost no other signs of masculinization.

There was nothing similar to the vasa deferentia. . . . As the external parts had more of the cow than the bull, the clytoris, which may also be reckoned an external part, was also similar to that of the cow. . . . Although I call these bodies testicles for the reasons given, yet they were only imitations of such. . . .[172]

But even though the testes had failed to stimulate the development of Wolffian duct derivatives, they had certainly succeeded in inhibiting the development of the Muellerian ducts, for "the vagina terminated in a blind end, and a little way beyond the opening of the urethra, beyond which the vagina and uterus were impervious" (Hunter). Short points out that true freemartins, such as the one Hunter obtained from a Mr. Arbuthnot, dissected and also had drawn by Mr. Bell, "invariably show some signs of masculinization; if the gonads have become testicular in appearance, the internal genitalia may show extensive masculinization and the clitoris may also have hypertrophied". On Hunter's first case (supplied by Mr. Wright), Short has this to say: ". . . there can be little doubt, that in his search for freemartins he had unwittingly stumbled across the first recorded case of testicular feminization"[173]. It is a tribute to his

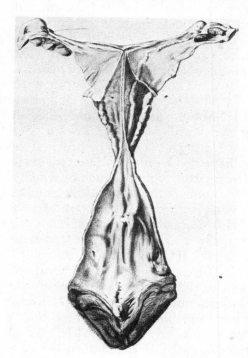

Figure 37 Mr Arbuthnot's freemartin

industry and meticulous attention to detail that we are able to give him full credit for this discovery, almost 200 years after the event.

Testicular feminization is well recognized in man: the individuals affected are genetically male (XY) and develop normal testicles, but become phenotypic females (with aplasia of the uterus), because the tissue of the target organ does not seem to respond to androgens. It has been assumed that this target organ defect may be due to the inability of the tissues to convert the secreted testosterone into its androgenically active metabolite, 5-alphadihydrotestosterone, which in normal individuals occurs preferentially in some target organs, but not in testicular feminization patients[172].

Short comes to the 'humbling' conclusion "that the true explanation of the condition continues to elude us . . . we still do not know what produces the gonadal sex-reversal in the first place[173]. . . . With the hormonal theory (proposed by Tandler and Keller[164] and Lillie[166]), untenable, and the cellular theory (Fechheimer, Herschler and Gilmore[172], and Goodfellow, Strong and Stewart[172]), unproven, what other alternatives are there to explain the freemartin condition?[174] . . . . The basic defect must be looked upon as the retention of medullary tissue in an XX gonad. The most likely reason for this would seem to be that male gonadal inductor substance has leaked across into the female's circulation via the placental anastomosis and interfered with ovarian development. Perhaps there is also a female gonadal inductor substance which could interfere with gonadal development in the male twin. There are a number of facts that argue against such an inductor substance hypothesis; the normal development of the chimaeric female marmoset is one of them . . . therefore it may be helpful to re-define the (freemartin) problem. It is essentially a question of the transfer of genetic information from a male to a female individual. More specifically, we must seek to explain how information, coded in the Y chromosome of a few cells in the genital ridge of a male foetus, is transferred to cells in the genital ridge of a female foetus. The problem becomes simpler if we accept Hamerton's thesis[175] that all the male-determining genes are in fact located on the X chromosome, and so are present, but latent, in normal female individuals. The Y chromosome of the male is postulated to act merely as a controlling centre, 'switching on' the male-determining genes of the X chromosome. In man, dizygotic twins almost invariably have separate placental circulations, even though there is gross fusion of the two placentae in about 40% of pregnancies.

Nevertheless there are on record three well-documented cases of opposite-sexed human twins with XX/XY blood chimerism, suggesting that foetal vascular anastomoses had developed. The girls showed no evidence of reproductive abnormalities, and in one instance both twins subsequently proved to be fertile[176].

Perhaps the anastomoses develop too late in gestation to interfere with the development of the reproductive tract.

Hunter's transplantation of the cock testis

There is no detailed report on these experiments, only hints, spread in Hunter's own writings and in those of his friends (see also Dr. Irvine's letter, p. 197). As we have seen, Hunter did consider the possible effect of the testis (of cocks) on secondary sex characteristics and sexual behaviour after transplantation into a hen. If he expected an almost complete reversal of sex in the case of a successful graft, he must have felt disappointed. It was not until 1924 that Pézard and co-workers showed that hens with functional testicular grafts develop combs and wattles as in the cock, but the spurs and plumage remain female[172].

Autotransplants of a cock's testicle into his own belly were also carried out by Hunter and the testicle adhered there and was nourished. This was reported, curiously enough, in his treatise on *The Natural History of Human Teeth* (London, 1771); but Hunter was especially interested in the powers of the union of the transplant and tissue into which it was grafted:

> By it the spurs of a young cock can be made to grow on his comb. . . .
> Teeth, after having been drawn and inserted into the sockets of another person, unite in the new socket, which is called transplanting; ingrafting and inoculation of trees succeed upon the same principle.

John Hunter performed his transplantation experiments to elucidate the properties of the 'vital principle'. He did not carry them out to study the action of the testes on secondary sex characters, nor to establish a clear concept of a humoral or hormonal or neuro-humoral mechanism. "He may have been satisfied when referring to the sympathies of the testis being exerted by the vital principle that he believed to pervade the organism"[178]. His preparations showing a tooth inserted into the cock's comb can still be seen at the Hunterian Museum of the Royal College of Surgeons[179]. Transplantation without the knowledge of bacteriology and its role in inflammation, of oxygen deficiency leading to atrophy of the transplant, and of immunological host reactions, is extremely difficult. It is surprising, therefore, that even a small number of such attempts was partially successful. In the years before Arnold Berthold's experiments, the

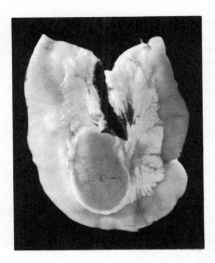

Figure 38 Cock testis transplanted by Hunter to the abdomen of a hen [Hunterian Museum]

causal influence of the gonads on the development of secondary sex characteristics was accepted without any attempts being made to elucidate functional interrelations. In the next chapter, "The Birth of Endocrinology", we shall have to begin, therefore, with the experiments of Adolf Berthold (1803–1861). However, we must mention here that, in 1799, Sir Everard Home (1756–1832) recorded that John Hunter had suggested artificial insemination in 1790. An actual (successful) artificial insemination was performed on Hunter's advice on a woman, whose husband had a hypospadias, by the husband using a syringe[180].

We conclude the present chapter with a brief note on William Cumberland Cruikshank's (1745–1800) experiments to discover the movements of the ova of rabbits. Cruikshank had been William Hunter's assistant and was Dr. Johnson's physician. The problem had been posed by William Harvey's observations in deer, that for a period of time after mating, there was no sign of any conceptus in the uterus. Cruikshank showed in rabbits that there was an interval following mating, when the fertilized ova were to be found in the Fallopian tubes. Later they would move into the uterus and there implant. His experiments were strongly encouraged by Dr. William Hunter, with whom he had discussed the problem as early as 1778.

1st.   The ovum is formed in, and comes out of the ovarium after conception.

2ndly.   It passes down the fallopian tube, and is some days in coming through it.

3rdly.   It is sometimes detained in the fallopian tube, and prevented from getting into the uterus.

4thly.   De Graaf saw one ovum only in the fallopian tube, 'in oviductus dextri medio unum!' I saw thirteen in one instance, five in another, seven in another, and three in another, in all twentyeight.

5thly.   The ovum comes into the uterus on the 4th day[181].

REFERENCES

1. Rolleston, Sir Humphry D.: The Endocrine Organs in Health and Disease, p. 16. Oxford University Press, 1936.
2. Bordeu, Théophile de: Recherches sur les Maladies Chroniques. VI. Analyse médicinale du sang. pp. 379, 382. Paris, Ruault, 1775.
3. Bordeu, Théophile de: Recherches Anatomiques sur la Position des Glandes et leur Action, pp. 142–144. Paris, G. F. Quillau, 1751.
4. ibid.: p. 161.
5. ibid.: p. 163.
6. ibid.: pp. 231, 232.
7. ibid.: pp. 398–399.
8. Neuburger, M.: Théophile de Bordeu als Varläufer der Lehre vou der iunereu Sekretion. Wien. Klin. Wschr. No. 39, 1367, 1911.
9. Biedl, A., Lehrbuch der Inneren Sekretion. Berlin and Vienna, 1910.
10. Richerand: Oeuvres Complètes de Bordeu, Paris, 1818, Tome premier, p. VII.
11. Henderson, J. R.: The Pancreas: Endocrine and Exocrine Functions. Chapter 1. Historical Introduction. p. 4. (unpublished).
12. Haller, Albrecht von: Bibliotheca Medicinae Practicae. 4 vols. Basle and Berne, 1776–88.
13. Haller, Albrecht von: Elementa physiologiae corporis humani. 8 vols. Lausanne, Berne, 1757–66.
14. Iason, A. H.: The Thyroid Gland in Medical History, p. 60. New York, Froben Press, 1946.
15. As 13: Vol. VIII, p. 30.
16. Meckel, Johann Friedrich, the younger: Tabulae anatomico-pathologicae. 4 parts, Lipsiae, I. F. Gleditsch, 1817–26.
17. Geoffroy Saint-Hilaire, Étienne, and Cuvier, Frédéric: Histoire naturelle des mammifères. 4 vols. Paris, Belin & Blaise, 1824–42.
18. Heister, Lorenz: Chirurgie, in welcher alles, was zur Wund-Artzney gehöret, nach der neuesten und besten Art. Nuernberg, J. Hoffman, 1718. (English translation: London, 1742.)
19. Vercelloni, J.: De Glandulis Oesophagi Conglomeratis. Asti, 1711.
20. Morgagni, Giovanni B.: De sedibus, et causis morborum per anatomen indagatis libri quinque. 2 vols. Venetiis, 1761.
21. Iason, A. H.: as 14: pp. 66–67.
22. Flajani, Giuseppe: Collezione d'osservazioni e riflessioni di chirurgia, Vol 3, pp. 270–273. Roma, 1802.
23. As 14, pp. 67–69.

24. As 14: pp. 62–64.
25. Lieutaud, J.: Précis de la médecine prat. Paris, 1759.
26. Zuckerman, Sir Solly: Lancet 1, 739–743, 789–795, 1954.
27. Lieutaud, J.: Essais Anatomiques, contenant l'histoire exact de toutes les parties qui composent le corps de l'homme, avec la manière de dissequer. Paris, Huart, 1742.
28. As 3: paragraph XXXVIII. Du corps qu'on nomme communement Glande pituitaire. pp. 141–146.
29. Henderson, J. R. and Daniel, P. M. Portal circulations and their relations to countercurrent systems. Q. J. Exp. Physiol. 63, 355–369, 1978.
30. Popa, G. T. and Fielding, U.: The vascular link between the pituitary and the hypothalamus. Lancet 2, 238–240, 1930.
31. As 14: p. 70.
32. As 14: p. 71.
33. Cooper, A. P.: Observations on the Structure and Diseases of the Testis. London, Long, Rees, Orme, Brown & Green, 1830.
34. As 14: p. 61.
35. As 1: p. 160.
36. As 14: p. 72.
37. CIBA Monographs, Number 10. The Development of Clinical Endocrinology. By R. Abderhalden. p. 309. Bombay, July 1951.
38. Garrison, F. H.: An Introduction to the History of Medicine. 4th ed., p. 334. Philadelphia, W. B. Saunders, 1929.
39. Burdach, E.: Beitrag zur mikroskopischen Anatomie der Nerven. Koenigsberg, 1837.
40. Vieussens, R.: Novum Vasorum Corporis Humani Systema. p. 242. Amsterdam 1705.
41. Baillie, M.: The Morbid Anatomy of some of the most Important Parts of the Human Body. 2nd ed., p. 451. London, 1797.
42. Petit, J. L.: Mem. Acad. R. Soc, Paris. p. 99, 1718.
43. Hedlund, T. H.: Års.-Berrätt. om Svens. Läk.-Sjukh. I., p. 20, Stockholm, 1833.
44. Frank, J. P.: De curandis hominum morbis epitome. Liber V, pp. 38–67. Mannheim, 1794.
45. Ettmueller, M. E.: Chemia experimentalis atque rationalis curiosa. edidit Aussfeld, 1684.
46. Latham, John: Facts and Opinions Concerning Diabetes. 1811.
47. Home, F.: Clinical Experiments. Edinburgh, 1780.
48. Papaspyros, N. S.: The History of Diabetes Mellitus, p. 16. London, 1952.
49. Cullen, W.: First Lines of the Practice of Physic. Edinburgh, 1787.
50. Dobson, Matthew: Experiments and observations on the urine in diabetes. Medical Observations and Inquiries by the Society of Physicians, Vol. V, p. 259, London, 1776.
51. Garrod, Sir Archibald: Trans. Med. Soc. Lond. p. 113, 1912.
52. Chevreul, E.: Note sur le sucre de diabètes. Ann. Chem. 95, 319–320, Paris, 1815.
53. Cawley, Thomas: A singular case of diabetes, consisting entirely in the quality of the urine; with an inquiry into the different theories of that disease. Lond. Med. J. 9, 286–308, 1788.
54. Recklinghausen, Friedrich von: Virch. Arch. XXX, p. 360, 1864.
55. Lancereaux, E.: Notes et reflexions à propos de 2 cas de diabète sucré avec altération du pancréas. Bull. Acad. Med. Paris, 2 sér., 6, 1215–1240, 1877.
56. Bright, Richard: Reports on Medical Cases Selected with a View of Illustrat-

ing the Symptoms and Cure of Diseases by a Reference to Morbid Anatomy, Vol. II, p. 262, London, Longman, 1827–31.
57. Bouchardat, Apollinaire: Mém. Acad. R Méd., Paris, XVI, 165, 1852.
58. Bouchardat, A.: De La Glycosurie ou Diabète Sucré; son Traitement Hygiènique. Paris, Germer-Baillière, 1875.
59. Frerichs, F. T. von: Ueber den Diabetes. Berlin, 1884.
60. As 1: p. 433.
61. Rollo, J.: Account of Two Cases of Diabetes Mellitus with Remarks as they Arose During the Progress of the Cure. London, C. Dilly, 1797.
62. Haugsted, F. C.: Thymi in Homine ac per Seriem Animalium, Hafniae, 1831.
63. As 37: p. 315.
64. As 37: p. 315.
65. Muller, W. H.: Exercitatio Anatomica de Thymo. Leyden, 1706.
66. Senac, J. B.: Traité de la Structure de Coeur, de son Action, et de ses Maladies. Vol. II, p. 687, Paris, 1749.
67. As 1: p. 440.
68. Kopp, J. H.: Denkwuerdigkeiten in der aerztlichen Praxis, Vol. I, p. 1, Frankfurt am Main, 1830.
69. Cooper, A. P.: The Anatomy of the Thymus Gland. London, Longman, Rees, Orme, Green and Brown, 1832.
70. Pozzi, G. I.: Commerciolum Epistolicum. Bologna, D. Petro Paulo Molinetto, 1732.
71. Hewson, Wm.: Philos. Trans. R. Soc., London, LXIII, 303, 1773.
72. Schenk, J. T.: Schola Partium Humani Corporis, p. 127. Jena, 1664.
73. Collins, S.: A System of Anatomy, p. 699. London, 1685.
74. Glisson, F.: Anatomia Hepatis, p. 443. London, 1654.
75. Charleton, W.: Excercitationes physico-anatomicae de economia animali, London, 1659.
76. Dionis, Pierre: L'anatomie de l'Homme, Paris, 1716.
77. Bellinger, F.: Tractus de Foetu Nutrito, London, 1717.
78. Caldani, F.: Nuovi Elementi di Anatomia, Naples, 1825.
79. Shumacker, Harris B.: The Early History of the Adrenal Glands. Bull. Inst. Hist. Med. **4,** 39–46, 1936.
80. Bell, John and Bell, Sir Charles: The Anatomy and Physiology of the Human Body, Vol 3, p. 354. London, 1829.
81. Coxe, J. R.: On the functions of the capsulae renales. Ann. J. Med. Sci. I, 40–49, 1827–28.
82. As 73: Book 1, Part 3, Chap. 21, pp. 472–473.
83. As 79: p. 41.
84. Goodsir, J.: On the supra-renal, thymus and thyroid bodies. Philos. Trans. R. Soc. **136,** 633–641, 1846.
85. As 79: p. 55.
86. Castellani, Carlo: Spermatozoan Biology from Leeuwenhoek to Spallanzani. J. Hist. Biol. **6,** No. 1, 37–68, 1975.
87. Buffon, G. L. L.: Histoire Naturelle, 44 Vols. Paris, 1749–1804.
88. Cole, F. J.: Early Theories on Sexual Generation, p. 183. Oxford University Press, 1930.
89. Needham, J. T.: An Account of Some New Microscopical Discoveries . . ., London, 1745.
90. Needham, J. T.: Observations upon the Generation, Composition and Decomposition . . . London, 1749.
91. As 87: p. 425.
92. As 87: p. 428.

93. As 86: p. 53.
94. As 87: p. 450.
95. Spallanzani, L.: Saggio di Osservazioni Microscopiche sul Sistema della Generazione de' Sigg. Needham e Buffon, in Dissertazioni due dell, Abate Spallanzani . . . Modena, 1765.
96. Needham, J. T.: Nouvelles Recherches sur les Dècouvertes Microscopiques et la Génération des Corps Organisès. Paris, 1769.
97. Spallanzani, L.: Lettres à M. L'Abbé Spallanzani (Ed. Castellani, C.) Milan, Episteme Editrice, 1971.
98. Spallanzani, L.: Epistolario (Ed. Biagi, B., Prondi, D.) Vol. I, letter No. 190, p. 302. Florence, 1958–64.
99. Spallanzani, L.: Osservazioni e sperienze intorno ai Vermicelli Spermatici in Opuscoli di Fisica Animale e Vegetabile, Modena, 1776.
100. Bracegirdle, B.: The performance of 17th and 18th century microscopes. Med. Hist. **22,** No. 4, 1978.
101. As 99: pp. 87–88.
102. As 99: p. 37.
103. Linnaeus, Carl von: (Linné, C.) Generatio Ambinega, p. 5. Upsala, 1759. (Transl. D. L. Hall.)
104. As 99, pp. 59–60.
105. As 99, p. 65.
106. As 99, p. 75.
107. Sandler, Iris: The Re-examination of Spallanzani's Interpretation of the Role of the Spermatic Animalcules in Fertilization. J. Hist. Biol. **6,** No. 1, pp. 193–223, 1973.
108. Fabricius de Aquapendente: De Formatione Ovi et Pulli Patavii ex. off. A. Bencÿ, 1621.
109. Harvey, Wm.: The Works of: Translated from the Latin, with a Life of the Author. By Robert Willis, M.D. London. Sydenham Society, 1847. p. 575: On Conception.
110. Bonnet, Charles: Considérations sur le corps organisés, in: Oeuvres D'histoire naturelle et de philosophie de Charles Bonnet; p. 363. Amsterdam, M. M. Rey, 1779.
111. Spallanzani, Lazzaro: Dissertazioni di Fisica Animale e Vegetabile. Vol. I (on gastric juice and action of saliva). Volume II. Part I: Della generazione di alcuni animali amfibi (On the generation of amphibians); Part II: Sopra la fecondazione artificiale in alcuni animali (Concerning the Artificial Fertilization of Certain Animals). Modena, Presso las Societá Tipografica 1780. (English translation in 1784). Dissertations Relative to the Natural History of Animals and Vegetables. Engl. version, Vol. II, Part I, Chap. i, p. 10.
112. ibid.: Part I, Chap. i, p. 14; Part II, Chap. i, p. 145.
113. Darlington, C. D.: Genetics and Man, p. 40. London, Allen & Unwin, 1964.
114. Spallanzani, L.: Dissertazioni, Part II, p. 202.
115. Spallanzani, Lazzaro: Fecondazione Artificiale, pp. 129–134. In: Prodromo Della Nuova Enciclopedia Italiana. Siena, 1779.
116. Koelliker, R. A. von: Ueber das Wesen der Sogenannten Samenthiere. N. Notiz., a.d. Gebiete der Natur und Heilkunde. Vol. **19,** pp. 4–8, Weimar, 1841.
117. Baer, E. von: De Ovi Mammalium et Hominis Genesi. Lipsiae, L. Vossius, 1827.
118. Baer, E. von: Ueber Entwicklungsgeschichte der Tiere, 3 volumes, Koenigsberg, Borntraegen, 1828–88.

119. Morgani, G. B.: De Sedibus and causis morborum. Epistola XLIV, 29, Venetiis, 1761.
120. Gosselin, L.: Arch. Gén. Méd. 4s., **XVI**, 24, 1848.
121. Davy, Sir Humphry: Philos. Trans. R. Soc. London, **104,** pp. 74, 587, 1814.
122. Gay-Lussac, L. J.: Mémoirs d'Iodide, Paris, 1814.
123. Courtois, Clement, Desormes: Ann. Chim. Paris **88,** 304–310, 1813.
124. Musitano, C.: Chirurgia Theoretica-Practica. Koeln, 1698.
125. Wilmer, Bradford: Cases and Remarks in Surgery; to which is subjoined, an appendix, containing the method of curing the bronchocele in Coventry. London, 1779.
126. Prosser, T.: An Account and Method of Cure of the Bronchocele or Derby Neck. London, W. Owen, 1769.
127. Coindet, J. F.: Découverte d'un Nouveau Remède Contre le Goitre, Bibliothèque Universelle, Ann. Chim. Phys. **14,** 190–198, 1820.
128. Coindet, J. F.: Ann. Chim. Phys. **15,** 49–59, 1820.
129. Coindet, J. F.: Observations on the use of iodine as a remedy for bronchocele. London Med. Phys. J. **44,** 1820.
130. Prout, W.: Chemistry, Meteorology, and the Function of Digestion considered with Reference to Natural Theology, p. 100. London, 1834.
131. Manson, A.: Medical Researches on the Effects of Iodine in Bronchocele, Paralysis, Chorea, Scrofula etc. London, 1825.
132. Inglis, J.: Treatise on English Bronchocele with a few Remarks on the Use of Iodine. London, 1838.
133. Rilliet, F.: Constitutional iodism, Bull. Acad. Méd., Paris **25,** p. 382, 1859.
134. Halsted, W. S.: Johns Hopkins Hosp. Rep. **19,** 71–257, 1920.
135. Giroud: J. Chirurgie, Paris III, **3,** 1792.
136. Green, J. H.: Lancer **2,** 351–352, 1828–29.
137. Porta, Luigi: Curra chirurgica, p. 126., Milano, 1849.
138. Quoted by A. Burns: Observations on the Surgical Anatomy of the Head and the Neck. pp. 202, 204, Edinburgh, 1812.
139. Coates, H.: Med. Chir. Trans., London, X, 312, 1812.
140. Earle, H.: London Med. Phys. J. **106,** 201, 1826.
141. Key, Aston: Lancet **2,** 358, 1824.
142. Dobson, J.: John Hunter. Edinburgh, E. & S. Livingstone, 1969.
143. Jørgensen, C. Barker: John Hunter, A. A. Berthold and the origins of endocrinology. Act. Hist. Sci. Nat. Med., Odense **24,** 1–54, 1971.
144. Hunter, J.: A Treatise on the Blood, Inflammation and Gunshot Wounds. p. 6, London, 1794 (Published posthumously).
145. Boerhave, H.: Institutions de Médecine, IV, p. 20, 1743–50.
146. Bordeu, Th. de: Recherches sur les maladres chroniques. Vol. I., Paris, 1775.
147. Withof, I. P. L.: De castratis. Commentationes quattuor. Duisburg, 1756.
148. Forbes, T. R.: Testis transplantation performed by John Hunter. Endocrinology **41,** 329–331, 1949.
149. Hunter, J.: Observations on Certain Parts of the Animal Oeconomy, London, 1786.
150. Burrows, H.: Biological Action of Sex Hormones, 2nd. ed. Cambridge University Press, 1949.
151. Hunter, J.: An experiment to determine the effect of extirpating one ovarium upon the number of young produced. Philos. Trans. R. Soc. London, **17,** 233–239, 1787.
152. Benson, B., Sorrentino, S., Evans, J. S.: Increase in serum FSH following unilateral ovariectomy in the rat. Endocrinology **84,** 369–374, 1969.

153. McLaren, A.: Regulation of ovulation rate after removal of one ovary in mice. Proc. R. Soc. B. **166,** 316–340, 1966.

154. Hunter, John: Essays and observations on Natural History, Anatomy . . . etc. (ed. Richard Owen) Vol. 1–2; London, 1861.

155. Hunter, John: On a secretion of the crop of breeding pigeons. 1786.

156. Riddle, O.: The preparation, identification and assay of prolactin – a hormone of the anterior pituitary. Am. J. Physiol. **105,** 191–216, 1933.

157. Riddle, O.: Prolactin in vertebrate function and organization. J. Natl. Cancer Inst. **31,** 1039–1110, 1963.

158. Irvine, W.: John Hunter's Experiments: Evidence of an Eye-Witness. Letter to Professor Thomas Hamilton, University of Glasgow, of 17 June 1771. Lancet I, 359–360, 1928.

159. Owen, R.: On the Anatomy of Vertebrates, Vol. 2: Birds and Mammals. London, 1866.

160. Owen, R.: Aves. Cyclop. Anat. Physiol. **1,** 265–358, 1836.

161. As 154: Vol. 1, p. 19.

162. Short, R. V.: New thoughts on sex determination and differentiation. The Glaxo Volume 39, p. 12, 1974.

163. Forbes, T. R.: The origin of the freemartin. Bull. Hist. Med. **20,** 461, 1946.

164. Tandler, J., Keller, K.: Ueber das Verhalten d. Chorions bei verschiedengeschlechtlicher Zwillings-graviditaet des Rindes und ueber die Morphologie d. Genitales der weiblichen Tiere, welche einer solchen Graviditaet entstammen. Dtsche tieraerzt. Wschr. **19,** 148, 1911.

165. As 162: p. 17.

166. Lillie, F. R.: The theory of the freemartin, Science **43,** 611, 1916.

167. Lillie, F. R.: The freemartin: a study of the action of sex hormones in the foetal life of cattle. J. Exp. Zool. **23,** 371, 1917.

168. As 162: p. 13.

169. Short, R. V.: Germ Cell Sex. Proc. Int. Symp. The Genetics of the Spermatozoon. p. 334, Edinburgh, Aug., 1971.

170. ibid.: p. 335.

171. Short, R. V., Smith, J., Mann, T., Evans, E. P., Hallett, J., Fryer, A. Hamerton, J. L.: Cytogenetic and endocrine studies of a freemartin heifer and its bull co-twin. Cytogenetics **8,** 369–388, 1969.

172. Short, R. V.: The bovine freemartin: a new look at an old problem. Philos. Trans. R. Soc. London **259,** 141–147, 1970.

173. ibid.: p. 142.

174. ibid.: p. 143.

175. Hamerton, J. L.: Significance of sex chromosome derived heterochromatin in mammals. Nature, London **219,** p. 910, 1968.

176. Race, R. R., Sanger, R.: Blood Groups in Man. 5th ed, p. 478. Oxford, Blackwell, 1968.

177. As 144: Vol. VIII, p. 256.

178. As 143: p. 17.

179. As 143: pp. 56–59.

180. Home, Sir Everard: Account of the dissection of an hermaphrodite dog. Philos. Trans. R. Soc. **18,** 157–178, 1799.

181. Cruikshank, Wm. C.: Experiments in which on the third day after impregnation, the ova of rabbits were found in fallopian tubes; and on the fourth day after impregnation in the uterus itself; with the first appearances of the foetus. Philos. Trans. **87,** 197–214, 1797.

182. Haighton, J.: An experimental inquiry concerning animal impregnation. Phil. Trans. R. Soc. London, **87,** pp. 159–196, 1797.

CHAPTER FIFTEEN

THE BIRTH OF ENDOCRINOLOGY – PART I

INTRODUCTION

IN 1820, the Viennese physiologist Georg Prochaska (1749–1820) proposed a general theory on the sympathetic mechanism of the gonads. It was inspired by the discoveries of the effects of electricity on the animal body. He identified electricity with the various kinds of vital principles that had been postulated to explain life[1]. He also assumed that interactions between organs were of an electrical nature.

> Die Organe wirken aber auch nur dynamisch ohne eine Materie zu ueberleiten, sondern nur um ihre Lebensprozesse zu bedingen, zu aendern, zu modifizieren, ohne dass man immer einen Zusammenhang durch Nerven zwischen ihnen nachweisen kann. Dieses wird einleuchtend in den Erscheinungen der Pubertaet, indem bey dem maennlichen Geschlechte die Ausbildung des Bartes, der Stimme, der Staerke und des Muthes von der Entwickelung der Hoden, und bey dem weiblichen Geschlechte die Ausbildung der Brueste, des Beckens und anderer Theile von der Entwickelung der weiblichen Geschlechtsteile besonders der Eyerstoecke abhaengen[2].

In this particular formulation of the testes being responsible not only for the development of the physical secondary characteristics, but also for strength and courage, whereas the ovaries produced only physical secondary sex characteristics, Prochaska would today be open to the accusation of being a male chauvinist pig.

He had also investigated the nature of reflex action. It was then thought that the harmonious interaction of several parts of the body, the so-called 'consensus partium', was under the exclusive control of the reflexes, either inherited or acquired in the course of individual existence.

A great variety of disorders were assumed to have a purely reflex basis. The effects of castration and the symptoms of the menopause were both considered to be due to nervous reflexes[3].

Hans Peter Schoenwetter pointed out, however, in his MD thesis[4] that it was not the ovaries, but the uterus which remained the focal issue in reproductive physiology up to the middle of the 19th century. We have already seen van Helmont's dictum: "Propter solumn uterum mulier est quod est", which was later paraphrased by Achille Chéreau (see p. 129) in favour of the ovary. Johann Wolfgang von Goethe, 1749–1832, perhaps the most famous German poet, who was also a statesman and no mean naturalist (he propounded a theory of colour vision and discovered the intermaxillary bone[5]), wrote: "Der Hauptpunkt der ganzen weiblichen Existenz ist die Gebaermutter" although he did stress the importance of the ovaries later in the treatise. The breasts, responsible for lactation, seemed to be directly connected with the uterus. Johann Heinrich Ferdinand Autenrieth (1772–1835) said in his *Handbuch der empirischen menschlichen* physiologie[6]:

> Wie haengen denn aber die Brueste, nicht mit den Bauchbedeckungen, sondern mit der Gebaermutter durch Gefaesse irgend auf eine Art zusammen?

> (In what manner are the breasts connected, not with the abdominal integuments, but with the womb by means of blood vessels?) . . . .

> The hair of the beard falls out if the testes are removed; they do not develop at all, if a man had been castrated before. In like manner, the monthly period does not appear if the womb is not present, in otherwise healthy persons; or the period will cease, even from the vagina, if the womb is surgically removed[7]. . . . Thus the beard will grow and the cartilages of the larynx increase by means of an hitherto unknown connection with the prior development of the sperm. Similarly, the secretion in the pregnant womb will produce as a consequence the secretion of milk[7]. [translation: V.C.M.]

Friedrich Hildebrandt (1764–1816) wrote in 1809 on similar terms, that the cause for the curious sympathy between the breasts and the womb is unknown; the anastomosis of the vasa epigastrica, from which there are branches to the uterus, and the vasa mammaria has no satisfactory explanation; nor is there any adequate nerve connection between the two organs[8]. As late as 1842, Friedrich Arnold (1803–1873) wrote in his *Lehrbuch der Physiologie des Menschen*[9],

> The relation of the milkglands to the womb is as well consensual, as it is antagonistic and vicarious. They swell somewhat at the time of the period and of conception, they wilt after abortion, they yield – as a rule – a lot of milk with ample menstruation, and they may show signs of disease in case of illness

of the womb. On the other hand, their activity is diminished with increased activity of the womb, e.g. when a nursing mother menstruates or becomes pregnant; in the same manner the opposite action occurs when there is marked activity of the milk glands: the functions of the womb appear diminished, because during the period of nursing there occurs – as a rule – neither a period nor pregnancy. These relations between the breast and womb are not based on a vascular or nervous connection, but are related to the physiology of reproduction. [translation: V.C.M.]

Witness to the change of opinion in this respect were Virchow's (see Section II) views. He was much impressed by Achille Chéreau's (1817–1885) paraphrase "Propter ovarium solum mulier est quod est"[10]. However, Chéreau is better remembered for his poetic interests! Virchow writes:

> Chéreau urges quite rightly that it has been completely wrong to regard the uterus as the characteristic organ and to say with Helmont: Propter solum uterum mulier est id quod est. The womb, as part of the sexual canal, of the whole apparatus of reproduction, is merely an organ of secondary importance. Remove the ovary, and we shall have before us a masculine woman ('Mannweib', in her 'its') ugly half-form with the coarse and harsh form (features), the heavy bone formation, the moustache, the rough voice, the flat chest, the sour and egotistic mentality and the distorted outlook[11].

and in the same vein:

> ... in short, all that we admire and respect in woman as womanly, is merely dependent on her ovaries.

Curiously enough, Giovanni Battista Morgagni (1682–1771), who described first a patient with missing gonads, called the old person 'muliercula'[4] (p. 31). Yet Virchow did not think of the role of the ovaries in terms of internal secretion, but rather in the then popular terms of guidance by the nervous system (see also p. 221). It was not until the end of the 19th century that Emil Knauer (1867–1935) and Josef Halban (1870–1937), both of Vienna, established the hormonal role of the ovaries.

In 1840, George Gulliver (1804–1882), assistant surgeon to the Royal Horseguards (Blues), a Fellow of the Royal Society (1839), and later an original Fellow of the Royal College of Surgeons of England (1843), Hunterian Orator (1863) – "a most unusual, if not unique combination"[12] – described the microscopic appearances of the adrenals and mentioned spheroidal bodies in the adrenals and in their veins. He said that the adrenals "poured into the blood a peculiar matter which has doubtless a special use, and is still an interesting and important subject for further inquiry". Accordingly, he added, the adrenal veins act as the excretory duct of the adrenals[13].

In 1856, Edme Félix Alfred Vulpian (1826–1887) published the observation that the adrenal medulla stains emerald-green with perchloride of iron and that a similar reaction can be obtained from the blood in the adrenal veins, but it does not occur in other organs or the blood elsewhere in the body. He also stressed that the substance thus stained seems to be connected with the function of the adrenals[14]. He thus discovered adrenaline in the adrenal medulla and in the adrenal veins (see also p. 231).

In 1841, Friedrich Gustav Jacob Henle (1809–1885) distinguished between glands with and without excretory ducts. In the latter, the blood absorbs the substances produced[15]. This view was confirmed by Johannes Mueller (1801–1858) in 1844[16] and by Rudolph Albert von Koelliker (1817–1905) (see also p. 223).

In 1801, Julien Jean César Legallois (1770–1814) submitted his thesis for the Paris doctorate of medicine, entitled: *Le sang, est-il identique dans tous les vaisseaux qu'il parcourt?* (= Is the blood identical in all the vessels it passes through?) By doing so, he anticipated even more definitely than de Bordeu the concept of internal secretion.

Legallois argued that the arterial blood remains unchanged in its composition, whereas the venous blood shows changes. He concluded:

> De l'identité du sang artériel et la diversité des sangs veineux, on peut conclure: . . . que le triomphe de la chimic animale serait de trouver des rapports entre le sang artériel, la matière de telle sècrètion et le sang veineux correspondant, tant dans l'état sain que dans l'état patholo-gique des divers animaux; de trouver des différences entre les divers sangs veineux; de trouver enfin ces différences proportionelles à celles des sécrétions correspondantes. Qu'arrivé à ce degré de perfection, il serait souvent possible qu'elle dégageât l'inconnu dans cette équation: sang artériel = telle sècrètion + sang veineux correspondant, c'est-à-dire que le premier membre étant donné, elle pourrait deviner à peu près ci qui doit être la sécrétion si elle connaissait le sang veineux . . .[17].

> From the identity of the arterial blood and the diversity of the venous bloods, one may conclude . . . that the triumph of animal chemistry would be to find relations between the arterial blood, the matter of such secretion and the corresponding venous blood, both in health and pathological conditions in different animals; to find the differences between the various venous bloods; and, in short, to find these differences proportional to those of the correspond-ing secretions. . . . Arrived at this degree of perfection, it would often be possible that the unknown was revealed by the equation: arterial blood = such secretion + corresponding venous blood – that is to say, the first number being given, it would be possible almost to guess at what ought to be the secretion, if one knew the venous blood. . . .

Legallois was, however, not aware of the difference between glands with external and those with internal secretion.

Legallois was an experimental physiologist and physician to the Bicêtre. He also made important contributions to the study of the respiratory system, to the location of the respiratory centre in the medulla oblongata and the role of the vagus nerve in the act of respiration[18]. Rolleston mentions that in his fatal illness, pneumonia, he refused to be bled[19].

BERTHOLD

So we arrive at the year 1849, when Arnold Adolph Berthold (1803–1861) of Goettingen (see also Section II) published his four-page paper on 'Transplantation der Hoden'[20], in which he showed that transplantation of a cock's testes to another part of the body prevented atrophy of the comb, the usual result of castration. Of four young, completely castrated cocks, two remained capons. Two, receiving ectopic transplants of their testicle in the abdomen, developed as normal cocks. He wrote:

> Da nun aber an fremde Stellen transplantierte Hoden mit ihren urspruengliche Nerven nicht mehr in Verbindung stehen koennen, und da es ... keine *specifischen*, der Secretion vorstehenden Nerven giebt, so folgt, dass der fragliche Consensus durch das productive Verhaeltniss der Hoden, d.h. durch deren Einwirkung auf das Blut, und dann durch entsprechende Einwirkung des Blutes auf den allgemeinen Organismus ueberhaupt, wovon allerdings das Nerven-system einen sehr wesentlichen Theil ausmacht, bedingt wird.

> Since the testes can no longer remain in connection with their original nerves after being transplanted to a strange place, and as there are no *specific* nerves producing secretion, it follows that the consensus in question must be effected through the productive relationship of the testes, that is to say, through their action on the blood, and then through the suitable ensuing action of the blood on the organism as a whole, of which, however, the nervous system forms a very substantial part.

Berthold's paper was forgotten until the beginning of this century when it was mentioned by Moritz Nussbaum[21], Artur Biedl (1869–1933)[22] and others. C. R. Moore said in 1932: "Berthold thus ... established the modern conception that the testis, wherever located, produces some substance that is distributed generally over the body by way of the blood stream". A similar view was expressed by many others, including Rolleston in 1936[23]. Although Berthold did not say in so many words that the testis maintains the main male secondary sex characteristics by means of a special substance manufactured in the gland and released into the blood circulation, that was the only possible conclusion which could be drawn from his experiments.

Berthold's communication has, according to Jørgensen, the character of a preliminary note. "He omits a mention of why he performed the experiments; nor does he discuss the results in relation to contemporary ideas on the relations between gonads and secondary sex characters." F. R. Forbes found, in 1949[24], a clue in Berthold's ideas on the nature of sex products, as he stated them in his *Lehrbuch der Physiologie fuer Studierende und Aerzte*[25]. Berthold compared the gonads with glands which extract their secretory products from the blood; he explained the resemblance of offspring with parents by the hypothesis that the gonads must extract specific matter which is given off to the blood from every tissue of the body, to be eventually incorporated into sperm and ova[26]. These represented thoughts that went back to Hippocrates and the Ancients (see Chapter 6).

In another paper, however, Berthold gave some indications for the reasons of his experiments: In the *Nachrichten von der G.A. Universitaet und der Koeniglichen Gesellschaft der Wissenschaften zu Goetingen* of 19 February, 1849, it says that Berthold made some special remarks on 8 February concerning the transplants of testicles. In an introductory paragraph he said:

> That the testes can be transplanted has already been demonstrated by John Hunter. The changes which the newly united or transplanted testicles will undergo, have not been examined in greater detail as yet.

Thus, Berthold was well acquainted with and inspired by Hunter's work on the transplantation of the testes, the results of which implied that even a transplanted gland could produce secondary male characteristics. He realized that – apart from the nervous system – there was only the circulating blood which was the mediator of 'sympathies' between the different parts of the body. In due fairness, however, it must be said that various highly skilled experimenters, including his friend and colleague in Goettingen, Rudolph Wagner (1805–1864), repeated his experiments unsuccessfully: both "the homo- and auto-transplanted testes consistently degenerated in castrated cocks"[27]. Berthold's own experiments, all of which – surprisingly – seem to have been successful, consisted only of six cocks. Wagner expressed in so many words that he had attempted to repeat Hunter's experiments which had been revived by Berthold; no doubt, his failure to reproduce the results of Hunter and Berthold was responsible for the latter's experiments lapsing into oblivion, especially as Berthold did not follow them up, even in his further reports. As Jørgensen points out, not only may Berthold have lost faith in his own results, but

> Transplantations of testis in the cock and other animals were resumed by several workers in the eighteen hundred and nineties, and continued well into the present century, largely with inconclusive results. The

investigators experienced great difficulties not only in obtaining survival of grafted testis, but also in securing complete castration of the cocks[28].

Testis transplants were equally unsuccessful in mammals[28] and amphibians[29].

Foges could say as late as 1903:

Die Annahme, dass die Entwicklung der sekundaeren Geschlechtscharactere durch die 'innere Sekretion' der Geschleschtsdruesen bedingt ist, wird in der einschlaegigen Literatur der letzten Jahre kaum mehr in Zweifel gezogen; es fehlt zwar bisher noch die einwandfreie experimentelle Beweisfuehrung, aber der Gedanke ist *a priori* so verstaendlich, so bestechend, dass er von Vielen schon als unbestreitbar richtig hingestellt wird. Der Gedanke ist auch nicht neu und findet sich schon in einer Arbeit Berthold's. . . .[29]

The assumption that the development of the secondary sex characteristics is due to the 'internal secretion' of the gonads, is hardly doubted in the relevant literature of the last years; the convincing experimental evidence for it is, however, still lacking; but the idea is so plausible *a priori*, so persuasive, that many regard it as irrefutably correct. The idea is not even new and can already be found in a paper by Berthold. . . .

As Jørgensen stresses, however, "in Berthold's time the idea of internal secretions as mediators, was not *a priori* the most comprehensible. Humoral integration was, at best, a theoretical possibility"[29]. This is why, as we shall discuss later, Sir Edward Sharpey-Schaefer (1850–1935) and his school attempted to lay the foundations of a 'New Physiology', of a sound endocrine science, by demonstration of the precise physiological effects of organ extracts. This was after 1893, when his attention had been drawn to the vasopressor effects of adrenal extract by George Oliver (1841–1915)[30].

Berthold also wrote a paper on the thyroids of green parrots and a lengthy treatise on the duration of animal and human gestation. In 1845, he published an observation of a case of a patient with true hermaphroditism[31].

There emerged other objections to Berthold's theory of the action of the testes on secondary sex characteristics by way of material carried by the blood. In certain hermaphrodite conditions part of the body is masculine and part is feminine. Such observations on insects and birds were known to Johann Friedrich Meckel the Younger (1781–1833)[32], to James Young Simpson (1811–1870)[33] and others. Birds wearing male plumage on one side of the body and female on the other, described very much later by O. Heinroth[34], and H. Poll[35] seemed of special importance in this connection. The male half of the plumage appeared to be always on the right side of the bird, the female plumage on the left side, with a sharp border between the two. This division seemed to be caused by the observed testicular development of the atrophic right ovary of the bird. Hunter had already studied this phenomenon, and Geoffroy Sainte-Hilaire (1772–1844) wrote about 'sur les femelles de faisans à plumages de mâles' etc. in 1825[36], as did W. Yarrell in 1827[37]. He recognized that the change to male plumage in female birds was apparently linked with a pathologically changed ovary. This sex change was regarded as a variant of hermaphroditism. One opinion was that the basic structure of the organism is hermaphroditic; under normal conditions one sex is dominant during growth, the characteristics of the other sex remain latent. (See also Ref. 38.)

If the gonad responsible for the existence of the secondary sex characters stops functioning, the latent characters become apparent. The actual mechanisms for this had a number of different explanations. According to A. Tichomiroff[39], the "Geshlechts-kraft" = sexual force, which makes the characteristics of one sex develop, has – at the same time – an antagonistic effect on the characteristics of the opposite sex. The celebrated Eugen Steinach (1861–1944) in 1894, held similar views concerning the mode of action of the gonads[40]. Others put forward Geoffroy Saint-Hilaire's hypothesis outlined above, but none of the explanations offered suggested humoral connections between the gonads and the secondary sex characters.

There were also observations of stags with unilateral atrophy of the antlers together with an atrophied testicle on the same side. Yarrell further described in 1857 a buck with a single antler on one side of the head with a scirrhous ovary on the opposite side[41]. Experimental removal of the right testicle in one buck, and of the left testicle in another four-year-old buck, resulted in no exceptional findings.

> Neither of these bucks cast either horn, nor was any lateral influence observable. They shed their horns as usual in the following spring, the new horns coming in due course. . . .

This experiment was, regrettably, overlooked and the hypothesis of gonads influencing secondary sex characteristics on the same side was pursued into the 20th century.

Rudolph Virchow (1821–1902) reported in 1848 on Siamese twin girls[42], who survived to the age of 22. They menstruated independently, yet after death the autopsy showed that their abdominal blood vessels anastomosed and the girls had a common circulation. This was striking evidence, in Virchow's opinion, against the theory of humoral maturation of the ova and "of course, also against humoral sympathies between ovaries and uterus"[42].

Instead, theories were gaining ground, suggesting nervous control of the functions of the gonads, including the development of secondary sex characteristics. These views were widely accepted and held valid until the turn of the century. These theories had their roots in treatises like that by Franz Joseph Gall (1758–1828) and Johann Caspar Spurzheim (1776–1832) on *Anatomie et physiologie du système nerveux en général, et du cerveau en particulier* (Paris, 1810–1819), in which they introduced a theory of localization of the cerebral function (on which later the popular science of phrenology was based). The work dealt in some detail with the role of the cerebellum, controlling gonadal function and sexual behaviour, as organ

de l'instinct de la propagation. . . . L'énergie de l'instinct de la propagation est, chez les adultes, dans un rapport direct avec le développement du cervelet.

His conclusions – in man and in animals – were the result of studies in agreement with Gall's general phrenological observations. To this, he also added the results of some experiments: castration inhibited the development of the cerebellum, the more so the younger the individual at the time of operation. Unilateral castration in rabbits caused contralateral atrophy of the cerebellum within eight months. There was also known atrophy of the testes, following lesions of the cerebellum (see also F. J. Gall and J. Vimont).

Jørgensen[43] also stresses the influence of M. Lallemand's monograph *Des pertes séminales involontaires* (Vols. 1–3, Paris, 1836–1842) on the later ideas of Brown-Sequard, on the general beneficial effects on the body of sperm stored in the vesiculae seminales: "Le séjour prolongé des zoospermes augmente . . . des fonctions génitales, la force et l'activité de toute l'économie" (Vol. 2, p. 439). This effect of stored sperm would affect the organism via the sympathetic nervous system.

Thomas Blizzard Curling (1811–1888), of London, in his *A Practical Treatise on the Disease of the Testis*[44] was of a similar opinion; according to him, the testes were controlled both by the brain and the sympathetic nervous system. Incidentally, Curling was one of the first to observe the clinical picture of cretinism, later named by Ord 'myxoedema'[45,46].

J. Obolensky reported that the testicle atrophied on cutting the spermatic nerve[47]. This fitted in well with the concept of trophic nerves, developed during the second half of the century[43]. Eugen Steinach (1861–1944) thought that the sexual activity of male frogs in the breeding season was caused by sensory nerve impulses in the maturing testis, and this also activated sexual centres in the brain[40]. As late as 1905, M. Nussbaum concluded that secretions from the transplanted testicle acted via the central nervous system, because he found that the thumb pads of frogs could be maintained by transplanted testis only when the thumbs were innervated; cutting the nerve supply produced regression of the thumbpads[43].

In the case of the ovaries, not only Virchow (see pp. 220 and 221) but Eduard Friedrich Wilhelm Pflueger (1829–1910) also assumed that the mechanism of the menstrual cycle is based on the reflexes[48]. He believed that swelling of the ovaries due to cell growth is accompanied by stimulation of nerve fibres terminating in the ovarian parenchyma. When a certain threshold of the nervous stimulation is reached, a powerful blood congestion of the external genitalia will result as a reflex action, which in consequence will produce the menstrual changes of the uterus and maturation of the larger follicles. He wrote:

> We observe, therefore in the bleeding and the release of the ovum two phenomena due to the same causation, namely the menstrual congestion. The constance of the latter's periodicity is founded in the fact that the weak stimulation of the nerves of the ovaries has to persist a certain time, until a sufficient threshold is reached in the spinal cord to produce the reflex action mentioned above.

Twenty years later, Ferdinand Adolf Kehrer's (1837–1914) observations on the results of ovariectomy seemed to support Pflueger's hypothesis[49]. Friedrich Leopold Goltz (1834–1902) (see also Section II) and A. Frensberg made observations to the contrary in 1874 when they succeeded in getting a bitch in heat and impregnated, giving birth to a normal pup, after the spinal cord had been severed at the level of the first lumbar vertebra[50]. Goltz concluded, therefore, that normal ovarian function and sexual behaviour cannot be mediated by the nervous system via the spinal cord to the brain. A pathway via the sympathetic nervous system still remained a possibility; but, he added:

> It would be possible, that the mysterious connection between the condition of the brain and that of the gonads is mediated by the blood. It is not unthinkable that during the heat peculiar substances are given off into the circulation from the active gonad and stimulate in the brain that particular reflex mechanism which forms the basis for the attraction of the sexes. I have to admit, that I am now more inclined towards that viewpoint. [translation: V.C.M.]

J. L. Brachet had already made, in 1837, similar observations on the effect of section of the spinal cord on the function of the gonads in cat and dog. In the tomcat, he was able to produce ejaculation several days after severing the cord. A bitch came on heat and was impregnated after transsection. He also quoted clinical examples of a man begetting children, and a woman having a successful delivery, although both had complete paraplegia of the lower part of the body. He concluded that it was the sympathetic nervous system which controlled gonadal function[51]. It was, however, Goltz who gave a correct analysis of his experiments and observations, adding his brilliant conclusions on neuro-endocrine inter-relations between the gonads and the brain and on the humoral control of the secondary sex characteristics.

Yet the promising beginnings, initiated by the ideas of Lower, of de Bordeu, Lieutaud, Wilkinson King, by the experiments of John Hunter and Arnold Berthold seemed to have been of no avail at that time. Thus, before 1855, we may regard as the precursors of the doctrine of internal secretion Lower (pituitary, 1670), de Bordeu (1775), John Hunter (testes, 1771), Legallois (1801), Wilkinson King (thyroid, 1836), Gulliver (adrenals, 1840), Berthold (1849), Carpenter (1852), and perhaps Hufeland (testes, 1797). Goltz's hunch eventually proved to be correct, but it took another forty years before experimental physiology, supported by the beginnings of biochemistry, provided the scientific basis for definitions like 'internal secretion' and 'endocrine function'.

The concept of internal secretion survived as a special property of the glands without excretory ducts, the ductless glands, the 'Blutgefaessdruesen' (= blood-vessel glands). In the first half of the 19th century these were the thymus, the lymphnodes, the thyroid, the adrenals and the spleen[52]. Johannes Mueller (1801–1858) restricted himself to the statement: "function unknown", when dealing with the adrenals and thyroid. Mueller was the founder of a famous medical team, the teacher and guide of Theodor Schwann, Gustav Jacob Henle, Albert von Koelliker, Rudolph Virchow, of Emil Du Bois Reymond, Hermann Ludwig Ferdinand von Helmholtz and Ernst Wilhelm von Brucke. Mueller's *Handbuch der Physiologie des Menschen*[16] (1834–1840) was one of the milestones of the time. In 1825, Mueller had published his researches on the development of the ova in the ovary of the 'phantom-grasshopper'[54] and the discovery of the Muellerian duct. As we have already said (see p. 216), Gustav Jacob Henle stated in his classic textbook *Allegemeine Anatomie des Menschen* in 1841[15] that, in the glands without excretory ducts, the blood undergoes a change and that the substances thus manufactured are absorbed by the blood-vessels or the lymphatics. He not only had the support of Johannes Mueller (in his *Handbook of Physiology* in 1844) but also in 1852 of Rudolph Albert von Koelliker in his *Handbuch der Gewebslehre des Menschen*[55], which was the first textbook of histology.

In 1830 Mueller had published his major study on glands and their mechanism of secretion: *De glandularum secernentium structura penitiori*[56] which became his most important histological work. In it he described the microscopic anatomy of a great number of secreting glands. He observed that the blood-vessels within the glands do not open up at the beginning of the excretory canals of the glands, but that the arteries form capillary nets over the elements of the glandular structure, which then become venous capillary nets.

> Omnium glandularum anatome demonstravimus, vasa sanguifera minima non in partes glandularum et fines ductuum secernentium continuo transire, sed vasa sanguifera ad parietes canalium secernentium ita sese habere, quam ad aliam quamcunque membranam secernentem. Itaque non apertis finibus in cavernulas canalium illorum hiant, sed arteriolae inter partes glandularum elementares qualescunque et super ipsas tenuissimis vasculorum retibus in venulas transeunt. . . . Vasorum sanguiferorum ramificationes concomitantur efflorescentiam canalium secernentium atque reticularis vasculis periphericis super partes elementares canaliumque secernentium fines vagantur.[57]

Yet in 1835, Mueller wrote in the first edition of his *Handbook of Physiology* that "the function of the thyroid gland is unknown"[58]. In his book on the structure of the glands, Mueller had stressed that the inside of all glands presents a maximal secreting surface in the smallest possible space:

> Omnes glandulae systemate ductuum secernentium permagnam intus superficiem secernentem offerunt, innumera vero varietas est formarum, quibus superficies secernens in minori spatio augetur. Quibus natura immensam diversitatem atque ubertatem fatetur, cum tamen in omnibus, iisdem circumscripta formationis legibus, commune quoddam, glandulis omnibus insitum aperiat.

In later editions of his *Handbuch der Physiologie des Menschen* he did take account of the results of recent research. He wrote about the glands:

> They are partly without excretory ducts, partly secreting and with excretory ducts. The glands without excretory ducts influence the juices which circulate within them and pass through them and return to the general circulation. They have no connection outside like the secreting glands. . . . These so-called glands without excretory ducts are of two entirely different types. 1. Possessing a rete mirabilis of the arteries, veins and lymphglands. These alone may be called vascular nodes. 2. The vascular glands or bloodvascular glands. The true bloodglands do not differ from other organs as regards blood and lymph vessels. To this group belong the spleen, the thyroid, the suprarenals, the thymus and the placenta[59].

The true function of the blood glands was unknown to Mueller. The anatomical and histological descriptions of the 'Bloodglands' by

Henle, von Koelliker and Alexander Ecker (in various editions up to 1866) still maintain that the purpose and functions of these glands are unknown.

THE YEAR 1855

The year 1855 could be regarded as a watershed in the history of endocrinology. Its three landmarks were the launching of the ideas of Professor Claude Bernard (1813–1878) of Paris; Thomas Addison's publication *On the Constitutional and Local Effects of Disease of the Supra-renal Capsules* and Professor Charles Édouard Brown-Séquard's (1817–1894) follow-up of Addison's observations in 1856.

Claude Bernard (see Section II) differentiated between the 'sécrétion externe' of the liver, namely, the discharge of the bile, and the 'sécrétion interne', by which he understood the giving-off of glucose into the blood. He deserves, therefore, the credit for introducing the term, even though he used it in a different sense from that customary today[60]. In the following years, Bernard and others analysed the extracts of other ductless glands, such as the thyroid and the adrenals. Yet, as F. G. Young has pointed out[61], the view that what we now call endocrine organs might pour their secretions directly into the blood stream, was current before Claude Bernard's writings about the liberation of sugar into the blood. The above-mentioned (p. 223) W. B. Carpenter (1813–1885) wrote in 1852:

> We refer to that elaborating agency, which is now generally believed to be exerted upon certain materials of the blood by the spleen, thymus and thyroid glands and the suprarenal capsules (which are sometimes collectively termed vascular glands) and which are ... unprovided with excretory ducts for the discharge of the product of their operation. These products, instead of being carried out of the body, are destined to be restored to the circulating current, apparently in a state of more complete adaptiveness to the wants of the nutritive function; in other words, these vascular glands are concerned in the assimilation of the materials that are destined to be converted into organised tissues, instead of being the instrument of the removal of the matters which result from the disintegration or decay of those tissues[62].

Although Carpenter also included fatty tissue with the ductless glands, his "conception clearly corresponds in general with the modern one of internal secretions"[63]. Another article, on the supra-renal capsules, written by Heinrich Frey (1822–1890), Professor in

Zurich, in the same *Cyclopaedia of Anatomy and Physiology* as Carpenter's, translated from the German, says as follows:

> Their contents [i.e. of the suprarenal capsules] are not exuded outwardly, as are those of the gland-vesicles previously described, but into the fibrous framework of the organ, in which they exist in the fluid form, and from which they are subsequently received into the vascular system either by immediate or mediate resorption. We are therefore correct in regarding the supra-renal capsules as glandular organs, and their function as secretory[63].

F. G. Young rightly assumes, therefore, that in describing the liberation of glucose into the blood, Claude Bernard was really applying to the liver a theory which was already accepted concerning 'vascular glands' in general, and the suprarenals in particular. Incidentally, Claude Bernard was the master of modern experimental medicine, which he himself defined as "induced observation". He said:

> With observation and experiment a fact is simply noted; the only difference is this – as the fact which an experimenter must verify does not present itself to him naturally; he must make it appear, i.e. induce it for a special reason and for a special object.

In the same year was published Thomas Addison's (1793–1860) (see Section II) book *On the Constitutional and Local Effects of Disease of the Suprarenal Capsules*[64].

Addison 'stumbled', as he said, on the bronzed disease while searching for the cause of pernicious anaemia. On 15 March 1849, he read a paper to the South London Medical Society, at the request of the president, John Hilton (1804–1878) entitled: 'On anaemia: disease of the suprarenal capsules'. He described the clinical symptoms of idiopathic anaemia (his main interest at the time), and he said that, in the three cases coming to necropsy, the suprarenals were diseased. In two of them, those were the only lesions in the body. Accordingly, he thought that the adrenals may be either directly or indirectly concerned with sanguinification and that the anaemia and the changes in the adrenals were not merely coincidental. He called the disease 'melasma suprarenale'[65] (see also p. 233). The significance of this observation was lost at the time, attention being focused on the anaemia. It was another six years before Addison was persuaded, mainly by Wilks, and published his monograph (see Figure 39) of 39 pages, which became one of the classics of medicine, the perfect description of an endocrine disease to which Armand Trousseau (1801–1867, the great clinician of the Hôtel-Dieu in Paris), gave the name Addison's disease[66]. Later (in 1909) pernicious anaemia was

ON THE

CONSTITUTIONAL AND LOCAL EFFECTS

OF

DISEASE

OF THE

SUPRA-RENAL CAPSULES.

BY

THOMAS ADDISON, M.D.,

SENIOR PHYSICIAN TO GUY'S HOSPITAL.

LONDON:

SAMUEL HIGHLEY, 32 FLEET STREET.

1855.

Figure 39   Title page of Addison's treatise on Addison's disease

given the additional name of 'Addison's anaemia' by William Hunter (in "Pernicious Anaemia . . .", of which only Volume 1 was published by Macmillan in 1909).

Rolleston records[67] that Gregorio Marañon (1887–1960), the leading Spanish endocrinologist (see Section II), in 1922, "retrospectively diagnosed Addison's disease, the illness of a priest in 1554–1557, described in the *Historia primitiva y exacta del Monasterio del Escorial*"[68]. Aran's case, recorded as a tuberculous abscess of the pancreas, was recognized as an undoubted case of Addison's disease by Sir Samuel Wilks (see Section II)[69]. François Amilcar Aran (1817–1861)[70] described in 1846 a young woman of 25, who had been admitted to the Hôpital de la Charité in Paris with a four year history of rheumatic pains, weakness and extreme tiredness. Her skin first turned yellow, in the last eight months the colour of bistre and eventually, she looked like a mulatto. There was severe vomiting, exhaustion and she soon succumbed. The post-mortem examination made the pathologists assume the diagnosis mentioned before. The

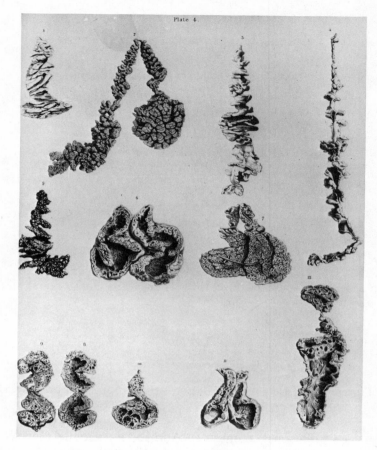

Figure 40   Plate 4 from Addison's treatise

connection with the suprarenal capsules never occurred to them. In April 1854, George Burrows (1801–1887) observed a case with necropsy at St. Bartholomew's Hospital in London, but the record remained unpublished until George Alexander Gibson (1854–1913) reported it in an address at Guy's Hospital in 1907[71].

Five of the eleven patients described by Addison had bilateral tuberculosis; one (No. 9) had unilateral tuberculosis (or, possibly, a growth, secondary to an uveal melanoma?); three showed evidence of secondary metastatic carcinoma, of which two were unilateral and one bilateral; one had a secondary carcinomatous nodule blocking the right suprarenal vein and causing a haemorrhage in that gland, but without any growth in either of them. Patient No. 4 showed apparently atrophy and fibrotic changes. Patient No. 5 was recorded by Richard Bright (1789–1858), of Bright's disease, as "Serous

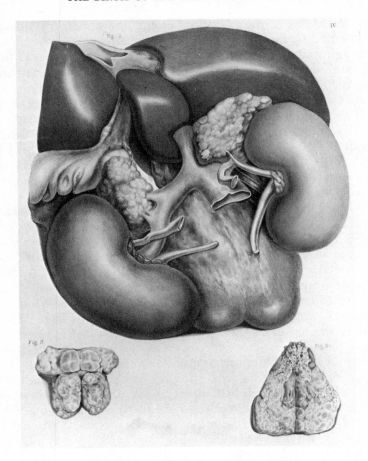

Figure 41   Plate IV from Addison's treatise

effusion under the arachnoid and into the ventricles in a case of emaciation with vomiting and diseased renal capsules" (see also Figures 40 and 41). The specimen of the suprarenals from the first patient in which any connection between pigmentation of the skin and disease of the suprarenals was thought to exist, is in Guy's Hospital museum.

Armand Trousseau (1801–1867) (see Section II) has, of course, special merit in other fields of endocrine diseases. In the second edition of his *Clinique Médicale de l'Hôtel-Dieu de Paris*, in 1865, there is also the first description of haemochromatosis under the heading of 'Glycosurie, diabète sucré' (Vol. 2, pp. 663–698). In the first edition of 1861, he had already described the observation in cases of tetany which bears his name as 'Trousseau's sign'[53].

Addison's classic monograph became the source of immediate experimental studies in animal and clinical work. At first, the physiological activity of the adrenal glands as a whole was investigated, to give way, later to the separate study of the cortex and the medulla. As usual, there arose opposition to the recognition of the new disease entity. In the first instance, Wilks himself accepted only four of the eleven cases.

Charles Hilton Fagge (1838–1883), another physician to Guy's and editor of the *Guy's Hospital Reports*, expressed doubts in his important textbook *The Principles and Practice of Medicine* about patients in whom only one adrenal was diseased[72], and so did George Neil Stewart (1860–1930), as late as 1929[73].

Brown-Séquard studied the effects of removal of the adrenals (see also p. 231). Some clinical and post-mortem observations were reported by (Sir) Jonathan Hutchinson (1828–1913) in the same year[74] (see also p. 232). At the Pathological Society of London, W. Baly showed a case on 18 November 1856, in support of Addison[75]. A special committee set up by the Society and consisting of J. S. Bristowe, Jonathan Hutchinson, J. W. Ogle, Samuel Wilks, S. W. Sibley and George Harley, reported in the Session of 1857–1858, that in four of the ten cases shown to the Society, bronzing and disease of the adrenals were associated; but George Harley (1829–1896), of paroxysmal haemoglobinuria fame, "vigorously contested the importance of the adrenals, and showed before the old Pathological Society white rats which had survived adrenalectomy" for months. This was in contradiction to Brown-Séquard's observations and was later explained by the presence of accessory cortical adrenal tissue (Marchand's adrenals) between the testes and epididymis, in the broad ligament and elsewhere in the abdomen. However, in 1933, R. Graunt[76] and in 1935, P. Schultze[77] showed that 80% of rats die after double adrenalectomy. Professor Charles Édouard Brown-Séquard came to the conclusion that the adrenals were essential to life[78]. Rolleston expressed it vividly as follows:

> In 1856, Brown-Séquard concluded from experimental removal of the adrenals that they were absolutely essential to life[79,80], that they removed from the blood a substance which developed into pigment, and that after their removal, pigment collected in the blood which became poisonous. Though the statements were disputed, the adrenals being regarded as unnecessary to life, and Brown-Séquard's results ascribed to operative trauma of the sympathetic, the hypothesis of their antitoxic function had a number of supporters and was not abandoned until Oliver and Schaefer in 1894 discovered the pressor principle (adrenaline) in the adrenal medulla (pp. 28–29).

In his first paper on 'Recherches expérimentales sur la physiologie et la pathologie des capsules surrénales'[79,80], Brown-Séquard concluded:

> . . . je me bornerai à dire: 1° Que les capsules surrénales paraissent être des organs essentiels à la vie, au moins chez les chiens, les chats, les lapins et les cochons d'Inde; 2° Que l'ablation de ces organes amène, en général, la mort plus rapidement, que l'ablation des reins. 3° Que les capsules surrénales ont avec le centre cérébrorachidien de nombreuses relations d'influence.

> (= 1. That the surrenal capsules appear to be organs essential for life, at least in dogs, cats, hares and guinea-pigs. 2. That ablation of these organs brings about death faster than removal of the kidneys. 3. That the surrenal capsules have with the brain centres numerous spheres of influence. [translation: V.C.M.]

Pierre Gratiolet attacked Brown-Séquard[81] that according to his own experimental results the fatalities after adrenalectomy were due to the close anatomical relations of the right adrenal to the liver, which caused hepatitis, peritonitis and death even after removal of the right adrenal alone. Brown-Séquard was then stung to a spirited reply[80], and proved that in *his* experiments hepatitis and peritonitis did not occur, nor was removal of the right adrenal alone fatal: "La mort dépend", he said, "surtout de l'absence des capsules surrénales, c'est-à-dire de l'absence de leurs fonctions." (= the death depends entirely on the absence of the surrenal capsules, i.e., the absence of their functions). And he repeated that the adrenals are "essentiels à vie".

It is of interest that, in the same volume of the *Comptes Rendus de l'Académie des Sciences* of Paris, was published the important paper by Edme F. A. Vulpian (1826–1887): 'Note sur quelques réactions propres à la substance des capsules surrénales', giving in barely three pages the description of the emerald-green colour which the medulla of the adrenals stains with perchloride of iron, a similar reaction being given by the blood in the adrenal veins, but not elsewhere in the body (see also p. 216). This applied to the adrenals of man, dog cat, sheep and a number of other animals. He concluded (p. 665):

> Il existe donc une matière spéciale, inconnu jusqu'ici, donnée de propriétés chimiques remarquables, qui se trouve exclusivement dans la substance médullaire des capsules surrénales, et qui, par conséquent, constitue le *signe particulier* de ces organes[82].

The view of the 'detoxicating role' of glands, the insufficiency of which would, therefore, lead to toxaemia, persisted for some time and was extended to other glands. As late as 1917, Noel Paton (1859–1928) and Findlay maintained that the main role of the parathyroids was the detoxication of guanidine[83]. This was in spite of the fact that, in the case of the thyroid gland, it had been established over forty years previously that the clinical and pathological symptoms of insufficiency were due to the lack of secretion of a substance or substances essential for and present in health.

The question of whether the whole adrenal tissue was necessary for survival was argued repeatedly and with the backing of experiments, the results of which were not always convincing[84]. The question whether hypertrophy of one adrenal follows the removal of the other has also given rise to contradictory and confusing views. However, H. Stilling's experiments seemed to confirm (in 1889) such a view of compensatory hypertrophy[85], as did T. R. Elliott's in 1913[86] the hypertrophy being in the cortex and the medulla remaining unchanged. E. M. and L. L. Mackay showed in 1926[87], that in albino rats the hypertrophy was due to increased size of the cortex, caused entirely by the size of the cells. This was the more remarkable because these rats are known to have accessory cortical adrenals. On the other hand, A. E. Boycott and E. L. Kennaway had maintained in 1924 that no compensatory hypertrophy occurs, either in the medulla or in the cortex[88]! Although in 1856 Sir Jonathan Hutchinson (1828–1913) analysed a collection of 27 patients in support, and Isaac E. Taylor of New York described patients with two autopsies[89], communications by various investigators (including Hutchinson) were published merely in the *Proceedings* of the Royal Medical and Chirurgical Society of London, but thought "not worthy of inclusion" in the *Transactions* of the Society[90]. This rebuff was keenly felt by Addison, "who had been President of the Society in 1849 and 1850 and had communicated the first of the rejected papers on suprarenal disease".

In France, as we have seen, it was Trousseau in particular who not only accepted Addison's findings, but honoured him by naming it Addison's disease and describing a case of tuberculous adrenals examined microscopically by Brown-Séquard[91]. Moreover, the celebrated Ernest Charles Lasègue (1816–1883), as editor of the *Archives Générales de Médécine*, discussed Addison's monograph and the cases reported in England by others[92]. But R. Mattei[93] in Italy, L. Martineau in France[94] and John Hughes Bennett (1812–1875) of Edinburgh[95] opposed the new disease entity of Addison's disease. As late as 1882, J. F. Goodhart (1845–1916) pronounced that Addison's disease was not due to any special pathological change in the adrenal glands alone, but to chronic inflammation which spreads to the abdominal sympathetic system and strangulates it[96]! The opinion that at least some of the symptoms of the disease might be caused by the spread of inflammation to the neighbouring semilunar ganglia and solar plexus was not new. S. O. Habershon (1825–1889) of Guy's had reported on such a spread in 1864[97], and so had F. S. Jaccoud of Paris in 1866[98].

E. H. Greenhow (1814–1888) published his book on Addison's Disease (London) in 1866, "in order, if possible, to dispel those doubts regarding the reality of its existence, which is still entertained by many members of the profession". He had collected 196 cases, which he analysed minutely and of which he accepted 128 as genuine; but even he was of the opinion that some of the features may be caused by encroachment of the sympathetic nervous system. After all, Addison himself said in a discussion at the Royal Medical and Chirurgical Society on 9 February 1858:

> We know that these organs (the suprarenals) are situated in the direct vicinity and in contact with the solar plexus and the semilunar ganglia, and receive of them a large supply of nerves, and who can tell what influence the contact of these diseased organs might have on these great nerve centres, and what share that secondary effect might have on the general health and in the production of the symptoms presented[99]?

Wilks, for one, was convinced that the adrenal lesion was not tuberculous, but a chronic inflammation like cirrhosis of the liver or a granular kidney. Even so, recognition was slow, and Wilks and Daldy, who edited Addison's collected papers in 1868[100], eight years after his death, remarked in the preface that "even now, it does not find a place in the nosology of some writers". In the first edition of the *Nomenclature of Diseases* in 1869 (Royal College of Physicians of London), there was an entry: "Morbus Addisoni, idem valet cutis aenea, melasma Addisoni".

The expression 'bronzed skin' was introduced by (Sir) Jonathan Hutchinson. This term was translated as 'cutis aenea' in *The Poet at the Breakfast Table* by Oliver Wendell Holmes (1809–1894).

> The Poet has a discoloration on the forehead and goes to consult Dr. Franklin, when the following dialogue ensues: 'The colour reminds me,' said Dr. Franklin, 'of what I have seen in a case of Addison's disease, Morbus Addisonii.'
> 'I said I thought the author of the *Spectator* was afflicted with a dropsy to which persons of sedentary and bibacious habits are liable.'
> 'The author of the *Spectator*!' cried out Dr. Franklin; 'I mean the celebrated Dr. Addison, the inventor, I would say, discoverer of the wonderful new disease called after him.'
> 'And what may this valuable invention or discovery consist in.' I asked, for I was anxious to know the nature of the gift which this benefactor of the race had bestowed upon us.
> 'A most interesting affection, and rare too. Allow me to look closely at that discoloration once more for a moment. Cutis aenea – bronze skin they call it sometimes – extraordinary pigmentation; a little more to

the light if you please. Ah! now I get the bronze-colouring admirably, beautifully. Would you have any objection to showing your case to the societies of medical improvement and medical observation?'
'May I ask if any vital organ is commonly involved in this interesting complaint?' I said faintly.
'Well, Sir,' the young doctor replied, 'there is an organ which is – sometimes – a little – touched I may say; a very curious and ingenious little organ or pair of organs. Did you ever hear of the capsulae suprarenales?'
'No,' said I, 'is it a mortal complaint?' getting nervous.
'It isn't a complaint – I mean they are not a complaint; they are two small organs, as I said, inside of you, and nobody knows what is the use of them. The most curious thing is that when anything is the matter with them, you turn the colour of bronze. After all I didn't mean to say I believed it Morbus Addisonii; I only thought of that when I saw the discoloration.'
'So he gave me a recipe which I took care to put where it could do no hurt to anybody, and paid him his fee (which he took with the air of a man in the receipt of a great income), and said good morning.'

It was Samuel Wilks in particular, whom credit is due for of the eventual acceptance of the new disease entity. He wrote:

Being also in accord with Goethe that discoveries are made by the age and not by the individual, I should consider the instances to be exceedingly rare of men who can be said to be living before their age, and to be the repository of knowledge quite foreign to the thought of the time. The rule is that a number of persons are employed at a particular piece of work, but one being a few steps in advance of the others is able to crown the edifice with his name, or, having the ability to generalise already known facts, may become in time to be regarded as their originator. Therefore it is that one name is remembered whilst those of coequals have long been buried to obscurity. . . . As regards Addison, however, the novelty of his discovery was complete, for although cases of melasma of a special form had been met with already, no one had hinted at their association with disease of the suprarenal bodies; and if any further proof were wanting of this statement, it is to be found in the scepticism with which almost up to the present day the discovery has been received, whilst there was a ready acceptance of the almost contemporaneous announcement of Bright, because it was quite in accordance with the knowledge of his time.

Apart from communicating numerous case histories in *Guy's Hospital Reports*, he also wrote a chapter on it in J. Russell Reynold's *System of Medicine* in 1869 (V, pp. 353–367). The aforementioned Greenhow collected and presented 300 patients in his 'Croonian Lectures on Addison's Disease' at the Royal College of Physicians of London in 1875, among them "those published before the appearance of

Addison's monograph", by Schotte (1823), Kirkes and Sibley (1854)[101]. In 1892, Lewin published the analysis of 683 case histories; P. H. Guttman in 1930 recorded 566 such cases between 1900 and 1929[102,103].

In a revealing and most interesting personal letter to Dr. (later Sir Humphrey) Rolleston of 1 January 1895, Sir Samuel Wilks discusses his own role in supporting the recognition of Addison's disease[104]. He says that he defined it in the chapter he wrote for Russell Reynold's *System of Medicine* (London, 1869) as follows:

> The disease is peculiar, uniform in character and primary in its nature
> . . . Three times, if not four times, was the subject of Addison's disease
> before the Medico-Chirurgical Society, but they would not publish
> any of the papers. After the refusal of the first, Addison was much
> vexed and therefore I worked up the case 18 (whose picture is in the
> pamphlet) especially for the Society. It was taken to the Society,
> discussed and refused publication[104].

It is often forgotten that (Sir) William Osler (1849–1919), when at the Johns Hopkins Hospital, had attempted to obtain clinical benefit from orally administering a glycerine extract to patients with Addison's disease. Success, however, escaped him in the case of a young girl of 21, who died during the treatment. Post-mortem examination showed extensive caseous destruction of the adrenals. Osler's glycerine extract was made of 54 fresh pigs' adrenals and given orally in a dose equal to half a gland's extract, three times daily. It is also interesting to note that the correct diagnosis was made (and confirmed by the post-mortem examination) first by Osler's chief, Dr. William Sydney Thayer (1864–1932), then by Osler himself, during the girl's observation both, as an out- and an in-patient, without the blood pressure being recorded even once! How this would upset a modern medical student, used to seeing a record of the patient's biochemistry (including a cortisol curve), often even before seeing the colour of the patient's skin[105].

One patient, however, did apparently derive temporary benefit from dried, whole adrenal glands. He is of special interest because, like Dr. Leonard Portal Mark of St. Bartholomew's Hospital in London, who was acromegalic (see also p. 310), he was a medical man, a professor of pharmacology, Dr. A. L. Muirhead, who described his own case: 'An autograph history of a case of Addison's disease'[106]. After the removal of his right kidney because of a calculus and infection in (?) 1918, Professor Muirhead had attacks of arthritis and gout. In March 1920, however, he developed unmistakable symptoms of Addison's disease, comparatively suddenly, with lowering of the blood pressure and bronzing of the skin. After various attempts of treatment with epinephrine, dried whole supra-renal gland and a similar preparation of pituitary gland by mouth – which all proved ineffective – he was admitted to the Mayo Clinic at Rochester, Minnesota, on 1 July 1920. His blood pressure was then 82/64 mmHg. From there, after the diagnosis had been confirmed, he was referred to Stanley Hospital under Dr. L. G. Rowntree, for treatment. Apart from a purin-free diet, his treatment consisted mainly of epinephrine injections hypodermically (1 cm³ of a 1:10 000 solution twice daily). Attempts were also made at giving rectal injections of dried whole suprarenal gland, 10 grains dissolved in sodium chloride and later with epinephrine, but rectal epinephrine caused severe tenesmus and the treatment was discontinued. The hypodermic administration led to an almost immediate and marked improvement, although the blood pressure did not improve much beyond 92/64 mmHg. The pigmentation of the skin disappeared almost completely, his strength and endurance increased so considerably that he could leave hospital after about eight weeks and after a month's further treatment at home, he was able to resume work as a university teacher. On his purin-free diet, he had no further attacks of gout. The improvement was, however, only temporary, and he died of the disease in the same year (1921)[107].

Recently, I have come across an account of the first description of Addison's disease at necropsy in Chile in 1878, in a woman patient, who was diagnosed by Francisco Mesa Henriquez. The account was published by his intern (student) Diego Baramonde Larenas. The story is related and reviewed by Dr. Claudio Costa-Casaretto, Professor of History of Medicine at the University of Chile[108]. Necropsy of the 46-year-old woman revealed enlargement of both adrenals, especially of the right adrenal, which was of hard consistency; the left was adherent to the walls of the stomach, and its external substance was replaced by, or converted into, a fibrous, dense sac, containing a caseous white mass. There was also genital tuberculosis present. Professor Costa-Casaretto also mentions that there were ten more reports of Addison's disease published in the Chilean medical literature up to 1900.

As well as other endocrine disorders which were identified in Chile during the XIX century. Paresis of the lower limbs produced by Basedow's disease and which was attributed to Charcot (1889), had already been described in our country 17 years before.

In 1660 Frans de le Boë, known as Sylvius (1614–1672) of Leyden had published his *De Lienis et Glandularum Usu*, in which he said:

His addi potest, cui libuerit, Genus tertium, ab utroque praedicto valde diversum, Glandularum Renalium, aut Succenturiatorum Renum nomine quibusdam venientium at notabilem in se cavitate habentium, atque in Venam proximam secundum appositam commissurae valvulam contenta sua affundentium.

One may add, if so desired, a third type, quite different from those previously described, namely the suprarenal glands with a remarkable cavity within them; they pass their secretion into the nearest vein through a valve. [translation: V.C.M.]

According to H. P. Schoenwetter (in his doctor-thesis)[4], it was Emil Huschke (1797–1858), anatomist and embryologist at Jena, who first made a clear anatomical distinction between the adrenal cortex and medulla. Huschke, like Antonio Maria Valsalva (1666–1723) before him thought that there was a connection between the adrenals and the gonads.

Hartman and Brownell, in their monograph on the adrenal gland (1949), stress that the name 'suprarenals', given to the organs found in man, is suitable only for mammals with an erect carriage. The term 'adrenals' is more generally applicable and will be used "Whenever interrenal and chromaffine tissues are combined into a single body"[109].

Johann Friedrich Meckel the Younger (1781–1833) (see also pp. 156 and 172) thought that the suprarenals have some influence on the gonads because in some cases of malformations at birth, both the sexual organs and the adrenal glands may be missing; because in guinea pigs, both the gonads and the adrenals are well developed; because in the case of mammals of the sea, both organs are very small; because in the case of birds and amphibia both organs are in close proximity; because there were cases in which the adrenals were diseased and so were the gonads[110].

When talking of any connection between the adrenals and the gonads, the hypertrophy of the adrenal cortex causing the adrenogenital syndrome must be mentioned. F. T. G. Prunty gave the Humphry Davy Rolleston Lectures at the Royal College of Physicians on 15 and 17 May 1956, on 'Chemical and Clinical Problems of the Adrenal Cortex'. He said about the hypertrophy "In the former group, the earliest association that I am able to find is the occurrence of a probable tumour in a virilized girl described by Henry Sampson in 1697"[111].

Dr. Michael Kelly of Melbourne, Australia, however, in a letter written on 15 September 1956[112], quotes a paper by Harry Keil: 'A note on antiquity of the adreno-genital syndrome'[113]. Keil found in the French translation of the writings of Hippocrates by Littré the clinical descriptions of two patients whose history sounds like an adreno-genital syndrome.

> At Abdera [a married woman] had had children previously; her husband having fled, her menses became suppressed for a long time; afterwards she had pains and redness in the joints . . . the body assumed a masculine appearance, the woman became hairy all over, a beard appeared on her, her voice became rough . . . and in spite of all that we could do to restore her menstruation, the menses did not come . . . [she] died not long after.

There was a second woman in Thasos who became masculine and lost her periods; the only hope of restoring her feminine appearance

> lay in the return of her menses but in her also, despite all measures, the menses did not return . . . this woman soon died[114].

Keil remarks:

> It may be noted also, that these protocols are found in a so-called spurious treatise in the Hippocratic corpus. However, the work is spurious only in the sense that it was probably not written by the shadowy Hippocrates himself. In every other respect the treatise is genuine, and its ancient vintage has been established beyond doubt. The manner in which the clinical data, particularly those of the first case, were recovered over 2000 years ago, is worthy of notice. It is equally interesting to realize that in its essential features the adreno-genital syndrome has remained fundamentally unchanged throughout the ages.

Keil also says that there were two translations of the sentence, . . . ". . . her husband having fled, . . ." and ". . . her husband having been banished . . .". Keil was inclined to accept the version that he fled, which would not be surprising, if he had to notice the change in the appearance of his wife! In an Addendum, Keil remarks: "The partial citations do not provide an adequate picture of the remarkable clinical knowledge exhibited by the ancient Greeks, and for this reason the complete translation is necessary for historical evaluation."

The occurrence of amenorrhoea and virilism was specifically noted by Ambroise Paré (1510–1590) (see also Section II), who wrote about it as follows:

> D'avantage aucune femmes ayant perdu leurs fleurs ou jamais n'ayants eu le cours d'icelles, dégénèrent en nature virile et sont appelées hommasses et des Latins viragines, parce qu'elles sont robustes, audaciennes et superbes, et ont la voix d'hommes et diviennent velues et barbuses, à raison que ce sang qu'elles perdent chacun mois est retenu.

> Some women, having lost their monthly flow, or having never had them, degenerate into a male type and are called masculine women or – in Latin – viragines, because they are robust, aggressive and arrogant, and have a man's voice and become hairy and develop beards, because the blood they (normally) lose every month, is retained[115].

Henry Sampson's patient, reported by him in 1698[116] (This reference differs from that given by Prunty, see p. 237, which I could not check because a copy of the volume was missing in the Library of the Royal Society of Medicine at the time) was a girl, who — originally sickly — became hale and hearty and strong when aged three. She also became fat. She further developed long and thick pubic and axillary hair and some hair on her chin like some old women. At six years she "was in face as large as a full grown woman" (? full-moon face?). She died quite suddenly with acute abdominal symptoms. At the autopsy there was (?) inflammation around the left kidney, which was double in size and "upon dissection there issued a vast quantity of blood". The "testes" were large and smooth. There was no mention of the adrenals. Henry Sampson (1629–1700) was a Fellow of Pembroke College, Cambridge, first as a cleric and later a physician.

Rolleston also quotes[117] the portrait of Eugenia Martinez de Games (Ragazza Gigantesca) by Juan Carreño (1614–1685) in the Prado (No. 646) in Madrid which "clearly suggests this condition". Again according to Rolleston[118] the earliest case confirmed by necropsy in this country is the one recorded by Wm. Cooke, surgeon, of Brentwood, in 1811, "under the heading of internal hydrocephalus, so that it has escaped notice, except perhaps by Linser (1903) whose reference to a case by a man of the same name (Phil. Trans. 1756) cannot be verified". A girl of four was, in 1806, fat, with a florid face, had precocious sexual development with dark pubic hair and pain in the right side of the abdomen. She died three years later of meningitis. Autopsy revealed a large necrotic tumour of irregular outline, speading from the right kidney across the spine towards the opposite kidney.

Another mid-19th century patient was a girl of 3 years, who was reported independently by three observers, in 1865 by J. W. Ogle (1824–1905), by H. Pitman (1808–1908), and in 1885 by William Howship Dickinson (1832–1913).

The skin was generally hyperaemic and of a gipsy coppery hue, though not bronzed, and covered with a remarkable growth of black hair. The eyebrows were thick and bushy, and there was a decided moustache. There was much curly hair about the external genitals which were large. Her language was that of a fishwife.

Interestingly enough, Rolleston and H. Marks were fortunate in examining the necropsy specimen in St. George's Hospital Museum microscopically and found it to be a cortical carcinoma[119].

A girl of nine years of age with virilism and precocious puberty most likely due to adrenocortical hyperplasia was reported in 1932 by J. Bauer and V. C. Medvei[120] (see Figure 24, p. 157).

As Rolleston points out[118], case histories with clinical manifestations, but without the proof of a necropsy, can be found dotted about in the older medical journals, usually among the collections of monstrosities as 'curiosities of precocious puberty'. In boys, cortical hyperplasia seems much rarer. Some of them were reported as the 'infant Hercules' type (see also p. 158). L. Guthrie and W. Emery suggested that the legends about young Hercules and Samson had their origin from the observation of such patients[121]; but records of such cases have existed since antiquity. According to Pliny, the son of one Enthymenes of Salamis was 4½ feet tall when aged 3 and developed puberty. Krateros, the brother of King Antigonos, "in seven years passed through Shakespeare's seven stages"[122]. He died at the age of seven. Charles Charlesworth was 4 feet 7 inches tall in 1734, when aged five, and weighed 87 lbs. and had every sign of puberty, a hairy body and worked with his father as a carrier; he died aged seven[123]. C. J. Geoffroy (1685–1752), membre de l'Académie des Sciences de Paris, reported in 1742 on a 'monstrous boy', aged 3 years and 2 months, whose size and strength made him a 'Prodigy of virility', with pubic hair, erectile penis (6 inches long), and there were a number of patients described as monstrosities[124].

As successful research on the structure of the adrenal cortex was delayed, because of the difficulty of the extirpation experiments and the production of a suitable cortical extract (whereas the main interest was centred on the easier study of the medulla, or, indeed, the whole adrenal, as the cortex was not recognized as being of specific importance), so was the knowledge of the effect of hypersecretion of cortical hormones. In 1902 P. G. Woolley compiled all the adrenal tumour cases available to him from the literature and from personal experience, and recorded only one case of "abnormally developed genitalia" among 22[125]. It occurred in a girl of 4½ years; she was one of the 11 females in the series, 16 of the tumours were diagnosed as 'carcinomas', but how many had cortical involvement is difficult to say [V.C.M.].

On the other hand, William Bulloch (1868–1941) and James Harry Sequeira (1865–1948)[126] and E. E. Glynn[127] both described classic cases of adreno-genitalism, Bulloch and Sequeira's description being the first of the syndrome under that name.

Somewhat later, Rogoff and Stewart reported, although there were no experimental animal models for their study, that dogs adrenalectomized during pregnancy or oestrus, survived for several weeks instead of one[128]. This was also confirmed by other observers. Robert Gaunt and H. W. Hays could, later, show that an injection of oestrogen (or follicular ovaries) reduced survival time after adrenal-ectomy in the ferret, whereas functional corpus luteum or (crystal-line) progesterone maintained life and good health during the period of pseudo-pregnancy. "Progesterone substitutes *standard* corticosteroids better in some species (hamster, ferret) than in others (rat, dog, man)"[129].

Gaunt adds in interesting quotation from Biedl's classical textbook[22] (p. 269 in the English translation of 1913): "Mulon even regards the corpus luteum verum as a temporary suprarenal cortex." Since then it has been established that the adrenal cortex normally produces a multitude of steroid hormones, including androgens and progesterone.

Bulloch and Sequeira mentioned[126] that one Otto had recorded a case of hypertrophy of the adrenals in 1816; this patient was also quoted by Lancereaux in the *Dictionnaire des Sciences Médicales*[130].

In contrast, J. Wiesel, who had worked with Biedl, described a girl of 18, who had no axillary hair, but one or two on the mons veneris, non-existent mammae, rudimentary nipples and infantile genitalia. Post-mortem examination revealed a striking hypoplasia of the adrenals[131].

Although hirsuties and virilism may be caused by excess androgen production from autonomous tumours of the adrenal cortex or congenital adrenal hyperplasia (CAH), from Cushing's disease, from ovarian tumours and, most commonly, from the polycystic ovary syndrome or even drug administration, there is a long history of the existence of marked hirsuties in women of familial or racial occurrence without menstrual disorders and com-pletely normal female sexual function. Julia Pastrana, of Sierra Madre in Mexico, died in childbed in 1860, aged 26, after the delivery of a son who died 36 hours after birth. The mother was $4\frac{1}{2}$ feet tall, well built, stoutish, of feminine appearance apart from a rough beard on her face and excessive hairiness of shoulders, hips, breasts and spine. Both, mother and son, were exhibited in a museum in Moscow, at least before the first War. They were also mentioned and discussed by Darwin (IV, vol. II, p. 434).

The celebrated Maphoon, 4th daughter of Shwé-Maong of Burma, was reported by Crawford in 1829 when she was $2\frac{1}{2}$ years old; she had been hairy since birth, and had delayed dentition. The mother was also hairy and also had abnormal dentition. Maphoon was seen again in 1855, when aged $28\frac{1}{2}$, by Colonel Henry Yule. She was then completely hairy, with hair on her nose "like the wisps of a fine skye terrier's coat and a beard, 4 inches long". At that time, she had two sons, the elder apparently being normal, then aged 4 or 5 years. The younger, aged 14 months, was hairy. When seen again in 1867, by

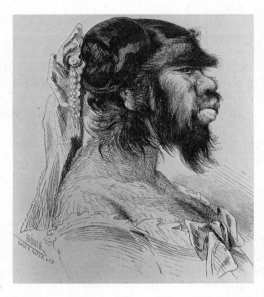

Figure 42   Julia Pastrana (after Alex. Ecker, Prof. Anat. (Freiburg))

Captain Houghton at the court of Ava, he seemed hairier than ever.

There is the portraiture of the hairy family (from Munich?) at Schloss Ambras in the Tyrol, father, mother son and daughter in 16th century dress (described by Siebold)[132]. Above all, there is the famous painting by José de Ribera (1591–1652): 'La mujer barbuda (Magdalena Ventura con su esposo e su hijo)' or 'The Bearded Woman (Magdalena Ventura with Husband and Son)', the bearded and moustachioed mother suckling her infant. It became widely known to the English public after the exhibition 'The Golden Age of Spanish Painting' at the Royal Academy of Arts in London in 1976.

The best documented hairy and bearded woman with normal female function was perhaps the 20-year-old young Swiss needle-woman, who presented herself at Charing Cross Hospital in London, when 5 months pregnant. There was a request to have a testimonial as to her sex as "she was under an engagement to marry, but that the masculine appearance of her face produced scruples in the mind of persons who would otherwise have performed the marriage ceremony". Her case was reported in full by W. D. Chowne, MD, physician to the Charing Cross Hospital, in *The Lancet* in 1852[133]. The report includes the information that the young lady was, in due course, confined at Charing Cross Hospital and was able to nurse her new-born daughter, who appeared

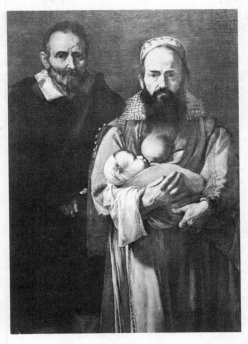

Figure 43 Ribera *La mujer barbuda* [by kindness of the Lerma Foundation at the Tavera Hospital, Toledo]

completely normal. The mother had an abundance of milk, "her mammae being even more than usually large." The child was fair.

As racial peculiarities, the writer, traveller and critic Max Nordau (1849–1923), wrote of the Provençal women in 1880:

> Das edle Gesicht der Provençalin wird durch eine ganz maennliche Behaarung grausam entstellt, die schon bereits beim zehnjaehrigen Maedchen als schwacher Flaum erscheint und bei der zwanzigjaehrigen bereits Husaren- und Sappeur-Dimensionen angenommen hat. . . . Allein hier handelt es sich . . . um einen richtigen Kinn-, Scnurr- und Backenbart, der nach dem Scheermesser schreit und namentlich im hoeheren Alter abstossend wirkt[134].

> Their noble features were cruelly distorted by an entirely virile hair growth, which begins already at the age of 10, and at the age of 20 has grown to a size, you expect to find on a hussar . . . it is a growth of true sidewhiskers, moustache and goatee, which needs the razor . . . at a higher age it becomes repulsive.

In France, hirsuties was observed to occur frequently in mental woman patients. Duflos, a pupil of Professor Dupré, found in 1901 among 1000 ordinary women patients in the hospitals of Paris, 290 with a beard, ten of whom had a strong beard. Among 1000 mental

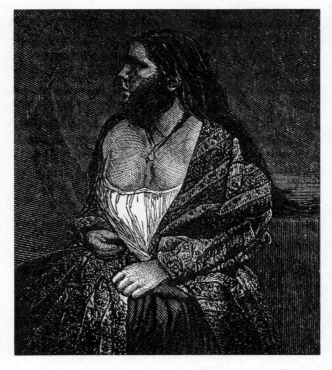

Figure 44   Chowne's case [*Lancet* **1,** 1852]

patients he found 497 bearded ones, 56 of whom had a strong growth of facial hair. Le Double found, among 1277 women in the mental asylums of the Touraine, 42 with a marked beard[135]. M. Laignel-Lavastine of the Hôpital Laennec in Paris, concluded in 1921:

> D'un mot, la fréquence des femmes à barbe dans les asiles d'aliénées s'explique par l'étude des correlations psycho-endocriniennes, et je dirai pour terminer, que les femmes à barbe gardent le vestibule de l'endocrino-psychiatrie[136].

> In one word, the frequency of bearded women in mental institutions is explained by the existence of the psycho-endocrine correlations, and, in fine, I would like to say that the bearded women guard the communication-corridors between endocrinology and psychiatry.

THE THYROID

It was in the case of the thyroid that it was first established that normal secretion of an endocrine gland is essential to good health, and that underfunction (hyposecretion) will lead to a picture of

XXXVII.—*On a Cretinoid State supervening in Adult Life in Women.* By Sir WILLIAM W. GULL, Bart., M.D. *Read October* 24, 1873.

THE remarks I have to make upon the above morbid state are drawn from the observation of five cases. Of two of these I am able to give many details, but the three others were only seen by me on one or two occasions.

CASE I.

Miss B., after the cessation of the catamenial period, became insensibly more and more languid, with general increase of bulk. This change went on from year to year, her face altering from oval to round, much like the full moon at rising. With a complexion soft and fair, the skin presenting a peculiarly smooth and fine texture was almost porcelainous in aspect, the cheeks tinted of a delicate rose-purple, the cellular tissue under the eyes being loose and

* See communication by me, ' Path. Soc. Trans.' vol. xvii. p. 186.

Figure 45 Gull's title page [by kind permission of the Royal Society of Medicine]

inefficiency, ill health and apparently toxic symptoms. It was another Guy's physician, Sir William Withey Gull (1816–1890) (see Section II), who gave in his paper 'On a cretinoid state supervening in adult life in women'[137] one of the first classic descriptions of myxoedema. He reported his observations of five patients. "Of two of these I am able to give many details, but the three others were only seen by me on one or two occasions". Case I:

Miss B., after the cessation of the catamenial period, became insensibly more and more languid, with general increase of bulk. The change went on from year to year, her face altering from oval to round, much like the full moon at rising. With a complexion soft and fair, the skin presenting a peculiarly smooth and fine texture was almost porcelainous in aspect, the cheeks tinted of a delicate rose-purple, the cellular tissue under the eyes being loose and folded, and that under the jaws and in the neck becoming heavy, thickened and folded. The lips large and of a rose-purple, alae nasi thick, cornea and pupil of the eye normal, but the distance between the eyes appearing disproportionately wide, and the rest of the nose depressed, giving the whole face a flattened broad character. The hair flaxen and soft, the whole expression of the face remarkably placid. The tongue broad and thick, voice guttural, and the pronunciation as if the tongue were too large for the mouth (cretinoid). The hands peculiarly broad and thick, spade-like, as if the whole textures were infiltrated. The integuments of the chest and abdomen loaded with subcutaneous fat. The upper and lower extremities also large and fat, with slight traces of oedema over the tibiae, but this not distinct, and pitting doubtfully on pressure. Urine normal. Heart's action and sound normal. Pulse, 72; breathing 18. Such is a general outline of the state to which I wish to call attention.

In his conclusions, Gull said:

In the cretinoid condition in adults which I have seen, the thyroid was not enlarged; but from the general fullness of the cutaneous tissues, and from the folds of the skin about the neck, I am not able to state what the exact condition of it was. The supra-clavicular masses of fat first described by Mr. Curling, and specially drawn attention to by Dr. Fagge [see p. 247] as occurring in cases of sporadic cretinism in children, did not attract my attention in adults. The masses of supra-clavicular fat are not infrequent in the adult, without any associated morbid change whatever.

Twenty-three years before, in 1850, Thomas Blizzard Curling (1811–1888), surgeon to the London Hospital, had reported on "Two cases of absence of the thyroid body and symmetrical swellings of fat tissue at the sides of the neck, connected with defective cerebral development"[138]. One patient was 10 years, the other 6 months old. Necropsies on these cases showed absence of the thyroid. Curling concluded:

Pathologists have been recently inclined to view the coincidence of these two conditions (the defective condition of the brain and the hypertrophy of the thyroid) as accidental, or as having no direct relation. In the foregoing cases we have examples of a directly opposite condition, viz., a defective brain, or cretinism, combined with an entire absence of the thyroid, which may be regarded as tending to confirm the more modern opinion respecting the connection between cretinism and bronchocele.

On 23 October 1877, William Miller Ord (1834–1902), read his paper "On myxoedema, a term proposed to be applied to an essential condition in the 'cretinoid' affection, occasionally observed in Middle-Aged Women'[139]. In it, he referred to the five patients described by Sir William Gull in 1873, and went on to record two of his own five patients of a similar kind whom he had had under his care during the previous 12 years. The description of the skin of the first patient, a woman of 54, was classic:

the skin over the whole body was singularly dry. On the limbs and trunk it was harsh and rough to the touch; the hairs were feebly developed and no trace of fatty secretion could be found. The skin was everywhere sensitive, but the limit of confusion in tactile discrimination was everywhere wider than average. The same sort of swelling observed in the skin was visible in the fauces.

The full report of the post-mortem examination by Dr. William

Smith Greenfield (1846–1919) was attached to the paper. The patient died aged 58, but Ord commented on a few important details:

1. There was oedema of the skin generally; but the cut surfaces yielded less fluid than their appearance would promise. 2. There was much serous effusion in the pleurae, pericardium and peritoneum. 3. The heart was of large size, weighing sixteen and a half ounces; the left ventricle hypertrophied, the wall being an inch thick; valves practically healthy. 4. The arteries were everywhere thickened, the larger ones atheromatous. . . . . 6. There was a firm, almost solid oedema in many parts, e.g. in heart, soft palate, larynx, stomach, and neck of bladder. 7. The brain showed very considerable degeneration of the larger arteries.

Dr. Ord continued:

The cases agree, in most respects, very closely with those narrated by Sir William Gull; in fact, I am inclined to think that two of them may have come under his observation. . . . As regards the class of cases immediately in question, my suggestion is that the whole collection of symptoms are related as effects to jelly-like swelling of the connective tissue, chiefly if not entirely consisting in an overgowth of the mucus-yielding cement by which the fibrils of the white elements are held together. Accordingly, I propose to give the name Myxoedema to the affection . . . but the name is only intended to represent the condition, and does not profess to involve an explanation of its causes. Whether the mucous oedema can be a degeneration, an arrest of development, or an introduction of new material, is not at present a question ripe for discussion; and though I should be grateful for suggestions on these points, I do not propose at present to express any opinion of my own.

The skin of one of the patients was chemically examined by Dr. Cranston Charles and was found to contain a substance "which corresponded in its reactions to the mucin of Scherer, Eichwald and Staedeler".

In his discussion, Ord referred to a paper published in 1871 by another Guy's man, Charles Hilton Fagge (1838–1883), who was his junior; 'On Sporadic Cretinism in England'[140]. Fagge described sporadic cretinism as distinct from the endemic one (see p. 252).

The relation between goitre and cretinism is ably and fully discussed by Dr. Hilton Fagge in a paper in Vol. 54 of the Transactions of this Society . . . this paper brought out more fully the principle which seemed likely to follow from Mr. Curling's observations, namely, that while goitre was more or less associated with endemic cretinism, the thyroid gland was actually absent or atrophied in sporadic cretinism occurring in this country; and that Dr. Fagge infers the existence of a direct antagonism between goitre and cretinism . . . it is obvious that the case of H. J. is one more in favour of them.

Gull's and Ord's observations received – as it were – a complement by the Swiss surgeon Emil Theodor Kocher (1841–1917) of Bern (see Section II), who first reported the result of 'Exstirpation einer Struma retro-oesophagea' in 1878[141]. Kocher was a pupil of Bernhard Rudolph Conrad von Langenbeck (1810–1887) and Christian Albert Theodor Billroth (1829–1894), and was professor of surgery in his native town from 1872 to 1917. He carried out thyroidectomy for goitre (a particularly difficult operation in his time) over 2000 times with only $4\frac{1}{2}$% mortality. In 1883, he published the description of 'cachexia strumipriva'.

In his paper 'Ueber Kropfexstirpation und ihre Folgen'[142], he found that condition as a sequel in 30 of his first 100 thyroidectomies, and coined the expression 'cachexia strumipriva' to describe the myxoedema following the operation.

As already mentioned (see p. 192), in England, Joseph Henry Green (1791–1863) of St. Thomas's and Guy's Hospital had reported on the removal of the enlarged right lobe of the thyroid gland in a young woman of 24, on 22 May 1829; the patient died *ca.* 2 weeks later (on 6 or 7 June).

> She had been in Guy's Hospital some months since and had there taken iodyne to a large extent. The tumour is now, she says, much smaller than at that time, and the integuments are quite loose over it. On Friday, 22nd of May, an operation having been determined on, at her own request, the patient was placed on the operating table ... it was found impossible (to remove) the whole of the gland, on account of the large vessels in the neighbourhood; the operation lasted 20 minutes; the wound was dressed with dry lint.

She seems to have died of septicaemia.

Jacques Louis Reverdin (1842–1929) and A. Reverdin (1849–1908) of Geneva reported on 'Accidents consécutifs à l'ablation totale du goître'[143], in 1882, in which they produced myxoedema by removal of the thyroid as a whole or in part. Probably unknown to them, Moritz Schiff (1823–1896) of Geneva had published a paper on his experimental total thyroidectomies in 1859[144] which he had carried out in 1856–1857 in dogs (often fatal after the first week) and in guinea pigs who survived a little longer. This fatal outcome could not be related to wound infection or to damage to the recurrent branch of the vagus or of the cervical sympathetic. Unfortunately, the title of his paper was 'Untersuchungen ueber die Zuckerbildung in der Leber und der Einfluss des Nerven-systems und die Erzeugung des Diabetes' (= 'Investigations on the formation of sugar in the liver and the production of diabetes'), which does not indicate the total range of his experiments. In a later communication[145], he proved that intra-abdominal transplantation of the thyroid will prevent the fatal effect of total thyroidectomy.

As well as Schiff, there were others who attempted similar experiments: Sir Astley Paston Cooper in 1836 (see p. 165), Wilhelm von Rapp (1794–1868) in 1840, and Heinrich Adolph von Bardeleben (1819–1895) in 1843, just to mention a few. Their results were inconclusive, mainly because the parathyroid glands, unknown at that time, were removed together with the thyroid. Finally, Sir Felix Semon (1849–1921) put forward the view, in the discussion of the paper 'A typical case of myxoedema' in 1883[146], that myxoedema, cachexia strumipriva and cretinism were all caused by loss of function of the thyroid, "a conclusion which at the time excited ridicule and was not published in the *Transactions of the Clinical Society of London*". It was, however, eventually fully confirmed in a report of a committee set up by the Clinical Society of London to investigate myxoedema, with W. M. Ord as chairman and W. B. Hadden as secretary.

One of the committee members was the professor and superintendent from 1884 to 1890 of the Brown Institution, (later Sir) Victor Alexander Haden Horsley (1857–1916) (see Section II), who was also in support. Semon, who was of German birth, was at that time one of the leading laryngologists in Britain. At that notable meeting, he called attention to Professor Kocher's report at the Twelfth Congress of German Surgeons, held in Berlin in April 1883, which was mentioned above: 'On the Extirpation of Goitre and its Consequences'[142]. He recalled the progressive deterioration into Kocher's cachexia strumipriva of those eighteen (out of 101 presented) cases of Kocher's patients, on whom total extirpation of the thyroid body had been performed. Semon continued:

> (Kocher) being himself unaware of the existence of myxoedema, he proposed for the affection he described the name of 'cachexia strumi-priva' (struma = goitre). Similar observations had been made by Professor Reverdin of Geneva.

He then quoted one of his own cases, in whom Professor Lister had removed the thyroid body *in toto* 3 years before. He (Dr. Semon) thought, however, that the identity of these changes with those met with in myxoedema, which he had found when reading through Professor Kocher's paper, was very evident.

> Not one symptom was present in myxoedema which was not met with in these cases of total extirpation; on the other hand, one symptom only had been observed in a certain number of these cases which was not present in myxoedema, viz., the arrest of the growth of the body after total removal of the gland in children. But the explanation of this

249

difference was obvious: myxoedema was essentially a disease of adult life. Looking upon the whole from a broad point of view, there appeared to be three conditions closely allied to each other, and having in common either absence or probably complete degeneration of the thyroid body: namely, cretinism, myxoedema, and the state after total removal of the thyroid body. In all three states, certain conditions of arrested development of mind and body were met with, which, looked upon in the new light thrown upon the subject by Professor Kocher's observations, could hardly be attributed to anything else but to the loss of the thyroid body, common to them all.

Between 1884 and 1886, Sir Victor Horsley produced experimental evidence that myxoedema, cretinism and surgical cachexia strumipriva are all, indeed, caused by deficient thyroid function[147-149], but some of the symptoms were due to the removal of the parathyroids. His careful experiments were carried out on monkeys. He found striking nervous symptoms after thyroidectomy: within 5 days tremors began and they persisted even after section of the motor nerves or the removal of the appropriate cortical centres. Inhalation of ether increased the tremor and reflex stimulation abolished it. Bulbar dyspnoea may appear, the salivary glands hypertrophied. Death occurred 1 or 2 months after thyroid extirpation. At post-mortem, the subcutaneous tissues were 'myxoedematous', i.e. swollen, sticky, jelly-like (especially in the neck). This was observed in other areas and along the course of the coronary arteries, but there were no changes in the synovial membranes. The membranes of the brain were distended with fluid, but no structural changes could be found in the nerve and brain tissues. In summary, his conclusions were (a) that the thyroid must be a regulator of the cerebral circulation; (b) that it must secrete a substance needed for the proper nutrition of the nervous system; (c) that the thyroid excretes a mucinous substance which is injurious to the nervous system; (d) that it is most likely also a blood-forming organ.

Thyroid atrophy during foetal life is virtually irreversible, and the complete cretin thus created is barely human. François Émmanuel Fodéré (1764–1835), the great authority in France on forensic medicine at the beginning of the 19th century, described these unfortunate people in his celebrated essay 'Essai sur le goître et le crétinage' (Turin, 1792), and in his 'Traité du Goître et du crétinism' (Paris, 1800) as follows:

Ici on ne reconnait pas l'homme. Frappé dans ses caractères distinctifs, la pensée et la parole, ce n'est plus ce maître de la terre, qui calcule l'immensité des cieux, et qui en décrit les mouvements; c'est le plus faible de tous les êtres vivants, puisqu'il est même incapable de pourvoir de lui–même à sa subsistance. Ce n'est plus cette physionomie animée, cet oeil superbe, où se peint la volonté; c'est un visage muet, semblable à ces vieilles pièces de monnaie, dont l'usage a effacé l'empreinte.

Here, one does not recognize a human being. Struck in his distinctive characteristics, the thought and the spoken word, this is no longer the lord of the earth, who calculates the immensity of the skies and describes their very movements; it is the weakest of all existing living beings, since he is even incapable to provide himself for his own subsistence. This is no more the animated countenance, the proud eye, which reflects the will; it is a dumb face, similar to those old pieces of coin, where (continuous) use has erased the imprint of the coin-face. [translation: V.C.M.]

Complete cretins cannot articulate. They are late in walking and are rarely capable of feeding themselves much before 10 years of age. Their height does not normally exceed five feet or so, and their skin tends to become brown. About them Fodéré said:

Le mot crétin vient lui-même de chrétien . . . titre qu'on donne a ces idiots, 'parce que', dit-on, 'ils sont incapables de commettre aucun péché.

The word 'cretin' itself is derived from 'Christian' . . . a title one gives these idiots because they are incapable of committing a sin. [translation: V.C.M.]

Fodéré, who hailed from the valley of La Maurienne, which was a goitre district, himself had a goitre. He believed that goitre was but the first step towards cretinism, and the latter was – in his opinion – invariably inherited, usually from the father's side.

Iason quotes George S. Blackie (1855–1895) on "Cretins and Cretinism"[150]:

The popular belief in many places lays the blame on the waters, and especially in Styria (Austria) wells from which inhabitants fear to drink, or having by accident drunk out of them, they rush to an antidotal well to counteract the bad effects. . . . We find the well to abound in iodine which would seem to be nature's specific for the complaint.

Later, Blackie continues:

there are five distinct classes of bronchocele to be met with arising probably from different causes but presenting the same phenomena. . . . Of these the cause of the first is tolerably well established, those of the second and third doubtful; and those of the two last unknown. These classes are: 1. Endemic bronchocele, caused by the waters being strongly impregnated with lime. 2. Weaver's bronchocele, caused by the mode of work and emanations of steeped flax. 3. Cardigenous bronchocele, arising from a functional derangement of the heart. 4. Congenital bronchocele, where an infant is born with the disease –

cause unknown. 5. Sporadic bronchocele, when an individual not residing in, or coming from a locality where the disease is endemic, is attacked by it, and where the causes of the second and third classes are inapplicable – cause also unknown.

Endemic cretinism occurs in certain areas (not limited necessarily to mountainous districts)[151]; in the districts affected, goitre is very often coupled with cretinism, although there are a few goitrous areas where cretinism is virtually absent, and some cretins have no goitre. Hermann Zondek drew a sharp distinction between endemic and spontaneous cretinism. Spontaneous cretinism, in Zondek's opinion, is congenital or infantile myxoedema (sporadic cretinism). The name (sporadic cretinism) is misleading,

> for by no means all children with thyroid deficiency are or become cretins, whilst true cretinism is an entirely different disease[152]. . . . In sporadic cretinism the thyroid is certainly the pathogenic centre of gravity; for endemic cretinism this has yet to be proved[153].

H. Norris, who described in 1848 apparently the only instance of endemic cretinism in England, wrote that in the village of Chiselborough in Somerset there were, out of a total population of 540, four complete cretins, 17 semi-idiots, five deaf-mutes, and the majority of the population were slow of speech and dull and all having a goitre[154]. Happily, Charles Hilton Fagge (1838–1883) of Guy's Hospital could report in 1871 that this endemic cretinism in Chiselborough had died out by 1870, in his report: 'On sporadic cretinism occurring in England'[155] in which he distinguished between sporadic cretinism in contrast to the endemic type.

It was, incidentally, Paracelsus (Aureolus Philippus Theophrastus Bombastus Ab Hohenheim, 1493–1541) in "De generatione stultorum"[156], who connected causally cretinism and goitre:

> Suadet hujus loci occasio, ut etiam de corporis deformitatibus et rebus illis connatis, ut sunt strumae et similia nonnihil differamus. Quae licet stultis quidem propria non sint, sed ipsis cum aliis communia; in stultis tamen eadem omnia frequentissima sunt.

(See also Chapter 12, p. 98.)

We have seen (in Chapter 14) that the discovery of iodine was put to use in the treatment of goitre. A further important contribution along that line was made by the long-lived Gaspard Adolphe Chatin (1813–1901), who showed in 1850 that iodine in plants of fresh ('sweet') water could prevent endemic goitre and cretinism. He was able to detect the presence of minute amounts of iodine in organic and inorganic matter, in watercress and all plants in fresh water, and pointed out that goitre and cretinism seem to occur where drinking water, soil, air and natural food are deficient in iodine[157].

Chatin found that iodine is universally present in nature, but that the amounts in different soils, plants, waters and animal and vegetable products vary. He discovered that the iodine content of food and water in goitre districts is low. In 1852, Chatin calculated that from all sources, the daily intake of iodine by a person living in goitre-free Paris was 1/100–1/200 mg; in Lyons and Turin, which were moderately goitrous places, the daily intake was 1/500–1/1000 mg; in highly goitrous Alpine valleys, there was a maximum of 1/2000 mg[158,159]. He recommended, consequently, that the water supply in goitrous districts should be supplemented with iodine.

> . . . il sera quelquefois facile d'approprier aux besoins des populations les eux minérales iodurées, qui, par une circonstance providentielle, jaillissent en grand nombre des contrées où les eaux potables sont le moins chargées d'iode[160].

That is, he recommends in those regions the utilization of the springs of mineral water which are rich in iodine, in contrast to the ordinary drinking water.

Attention to those facts had been drawn before him by Prevost and Maffoni[161] and J. Inglis in England in 1831–1832[162]. The French Academy of Science appointed a commission for the study of goitre; they decided that they could not accept the idea that small amounts of iodine could produce any physiological effect on the animal body. As a result of this and the criticism of the chemists, Chatin's work fell into discredit and oblivion, until von Fellenberg rediscovered it in 1923[163].

This reminds one of the fate of the recommendation of the Goitre Subcommittee of the Medical Research Council of 1944 and 1948 on the iodization of salt in the United Kingdom: "the adoption of a national policy of adding a trace of iodine to all common salt consumed in this country (one part of KI to 100 000 parts of salt)". An attempt was made to put the recommendation into effective action in 1960, but this failed.

In 1845, a Commission of 19 members was appointed by King Carlo Alberto of Sardinia to investigate the extent, nature and causes of endemic goitre throughout the Kingdom (i.e. Savoy, Nice, Piedmont, Genoa and the Island of Sardinia). In 1855, F. Koestl[164] suggested the use of iodized salt in Austria, and Cesare Lombroso (1836–1909) recommended in 1859 that all goitrous persons of marriageable age should be treated with iodine to prevent cretinism, and that iodine should also be administered to farm animals.

A French experiment carried out in 1860, at the instigation of J. B.

Boussingault, failed. Boussingault had lived for many years in Colombia, where he learnt about the experience of the local people on the therapeutic effect of the salt from an abandoned mine in Guaca (Department of Antioquia). In 1825, he analysed the salt and found that it contained large quantities of iodine. In 1833, he suggested iodization of salt for the prevention of goitre[165]. This was subsequently supported by Jean Louis Prévost (1790–1850)[165,166], and by G. A. Chatin. This first known experiment in goitre prevention was carried out by the Departments of Bas-Rhin, Seine-Inférieure and Haut-Savoie. Goitrous families received salt fortified with 0.1–0.5 g of potassium iodide per kilogram of salt. Schoolchildren with goitre received daily tablets or a solution of 0.01 g of potassium iodide.

> Open bottles containing iodine were placed in bedrooms. In view of the high doses of iodide, it is small wonder that toxic symptoms of iodism and Jod-Basedow were frequent and that, consequently, iodide prophylaxis was discredited and abandoned.

It was not successfully revived until David Marine and O. P. Kimball's large scale experiment in Akron, Ohio, U.S.A. in 1917[167] (see also p. 514). The results were so convincing and striking that Marine's well-known aphorism cannot be quoted too often:

> Simple goitre is the easiest of all known diseases to prevent. . . . It may be excluded from the list of human diseases as soon as society determines to make the effort. (David Marine, 1880–1976; see also Section II.)

The Lancet, commenting on the situation in the United Kingdom, gave in its Editorial of 12 April 1958, the conclusive answer: "So far, this country has made no attempt to eliminate goitre." (In October 1948, the Medical Research Council Memorandum No. 18 estimated that there were some 500 000 people in England, Wales and Scotland between 5 and 20 years of age who had simple goitre.) The recommendation for iodized salt was repeated. It was established that potassium iodate could be used instead of iodide, which eliminated certain technical difficulties raised by the salt manufacturers.

Ernest H. Starling referred to Marine and Kimball's successful experiment in his Harveian Oration to the Royal College of Physicians 'On the Wisdom of the Body', given in London on St. Luke's Day, 1923:

> It has been shown by Marine and others that goitre can be practically eliminated from these districts (especially in Switzerland and certain parts of the United States) by the occasional administration of small doses of iodine or iodides. These results were communicated in 1917 to Dr. Klinger, of Zurich, and as a result of his experience the Swiss

Goitre Commission has recommended the adoption of this method of goitre prevention as a public health measure throughout the entire state. Already great progress has been made in the abolition of this disease from the country. Thus the incidence of goitre among all the school-children of the canton of St. Gallen has been reduced from 87.6% in January 1919, to 13.1% in January 1922[168].

David Marine (1880–1976), called in one of his obituaries the 'Nestor of Thyroidology', made – according to James H. Means, who also coined the above eponym in 1961 – four major contributions to thyroid research:

(1) He established, in 1907, that iodine is necessary for thyroid function.

(2) In 1911, he proposed treatment of Graves' disease with iodine, which was taken up by Henry Stanley Plummer (1874–1937) 12 years later.

(3) He introduced goitre prevention with iodine in 1917.

(4) In 1932, he described cyanide goitre[169,170].

Actually, in 1909, Marine rejected the idea of iodine deficiency as the sole linear cause of goitre, in favour of a multiple causation, of a complex nature[171]. Eventually, he proposed iodization of all salt for the entire population, but – in order to avoid side effects from excessive iodine intake (especially Jod-Basedow) – he insisted on a general prophylaxis with 1: 100 000 parts of iodine of all salt rather than the original 1: 10 000 of iodized table salt only. In his paper with Lenhart, in 1909, he wrote: ". . . it is our belief that one or more chemical substances will be found which are antagonistic to or inhibit the normal absorption or assimilation of iodine"[171]. He elaborated this statement later: ". . . goitre may develop because of relative iodine deficiency caused by factors which interfere with the absorption or utilization of iodine". Three years later such a goitrogenic factor became the subject of intensive inquiry. It was eventually established that the thiocyanates of the Brassica plants (cabbage, cauliflower, turnip) were goitrogenic; the effect could be prevented when cabbage and iodine were given simultaneously[172] (see also p. 514).

In 1850, Fréderic Rilliet (1814–1861) (see also p. 191), presented to the Academy of Medicine in Paris the classic description of the effects of overdosage of iodine[173]. Before him, it had been mentioned by Jean François Coindet (1774–1834) of Geneva in 1821[174]. It was Ernst Theodor Kocher (1841–1917) who coined the expression 'Jod-Basedow' for the condition, in 1910; this term was refused recognition by many workers in the field, until John B. Stanbury and his team, working in Mendoza, Argentina, confirmed that Jod-Basedow can occur if the therapeutic dose of iodine is much larger than the daily requirement of an individual patient[175]. Iodine thus does not cause, but conditions the development of, the disease. Hyperthyroidism developing during treatment with 200–300 μg of iodine suggests (Plummer's) toxic adenoma; hyperthyroidism developing on prolonged treatment with larger doses (much larger than the daily, individual requirement) of iodine, suggests Jod-Basedow, the symptoms of which usually disappear spontaneously a few weeks after discontinuing iodine treatment[176]. Coindet[177] and later others, noticed that occasionally, on about the seventh day of iodine therapy, a painful enlargement of the goitre may occur, if large doses of iodine are given[178]. After discontinuing iodine therapy, there is a spontaneous decrease of the goitre. This transient, harmless condition is known as iodine thyroiditis, caused perhaps by a temporary hypersecretion of the thyrotropic hormone, causing the sudden formation of iodine-containing colloid in the follicles.

Although Hermann Lebert (1813–1878) suggested chemical investigation of the thyroid in 1862[179], this was not begun until 1882 (by Bubnow)[180]. Bubnow carried out a systematic biochemical examination of the gland. Although he confirmed the existence of xanthines and creatinine, he turned his main attention to the proteins in the thyroid, assuming that the 'colloid' in the follicles of the normal gland was perhaps protein in nature and a significant constituent. He eventually isolated three 'thyroproteins' (I, II and III), which were all soluble in acetic acid and thus not identifiable as mucin. Kocher predicted in 1893 that iodine might occur in the thyroid, but it was Eugen Baumann (1846–1896) of Freiburg-im-Breisgau, who demonstrated the presence of iodine in organic combination as a normal constituent of the thyroid gland, and that the amount varies, usually being in the range of 0.05–0.45%. Baumann succeeded after several others (Tschirsch, 1895; Drechsel, 1895–6 and Fraenkel, 1895) had failed. Baumann named the new product 'thyroiodin' and later 'iodothyrin'; the discovery surprised him, as he himself expressed: "... als ich diese Beobachtung zuerst machte, glaubte ich an alles Andere eher, als dass das Iod meiner Substanz angehoere"[181–183] ("When I first made this observation, I could believe anything rather than that the iodine belonged to my substance".)

Incidentally, (Sir) Charles Robert Harington, himself one of the most brilliant biochemists of modern times (1897–1972), who occupies a very special position in the investigation of the chemistry and physiology of the thyroid, described the efforts to elucidate and clarify the chemistry of the thyroid vividly and dramatically in his magnum opus *The Thyroid Gland, Its Chemistry and Physiology*[184], which is a classic from every point of view. It is also of interest that Harington himself accepted the existence of 'Jod-Basedow', because — as he said:

> At first sight the discovery of iodine in the thyroid by Baumann (1896), and the suggestion which followed that iodine was an essential constituent of the active secretion of the gland seemed to afford a rational explanation of the injurious effect of iodine in Graves' disease . . .

and

> The fear of iodine seemed in fact to be justified by the undoubted effect of iodine in causing occasional exacerbations of Graves' disease, and still more by its apparent power of causing a patient with simple goitre to develop Graves' disease.

The latter phenomenon has already been referred to when discussing the early work on the iodine therapy of simple goitre. Graves' disease was not at that time recognized, but the description by Wm. Gairdner (1824) of the condition of goitrous patients after over-vigorous treatment with iodine leaves no doubt that the syndrome of Graves' disease had been elicited or at least precipitated in them by the use of the drug. He said[185]:

> I have seen more than one physician seriously injured in his reputation, and many patients irrecoverably injured in their health by this subtle and powerful medicine . . .

Simultaneously with Baumann's investigations, R. Hutchison studied the proteins of the thyroid gland[186]. The active protein-free digestion product he obtained seemed closely related to Baumann's iodothyrin, although the iodine content was lower. Hutchison's results showed, however, that Baumann's view that iodothyrin contained the whole of the iodine of the thyroid was not correct. This was also confirmed by the work of R. Tambach[187]. The researches of these investigators (Baumann, Hutchison, Tambach, and D. Hellin in 1898) were carefully repeated, developed and extended by A. Oswald, and published in numerous original papers between 1897 and 1925[188,189]. Oswald also investigated the various factors influencing the iodine content of the thyroid gland, such as disease, diet, seasonal variations and age. These factors were also on the research programme of other workers. The distribution of iodine in the thyroid was studied later by A. L. Tatum[190]. In spite of all these efforts the only iodine-containing protein was limited to 'gorgonin', a protein derived from the axial skeleton of the coral, isolated by E. Drechsel[191]. This was shown in 1905 by H. L. Wheeler and G. S. Jamieson really to be 3:5-diiodothyrosine[192]; but diiodothyrosine is devoid of thyroid activity. The isolation of a physiologically active iodine compound from the products of alkaline hydrolysis of the thyroid will be described later.

The *excessive function* of the thyroid cells has now to be considered. The idea that hypersecretion of a ductless gland, such as the thyroid, might cause disease in the form of exophthalamic goitre was first put forward in 1886 by Paul Julius Moebius (1853–1907) (see Section II) in a review of 'Vom Verhaeltnisse der Poliomyelencephalitis zur Basedowschen Krankheit'[193] (see also p. 266), and supported by Wm. Smith Greenfield (1846–1919). Greenfield described hyperplasia of the thyroid at the Bradshaw Lecture at the Royal College of Physicians in 1893[194]; this was regarded as being responsible for "exaggerated but probably perverted function" by N. W. Janney in 1922[195]. As Rolleston put it in 1936[12] (p. 30):

The conception of disease due to excess of a normal hormone now appears to be a natural corollary of the proof that absence or diminution in the normal activity of a gland (the thyroid) causes morbid results. But although the causation of myxoedema was clear before 1890, the general recognition of excessive glandular activity was established slowly. It was first suggested by Ludwig Rehn (1847–1930), well known for his work in thyroid surgery[196], in 1884 in the case of Graves' disease, and was built up gradually by the following considerations: the enlargement of the thyroid in Graves' disease; the production by excessive doses of thyroid gland substance of symptoms (thyroidism) more or less resembling those of Graves' disease, an extreme example being von Notthaft's patient in 1898 who, after taking a thousand tablets of thyroid gland substance in 5 weeks, developed the complete picture of Graves' disease which gradually disappeared after this treatment was discontinued[197]; to some extent Wm. Smith Greenfield's demonstration of histological hyperplasia [see p. 247] and overactivity of the thyroid in Graves' disease in 1893; the correlation in 1894 by Augusto T. Tamburini (1848–1919) of Modena of acromegaly with hypertrophy and over-activity of the pituitary[198], and the occurrence in acromegaly of hyperplasia of the eosinophil cells in the anterior lobe of the pituitary by Benda in 1900[199], and Dean Lewis in 1905[200]. It was therefore not until well in this century that hyperthyroidism (exophthalmic or toxic goitre) and hyperpituitarism (acromegaly) were generally accepted[201].

At the same time (1893), Friedrich von Mueller (1858–1941) demonstrated that the wasting in Graves' disease was accompanied by a great increase in nitrogenous catabolism[202].

Mueller was the first to examine the metabolism of a female patient with exophthalmic goitre and found a negative nitrogen balance. From this he concluded that in that disease the oxidation rate increases to such a degree that even an increased intake of food cannot compensate for it. Two years later, Adolf Magnus-Levy (1865–1955) confirmed Mueller's assumption. He showed that in such patients oxygen consumption is increased, but returns to normal on cure. Moreover, he later showed that oxygen consumption is reduced in myxoedema[203]. His investigations were to become the fundament for the modern concept of the assessment of thyroid function. All these findings confirmed Moebius' hunch, based solely on clinical features, that exophthalmic goitre was the opposite of myxoedema.

In the previous chapter was discussed the first classic account of exophthalmic goitre by Caleb Hillier Parry (1755–1822) in 1825. Before him, Giuseppe Flajani of Ascoli (1741–1808) had reported from Rome in 1802, on his successful treatment of two patients with exophthalmic goitre, without obviously realizing the significance of the three main symptoms, goitre, exophthalmos and palpitation[205]. Nor did Antonio Testa's (1756–1814) reference in 1800 to the coincidence of prominent eyes and disease of the heart seem to have any special significance to him. Testa, Professor of Medicine and Surgery at Ferrara and also Professor of Medicine at Bologna, "a learned theorist, but a mediocre clinician"[204] was, in his own writings, "prone to digressions more curious than useful"[204]. Flajani's first patient was a young Spaniard of 22, living in Rome, who developed protrusions of the eyes and a tumour in the front of the neck,

which in the course of four months increased to a considerable size, so that it occupied the anterior and lateral part of the neck. He remained under treatment for seven months, not so much on account of the tumour as on account of the difficulty which he had in breathing and on account of an extraordinary palpitation in the region of the heart. The above-mentioned symptoms compelled him to abandon his occupation as a painter . . . [The patient] applied for relief regarding reduction or removal of the tumour, as it seemed to him that the pressure of the tumour on the subjacent parts was increasing the difficulty he had in breathing. . . . The trouble being such, the curative treatment had to be directed to the resolution of the stagnant tumour. For this purpose I applied a double compress saturated with cold vinegar, strengthened by a dose of sal ammoniae. This, after twenty days, visibly decreased the size of the tumour, by at least one third; the patient breathed with less difficulty and the monthly withdrawal of blood (which had emaciated him), was not necessary. In addition, a strip of linen with white ointment and camphor was applied, and complete resolution of the tumour was achieved in four months. The palpitation disappeared and he took up his occupation as a painter, which he still carried on, on leaving Rome, five years after the cure[205].

In the second case, of a young woman, he used a similar local application, to which he added 2 ounces of bitter herb-juice every morning on an empty stomach plus a cupful of milk with an infusion of dogwort; but in this account, Flajani does not speak of protrusion of the eyes, only of swelling of the thyroid and of palpitation.

The next patient with exophthalmic goitre – according to John Wickham Legge (1843–1921) (see also p. 265) was described by a nameless writer in the *Medico-Chirurgical Journal and Review* for 1816 (Vol. I, p. 179), in the shape of a 22-year-old lady with palpitations of the heart and a swelling on each side of the neck as large as a goose's egg. The eyes had a prominence as though they were about to start from their sockets. She was very nervous, tall and extremely plethoric. Fortunately, after – or in spite of – polypragmatic treatment, her condition improved considerably after 7 months.

After Parry, there followed two more accurate classic descriptions of exophthalmic toxic goitre: in 1835, Robert James Graves (1796–1853) (see Section II) of Dublin, published a short paper: 'Palpitation of the heart with enlargement of the thyroid gland'[206].

> A lady, aged 20, became affected with some symptoms which were supposed to be hysterical. . . . After she had been in this nervous state about three months, it was observed that her pulse had become singularly rapid. This rapidity existed apparently without any cause and it was constant, the pulse being never under 120 and often much higher. She next complained of weakness on exertion and began to look pale and thin. Thus she continued for a year. . . . It was now observed that her eyes assumed a singular appearance for the eyeballs were apparently enlarged, so that when she slept or tried to shut her eyes they were incapable of closing. When the eyes were opened, the white sclerotic could be seen to a breadth of several lines around the cornea.

Graves was definite that enlargement of the thyroid was caused by hypertrophy, in contrast to simple goitre.

> I have lately seen three cases of violent and long continued palpitations in females in each of which the same peculiarity presented itself, viz., enlargement of the thyroid gland. The size of the gland, at all times considerably greater than natural, was subject to remarkable variations in every one of these patients. When the palpitations were violent, the gland used notably to swell and became distended, having all the appearance of being increased in size, in consequence of an interstitial and sudden effusion of fluid into its substance. The swelling immediately began to subside as the violence of the paroxysm of palpitation decreased and during the intervals the size of the gland remained stationary.

the stomach, this remains in the stomach for some time and coagulates, the secretions of that organ act on it, and change it to a black colour, in which state it is thrown up. This is the case in yellow fever, and such also was the origin of the black vomit in the fever of 1827.

I may observe that in that epidemic, as well as in the present, a close inquiry into the history of numerous cases has convinced me that the gastro-typhus of this country, as well as the yellow fever of warmer latitudes, may arise spontaneously, and be propagated by contagion. This, I believe, is a fact which every physician who has seen much of fever has not the slightest doubt of. We have all repeatedly seen instances of persons catching cold while the system was in a relaxed or debilitated state; we have seen this cold followed by violent feverish symptoms, and we have observed these symptoms pass gradually into fever of a typhus character, and capable of being propagated by contagion. So many examples of this have now occurred, that there can be no doubt that fever may arise spontaneously, that it may become in this way sporadic, and, finally, epidemic. At certain periods it appears to be a matter of very little consequence, with regard to the mass of society in general, how many sporadic cases of this description may occur, but at other periods, and under a certain state of atmosphere, the disease becomes extensively diffused, and assumes the character of an epidemic. Here each individual case proves a centre of contagion, from which the disease spreads on every side. On the other hand, fever may originate spontaneously, assume a typhoid character, and yet produce no contagion. Recollecting these circumstances, you will be able to reconcile the conflicting opinions of those who have argued so hotly respecting the nature of yellow fever, some asserting that it is always contagious, others never. The fact is, that both are right and both wrong; fever may originate spontaneously and without contagion, but it may also be produced by contagion, and it may, under one class of circumstances, run through its course without being communicated to others, whereas under a different state of things each case becomes a centre from which the disease spreads on every side. In the present epidemic of maculated or spotted fever, the contagious nature of the disease was strongly exemplified, for more than twenty of the students who were in the habit of visiting the fever wards in the Meath Hospital were attacked with spotted fever in the course of two months. Although the disease was very violent in many, and serious in all, Dr. Stokes and I lost but one of these students; we had every reason, therefore, to congratulate ourselves on the success of the treatment we employed. I shall return to this subject hereafter.

I have lately seen three cases of violent and long continued palpitations in females, in each of which the same peculiarity presented itself, viz. enlargement of the thyroid gland; the size of this gland, at all times considerably greater than natural, was subject to remarkable variations in every one of these patients. When the palpitations were violent the gland used notably to swell and become distended, having all the appearance of being increased in size in consequence of an interstitial and sudden effusion of fluid into its substance. The swelling immediately began to subside as the violence of the paroxysm of palpitation decreased, and during the intervals the size of the gland remained stationary. Its increase of size and the variations to which it was liable had attracted forcibly the attention both of the patients and of their friends. There was not the slightest evidence of any thing like inflammation of the gland. One of these ladies, residing in the neighbourhood of Black Rock, was seen by Dr. Harvey and Dr. William Stokes, another of them, the wife of a clergyman in the county of Wicklow, was seen by Dr. Marsh, and the third lives in Grafton-street. The palpitations have in all lasted considerably more than a year, and with such violence as to be at times exceedingly distressing, and yet there seems no certain grounds for concluding that organic disease of the heart exists. In one the beating of the heart could be heard during the paroxysm at some distance from the bed, a phenomenon I had never before witnessed, and which strongly excited my attention and curiosity. She herself, her friends, and Dr. Harvey all testified the frequency of this occurrence, and said that the sound was at times much louder than when I examined the patient, and yet I could distinctly hear the heart beating when my ear was distant at least four feet from her chest! It was the first or dull sound which was thus audible. This fact is well worthy of notice, and when duly considered appears to favour the explanation lately given by Magendie of the causes of the sounds produced during the heart's action, for none of those previously proposed seem to me capable of accounting for a sound so loud and so distinct. But to return to our subject. The sudden manner in which the thyroid in the above three females used to increase and again diminish in size, and the connexion of this with the state of the heart's action, are circumstances which may be considered as indicating that the thyroid is slightly analogous in structure to the tissues properly called erectile. It is well known that no part of the body is so subject to increase in size as the thyroid gland, and not unfrequently this increase has been observed to be remarkably rapid, constituting the different varieties of bronchocele or goitre. The enlargement of the thyroid, of which I am now speaking, seems to be essentially different from goitre in not attaining a size at all equal to that observed in the latter disease. Indeed this enlargement deserves rather the name of hypertrophy, and is at once distinguishable from bronchocele by its becoming sta-

Figure 46 Graves' description of "three cases of violent and long continued palpitations in females, in each of which the same peculiarity presented itself, viz. enlargement of the thyroid gland" – exophthalmic goitre

Graves did not mention tremor; this was described with emphasis by Jean Martin Charcot (1825–1893) who gave the first account of toxic goitre in France in 1856[207].

A fourth case with exophthalmos, Graves observed in 1838. It was in his honour that Armand Trousseau (1801–1867) used the term 'Graves' disease' in his lectures in 1860. It has become the current name of the condition in English-speaking countries. In fact, in 1933 Harington urged that

> In view of the doubtful position occupied by the thyroid in the production of the condition, it seems preferable to avoid the term exophthalmic goitre so far as possible, more especially since exopthalmos and goitre (in the sense of a conspicuous swelling of the thyroid gland) need not by any means be the most prominent symptoms; throughout this discussion, therefore, the term Graves' disease will be employed[208].

In 1837, F. P. Pauli of Heidelberg reported a case[209]; but the most important accurate account of the disease in Europe was given in 1840 by Carl Adloph von Basedow of Merseburg (see Section II) (1799–1854), in a paper with the title: "Exophthalmos durch Hypertrophie des Zellgewebes in der Augenhoehle"[210] (= Exophthalmos caused by hypertrophy of the cellular tissue in the orbit). His description of three women and one man with exophthalmos, goitre and palpitations gave rise to the phrase: "Das Merseburger Triad" (The Merseburg Triad).

The term 'hyperthyroidism', first used by Charles Horace Mayo of Minnesota in 1907, has been employed

> to include the two conditions of (1) primary exophthalmic goitre, and (2) the more recently recognised secondary exophthalmic goitre, toxic adenoma, or adenomatous goitre with hyperthyroidism, which Henry Stanley Plummer (1874–1937) and Walter Meredith Boothby (1880–1953)[211] regarded as distinct from primary exophthalmic goitre . . .[212].

Von Basedow also mentioned emaciation, amenorrhoea, excessive perspiration, diarrhoea, nervous restlessness, air-hunger and tremor. He also noted a brawny, non-oedematous swelling of the legs (local myxoedema). In 1848, he discussed the necropsy of the man among his four originally presented patients, and remarked on the resemblance to chlorosis. In 1840 Basedow reviewed the available literature, mentioning Charles de Saint-Yves' (1687–1733) paper in his 'Nouveau traité des maladies des yeux' (Paris, 1722) (see also p. 159). Basedow's paper appeared in the same volume of the *Wochenschrift fuer die gesamte Heilkunde* as Bernhard Mohr's (1809–1842) first description of a patient with pituitary obesity with infantilism (Froehlich-Babinski)[213] (see also p. 320).

WOCHENSCHRIFT
für die
g e s a m m t e

HEILKUNDE.

Herausgeber: Dr. *Casper*.
Mitredaction: Dr. *Romberg*, Dr. *v. Stosch*.

Diese Wochenschrift erscheint jedesmal am Sonnabende in Lieferungen von 1, bisweilen 1½ Bogen. Der Preis des Jahrgangs, mit den nöthigen Registern ist auf 3⅓ Thlr. bestimmt, wofür sämmtliche Buchhandlungen und Postämter sie zu liefern im Stande sind.

A. *Hirschwald.*

№ 13.　*Berlin, den* 28ten *März*　1840.

Ueber den Exophthalmos. Vom Dr. v. Basedow. — Die psychische Mitwirkung des Kranken zur Heilung gelähmter Glieder. Vom Dr. Reinbold. — Vermischtes. Von den Wundärzten Roscher und Rasch. — Krit. Anzeiger.

Exophthalmos durch Hypertrophie des Zellgewebes in der Augenhöhle.

Mitgetheilt

vom Dr. *v. Basedow*, pract. Arzte in **Merseburg**.

Exophthalmos ist, unterscheidet man den *Prolapsus bulbi* durch Lähmung des muskulösen Retentions-Apparates, immer nur Symptom einer mit Anschwellung verbundenen Erkrankung der benachbarten weichen und harten Umgebungen des Augapfels, der *Osteomalacie*, *Periostitis*, *Exostosis*, der polyposen Erkrankung der Stirn-, Oberkiefer- und Nasen-Höhle, der *Tumores* im Gehirn, der Balggeschwülste in der *Orbita*, der Scirrhen der *Glandula lacrymalis*, der traumatisch-ecchymotischen und inflammatorischen Anschwellung des Zellgewebes der *Orbita*.

Ich habe aber Gelegenheit gehabt, mehrmals *Exoph*-
Jahrgang 1840.　　　　14

Figure 47 Title page of von Basedow's description of exophthalmic goitre (1846) [By kind permission of the Institute for the History of Medicine, University of Vienna, Austria]

As Rolleston has pointed out, few diseases can have had more synonyms and none more eponyms. G. Dock[214], and C. P. Howard[215] collected more than twenty. Meanwhile, it may suffice to say, that whereas 'Graves' disease' is used in the English speaking countries, (although Osler preferred talking of Parry's disease in 1898), on the continent of Europe 'Basedow's disease' is popular; in Italy, 'Morbo di Flajani' seems now superseded by 'Morbo di Basedow'.

Although in 1889 Wilks regarded Basedow's description "as so complete that little had since been added to it", it received the usual resistance and criticism. It was soon followed by an account of five

— 565 —

darin nur eine durch locale und nationale Einflüsse her-
beigeführte Modification in den Erscheinungen.

Möglich ist es, dass diese Modification einen Antheil
gehabt an der grössern Bösartigkeit der Nachkrankheit
in der Londoner Epidemie. Uns starb nicht Einer von
den vielen Kranken, die wir an Wassersucht nach dem
Scharlach behandelt haben.

Mittheilungen für neuropathologische Studien.

Vom

Dr. *Mohr*, Privatdocenten in Würzburg.

(Schluss.)

4. Hypertrophie (markschwammige Entartung?) der
Hypophysis cerebri und dadurch bedingter Druck
auf die Hirngrundfläche, insbesondere auf die
Sehnerven, das *Chiasma* derselben und den link-
seitigen Hirnschenkel.

(Aus der medic. Klinik des Julius-Hospitals.)

Moser, *Elisa*, 57 Jahre alt, Gärtnersfrau, wurde am
22. October 1839 in die Anstalt aufgenommen. Von der
Kranken selbst war wegen Gedächtnissschwäche wenig
bezüglich auf ihrer Anamnese zu ermitteln, von ihrer Umge-
bung aber brachte man Folgendes in Erfahrung. *M.* leidet
seit beiläufig 6 Jahren (ob seit Cessation ihrer *Menses?*)
an Schwindel und periodischem Kopfweh. Vor 3 Jahren
verfiel sie in einen Zustand von Geisteszerrüttung, welcher sich nach einer Dauer von mehrern Wochen auf
Blutentziehungen und ausleerende Mittel zwar verlor,
aber von Gedächtnissschwäche, allmählig sich einstellen-
der Schwerfälligkeit in den Bewegungen und verminder-
ter Sehkraft gefolgt wurde, Erscheinungen, die wie Kopfschmerz und Schwindel periodische Zu - und Abnahme

Figure 48 B. Mohr's description of pituitary obesity (Froehlich-Babinski), 1840 [By kind permission of the Institute for the History of Medicine, University of Vienna, Austria]

cases by A. T. Brueck, a court physician at Bad Driburg, who presented them as hysterical – he called the disease 'buphthalmus hystericus' – making sarcastic remarks about the colour of the girls' eyes and their influence on susceptible male admirers, ridiculing von Basedow's description. E. H. Henoch (1820–1910) in 1848[216],

went out of his way ... to declare, in the journal which had published von Basedow's paper, that "nowhere have German medical men mentioned this striking symptom complex"[217].

John Wickham Legge (1843–1921), a physician at St. Bartholomew's Hospital in London, was, in 1882, very critical of von Basedow[218].

The impression which a careful reading of his article gives me is that he took a retrograde step rather than one in advance, fixing the attention upon the prominent eyes, and leaving the heart and the thyroid too much in the background. There is no doubt that he made a great point of the exophthalmos, of which Graves spoke only incidentally, but I do not see that it was an advantage to raise the exophthalmos to the rank of the one pathognomic sign, to the disparagement of the two. . . . The thyroid is as accidental to von Basedow as the eyes to Graves. Von Basedow never seems to have grasped the threefold character of the symptoms. . . .

Legge concluded:

If we are to search for the true founders of our knowledge of exophthalmic goitre, it seems that we must look to Dublin – to Graves, to Marsh and to Stokes; not to Merseburg.

Legge was more than somewhat unfair to von Basedow, who introduced the term 'Merseburg triad' in full recognition of the main symptoms. Numerous papers and observations followed Graves' and von Basedow's accounts. They included papers by Sir Henry Marsh (1790–1860), when he was president of the Pathological Society in Dublin, in January 1841[219,220]; James Begbie (1798–1869) read a paper to the Medico-Chirurgical Society of Edinburgh in January 1849 on "Anaemia and its consequences, enlargement of the thyroid gland and eyeballs; anaemia and goitre, are they related?"[221] in which he argued that anaemia was the primary disorder. Also in 1849, the oculist W. White Cooper (1816–1886) wrote "On protrusion of the eyes in connexion with anaemia, palpitation and goitre"[222], and William Mackenzie spoke in his 'Practical Treatise on Diseases of the Eye'[223] of "anaemic exophthalmos"! Friedrich Wilhelm Ernst Albrecht von Graefe (1828–1870) described his sign much later, in 1864[224]. Basedow himself had assumed that the exophthalmos was caused by an increase of the connective tissue in the orbits, which he equated with a masked scrofulous dyscrasia.

In France, the first description was given by Jean Martin Charcot (see also p. 268) (1825–1893) in May 1856[207], reporting on one patient, on seven necropsies, and connecting palpitation, goitre, exophthalmos and tremor; he called it 'cachexia exophthalmica'. P. Fischer of Paris also used that name in 1859[225], and then Armand Trousseau (1801–1867) became involved[226,227]. He reported on a paper by François Amilcar Aran (1817–1861)[228] (of Aran-Duchenne disease fame), in which the exophthalmos was ascribed to contraction of the small muscular fibres described by Heinrich Mueller (1809–1875)[229]; he gave two lectures at the Hôtel-de-Dieu in December 1860, on Graves' disease, as he called it. The French school laid particular emphasis on the nervous symptoms of Graves' disease; the whole syndrome was regarded by them (Charcot, 1856, 1859; Trousseau, 1867; and Pierre Marie, 1883), as being of nervous origin, either a type of hysteria, or associated with a definite nervous lesion; the enlargement of the thyroid – not always very conspicuous – was thought to be a secondary phenomenon. It was Paul Julius Moebius, oculist (1853–1907) in Leipzig, who had put forward the view in 1886, that the primary factor responsible for the disease was the thyroid gland (see p. 258). Curiously enough, Moebius, a brilliant eye surgeon and outstanding medical man, later became involved in a heated international controversy, after publishing a book *Ueber den physiologischen Schwachsinn des Weibes* ("On the physiological mental deficiency of woman"). This was originally published *ca.* 1900 (by Carl Marhold in Halle an der Saale) and went into numerous editions (the author's own copy is the seventh edition of 1905 of 140 pages). In the original pamphlet, which was only 24 pages long, Moebius attempted to present scientific evidence that woman's brain and general intellectual capacity is less developed than man's. He argued that it is almost akin to some natural mental defect, although he found it difficult to give a precise definition of natural mental deficiency, except in relation to man's intellect. The later editions expand somewhat on his original thesis, but are mainly enlarged by adding, honestly, all the correspondence, criticisms, reviews – in agreement or against this thesis; a most remarkable effort!

The description of *Increased Action of the Heart and of the Arteries of the Neck followed by Enlargement of the Thyroid Gland and the Eyeballs* in William Stokes (1804–1878) of Dublin's book on *Diseases of the Heart and Aorta*[230] was much more complete than that of his teacher and predecessor, Graves (see Section II).

By 1880, when H. Sattler presented the first comprehensive review: 'Die Basedow'sche Krankheit'[231], he could already record 274 communications on the subject. Moebius's opinion that the thyroid was the main cause of Graves' disease found, of course, particular support by the observation of George Redmayne Murray, in 1891, of the results of the replacement therapy of myxoedema[232]. It soon became obvious that careless administration of excessive amounts of thyroid extract during the course of that successful treatment could produce tachycardia, nervous and other symptoms characteristic of Graves' disease. Henry Stanley Plummer of the Mayo Clinic (1874–1937) defined toxic adenoma of the thyroid and discriminated between it and Graves' disease in 1914.

Before leaving this subject, it should be mentioned that William Heberden the Elder (1710–1801) must have seen cases of Graves' disease, because in the chapter on 'Aneurysma' in his posthumously published *Commentarii de Morborum Historia et Curatione* (London,

1802), he wrote: "... many tumours of the neck, apparently of this sort, from having a strong pulsation in them, have after several years spontaneously decreased till at last they have almost disappeared" (but in the chapter on 'Bronchocele', he does not mention them).

As we have seen before, Aetios (500 AD) and Ambroise Paré (1561) regarded patients with exophthalmic goitre erroneously as cases of aneurysm (see also p. 112).

In 1896, Vaughan Pendred (1869–1946), drew attention to the association of goitre with deaf-mutism[233]. The aetiology of toxic goitre gave rise to many speculations and theories. In the first place, it was soon established that it was much more frequent in women than in men (Hector Mackenzie, G. R. Murray, J. M. H. Campbell, etc.[234]). It was also soon established that it often occurred in families (W. B. Cheadle, 1875; Hector Mackenzie, 1890; the latter also quoting Oesterreicher's report of its occurrence in eight out of ten sisters[235]).

The nature of toxic goitre has not been definitely settled to this day. Of the early theories just a few should be mentioned. In 1860 Trousseau thought it to be a neurosis analogous to hysteria[236]. C. Handfield Jones (1819–1890) suggested in a paper to the Royal Medical and Chirurgical Society (November 1860) that the exophthalmos was due to effusion of fluid in the cellular tissue in the orbit and that the disease was mainly an affection of the vasomotor nervous system[237,238]. Others (Koeben[239] in 1865) thought that the symptoms of toxic goitre were caused by the thyroid pressed on the sympathetic in the neck. Yet others thought that nervous stress may be one of the underlying causes. The occasional presence of thymus enlargement made some regard this as an aetiological factor, as did improvement after thymectomy, which was fashionable around 1914. The adrenal cortex was also implicated, and, especially, the anterior pituitary; the experimental production of toxic goitre introduced even more confusing factors: in 1879 Fihlene transected the restiform bodies, in 1915 Cannon and Binger sutured the superior cervical sympathetic to the phrenic nerve in a cat, producing the symptoms, which were stopped by removal of the thyroid (all references cited in pp. 233–234 of Ref. 12). Osteoporosis at necropsy was reported by Friedrich Daniel von Recklinghausen (1833–1910), and confirmed by Koeppen in 1892 and Kummer in 1917 (references cited in Ref. 12, pp. 233–234). Of the most important clinical signs, the time-table of description is as follows: Dalrymple's sign before 1849 (John Dalrymple, FRS (1803–1852), surgeon to the Royal Ophthalmic Hospital, never published this observation, but it was reported in 1849 by his friend W. White Cooper (1816–1886). Stellwag's sign, described in 1869 by Carl Stellwag von Carion

(1828–1904); von Graefe's sign, described in 1864 by Albrecht von Graefe (1828–1870), which nowadays is simply called lid-lag, due perhaps to spasm of the superior levator palpabrae muscle[240]. Joffroy's sign, described in 1893 by Alexis Joffroy (1844–1908) of Paris. Rosenbach's sign, fine tremor of the eyelids, described by Ottomar Rosenbach (1851–1907) of Berlin, also ascribed to the spasm of the superior levator muscle[240]. Tremor was originally mentioned by Basedow in 1840, but its importance was stressed by Charcot, who said that it may appear as one of the early signs of the disease.

F. E. Féréol talked of 'cardio-vascular ataxia' and Guéeau de Mussy (1814–1892) also wrote on tremor in 1881. Pierre Marie regarded tremor as one of the cardinal signs and described it in 1883 as a fine tremor, on an average 8½ per second, twice as frequent as in paralysis agitans and faster than senile tremor and not affecting individual fingers separately, in contrast to the rapid tremor of alcoholics and in general paralysis of the insane[241]. This was later confirmed by (Sir) Byrom Bramwell (1847–1931), in 1890[242]. W. B. Cheadle of St. George's Hospital, London, recorded a (comparatively rare) case of hemiplegia in toxic goitre and also the important occurrence of amenorrhoea which may precede and accompany the illness; the periods returning on recovery[243]. Impotence also was reported in men.

In 1860 Trousseau described 'formes frustes' or incomplete forms, which may be very difficult to diagnose. This was confirmed by Pierre Marie in his 'Thèse de Paris' in 1883, Charcot in 1885 and František Chvostek (1835–1884) the Elder, of 'Chvostek's sign' in latent tetany; in 1887 he described forms with one symptom only.

Although it was A. A. Bowlby (1855–1929) who first reported on an 'infiltrating fibroma' of the thyroid in a woman of 42, in 1885[244], the second man to describe the enlargement of the thyroid due to dense fibrous tissue deposition had the honour of having the disease named after him. It was called 'Riedel's thyroiditis' after Bernhard Moritz Karl Ludwig Riedel (1846–1916)[245].

To illustrate the confused terminology relating to exophthalmic goitre in the 19th century, Alfred H. Iason presents the following collection[246]: 1. Exophthalmus hystericus (Brueck), 1835. 2. Exophthalmic bronchocele (Laycock), 1838. 3. Die Glotzaugen (Basedow), 1848. 4. Glotzaugencachexie (Basedow), 1848. 5. Cachexie exophthalmique (Charcot), 1856. 6. Exophthalmus anemicus (Prael), 1857. 7. Cachexia exophthalamica (Withuisen), 1858. 8. Cardiogmus strumosus s. Morbus Basedowii (Hirsch), 1858. 9. Maladie de Basedow (Charcot), 1859. 10. Goitre exophthalmique (Trousseau), 1860. 11. Morbus Gravesii (Mannheim), 1864.

12. Exophthalmic goitre (Hamill), 1861. 13. Nevrose thyro-exophthalmique (Corlieu), 1863. 14. Struma exophthalmica (Begbie), 1868. 15. Tachycardia strumosa exophthalmica (Lebert), 1872. 16. Morbo del Flajani (Pensutti), 1887. 17. Morbo di Flajani (Bacelli and De Renzi), 1887. 18. Cachexie thyroidienne (Gauthier), 1888. 19. Hystérie thyroidienne (Pader), 1899. 20. Parry's disease (Osler), 1898.

Iason also collected an amusing list of some of the theories suggested for the causation of thyroid diseases[246]: Graves considered exophthalmic goitre a dyscrasia of scrofulous and circulatory origin; Basedow, a general dyscrasic malady; Marsh, Prael and Hensinger a disease of the heart; Friedrich, an enlargement of the coronary arteries; Eulenberg, Panas and others, a neurosis of central origin; Stokes a cardiac neurosis; Tedeschi, Warburton, Filehne, of bulbar origin. Gaylor, Lane, Reveno, Halsted, due to the function of the thyroid as a detoxicating organ; Gautier and others, thyroid insufficiency. Trousseau, Charcot, Jaboulay, Aran, Kolber, sympathetic (cervical) involvement; Bircher, Hart, Matti, Haberer, Basch, Hammer, thymus causation; Cannon, adrenal causation; Gley, parathyroid causation; Salmon, pituitary involvement; Delstre, gonad theory; Moebius, Renaut, Mario, Béclère, hyperthyroidism; Janney, Halverson, Hawk, dysthyroidism; Plummer, dysthyroidism plus hyperthyroidism; Eppinger, Hess, vagotonia and sympathicotonia; Sajous, toxic-neurogenic; Crile, kinetic theory; Moseley, rupture of the jugular vessels from drinking snow and ice water (1804); Claude, Eppinger, Stengel, Gougerot, Falta, Rudinger, multiglandular insufficiency; Rush, Liebermeister, vascular shunt; and many others!

THE OVUM, THE SPERM, FERTILIZATION AND GENETICS

The 19th century also showed progress in unravelling the dynamics of maturation, fertilization and segmentation of the ovum, a field in which no real progress had been made since William Harvey's time. This did not mean that the recognition, isolation, chemical analysis and synthesis of the hormones of the ovary showed signs of speedy development. In fact, it is remarkable – as Professor George Washington Corner (b. 1889) (see Section II) pointed out in his Sir Henry Dale Lecture for 1964, at the Middlesex Hospital in London – that the clues for their discovery remained so obscure for such a long time[247]. Although animal (and human) female castration and some of its effects have been known since ancient times, the phenomenon of castrate atrophy did not get into the medical literature until after the middle of the 19th century.

In 1826, Jean Louis Prévost (1790–1850) and Jean Baptiste André Dumas (1800–1884) (both of early successful experiments of animal blood-transfusion fame in 1821), gave the first description of their observations of the segmentation of the frog's egg[248]. A year or so before, Johannes Mueller (1801–1858) had published his discovery of the Muellerian duct[249]. Next followed the discovery of the mammalian ovum by Carl Ernst von Baer (1792–1876)[250] (see also pp. 187 and 188).

In 1861, Carl Gegenbauer (1826–1903), the great German comparative anatomist, demonstrated that the ovum of all vertebrates was unicellular[251]. It has already been mentioned that it was Antonj van Leeuwenhoek who, in 1677, first described the spermatozoa; originally pointed out to him by the student Hamen in 1674[252]. Then Spallanzani showed, in a filtration experiment in 1786 that the spermatozoon is essential for fertilization. Its cellular origin was demonstrated by Rudolph Albert von Koelliker (1817–1905)[253] in 1841.

In 1865, Franz Schweiger-Seidel (1834–1871) demonstrated proof that the spermatozoa are cells, possessing a nucleus and cytoplasm[254]. The union of the spermatozoon with the ovum was first observed in the rabbit by Martin Barry in 1843[255]. Rudolf Ludwig Karl Virchow (1821–1902) clearly stated in 1853 that the ovum is derived, in continuous line of descent, from pre-existing fertilized ova[255]. Oscar Hertwig (1849–1922) was able to show, in 1875, that the sperm enters the ovum, followed by the union of the nuclei of the male and female gametes, which act thus accomplishes fertilization[256]. In 1880, Walther Fleming (1843–1905) gave a classic description of cell division and karyokinesis[257].

In 1883, Édouard van Beneden (1846–1910) discovered that the associated male and female nuclei in the fertilized ovum each contain half as many chromosomes as the normal body cells of the same species[258]. Genetics and the problem of heredity cannot be discussed in detail within the framework of the present book; but it cannot be entirely omitted or divorced from the field of endocrinology. It has to be mentioned – in passing – that August Friedrich Leopold Weisman (1834–1914) of Frankfurt-am-Main made a major contribution to the theory of evolution with his theory of the immortality of the germ-plasm, a complex structure contained in the nuclei of the cells of reproduction. The union ('amphimixis') of two germs is the main agent in evolution. The germ-plasm of the sex-cells is in the chromosomes, and Weisman predicted the 'reduction division' (by one half) in the mature sex-cells. He also assumed, correctly, that the

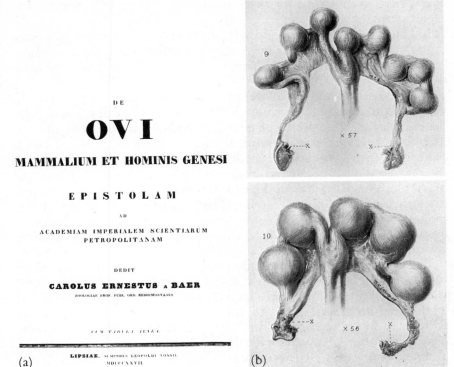

DE

OVI

MAMMALIUM ET HOMINIS GENESI

EPISTOLAM

AD

ACADEMIAM IMPERIALEM SCIENTIARUM
PETROPOLITANAM

DEDIT

CAROLUS ERNESTUS A BAER

ZOOLOGIAE PROF. PUBL. ORD. REGIOMONTANUS

CUM TABULA AENEA

LIPSIAE, SUMPTIBUS LEOPOLDI VOSSII.
MDCCCXXVII.

(a)

(b)

Figure 49   Von Baer's paper on the mammalian ovum: (a) frontispiece and (b) plate

determinants in the chromosomes are arranged in a linear series. He also produced experimental proof for his theory that acquired characteristics are not directly transmitted. Weisman's main work was published between 1891 and 1904[259–261].

Needless to say that in the Hippocratic Writings, there is reference to heredity:

> ... The semen is produced by the whole body, healthy by healthy parts, sick by sick parts. This means that usually bald people produce bald people, blue-eyed other blue-eyed ones and squinting ones others who are squinting. If this law prevails for other diseases, it should be expected, that long-headed (macrocephalic) people are begotten by long-headed ones. It is, however, also said that 'the chief cause of the length of their heads was at first found to be in their customs, but nowadays nature collaborates with tradition and they consider those with the longest heads the most nobly born'[262].

The 'pangenesis' theory, that the sperm is produced by all parts of the body (it contains something of and, therefore, can reproduce every part), was probably first put forward in the 5th century by Democritus[263].

In 'The seed' (Περί σπέρματος) of the Hippocratic Writings, it is said; ". . . (the child) must inevitably resemble each parent in some respect, since it is from both parents that the sperm comes to form the child"[264].

Both Aristotle and Plato stressed the importance of heredity[265]. Plato, in the *Republic*, demands that "the best" of both sexes should beget children, who are to be educated with great care. The idea of 'the best (ἄριστοι) is underlying the idea that the Republic (Plato's *State of Utopia*) should be guided by an 'aristocracy', not by a dictator (= tyrant) nor by an oligarchy (= reign of a few) of the left or right. The 'Guards' of Plato's Utopia are one of the highest categories in his social hierarchy. The idea of a dictatorship of the crowds (= rule of the people or 'democracy') by means of anonymous committees, as discussed much later by Gustave Le Bon[266], was totally alien to Plato.

The Spanish physician Mercado published *De Morbis Hereditariis* in 1605[267], in which he maintained that both parents contribute to the seed of the child. Malphighi (1628–1694) was the originator of the 'preformation theory', that in the ovum the whole individual is preformed in complete and final shape, and this theory was maintained long after Leeuwenhoek's discovery of the sperm and brought to an end only by C. F. Wolff's (1733–1794) critical attack in 1769. Experimental research on heredity in plants was carried out by Gaertner (1772–1850) and Koelreuter (1733–1806), preparing the ground for Mendel's experiments in the mid-19th century.

One of the most important forerunners of modern human geneticists was, however, the English physician Joseph Adams (1756–1818) (see also Section II). In 1814 he published *A Treatise on the Supposed Hereditary Properties of Diseases*[268], which was intended to provide a basis for genetic counselling. Adams differentiated between 'familial' (recessive) and 'hereditary' (dominant) occurrences and appreciated that in familial conditions parents are often inter-related. He also said that hereditary illness may not be evident at birth, but become manifest at a later age. Predisposition to illness may be latent, but leading to manifest disease when certain environmental factors also become present. Accordingly, illnesses which may appear clinically identical may have a different underlying genetic cause. Although reproduction of people suffering from inherited disease is often diminished, and such diseases would perhaps die out in due course, new mutations emerging in children of healthy parents may perpetuate them. An increase in hereditary disease frequency in isolated areas could be caused by inbreeding. The

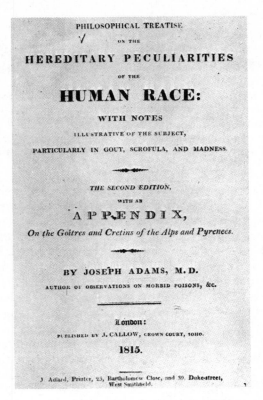

Figure 49(c) Front page of the Second Edition of Adams' book with a modified title and an important Appendix

knowledge of diseases occurring in families and their age of onset may form a basis of what is to-day called genetic counselling. Adams, therefore, suggested the setting up of registries for families with inherited diseases – a very modern idea!

Christian Frederick Nasse (1778–1851) in Germany, described haemophilia in 1820[269] and pointed out the apparent immunity of women, in spite of the fact that they are capable of transmitting the disease ('Nasse's Law'). He also made the observation that some of the male offspring of such women were normal.

The truly scientific foundation of genetics was only achieved by Gregor Mendel (see Section II). In 1865, Gregor Johann Mendel (1822–1884), abbot of the Augustinian monastery in Bruenn, Austria, reported on the results of certain experiments of his on hybridization in peas, which was the discovery of the law governing the inheritance of dominant and recessive characters in hybrids[270]. It

273

remained overlooked and forgotten for 35 years until re-discovered by Hugo Marie de Vries (1848–1935) in 1900[271].

In 1870, Karl Ewald Konstantin Hering (1834–1918), a Saxon professor, produced his psycho-physical theory of heredity:

> that facultative memory, the automatic power of protoplasm to do what it has done before, is the distinctive property of all living matter. The transmission and reproduction of parental characters are supposed to be the result of the organism's unconscious memory of the past, the mechanism being . . . the persistence of Wave motions of molecules[272,273].

Sir Francis Galton (1822–1911), incidentally a cousin of Charles Darwin, began experimenting in 1871 to investigate the laws of heredity by statistical induction, with remarkable results. He was also the founder of the Eugenics Laboratory in London in 1904, to further the doctinre of Eugenics (a term invented by him). He established[274] the 'Law of Filial Regression', i.e. that the offspring of parents who are unusual in talent, height, etc. regress to the average of the line; also the 'Law of Ancestral Inheritance', that is that each parent contributes $(\frac{1}{2})^2 = \frac{1}{4}$ of the total inheritance, each of the four grandparents $(\frac{1}{2})^4 = \frac{1}{16}$, and – in general – the ancestors n degrees removed: $(\frac{1}{2})^{2n}$. Most important, however, proved the investigations of Thomas Hunt Morgan (1866–1945) on the fruit-fly (*Drosophila melanogaster*). With his collaborators Bridges, Muller and Sturtevant, he achieved over 200 mutations in *Drosophila* and showed the mechanism of heredity to be definitely allocated to the genes within the chromosomes. In their long and patient experiments they discovered the phenomena of coupling, linkage, sex-linked inheritance, crossing-over, and the plotting of genes on chromosome maps. Their findings also confirmed Mendel's results, and had the most profound influence on modern ideas on inheritance and, of course, formed a connecting link to the endocrinology of reproduction, and sex determination[275–277].

These investigations stimulated Richard Benedict Goldschmidt's (1878–1958) work on the determination of sex[278]. Far more important, however, Morgan's work leads and links up eventually (although, admittedly, the conditions in insects are not identical) with problems such as the freemartins (Lillie and, especially, R. V. Short, who also discussed germ cell sex in mammals, and the influence of hormones along the line of development; see Chapter 14).

Koelliker (see p. 270) made another important contribution to his previous studies on the cellular origin of the spermatozoa: in 1885, he suggested that inherited characteristics were transmitted by the cell nucleus: "Die Bedeutung der Zellkerne fuer die Vorgaenge der Vererbung"[279]. This was confirmed in 1903 by two other research workers, Theodor Boveri (1862–1915)[280], and by Walter Stanborough Sutton (1877–1916)[281]. They both suggested that the hereditary particles (genes) in the cell are borne by the chromosomes (Sutton–Boveri hypothesis). Weisman (see p. 270) believed that the object of the partition of the chromosomes in the cells of the gonads was to keep the number of chromosomes constant in a given species[282].

An anonymous contributor to *The Lancet* expressed it in March 1957 very aptly and wittily[283]:

> The dominant gene, the dominant gene
> Is the happiest creature that ever was seen;
> We mortals can only admire at a distance
> The joys of chromosomatic existence –
> Or marvel how Nature determines the sexes
> By cunningly mixing the Y's and the X's
> (For, as Mendel has proved, it is only statistics
> That settle our primary characteristics).
> Just imagine the life of ineffable bliss you
> Could spend as a speck in the nuclear tissue!
> Fraternally twinned with a charming recessive –
> Your relationship tender, but firmly possessive;
> Dictating the pigment, the shape of the nose,
> Or whether your host shall have suckers for toes.
> Do you find immortality's promise seductive?
> Make your home in a cell that is marked "Reproductive".
> A short life, but merry? You dread being static?
> Your calling is plain – you are clearly Somatic –
> For you cannot grow stale, with your every ambition
> Fulfilled by perpetual cellular fission.
> So banish your doubts, your neuroses, and revel
> In life as it's lived at molecular level!
> ENVOI Princess! You discover the key to my riddle
> By shuffling two chromosomes – split down the middle.

Nearly forty years after Mendel, (Sir) Archibald Garrod's (1857–1936) paper in 1902 on 'The incidence of alkaptonuria: a study in chemical individuality'[284], followed in 1909 by his book *Inborn Errors of Metabolism*[285], applied Mendel's gene concept for the first time to a human characteristic and, thus, introduced Mendel's rules into research into human genetics. Vogel and Motulsky stress that Garrod's paper put forward the "following new insights": whether a person has alkaptonuria or not, is a matter of "a clear alternative", there are no transient forms[286]. This fact becomes the condition for the straightforward pattern of simple forms of inheritance. It is a congenital abnormality and can be observed in siblings and not in parents, but the parents are often first cousins. These latter two features can be explained by a recessive mode of inheritance, according to Mendel. The significance of first cousin marriages especially applies to rare conditions and may be a foreboding of population genetics. Alkaptonuria may be an example for other inborn errors of metabolism, e.g. cystinuria (1908).

(Sir) Archibald Edward Garrod had been on the staff of St. Bartholomew's Hospital, London, from 1904 onwards, since 1912 as a physician. In 1919, he was elected the first full-time professor of the Medical Clinic, which he had planned himself. Before he could take up his duties, however, he was appointed successor to Sir William Osler, as Regius Professor of Medicine at Oxford. He was one of the first to recognize the importance of the science of biochemistry for medicine.

Finally, the discovery of the ABO blood group system by Karl Landsteiner (1868–1943) of Vienna[287], and the proof that these blood types are inherited according to Mendelian laws, by Emil von Dungern (1876–?) and Ludwik Hirszfeld (1884–1954), was an outstanding example of the principles of Mendelian inheritance applied to human characteristics[288].

Vogel and Motulsky point out that the recent giant strides in the development of genetic research and its clinical application to human problems may mean a "succession of victories". The histocompatibility gene complex, studied in the 1960s and 1970s, has become important for the understanding as to why several genes with related function might occur in closely linked clusters. This may be of importance to understanding susceptibility to many auto-immune diseases. Yet, will all these achievements be recognized as such by our descendents? That is the question.

THE PANCREAS AND PARATHYROIDS

For the sake of completeness, two endocrine glands must be mentioned briefly; they were discovered, but not understood, *after* Berthold's experiments in 1849. In 1869, there was published in Berlin an MD thesis of a young medical student, aged 22, one Paul Langerhans (1847–1888) (see Section II), entitled: 'Beitraege zur mikroskopischen Anatomie der Bauchspeicheldruese' (Contributions to the microscopical anatomy of the pancreas)[289]. It contained the first account of islands of cells in the body of the pancreas, which differed from the cells of the tissue; but Langerhans did not suggest any function for them.

John R. Henderson[290] is in his account less kind to Paul Langerhans. He writes:

> His thesis was tiny, and full of self-deprecatory remarks; it was an histological investigation of the rabbit's pancreas, using a variety of stains and injection techniques. His conclusions were that he had found nothing new, and he hoped that his examiners would look tolerantly on his efforts. But in it, he refers to islands of clear cells scattered throughout the gland, whose staining properties were quite different from the surrounding tissue. He noticed that these areas were more richly innervated than the surrounding tissue, but could suggest no function for the areas except that they might be lymph nodes.

Langerhans later showed that similar tissue was present in the gut wall of lower chordates, which cells were later called the 'follicles of Langerhans'. His areas of clear cells in the pancreas aroused no interest at the time.

In 1893, Gustave-Édouard Laguesse (1861–1927), who had already suspected that those cells had an important endocrine function, called them the 'islets of Langerhans'[291] (see also p. 457 and p. 605). Langerhans, who had died in 1888, was not aware of the honour bestowed on him, nor of the function of the cells he had discovered. Eleven years before, in 1882, Willy Kuehne (1837–1900) and A. S. Lea (1853–1915), had described the islands as collections of lymphoid tissue, only to be corrected by Laguesse and others[292]. They had designed a remarkable apparatus for investigating pancreatic circulation in the living rabbit[293]. With the help of Berlin Blue injections he produced extraordinarily accurate drawings of the injected segment of blood circulation[294]. The dilated 'glomerular' vessels, he shows, undoubtedly represent islets, but

> although he noticed them and spent nearly two pages of his paper ruminating on their nature, he had no knowledge of the clear areas that Langerhans had described 23 years previously, and so had no reason to associate the 'glomerular' vessels that he saw with islets.

It was not until Laguesse investigated the embryology of the pancreas, that he saw that in the foetal tissue were large areas of palely staining cells, and that there was a proportionately greater mass of these cells in the foetal tissue than in that of the adult. Laguesse had, in some extraordinary way, seen Langerhans's thesis; remembering the original observation, he suggested with 'fine charity'[290] that they should be called the 'Islets of Langerhans'.

The *parathyroids* were also slow starters. Like toxic goitre, they have several synonyms. The term 'parathyroid' is, in Rolleston's (and others') view "unfortunate", as it may be thought to imply not only an anatomical relation, but also a close physiological resem-

CARL M. SEIPEL

ON A NEW GLAND IN MAN AND SEVERAL MAMMALS[1]

IVAR SANDSTRÖM

About three years ago [1877] I found on the thyroid gland of a dog a small organ, hardly as big as a hemp seed, which was enclosed in the same connective tissue capsule as the thyroid, but could be distinguished therefrom by a lighter color. A superficial examination revealed an organ of a totally different structure from that of the thyroid, and with a very rich vascularity. Therefore I thought it could possibly be a vascular gland like the *Gl. carotidea*. Even in the cat and the rabbit similar glands were found. However, time and material did not allow me to continue the investigations, and it was not until this winter [1880] that I have been able to take the problem up again. The existence of a hitherto unknown gland in animals that have so often been a subject of anatomical examination called for a thorough approach to the region around the thyroid gland even in man. Although the probability of finding something hitherto unrecognized seemed so small that it was exclusively with the purpose of completing the investigations rather than with the hope of finding something new that I began a careful examination of this region. So much the greater was my astonishment therefore when in the first individual examined I found on both sides at the inferior border of the thyroid gland an organ of the size of a small pea, which, judging from its exterior, did not appear to be a lymph gland, nor an accessory thyroid gland, and upon histological examination showed a rather peculiar structure. After several examinations not only was I convinced of the constancy of its appearance but I was also able to show that two such glands in most cases occur on each side. Since then my interest has been so predominantly centered on a deeper study of the structure and importance of these glands in man, that examinations of animals have been limited to dog, cat, rabbit, ox, and horse, and even there they have been rather scanty. However, I hope to complete a comparative study and description on some other occasion.

[1] A translation from the Swedish by Dr. Carl M. Seipel of Stockholm. From *Upsala Läkareförenings Förhandlingar*, 1879-80, 15, 441-471.

Figure 50 Title page of Sandstroem's paper [Bull. Inst. Hist. Med. Johns Hopkins Univ. **6**, 192, 1936]

blance to the thyroid[295]. The existence of the parathyroids was noted in 1855 by Robert Remak (1815–1865) of Berlin, the first Jew to be given an academic appointment at a Prussian university[295] and by Sir Richard Owen (1804–1892), superintendent of the Natural History Department of the British Museum, who – in 1852 – described in an Indian rhinoceros "a small, compact, yellow, glandular body, attached to the thyroid where the veins emerge"[296] and by Virchow in 1863, in man[297].

The first complete and systematic description, however, was given in 1880 by Yvar Victor Sandstroem (1852–1889) of Upsala (see Section II). He described two parathyroid bodies in man, on each side of the neck, which he managed to obtain in 43 out of 50 necropsies[298]. In the same year, Anton Woelfler (1850–1917), Billroth's first assistant (later professor of surgery in Graz and Prague), noticed areas of "young tissue" with colloid in the thyroid, which he called "foetal rests", but which might have been intrathyroid inclusion of parathyroid tissue[299]. These and other similar accounts (Baber, E. Cresswell, in 1881)[300] were heeded little, until in 1891, Eugène Gley (1857–1930) of Paris (see Section II) discovered, or rediscovered, the external or lower parathyroids in rabbits ("Sur les fonctions du corps thyroide")[301,302]. He then came across Sandstroem's description, to which he referred. Suspecting the importance of his discovery, he set about investigating their physiological and pathological significance. His work showed that the parathyroids are essential for the maintenance of life.

REFERENCES

1. Prochaska, Georg: Disquisitio anatomico-physiologica organismi corporis humani ejusque processus vitalis. Viennae, 1812.
2. Prochaska, Georg: Physiologie oder Lehre von der Natur des Menschen, pp. 64–66. Wien, 1820.
3. Abderhalden, R.: From the History of Endocrinology. CIBA Monographs, No. 10, 317. Bombay, 1951.
4. Schoenwetter, Hans Peter: Zur Vorgeschichte der Endokrinologie, Zuercher Medizingeschichtliche Abhandlungen, Neue Reihe Nr. 61. Juris Druck und Verlag, 1968.
5. Goethe, J. W. von: Uber den Zwischenkiefer des Menschen und der Thiere. Acta Acad. Leopold-Carol, Halle **15**, 1–48, 1831.
6. Autenrieth, J. H. F.: Handbuch der empirischen menschilichen Physiologie. Vol. III, p. 257. Tuebingen, 1802.
7. Ibid.: para. 752.
8. Hildebrandt, F.: Lehrbuch der Physiologie, 4th ed. paras 721, 813, 838, 848. Erlangen, 1809.
9. Arnold, F.: Lehrbuch der Physiologie des Menschen. para 1001, Zuerich, 1842.
10. Chéreau, A.: Propter ovarium solumn mulier est quod est. In Maladies des Ovaries, 72–91, Paris.
11. Virchow: Gesammelte Abhandlungen zur wissen schaftlichen Medizin. p. 747, 1856.
12. Rolleston, Sir Humphry D.: The Endocrine Organs in Health and Disease with an Historical Review. p. 19. London, Oxford University Press, 1936.
13. Gulliver, George: Dublin Med. Press III, 11, 1840.
14. As 82.
15. Henle, Friedrich G. J.: Allgemeine Anatomie des Menschen. Leipzig, 1841.
16. Mueller, Johannes: Handbuch der Physiologie der Menschen. Coblenz, 1844.
17. Legallois, Julien J. C.: Oeuvres de Legallois, Vol. 2, p. 209. Paris, 1830.
18. Legallois, Julien J. C.: Expériences sur le principe de la vie. Paris, D'Hautel, 1812.

19. As 12: p. 18.
20. Berthold, Arnold A.: Transplantation der Hoden. Arch. Anat., Physiol., Wiss. Med. 42–46, 1849 (The transplantation of testes. Translation by Quiring, D. P. Bull. Hist. Med. **16**, 399–401, 1944.
21. Nussbaum, Moritz: Innere Sekretion und Nerveneinfluss. Merkel-Bonnet Ergebn. **15**, 39–89, 1905.
22. Biedl, Artur: Innere Sekretion. Berlin, Wien, Urgan & Schwarzenberg, 1910.
23. As 12: p. 20.
24. Forbes, F. R.: A. A. Berthold and the first endocrine experiment: some speculation as to its origin. Bull. Hist. Med. **23**, 263–67, 1949.
25. Berthold, A. A.: Lehrbuch der Physiologie fuer Studierende und Aerzte. Goettingen, 1829, 1837, 1848.
26. Ibid.: Vol. 2, p. 569, 1848 edition.
27. Wagner, Rudolph: Mittheilung einer einfachen Methode zu Versuchen über die Veraenderungen thierischer Gewebe . . . etc., Nachr. Kgl. Ges. Wiss. Goettingen, pp. 97–109, 1851.
28. Jørgensen, C. Barker: John Hunger, A. A. Berthold and the origins of endocrinology. Acta Hist. Scient. Nat. Med., Odense, U.P. **24**, 1–54, 1971.
29. Ibid.: p. 32.
30. Borell, Merriley: Setting the standards for a new science: Edward Schaefer and endocrinology. Med. Hist. **22**, 282–290, 1978.
31. Berthold, A. A.: Seitliche Zwitterbildung (Hermaphroditismus lateralis) beim Menschen beobachtet. Abhandl. Kgl. Ges. Wiss. Goettingen. **2**, 97–104, 1845.
32. Meckel, Johann Friedrich, the Younger: Ueber Zwitterbildungen. Reils. Arch. Physiol. **11**, 263–340, 1812.
33. Simpson, James Young: Hermaphroditism. In Cyclop. of Anatomy and Physiology (Ed. Todd, R. B.) Vol. 2, pp. 684–738, 1839.
34. Heinroth, O.: Ein lateral hermaphroditisch gefaerbter Bimpel, (Pyrrhula pyrrhula europea Vieill.) Sitzungsber. Ges. Naturf. Freund., Berlin: pp. 328–330, 1909.
35. Poll, H.: Zur Lehre von den sekundaeren Sexualcharacteren. Sitzungsber. Ges. naturf. Freund. Berlin, pp. 331–358, 1909.
36. Sainte-Hilaire, Geoffroy: Sur les femelles de faisans à plumages de mâles; etc. Mém. Mus. Hist. nat. **12**, 220–231, 1825.
37. Yarrell, W.: On the change of the plumage of some hen-pheasants. Philos. Trans. 268–275, 1827.
38. Darwin, C.: The Variation of Animals and Plants under Domestication. London, 1868.
39. Tichomiroff, A.: Androgynie bei Voegeln. Anat. Anzeiger **3**, 221–228, 1888.
40. Steinach, Eugen: Uentersuchungen zur vergleichended Physiologie der maennlichen Geschlechtsorgane, insbesondere der accessorischen Geschlechtsdruesen. Arch. ges. Physiol. **56**, 304–338, 1894.
41. Yarrell, W.: On the influence of the sexual organ in modifying external character. J. Proc. Linn. Soc. Zool. **1**, 76–82, 1857.
42. As 28: p. 34.
43. As 28: p. 35.
44. Curling, T. B.: A Practical Treatise on the Diseases of the Testis. 2nd ed., London, 1856.
45. Ord, W. M.: Med.-chir. Trans. **33**, 303-306, 1850.
46. Ord, W. M.: Med.-chir. Trans. **61**, 37–78; 1878 [On myxoedema].
47. Obolensky, J.: Die Durchschneidung. d. Nervus spermaticus u. deren Einfluss auf d. Hoden. Centralbl. med. Wiss. 497–500, 1867.

48. As 28: p. 36.
49. Kehrer, F. A.: Versuche ueber Castration u. Erzeugung v. Hydrosalpinx. Beitr. klin, u. exp. Geburtsk. u. Gynaek. **2**, 282–292, 1887.
50. Goltz, F. u. A. Frensberg: Ueber d. Einfluss d. Nervensystems auf d. Vorgaenge wd. d. Schwangerschaft u.d. Gebaerakts. Pfleuger's Arch. **9**, 552–565, 1874.
51. Brachet, J. L.: Recherches expérimentales sur les fonctions du système nerveux ganglionaire. 2nd éd., Paris, 1837.
52. Ecker, A.: Blutgefaessdruesen. In Handwoerterbuch d. Physiol. (ed. Wagner, R.) Vol. 4, pp. 107–166. Braunschweig, 1853.
53. Trousseau, A.: Clinique médicale de l'Hôtel-Dieu de Paris, vol. 2, pp. 112–114: 1861.
54. Mueller, J.: Ueber die Entwickelung der Eier im Eierstock bei den Gespenstheuschrecken. Nova Acta phys.-med. Acad. Caes. Leopold nat. curios., Bonn **12**, 553–672, 1825.
55. Koelliker, R. A. von: Handbuch der Gewebslehre des Menschen. Leipzig, W. Engelmann, 1852.
56. Mueller, J.: De Glandulanum secernentium structura penitiori, Lipsiae, Sumpt. L. Vossii.
57. Ibid.: p. 111.
58. As 16: Section IV, No. 17, Chapter C: On the thyroid gland.
59. As 16: 4th ed., Vol. I, p. 346, 1844.
60. Bernard, C.: Leçons de Physiologie Expérimentale Appliquée à la Médecine. 2 Vols. Paris, J. B. Baillière, 1855–1856.
61. Cited from F. G. Young: Ideas About Animal Hormones, p. 137, in The Chemistry of Life (ed. Needham, Joseph) London, 1970.
62. Carpenter, W. B.: Cyclopaedia of Anatomy and Physiology (ed. Todd, R. B.), Vol. IV, p. 440, London, 1852.
63. As 12: p. 21.
64. Addison, T.: On the Constitutional and Local Effects of Disease of the Suprarenal Capsules. London, S. Highley, 1855.
65. Addison, Thomas: London med. Gaz. **43**, 517–518, 1849.
66. Trousseau, Armand: Bronze Addison's Disease. Arch. Gén. Méd. **8**, 478, 1856.
67. As 12: p. 332.
68. Marañon, G. P. D.: Siglo méd., Madrid **70**, p. 605, 1922.
69. Wilks, Sir Samuel: Hist. Notes on Bright's, Addison, and Hodgkins Disease, Guy's Hosp. Rep. 3rd Series **22**, 259, 1877.
70. Aran, A. F.: Arch. Gén. Méd. Paris, 4 s, XII, 61; 1846.
71. Burrows, G.: Guy's Hosp. Gaz. XXI, 429, 1907.
72. Fagge, C. H.: The Principles and Practice of Medicine, 2 Vols. London, J. & A. Churchill, 1886.
73. Stewart, G. N.: Arch. Intern. Med. **43**, p. 733, Chicago, 1929. insufficiency (Addison's Disease). J. Am. Med. Assoc. **92**, 1569–1571, 1929.
74. Hutchinson, Sir Jonathan: Med. Times Gaz. **32**, 593, 623, 648 in 1855; **33**, 60, 518, 646, 1856; Trans. Path. Soc. **7**, 270, 1856; Proc. Roy. Med. Chir. Soc., London **2**, 36, 1858.
75. Baly, W.: Trans. Path. Soc. London **8**, 325, 1856–1857.
76. Graunt, R.: Am. J. Physiol. Boston **103**, 494, 1933.
77. Schultze, P.: J. Physiol. London **84**, 70, 1935.
78. Brown-Séquard, Charles Édouard: Arch. Gén. Méd. Paris 5 s, VIII, 385, 372, 1856.
79. Brown-Séquard, Charles Édouard: C. R. Acad. Sci. Paris **43**, 422–425, 1856.

80. Ibid.: pp. 542–546.
81. Gratiolet, P.: C.R. Acad. Sci., Paris, **43,** 468–470, 1856.
82. Vulpian, Edme F. A.: Note sur quelques réactions propres à la substance des capsules surrénales. C.R. Acad. Sci., Paris **43,** 663–665, 1856.
83. Paton, Noel and Findlay: Q. J. Exp. Physiol., London **10,** 203, 315, 1917.
84. Nothnagel, Carl Wm. H.: Ztschr. klin. Med., Berlin **1,** 77, 1879.
85. Stilling, H.: Virch. Arch., Berlin **118,** 569, 1889.
86. Elliott, T. R.: J. Physiol. **46,** 285, 1913.
87. Mackay, E. M., Mackay L. L.: J. Exp. Med. **43,** 393, 1926.
88. Boycott, A. E., Kennaway, E. L.: J. Pathol. Bacteriol. **27,** 171, 1924.
89. Taylor, Isaac E., N.Y. J. Med. 3 s, **1,** 145, 1856.
90. As 12: pp. 337–338.
91. Trousseau, A.: Bull. Acad. Impér. Méd. **21,** 1036, Paris, 1855–1856.
92. Lasègue, E. C.: Arch. Méd. Paris 5 s, **7,** 257, 1856.
93. Mattei, R.: Sperimentale **11,** 3, 1863.
94. Martineau, L. De la Maladie D'Addison. Paris, 1864.
95. Bennett, John H.: Clinical Lectures on the Principles and Practice of Medicine. Edinburgh, 1865.
96. Goodhart, J. F.: Trans. Pathol. Soc. London **33,** 340, 346, 1882.
97. Habershon, S. O.: Guy's Hosp. Rep. 3 s, **10,** 78, 1864.
98. Jaccoud, F. S.: Nouv. dict. de méd. et de chir. prat., Vol. 5, p. 676, Paris, 1866.
99. As 12: p. 340.
100. Addison's collected papers: Edited with introductory prefaces by Wilks and Daldy, New Sydenham Society, London, 1868.
101. As 12: p. 339.
102. Guttman, P. H.: Arch. Pathol., Chicago. **10,** 742, 1930.
103. Ibid., p. 895.
104. As 12: pp. 340–342.
105. Osler, Wm.: Case of Addison's Disease – death during treatment with the suprarenal extract. Bull. Johns Hopkins Hosp. **7,** 208–209, 1896.
106. Muirhead, A. L.: An autograph history of a case of Addison's disease, J. Am. Med. Assoc. **76,** 652–653, 1921.
107. As 12: p. 355.
108. Costa-Casaretto, Claudio: Rev. Med. Chile, **106,** No. 12, 1034–1044, 1978.
109. Hartman, Frank A. and Brownell, K. A.: The Adrenal Gland, note on p. 17, London, H. Kimpton, 1949.
110. Meckel, J. F. the younger: Abhandlungen aus der menschlichen und vergleichenden Anatomie und Physiologie. Halle, 1806. In the section on "Ueber die Schilddruese, Nebenniere, und einige ihnen verwandte Organe". (Essays on Human and comparative anatomy and physiology, section on "the thyroid, suprarenals and some related organs".)
111. Sampson Henry: Philos. Trans. B. **19,** 7, 1697 (see also reference 116).
112. Kelly, Michael: Br. Med. J. **2,** 1301–1302, 1956.
113. Keil H.: Bull. Hist. Med. xxIII, 201–202, 1949.
114. Littré, M. P. E.: 'Oeuvres Complètes d'Hippocrate. Traduction nouvelle avec le texte grec en regard . . .' 10 Vols. Paris, J. B. Baillière, 1839–1861. Vol. V, p. 357, referring to Epid VI, Sect. 8, 32.
115. Paré, Ambroise: Les causes pourquoi le flux menstrual est retenu aux femmes. Vingt-troisième livre, Chap. LX.
116. Sampson, H.: Philos. Trans. R. Soc. xx, 80, 1698.
117. As 12: p. 362.
118. As 12: p. 364.

119. Rolleston, Sir Humphry D. and Marks, H.: Am. J. Med. Sci., Philadelphia, **116,** 383, 1898.
120. Bauer, J. and Medvei, V. C.: Ueber Interrenalismus und die geschlechtsumstimmende Wirkung der Nebennierenrinde. Dtch. med. Wschr. No. 41–42, 1–14, 1932.
121. Guthrie, L. and Emery, W.: Trans. Clin. Soc. Lond. **40,** 175, 1907.
122. As 12: p. 366.
123. Wood, E. J.: Giants and Dwarfs, p. 140, 1868.
124. Geoffroy, C. J.: Philos. Trans. **42,** 627, 1742–1743.
125. Woolley, P. G.: Adrenal Tumours. Am. J. Med. Sci. **125,** 33–46, 1902.
126. Bulloch, Wm. and Sequeira, J. H.: On the relation of the suprarenal capsules to the sex organs. Trans. Path. Soc. London **56,** 189–208, 1905.
127. Glynn, E. E.: The adrenal cortex, its rests and tumours, its relation to the other ductless glands, and especially to sex. Q. J. Med., Oxford **5,** 157–192, 1911/12.
128. Rogoff, J. M., Stewart, G. N.: Studies on adrenal insufficiency. Influence of 'heat' on the survival periods of dogs after adrenalectomy. Am. J. Physiol. **86,** 20–24, 1928.
129. Gaunt, R. and Hays, H. W.: Role of progesterone and other hormones in survival of pseudo-pregnant adrenalectomised ferrets. Am. J. Physiol. **124,** 767–773, 1938.
130. Lancereaux: Dictionnaire des Sciences Médicales, Vol. III, Sér. III, p. 157, 1876.
131. Wiesel, J.: Zeitschr. f. Heilk. xxiv, 1903.
132. Siebold, C. Th. von: Virchow's Arch. Pathol. Anat. Physiol. **100,** 66, 1885.
133. Chowne, W. D.: Remarkable case of hirsute growth in a female. Lancet I, 421–422, 1852; 514–516, 1852; II, 51–53, 1852.
134. Nordau, Max: Vom Kreml zur Alhambra; Kulturstudien, Leipzig II, 228, 1880.
135. Le Double et Houssay: Les Velus. Vigot éd. 1901.
136. Laigne-Lavastine, M.: Femmes à barbe et endocrino-psychiatrie. Paris méd. T11, 325, 1921.
137. Gull, Sir Wm. Withey: Trans. Clin. Soc. Lond. **7,** 180–185, 1873–1874 (Read: 24 Oct 1873).
138. Curling, Thos. B.: Med. Chir. Trans. **33,** 303–306, 1850.
139. Ord, Wm. M.: Med. Chir. Trans. **61,** 57–78, 1878.
140. Fagge, Charles Hilton: On sporadic cretinism in England, Med. Chir. Trans. **54,** 155–170, 1871.
141. Kocher, Emil Theodor: Exstirpation einer Struma retrooesophagea. Korresp. Blatt schweiz. Aerzte, **8,** 702–705, 1878.
142. Kocher, Emil Theodor: Ueber Kropfexstirpation und ihre Folgen. Arch. Klin. Chir. **29,** 254–337, 1883.
143. Reverdin, A.: Accidents consécutifs à l'ablation totale du goître. Rev. Méd. Suisse Rom. **2,** 539, 1882.
144. Schiff, Moritz: Schweiz. Mschr. prakt. Med. **4,** 267–275, 1859.
145. Schiff, Moritz: Arch. Exp. Pathol., Pharmakol. **18,** 25, 1884.
146. Semon, Sir Felix: A typical case of myxoedema. Br. Med. J. **2,** 1072, 1883.
147. Horsley, Sir Victor: On the function of the thyroid glands. Proc. R. Soc. London **38,** 5–7, 1884–1885.
148. Horsley, Sir Victor: Proc. R. Soc. London **40,** 6–9, 1886.
149. Horsley, Sir Victor: A recent specimen of artificial myxoedema in a monkey, Lancet **2,** 827, 1884.

150. Iason, A. M.: The Thyroid Gland in Medical History. New York, p. 92, 1946.
151. Zondek, Hermann: The Diseases of the Endocrine Glands, 2nd English Ed. London, Edward Arnold, p. 210, 1944.
152. Ibid.: p. 203.
153. Ibid.: p. 210.
154. Norris, H.: Notice of a remarkable disease, analogous to cretinism, existing in a small village in the West of England. Med. Times **17,** 257, 1848.
155. As 140.
156. Paracelsus, A. P. T. Bombastus ab Hohenheim: De generatione stultorum, in Opera **2,** 174–182, Strassburg, 1603.
157. Chatin, Gaspard A.: Existence de l'iode dans les plantes d'eau douce . . . C. R. Acad. Sci., Paris **30,** 352–354, 1850.
158. Chatin, G. A.: Recherche comparative de l'iode et de quelques autres principes dans les eaux (et les égouts) qui alimentent Paris, Londres et Turin. C. R. Acad. Sci., Paris **35,** 127, 1852.
159. Chatin, G. A.: Recherche de l'iode dans l'air, les eaux, le sol et les produits alimentaries des Alpes de la France et du Piémont. C. R. Acad. Sci., Paris **34,** 14; **51,** 409, 1852.
160. Chatin, G. A.: C. R. Acad. Sci., Paris **38,** 83, 1854.
161. Prévost and Maffoni: Atti dell'acad. med.-chir. di Torino, 1846.
162. Inglis, J.: Treatise on English Bronchocele, with a Few Remarks on the Use of Iodine and its Compounds, London, 1838.
163. Fellenberg, T. von (Swiss): Mitt. Lebensmitt **24,** 123, 1923.
164. Koestl, F.: Der endemische Kretinismus als Gegenstand der oeffentlichen Fuersorge. Wien. 1855.
165. Boussingault, J. B.: Ann. Chim. Phys. **54,** 163, 1833.
166. Quervain, F. de: Schweiz. med. Wochenschr, **52,** 857, 1922.
167. Marine, David and Kimball, O. P.: Arch. Int. Med. **25,** 661, 1920; J. Am. Med. Assoc. **77,** 1068, 1921; Am. J. Med. Sci. **163,** 634, 1922.
168. Starling, E. H.: The Wisdom of the Body. The Harveian Oration, delivered to the R. Coll. Physicians London on St. Luke's Day, 1923. H. K. Lewis & Co., 1923.
169. Means, J. H.: The Tree of Thyroidology. A Drawing, 1946.
170. Means, J. H.: The Association of American Physicians: its First Seventy-Five Years. New York; McGraw-Hill, 1961.
171. Marine, D. and Lenhart, C. H.: Arch. Intern. Med. **4,** 440, 1909.
172. Chesney, A. M., Clawson, T. A. and Webster, B. P.: Bull. Johns Hopkins Hosp. **43,** 261 and 278, 1928.
173. Rilliet, Frédéric: Mém. Acad. Méd. Paris **24,** 23, 1858–1859.
174. Coindet, François: Bibl. Universelle Sci. Arts. Genève, **16,** 140, 1821.
175. Stanbury, John B.: Endemic Goitre. The Adaptation of Man to Thyroid Deficiency. p. 66, Cambridge, Ma, 1954.
176. Kocher, Emil Th.: Arch. klin. Chir. **92,** 1166, 1910.
177. As 174.
178. Marine, D.: Medicine, Baltimore, **6,** 127, 1927.
179. Lebert, H.: cit. from Iason, A. H.: The Thyroid Gland in Medical History. p. 83, New York, Froben Press, 1946.
180. Bubnow, N. A.: Z. Physiol. Chemie **8,** 147, 1884.
181. Baumann, Eugen: Ueber das normale Vorkommen von Jod im Thierkoerper. Z. Physiol. Chemie **21,** 319, 1896.
182. Baumann, Engen: Ueber das Thyrojodin, Muenchn. Med. Wochenschr. **43,** 309, 1896.

183. Baumann, Eugen and Goldman, E.: Ist das Iodothyrin (Thyrojodin) der lebenswichtige Bestandteil der Schilddruese? Muenchn. Med. Wochenschr. **43,** 1153, 1896.
184. Harington, Sir Charles Robert: The Thyroid Gland, Its Chemistry and Physiology, Oxford University Press, London, 1933.
185. Gairdner, Wm.: Essay on the effects of iodine on the human constitution; with practical observations on its use in the case of Bronchocele, Scrophula and Tuberculous Diseases of the Chest and Abdomen. London, T. & G. Underwood, 1824.
186. Hutchison, R.: J. Physiol. (London), **20,** 474–496, 1896.
187. Tambach, R.: Zur Chemie des Jods in der Schilddruese. Z. Biol. **36,** 549–569, 1898.
188. Oswald, A.: Ueber den Jodgehalt der Schilddruese. Hoppe-Seyler's Z. Physiol. Chem. **23,** 265, 1897.
189. Oswald, A.: Zur Kenntnis der Thyreoglobulinus. Z. Physiol. Chem. **32,** 121, 1901.
190. Tatum, A. L.: A study of the distribution of iodine between cells and colloid in the thyroid gland. J. Biol. Chem. **42,** 47, 1920.
191. Drechsel, E.: Beitraege zur Chemie einiger Seethiere. Z. Biol. **33,** 85, 1895.
192. Wheeler, H. L. and Jamieson, G. S.: Synthesis of iodogorgonic acid. Am. Chem. J. **33,** 365–372, 1905.
193. Jendrassik, E.: Arch. Psychiatrie **17,** 301–321, 1886.
194. Greenfield, Wm. Smith: Br. Med. J. **2,** 1493; 1553, 1893.
195. Janney, N. W.: Endocrinology **6,** 633, 1922.
196. Rehn, Ludwig: Berlin Klin. Wochenschr. **21,** 163, 1884.
197. Notthaft, A. von: Centralblatt Inn. Med. **19,** 353, 1898.
198. Tamburini, A.: Riv. Sper. di freniat., Reggio-Emilia, **20,** 559, 1894.
199. Benda, Carl: Beitraege zur normalen und pathologischen Histologie der menschlichen Hypophysis cerebri. Berlin. Klin. Wochenschr. **37,** 1205–1210, 1900.
200. Lewis, Dean: Bull. Johns Hopkins Hosp. **16,** 554, Baltimore, 1905.
201. As 12: p. 30.
202. Mueller, Friedrich von: Beitraege zur Kentniss der Basedow'schen Krankheit. Dtsch. Arch. Klin. Med. **51,** 335–412, 1893.
203. Magnus-Levy, A.: Ueber den Respiratorischen Geswechsel unter dem Einfluss der Thyreoidea Sowie unter Verschiedenen Pathologischen Zustaenden. Berlin, Klin. Wochenschr. **32,** 650–652, 1895.
204. As 12: p. 211.
205. Flajani, Giuseppe: Sopra un tumor freddo nell'anterior parte dell collo detto broncocele. Collezione d'osservazioni e riflessioni di chirurgia, Roma, **3,** 270–273, 1802.
206. Graves, Robert J.: Lond. Med. Surg. J. (Renshaw's) **7,** 516–517, 1835.
207. Charcot, Jean M.: Gaz. Méd. Paris, 3 s, **11,** 599, 1856.
208. As 184: p. 172.
209. Pauli, F. P.: Med. Ann. Heidelberg, **3,** 218, 1837.
210. Basedow, Carl A. von: Wochenschr. Ges Heilk. **6,** 197–204, pp. 220–228. Berlin, 1840; idem, ibid., **14,** p. 769, 1848.
211. Plummer, H. S. and Boothby, W. M.: J. Iowa State Med. Soc. **14,** 66, 1924.
212. As 12: p. 209.
213. Mohr, B.: Wochenschr. Ges. Heilk. **6,** 565–571, 1840.
214. Dock, G.: J. Am. Med. Ass. **51,** 1119, Chicago, 1908.
215. Howard, C. P.: Endocrinol. and Metab. (Ed. L. F. Barber), Vol. I, 304, 1922.
216. Henoch, E. H.: Wochenschr. Ges. Heilk. **14,** 609–625, 1848.

217. As 12: p. 215.
218. Legge, John W.: Note on the history of exophthalmic goitre. St. Bartholomew's Hosp. Rep. **18,** 7, 1882.
219. Marsh, Sir Henry: Dubl. J. Med. Sci. **20,** 471, 1841.
220. Marsh, Sir Henry: Proc. Pathol. Soc. Dublin, 3rd rep. p. 25, 1840–1847.
221. Begbie, J.: Month. J. Med. Sci., London, Edinb. **9,** 495, 1849.
222. Cooper, W. White: Lancet **1,** 551, 1849.
223. Mackenzie, W.: Practical Treatise on Diseases of the Eye. London, 1854.
224. Graefe, F. Wm. E. A. von: Ueber Basedow'sche Krankheit. Dtsch Klinik **16,** 158–159, 1864.
225. Fischer, P.: Arch. Gén. Méd., 5 s, **14,** 521, 652, 1859.
226. Trousseau, A.: Gaz. d'Hôp., Paris **33,** 553, 1860.
227. Trousseau, A.: Lancet **2,** 575–598, 1860.
228. Aran, F. A.: Bull. Acad. Impér. Méd. Paris **26,** 122, 1860.
229. Mueller, Heinrich: Verhdlg. Phys.-Med. Ges. Wuerzburg, **9,** 244, 1859.
230. Stokes, W.: Diseases of the Heart and Aorta. pp. 278–297. Dublin, 1854.
231. Sattler, H.: Die Basedow'sche Krankheit, in Hdbuch. Ges. Augenhlkde von A. Graefe & Th. Saemisch, Vol. VI, **2,** p. 949, 1880.
232. Murray, George Redmayne: Note on the treatment of myxoedema by hypodermic injections of an extract of the thyroid gland of sheep. Br. Med. J. **2,** 796–797, 1891.
233. Pendred, V.: Deaf-mutism and goitre. Lancet **2,** 532, 1896.
234. As 12: p. 219.
235. As 12: pp. 222, 223.
236. Trousseau, A.: Gaz. d, Hôp., Paris **33,** 553, 1860.
237. Jones, C. Handfield: Proptosis, goitre and palpitation, Lancet **2,** 562, 1860.
238. Jones, C. H.: Proc. R. Med. Chir. Soc. **3,** 298, 1861.
239. As 12: p. 228.
240. As 12: p. 237.
241. Marie, Pierre: Arch. Neurol. **6,** 79, 1883.
242. Bramwell, Sir Byrom: Studies in Clinical Medicine, Vol. I, p. 290. Edinburgh, 1890.
243. Cheadle, W. B.: St. George's Hosp. Rep. **4,** 175, 1869.
244. Bowlby A. A.: Trans. Pathol. Soc. London **36,** 420, 1885.
245. Riedel, B. M. K. L.: Die Chronische, zur Bildung Eisenharter Tumoren fuehrende Entzuendung der Schilddruesse. Verh. Dtsch. Ges. Chir. **25,** 101–105, 1896.
246. Iason, A. H.: The Thyroid Gland in Medical History. New York. pp. 85–86: 1946.
247. Corner, George Washington: The early history of the oestrogenic hormones. Proc. Soc. Endocrinology, pp. iii–xvii, in J. Endocrinol. **31,** (2), London, Cambridge Univ. Press, 1965.
248. Prévost, J. L. and Dumas, J. B. A.: Memoire sur le développement du poulet dans l'oeuf. Paris. Ann. Sci. nat. **12,** 415–443, 1827.
249. As 54.
250. Baer, Carl Ernst von.: De ovi mammalium et hominis genesi. Lipsiae, L. Vossius, 1827.
251. Gegenbauer, Carl: Ueber den Bau und die Entwickelung der Wirbelthiereier mit partieller Dotterteilung. Arch. Anat. Physiol. Wiss. Med. 491–529, 1861.
252. Garrison, F. H.: An Introduction to the History of Medicine. 4th ed. Repr. p. 254. Philadelphia, W.B. Saunders, 1929.
253. Koelliker, A. von: N. Notiz, Geb. Natur u. Heilkde. Weimar. **19,** 4–8, 1841.

254. Schweiger-Seidel, F.: Ueber die Samenkoerperchen u. ihre Entwicklung. Arch. Mikr. Anat. **1,** 309–335, 1865.
255. Barry, Martin: cit. after Garrison, as 252, p. 258.
256. Hertwig, Oscar: Morph. Jahrb. Leipzig, ı, 347–434, 1875/76.
257. Fleming, W.: Arch. Mikr. Anat., **16,** 302–436, 1880; **18,** 15–259 (transl. of Part II in J. All. Biol. **25,** No. 1, pt. 2, pp. 3–69, 1965).
258. Beneden, É. van: La maturation de l'oeuf, la fécondation et les premières phases du developpement des mammifères. Bull. Acad. R. Sci. Belg., 2nd Sér. **40,** 686–736, 1875.
259. Weisman, A. F. L.: Amphimixis, oder die Vermischung der Individuen. Jena, G. Fischer, 1891.
260. Weisman, A. F. L.: Das Keimplasma. Jena, G. Fischer, 1892.
261. Weisman, A. F. L.: Aufsaetze ueber die Vererbung und Verwandte Biologische Fragen. Jena, G. Fischer, 1892.
262. Lloyd, G. E. R. Ed, Hippocratic Writings, in Airs, Waters, Places, pp. 161–162, Pelican Classics, Penguin Books, 1978.
263. Ibid.: in Introduction, p. 46.
264. Ibid.: in The Seed and The Nature of the Child, pp. 317–347.
265. Vogel, F. and Motulsky, A. G.: Human Genetics. Problems and Approaches. Chapter 1: History of Human Genetics, pp. 8–17; Berlin, Springer-Verlag, 1979.
266. Le Bon, Gustave: The Crowd. First English edition, London, Ernest Benn, 1896.
267. As 265: p. 9.
268. Adams, Joseph: A Treatise on the Supposed Hereditary Properties of Diseases. London, J. Callow, 1814.
269. Nasse, Chr. F.: Von einer erblichen Neigung zu toedtlichen Blutungen. Arch. med. Erfahr, ı, 385–434, 1820.
270. Mendel, Gregor J.: Versuche ueber Pflanzen-Hybriden. Verh. naturf. Vereines Bruenn **4,** 3–47, 1865.
271. de Vries, Hugo M.: Die Mutationstheorie, Leipzig, Veit & Co., 1901/3.
272. As 252: p. 516.
273. Hering, K. E. K.: Ueber das Gedaechtnis also eine allgemeine Funktion der organisierten Materie. Abh. k. Akad. Wiss., Wien **20,** 253–278, 1870.
274. Galton, F.: Natural Inheritance. London, Macmillan, 1889.
275. Morgan, T. H., Sturtevant, A. H. *et al*: The Mechanism of Mendelian Heredity. New York, H. Holt, 1915.
276. Morgan, T. H.: Sex-linked inheritance in *Drosophila*. Science **32,** 120–122, 1910.
277. Sturtevant, A. H.: The linear arrangement of six sex-linked factors in *Drosophila*, as shown by their mode of association. J. Exp. Zool. **14,** 43–59, 1913.
278. Goldschmidt, R. B.: Geschlechtsbestimmung, Berlin, 1921; English translation 1923.
279. Koelliker, A. von: Z. Wiss. Zool. **42,** 1–46, 1885.
280. Boveri, Th., Ueber mehrpolige Mitosen als Mittel z. Analyse d Zellkerns. Verh. Phys.-Med. Ges. Wuerzburg, **35,** 67–90, 1903.
281. Sutton, W. S.: The chromosomes in heredity. Biol. Bull. **4,** 231–251, 1903.
282. As 260.
283. In England now: a running commentary by peripatetic correspondents, Lancet ı, 476, 1957.
284. Garrod, Sir Archibald E.: The incidence of alkaptonuria: a study in chemical individuality. Lancet, ıı, 1616–1620, 1902.

285. Garrod, Sir Archibald: Inborn Errors of Metabolism. H. Frowde, London, 1909.
286. As 265: p. 12.
287. Landsteiner, K.: Zur Kenntnis der antifermentativen, lytischen und agglutinierenden Wirkungen des Blutserums und der Lymphe. Zentralbl. Bakteriol. **27,** 357–362, 1900.
288. Dungern, Emil von and Hirszfeld, L.: Ueber Vererbung gruppenspezifischer Strukturen des Blutes (= On the inheritance of group-specific structures of the blood). Z. Immunitaetsforschung. **6,** 284–292, 1910.
289. Langerhans, P.: Beitraege zur mikroskopischen Anatomie der Bauchspeicheldruese (Contributions to the Microscopical Anatomy of the Pancreas); Inaugural-Dissertation. Berlin, Gustave Lange, 1869.
290. Henderson, John R.: The Pancreas, Chapter 1, Historical Introduction, p. 9. Unpublished manuscript.
291. Laguesse, G.-É.: C. R. Soc. Biol., Paris **14,** 819, 1893.
292. Kuehne, Willy and Lea, A. S.: Verhdl. Naturhistor.-Med. Ver., Heidelberg, n.F. **1,** 194, 1874–1877.
293. As 290: p. 10 and Figure 6.
294. As 290: Figure 7.
295. As 12: p. 275.
296. Owen, Sir Richard: On the anatomy of the Indian rhinoceros, *Rh. unicornis* L. Trans. Zool. Soc., Lond. **4,** 31–58, 1852.
297. Virchow, R.: Die Krankhaften Geschwuelste. Berlin, Vol. III, p. 13, 1867.
298. Sandstroem, Ivar V.: Om en ny körtel hos menniskan och åtskilliga Däggdjur. Upsala Läkaref. Förh. **15,** pp. 441–471; 1880. (First systematic account of the parathyroids. Translation in: Bull. Inst. Hist. Med. Baltimore. Johns Hopkins University **6,** 192–222, 1938.
299. Woelfler, Anton: Ueber die Entwickelung und den Bau der Schilddruese. Berlin 1880.
300. Baber, E. Cresswell: Phil. Trans. R. Soc. London **172,** 600, 1881.
301. Gley, Eugène: Sur les fonctions du corps thyroide. C. R. Soc. Biol., Paris **43,** 841–847, 1891.
302. Gley, Eugène: Arch. Physiol. Norm. Pathol., Paris **24,** 135, 1892.

CHAPTER SIXTEEN

THE BIRTH OF ENDOCRINOLOGY – PART II

BROWN–SÉQUARD AGAIN AND HIS ORGANOTHERAPY — MURRAY

LAST first of June I sent to the Society of Biology a communication, which was followed by several others, showing the remarkable effects produced on myself by subcutaneous injection of a liquid obtained by the maceration on a mortar of the testicle of a dog or of a guineapig to which one has added a little water[1].

Thus did Charles Édouard Brown-Séquard (1817–1894) (see Section II), the French neurologist and physiologist, address himself to his professional audience in the autumn of 1889. We had come across him in 1856, when he carried out his experimental studies to prove that the adrenals are essential to life, following Addison's monograph (see pp. 230–231). He was now 72 years of age and still actively engaged in research. In June 1889 he had suggested to the Society of Biology in Paris that the testes contained an active, dynamogenic, invigorating substance, which he thought he could obtain from animals and inject into men and rejuvenate them. He put forward this suggestion again in another, contemporary paper: 'Du rôle physiologique et thérapeutique d'un suc extrait de testicules d'animaux d'après nombre de faits observés chez l'homme'[2].

Dr. Merriley Borell has made the historical developments in the endocrine field between 1880 and 1930 her special subject of study[3]. Her painstaking and meticulous researches have made my task in discussing this complex, difficult, but fascinating period much easier. In referring to the second paper, she says: "In this paper, Brown-Séquard evaluated the world-wide response which has been provoked by his experiments on the function of the testes." The term 'world-wide' in this connection is of importance, because Brown-Séquard's experiments had important repercussions not only in France, but also in Britain and in the United States, and not only among his contemporaries, but among his medical and scientific successors, whether followers or opponents, and among the lay public.

The title of the paper submitted to the Society of Biology was: "Des effets produits chez l'homme par des injections souscutanées d'une liquide retiré des testicules frais de cobaye et de chien." Dr. Borell says:

> Within weeks, testicular extract was being given to patients with every kind of illness. Within two years, many physicians thought that not only the testes, but every organ of the body possessed some active principle which might be of immediate therapeutic value. Organo-therapy, or the method of Brown-Séquard, as it was often called, came to be the therapeutic hope of physicians from Cleveland to Bucharest.[3] (See p. 301.)

Although the interest in Brown-Séquard's testicular therapy waned, adrenal and thyroid extracts emerged within the next 10 years and the attention of the physiologists had been directed to the idea of 'internal secretion', a term coined by (Sharpey-)Schaefer. In Brown-Séquard's opinion, "the feebleness of old men is in part due to the diminution of the function of the testicles"[4]. He had, in 1869, already suggested that "if it were possible to inject, without danger, sperm into the veins of old men, one would be able to obtain with them some manifestation of rejuvenation at once with respect to intellec-tual work and physical powers of the organism"[4].

Brown-Séquard was well known both in England and in the United States. He had been elected to the Royal Society (of London) in 1860, to the American Academy of Arts and Sciences in 1867, to the National Academy of Sciences in 1868. He had lectured in both countries, in the U.S. in Boston, in Philadelphia and in New York, and had taught at the Harvard Medical School in the 1850s and 1860s[3]. Some of his preliminary experiments were performed near Boston during a stay in America, in 1875, when he tried to graft "either entire guinea-pigs or parts of guinea-pigs onto old dogs, but it is not clear how this was done"[3].

What Dr. Borell's studies brought out is of particular interest. Namely the different reaction to Brown-Séquard's new ideas, auto-experiments and experiments in general, in Britain and America.

(a) Britain

Brown-Séquard, who was British by birth (in 1817), became French in 1878 when he became Professor of Medicine at the Collège de France. He was also one of the first physicians to the National Hospital for the Paralysed and Epileptic in London in 1860 and 1863; in 1860 he also became an FRCP London, as well as being a Fellow of the Royal Society. After 1863, he taught and lectured in the United States and, occasionally, in Britain. Cambridge conferred upon him an honorary LLD in 1881, and he received the Baly Medal of the Royal College of Physicians of London. His third wife, Emma Dakin, was English.

Three weeks after Brown-Séquard's first communication on testicular extract, the *British Medical Journal* published an article: 'The pentacle of rejuvenescence'[5], reporting on the experiments. The account was strictly factual, but as Borell points out

> preliminary comments in the report suggest that the popular reaction to the public announcement of Brown-Séquard's 'discovery' had been quite unsettling to the medical profession. . . . 'The statements he (B-S) made – which have unfortunately attracted a good deal of attention in the public press – recall the wild imaginings of mediaeval philosophers in search of an elixir vitae'. The choice of the title is itself an indication of the disbelief with which Brown-Séquard's results were received. 'Pentacle' refers to a symbol used in magic, a 'five pointed star'.[6]

On 6 July 1889, the *British Medical Journal* published a thirteen line report on the results of G. Variot's (of Paris) successful use of Brown-Séquard's method in three men with senile debility[8]. Whereas Variot's observations confirmed those of Brown-Séquard, that his own treatment results were not due to autosuggestion, Borell stresses "there was no indication that the editors of the British Medical Journal shared this view"[7]. Brown-Séquard said:

> . . . I hope that other physiologists of advanced age will repeat these experiments and will show whether the effects which I have obtained on myself depend on my personal idiosyncrasy or not. As for the question of knowing whether it is a kind of autosuggestion without hypnotism to which must be attributed entirely the very considerable changes which have been produced in my body, I do not wish to discuss that today . . . in the account which I shall give now (in this number) of a considerable number of cases in which injections similar to mine have been given, without the individuals concerned knowing that we were seeking to learn whether they would increase in strength, this result has been obtained. It is, therefore, clear that it is not as the result of a kind of autosuggestion that the vigour of the nerve centres is

increased and that it is in fact to a particular action of the injected liquid that this effect is due.[1]

On 29 August 1889, the *British Medical Journal* (II, 446), commented in only eight lines on a report from Indianapolis that Brown-Séquard rejuvenating fluid had invigorated a "decrepit old man", under the (*B.M.J.*) heading: 'The new elixir of youth', with the acid comment that no "medical authority" had been given. The Brown-Séquard method also outraged the anti-vivisectionists, who feared that the use of animal extracts would cause increased suffering. Some medical men voiced concern that such treatment might involve masturbation, not to mention the castration of animals[6]. Brown-Séquard's offer to write an article for *The Lancet* was accepted. The article, 'Note on the effects produced on man by subcutaneous injections of a liquid obtained of the testicles of animals', was sent from Brighton, where Brown-Séquard was visiting in the summer of 1889. In January 1890, *The Lancet*'s New York correspondent wrote somewhat disparagingly on the reception of the "method of Brown-Séquard" in the United States[6].

> In the hands of one experimenter, the paralysed immediately walk, the lame throw aside cane and crutches, the deaf hear and the blind see. The same experiments failed altogether in the practice of another. . . . No British reports on the testing of the testicular extracts were published in the Lancet, either in 1890 or in 1891.[6]

He soon sent testicular extract, on request, to friends or followers in London, or asked his co-worker and assistant Jacques Arsène d'Arsonval (1851–1940) to do so on his behalf. Among the recipients were a Dr. Fanton-Cameron, about whom nothing more is known[6], Robert Brudenell Carter, FRCS (1828–1918), the eye surgeon, and Sir Victor Horsley (1857–1916); finally his old friend and his wife's cousin, Dr. W. D. Waterhouse of London, whose report on the use of the extract finally appeared in the *British Medical Journal* of 30 January 1892[9]. "At which time," Borell writes, "organotherapy was becoming an acceptable mode of therapeutics in Britain." The reason for this respectability was the work on the thyroid gland, in which Horsley played an important role, especially from 1884 to 1886 (see pp. 249–250). In February 1890, Horsley had suggested grafts of thyroid tissue as a treatment for myxoedematous patients. This idea was modified and successfully put into action by his former student at University College Hospital (from 1886 to 1889), George Redmayne Murray (1865–1939) (see Section II), who injected thyroid extract[10] into such patients, after he had toured medical clinics in Berlin and Paris between 1889 and 1890. It was perhaps in Paris that he learned about the therapeutic experiments with (testicular) organ extracts. On return, he became pathologist to the Hospital for Sick Children in Newcastle and later Professor of Comparative Pathology in the University of Durham and Physician to the Royal Infirmary in Newcastle. He wrote to Horsley about his idea of experimenting with thyroid extract. Although Horsley was slightly sceptical, he did not discourage the young man from making the attempt[6]. (Letter of 3 December 1890: "However, it cannot do any harm, and I think it would be worth trying, as it is possible from Schiff's results of imperfect transplantation that an emulsion of the gland might possess some of its active properties.") Moritz Schiff, 1823–1896, had also made important experiments on the production of artificial diabetes.

In a later letter of 22 June 1891, Horsley appeared more encouraging, quoting recent thyroid literature, but without mentioning a paper which Brown-Séquard had published in April with d'Arsonval[11]. In it, they had argued that potent substances must exist in animal tissues, the process (and the result) of "internal secretion". These substances could be discovered by using extracts obtained from specific tissues for the treatment of certain diseases which are perhaps due to deficiency of an internal secretion, and they outlined a programme for such an experimental therapy. This was the method which became known as 'organotherapy'.

Horsley wrote:

. . . The clinical reference is as follows – Bettencourt and Serrano (*Progrès Medical*, 1890, Vol. XII, p. 170). These authors, who had adopted the suggestion of grafting the thyroid, suggest that the benefits obtained therefrom are due to absorption of material from the gland, and the same idea had occurred to Schiff and others. Hoping this is not too late for your wants, and that you will publish at once . . . I am Yours very sincerely . . .[6]

Murray had in fact suggested at the meeting on 12 February 1891 of the Northumberland and Durham Medical Society (with Dr. Drummond in the chair), that myxoedema was not due to a failure of excretion but to loss of an active internal secretion. He, therefore, proposed to attempt a replacement therapy of extract from sheep's thyroid, especially as implants of such thyroid tissue had proved temporarily beneficial according to reports from Portugal. Sir Walter Langdon–Brown related in his Presidential Address in 1946 to the newly formed Section of Endocrinology of the Royal Society of Medicine:

I heard the story of what followed from Murray's own lips. A senior member of the Society said, that it would be just as sensible to treat a case of locomotor ataxia with an emulsion of spinal cord!

Undeterred, Murray pursued his idea once he had made arrangements with the slaughterhouse to obtain supplies of fresh sheep's thyroid, although the medical college of Newcastle refused to grant him any facilities. The patient, on whom Murray reported in October 1891, was a woman of 46, who lived until the age of 74 with her hypodermic injections of glycerin extract of sheep's thyroid; during the following 28 years she received the equivalent of 870 sheep's thyroids!

Murray reported his observations on the treatment of myxoedema with thyroid juice within a month of Horsley's letter[10]. His 'Note on the treatment of myxoedema by hypodermic injections of an extract of the thyroid gland of a sheep'[10] had actually been read in the Section of Therapeutics at the Annual Meeting of the British Medical Association in Bournemouth in July 1891. Murray made no reference to Brown-Séquard and d'Arsonval, but credited Horsley with the suggestion. The French claimed, however, that Charles Bouchard (1837–1915), Professor of General Pathology at the Faculty in Paris, had already recommended this treatment in 1887[6]. Murray concluded that myxoedema "is due to the loss of function of the thyroid gland"[10]. Apart from references to Kocher's observations and Horsley's experiments, he also quoted the work of (Baron) Anton von Eiselsberg (1860–1939), the Viennese surgeon, who had shown that transplantation of the thyroid into the abdominal integument of a cat prevented myxoedema; but the early experiments of von Eiselsberg were confusing, because removal of the thyroid involved also removal of the parathyroids, thus causing tetany[12].

Bettencourt and Serrano's (of Lisbon) experiment mentioned by Horsley in his letter, had proved that

> as the improvement commenced the day after the operation, it could not be due to the gland becoming vascularized and so functional, but suggested that it was due to the absorption of the juice of the healthy thyroid gland by the tissues of the patient.[10]

Murray's final conclusion was, that if myxoedema and cachexia strumipriva are caused by the lack of some substance (produced and) present in the normal thyroid, necessary to maintain the body in health, "it is at least rational treatment to supply that deficiency as far as possible by injecting the extract of a healthy gland"[10].

Transplants or grafts were also carried out by H. Bircher[13] in 1890, by H. Fenwick and W. J. Collins[14], G. A. Wright[15] and by J. MacPherson[16]. However, improvement was only temporary and most likely due to the absorption of the graft. When Albert Kocher revived the treatment by grafting in 1923, he wisely kept the patient

DISEASES

OF THE

THYROID GLAND

PART I.
MYXŒDEMA AND CRETINISM

BY

GEORGE R. MURRAY
M.A., M.D. CAMB., F.R.C.P.
GRATE PROFESSOR OF COMPARATIVE PATHOLOGY IN THE UNIVERSITY OF DURHAM
PHYSICIAN TO THE ROYAL INFIRMARY, NEWCASTLE

WITH ILLUSTRATIONS

LONDON
H. K. LEWIS, 136 GOWER STREET, W.C.
1900

NORTHUMBERLAND AND DURHAM

MEDICAL SOCIETY.

SESSION 1890-91

FEBRUARY MEETING.

THE FIFTH MONTHLY MEETING of this Society was held in the Library of the Royal Infirmary, Newcastle-upon-Tyne, on the evening of Thursday, 12th February, 1891—Dr. Drummond (President) in the chair. Fifty-four members present.

MYXŒDEMA

Dr. GEORGE MURRAY : I have brought this patient before you this evening as a good typical case of myxœdema, and also because I wish to have your opinion upon a mode of treatment which I believe to be new, and which I propose to try in this case.

The patient is a woman of 46, she has had a family of nine children, of whom six are living. Four or five years ago, her relations first noticed that her speech and actions were becoming very slow, and she, herself, began to feel that it was a great effort to do her ordinary housework. Her features gradually became enlarged and thickened. The hands and feet also increased in size and altered somewhat in shape. At the present time she presents most of the characteristic symptoms of myxœdema. She complains of langour, great sensitiveness to cold, and a disinclination to see strangers. The features are notably thickened. This change is well seen in the alæ nasi and lips. The connective tissue of the eyelids and beneath the eyes is swollen and œdematous in appearance. It, however, does not "pit" on pressure being made, nor would any fluid exude if it were pricked as in the œdema of Bright's disease. The cheeks have the characteristic pink colouration in the centre. The tongue is not unusually large, at the present time, though the patient tells me that it was enlarged at an earlier period of her illness. The hands and feet are both enlarged ; the former have that peculiar shape which has been described as "spade-like." The skin is dry, and the superficial layers of the epidermis are constantly being shed. The hair is very

It has occurred to me that it would be worth while to try the hypodermic injection of an emulsion or extract of the thyroid gland of a sheep. This treatment appears to be rational, and, at any rate, would not harm the patient. We may, I think, by this means hope to produce as much improvement in a case of myxœdema as was brought about by the absorption of the juice of a piece of the gland which had been introduced beneath the skin, and it has the advantage of being a much simpler proceeding.

secretion. To emphasise his faith in his hypothesis, he showed a case of myxœdema at a meeting of the Newcastle and Northumberland Medical Society, and said that he proposed to treat it by an extract of thyroid gland. I had the story of what followed from Murray's own lips. A senior member of the Society said that it would be just as sensible to treat a case of locomotor ataxy with an emulsion of spinal cord! Undeterred, Murray made arrangements with a slaughterhouse to be allowed to dissect out sheep's thyroids under antiseptic precautions. The Medical School at Newcastle refused him any facilities, but Armstrong College came to his assistance and gave him a room in which to prepare his extracts. A year later he triumphantly showed the case of myxœdema which had been curéd by his extracts before the same Society. When Hector

Figure 51 George R. Murray's paper [by kind permission of the University of Newcastle-upon-Tyne (Dr. C. N. Armstrong)]

on thyroid extract before and after the operation, otherwise the graft would be "simply eaten up" by the subthyroid patient[17]. Curiously enough, Henry Fenwick, one of whose papers appeared in the *British Medical Journal* in the same issue as Murray's second paper[18–20], reported on a patient, treated by injections, merely a diuretic effect and assumed that myxoedema was somehow linked to disturbance of the function of the kidney. In his next report on two patients, in 1892[21], he came to similar conclusions. Soon after, Hector Mackenzie (1856–1929) and E. L. Fox reported, independently, on patients in whom the oral administration of thyroid preparations had been quite successful[22,23], whereas F. Howitz (1828–1912), Professor of Clinical

Surgery in Copenhagen, in the same year (1892) claimed similar results by feeding patients on lightly cooked thyroids of sheep[24]. Murray did not seem to know of Eugène Gley's (1857-1930) (see Section II) study[25] and thus was convinced that he was the first in the field to use this treatment in humans. As Borell puts it, the use of thyroid extract as treatment was "in the air" in the winter of 1890–1891. She took the phrase from one of Brown-Séquard's letters to d'Arsonval, urging him to present a communication to the Society of Biology, because "the thing is in the air – especially in Italy"[6].

Thus, Murray's treatment of myxoedema by the subcutaneous injection of thyroid juice in 1891 became the first generally recognized success of organotherapy. The study of thyroid pathology had also become the first indicator of the research problems to which the new idea of internal secretion was applicable. Numerous reports on patients so treated appeared in Britain. A leading article of the *British Medical Journal* of 29 October 1892[26] declared that a rational therapy for myxoedema had been discovered. Moreover, the gland extract could now be fed successfully by mouth. In France, the brilliant and celebrated Jean Martin Charcot (1825–1893), Pierre Marie's teacher, made an equally important contribution to the subject, entitled: 'Myxoedème, cachexie pachydermique en état crétinoide'[27].

Soon, the same reasoning was applied to the treatment of diabetes mellitus by pancreatic extract. A paper was presented by Vaughan Harley (1863–1923) 'The pathogenesis of pancreatic diabetes mellitus' in 1892[28], at the same meeting of the British Medical Association to which Murray gave an enlarged version of his experience of the treatment of myxoedema by hypodermic injections of thyroid gland extract[29]. To the suggestion that pancreatic juice should be used in the treatment of diabetes, Harley could point out that such attempts had been made over the last 2 years, in England and abroad, but without success. Such a parallel between thyroid and pancreatic function had been considered by Brown-Séquard and d'Arsonval 18 months earlier, but only now did such views on glandular function and the application of organotherapy become acceptable. The three patients with paralysis, treated with Brown-Séquard's testicular extract and presented at the 'Clinical Evening of the Harveian Society of London' on 7 January 1891 (see p. 292, W. D. Waterhouse), were now reported briefly in the *British Medical Journal* on 30 January 1892[6], and a letter was printed by a Dr. Ambrose on the method of preparing Brown-Séquard's extract, a sign of the change of attitude. The idea of treating diabetes by pancreatic extracts was encouraged again and several clinical research workers took up the challenge[30,31]: Hector W. G. Mackenzie; Neville Wood of the Victoria Hospital for Children, but especially William Hale White

(1857–1949) of Guy's Hospital[30,31]. The basis for these ideas was given by the experimental work of Joseph von Mering (1849–1908) of Cologne, a pupil of Frerichs and Hoppe-Seyler, who had investigated phloridzin diabetes in 1886[32]. Friedrich Theodor Frerichs (1819–1885), who was Professor of Pathology in Berlin, pronounced in 1884 that 20% of diabetics showed gross changes of the pancreas[33]. The most important experimental work was the extirpation of the pancreas of a dog by J. von Mering and Oscar Minkowski (1858–1931)[34] followed by diabetes. At that time, Oscar Minkowski was an assistant to Bernard Naunyn (1839–1925) at the Medical Clinic of the University of Strasbourg. Naunyn had devoted his life to the study of diabetes and was the leading authority of his time on that subject. His work was summarized in his book: *Der Diabetes Mellitus*[35].

According to a letter written by Minkowski in 1926 and published by Houssay in 1952[36], von Mering was working in April 1889 in Hoppe-Seyler's Institute, which Minkowski visited to look at some chemical periodicals in the library. (Ernest Felix Immanuel Hoppe-Seyler, 1825–1895, was professor of physical chemistry in Strasbourg from 1872 to 1895, and had first obtained haemoglobin in crystalline form.) Minkowski accidentally met von Mering there and talked to him about 'Lipanin', which the latter had recommended for the treatment of some digestive disturbances, because of the free fatty acid content of the oil (of 6%). Minkowski was critical of that recommendation; some discussion developed as to whether the pancreas had a really important role in splitting fatty acids in the gut. As a result of that discussion, the two men began an investigation on the digestion of fat, and of the surgically difficult operation of the removal of the pancreas from a dog. The dog was supplied by von Mering, who also assisted at the operation. The next day, von Mering had to go away for a time and the dog was kept by Minkowski tied up in the laboratory, as there was no cage available. Although the dog had been house-trained and was frequently taken out by the laboratory assistant, it developed polyuria. Minkowski, trained by Naunyn always to test for sugar in the urine in any case of polyuria, found that the dog excreted 12% of sugar and was suffering from diabetes mellitus. The story that glycosuria was first suspected because the laboratory assistant noticed that flies settled wherever the dog had passed urine has been contradicted by Minkowski, but F. G. Young[36] thought that such an observation might have been made independently. This unexpected result was – according to Minkowski – of little interest to von Mering, although he did assist with the removal of the pancreas in a few more dogs and also carried out some determinations of glycogen in liver tissue. The publication of this very important observation was by von Mering and Minkowski in alphabetical order, and also because von Mering was the senior of the two.

Later followed Laguesse (1861–1927) and Edouard Hédon (1863–1933), who in 1893 ascribed an internal secretion to the islands of Langerhans. Hédon also showed that if the major part of the pancreas was removed, but a small piece of the tissue was transplanted, with its circulation intact, to the surface of the abdomen, diabetes did not develop.

> But a severely diabetic condition immediately appeared if the pancreatic graft was excised in circumstances in which the abdomen was not opened. Moreover, since there was no nerve supply to the graft, the control of secretion of the assumed hormone (insulin) appeared not to depend upon nervous stimuli.[36]

Finally, Eugène Lindsay Opie (1873–1971) established the association between the failure of the islets of Langerhans and the occurrence of diabetes[37]. He described an interlobar form of chronic pancreatitis, where the islands of Langerhans are rarely affected, and an interacinous form, where diabetes is frequent. Later, he described hyaline degeneration of the islands, which is common in diabetics, but may also exist in old people without clinical diabetes. Opie made his observations while working at the Institute of Pathological Anatomy of the Johns Hopkins University. Unknown to him, in St. Petersburg Leonid Wassilyevitch Ssobolew (1876–1919), found at the same time that ligation of the excretory ducts of the pancreas led to atrophy of the acinous tissue with the islets of Langerhans remaining intact[38].

In 1909 William George MacCallum (1874–1944) of Dunnville, Ontario, proved that tying the pancreatic ducts produced atrophy of the pancreas, but without influence upon the islet cells, unless they were also damaged, in which case diabetic symptoms promptly occurred[39]. Incidentally, Naunyn in his above-quoted monograph, stressed the importance of the hereditory factor in diabetes ('diabetische Anlage'), which had already been noted by the Indian medical writers of the 7th century AD, mentioned by Guillaume Rondelet (Rondeletius), 1507–1566, zoologist and physician of Montepellier ('Methodus curandorum omnium morborum corporis humani in tres libros distincta . . .')[40], and by Richard Morton (1637–1698), who was also the first to describe anorexia nervosa (see p. 616). Friedrich Theodor Frerichs (1819–1885), who was Professor of Pathology in Berlin and one of the pioneers of scientific clinical teaching in Germany, also said that he found a family history in 10% of his diabetic patients. Graham Lusk (1866–1932), of Bridgeport,

Conn., U.S.A. made the original observation that a completely diabetic patient will excrete not only the carbohydrate he has ingested, but also sugar equal to half the protein molecule[41].

Brown-Séquard published in June 1893 a two-part article in the *British Medical Journal*: 'On a new therapeutic method consisting in the use of organic liquids extracted from glands and other organs'[42]. He summed up:

> When a morbid state, as myxoedema, or a series of symptoms, such as we see in cases of deficiency to the internal secretion of any gland, exists, it is very easy to understand how the cure is obtained when glandular liquid extracts are used: we simply give to the blood the principle or principles missing in it. . . . The great movement in therapeutics as regards the organic liquid extracts, has its origin in the experiments which I made on myself in 1889, experiments which were at first so completely misunderstood[43].

At the end of Brown-Séquard's publication, the *British Medical Journal* summed up the situation in a leading article entitled: 'Animal extracts as therapeutic agents'[44]. In it, it was admitted "that there is, after all, something in Brown-Séquard's testicular extract experiments, especially after the success of the treatment with thyroid extract". It was also admitted, that

> many organs do more than what was formerly regarded as their functions. The experiments . . . have led to the introduction of the expression 'internal secretion'. We think that this term is a rather unfortunately chosen one: but it, nonetheless, expresses that the organs in question have some action on the blood, and through it on the tissues generally, which influences their metabolic changes.

The editors felt, however, sceptical and – while admitting the method of treatment in myxoedema – they were "compelled to doubt many of the other so-called cures". Many of these extracts proved very poisonous when injected, to which objection Brown-Séquard replied that they must be properly prepared[45]. The editors of the *British Medical Journal* sided with Massalongo, who repeated some of Brown-Séquard's experiments and found that it was merely "A New Phase of Suggestive Therapeutics", as published in the *Riforma Medica* in February 1893. He found

> that in organic disease the improvement is due to suggestion and the influence of the imagination; and that such curative effects are best marked in cases of hysteria and neurasthenia . . . and that equally good results were here obtained by inert substances. . . .[6]

This scepticism could only be changed if methods could be found which would permit reliable measurement of physiological effects of the products of 'internal secretions' or of the 'organ extracts'. This occurred in the autumn of 1893, as a result of the meeting of a Harrogate physician, George Oliver, and the London physiologist Edward Albert Schaefer, followed by a collaboration which was to be as happy as important for the future development of endocrinology.

(b) America

The response to Brown-Séquard's paper in autumn 1889, 'On the physiological and therapeutic role of a juice extracted from the testicles of animals according to a number of facts observed in man'[46], was discussed by Dr. Merriley Borell in her thorough and excellent study of the development and the history of the field of endocrinology during that period[3].

Early in 1889, Brown-Séquard and d'Arsonval, who later succeeded him at the Collège de France, experimented by giving subcutaneous injections of liquid extract of testicles of vigorous young mammals to male rabbits. Finding no harmful side effects, Brown-Séquard, then 72, gave himself a series of subcutaneous injections of a watery extract of ground dog-testicle in May 1889. He put forward as motivation for his experiments that "the physiological and clinical history of the testicles is full of interesting facts which everyone knows and which leave no doubt on the role of these organs on the individual who carries them"[1]. It was generally assumed that loss of semen meant loss of strength and that sexual excess – including masturbation in excess – causes debility. Conversely, he argued, perhaps strength could be gained by retention of semen. There might be some substance absorbed by the blood from the semen, resulting in increased vigour and power for those who abstained from ejaculation[3]. This was perhaps not so different from some of Aristotle's ideas (pp. 47–48). Interestingly enough, Brown-Séquard said about his auto-injections with testicular fluid-extract: "I have made this experiment with the conviction that I would obtain with it a notable augmentation of the powers of action of the nervous centres and especially those of the spinal cord"[1]. He also believed, therefore, that there was a specific action on the nervous centres. He himself felt that after receiving eight injections between 15 and 30 May 1889, his strength, vigour and mental activity improved and that there was increased contractility of the bladder and of the intestine, an added proof that "la puissance dynamogénique" was in the spinal cord itself[1]. The extract was prepared as follows: each dog-testicle, with its blood and sperm, was crushed in $2.3\,cm^3$ of water, then filtered through a Pasteur filter. About 1.0 cm^3 of the extract (equal to $\frac{1}{4}$ to $\frac{1}{3}$ of testicle) was injected subcutaneously[4].

In his paper in the autumn 1889[2], Brown-Séquard was able to append a summary of a number of studies on the use of testicular extracts mainly on debilitated people, from France (Variot and Dehoux from Paris; Villeneuve from Marseille), from the United States (H. P. Loomis of New York; W. A. Hammond from Washington; Brainerd from Cleveland); from Roumania (Grigorescu from Bucharest) and others. But Brown-Séquard was not amused that in the United States, in contrast to the cautious reception in Britain, the extract was described as "Elixir of Life". He complained:

> In the United States especially and often without knowing what I did or the most elementary rules regarding subcutaneous injections of animal materials, several physicians or rather the medicasters and charlatans have exploited the ardent desires of a great number of individuals and have made them run the greatest risks, if they have not done worse.[2]

Proof of this was a publication by Newall Dunbar in Boston in 1889, entitled: 'The Elixir of Life – Dr. Brown-Séquard's own Account of his Famous Alleged Remedy for Debility and Old Age, Dr. Variot's Experiments and Contemporaneous Comments of the Profession and the Press"[47]. The risk of infection and side-effects thus being made real, Brown-Séquard and d'Arsonval undertook to supply their extract free of cost to reputable physicians who wished to test it, although the arrival of sterilized commercial preparations improved the situation. Most criticisms were directed at the possible auto-suggestive basis of the so-called cures which were reported (see also the discussion in the leading article of the *British Medical Journal* of 17 June 1893[44] mentioned on p. 299). At the same time, however, many physicians throughout the West became interested in testing the effects of all sorts of organ extracts (from the spinal cord, the spleen, the thymus and the liver). As d'Arsonval remarked sarcastically: "The testicular fluid has put them in the mood[48]." Testicular fluid extract was now being tested in the treatment of a variety of diseases. In tuberculosis it was tested side by side with Koch's lymph. At a time when tetanus and diphtheria antitoxin were also discovered, the air was pregnant with ideas on the use of organ products in treatment. In March 1891, he wrote to d'Arsonval:

> . . . all the glands of 'external' secretion are at the same time glands of 'internal' secretion, like the testicles. The kidneys, the salivary glands, the pancreas, are not solely eliminating organs. They are, like the thyroid, the spleen, etc., organs giving to the blood important principles, either in a direct manner or by resorption after external secretion.

Thus he suspected powerful 'internal secretions' in every tissue[48].

Dr. Borell finally indicates, in her paper, how injections of organ extracts "came to be recognised as a general form of therapy by 1891"[3]. She also suggests "that the rise of organotherapy and the rise of serotherapy were closely related phenomena". She uses the account of the foundation in 1893 and the work of the New York Pasteur Institute by the French physician Dr. Paul Gibier, who had worked with Pasteur in 1886 and emigrated to the United States in 1889, to set up a clinic for the treatment of hydrophobia. Gibier had also been a member of the French commission which had studied Koch's work in Berlin. His New York Pasteur Institute eventually had a laboratory and a biological supply centre attached to it. 'The New York Pasteur Institute for the Preventive Treatment of Hydrophobia and for the Study of Contagious Diseases' was incorporated as the 'Bacteriological Institute'[3]. Gibier later published *The New York Therapeutic Review*, after a time renamed *Bulletin of the Pasteur Institute*, which had a circulation of 100 000. Articles like 'Injection of organic fluids according to professor Brown-Séquard's Method' were published in *The New York Therapeutic Review*. After Gibier's death, his nephew, George Gibier Rambaud, succeeded him and was praised for his work on vaccines and sera in 1913. No reference was made to the organ extracts supplied by the laboratory,

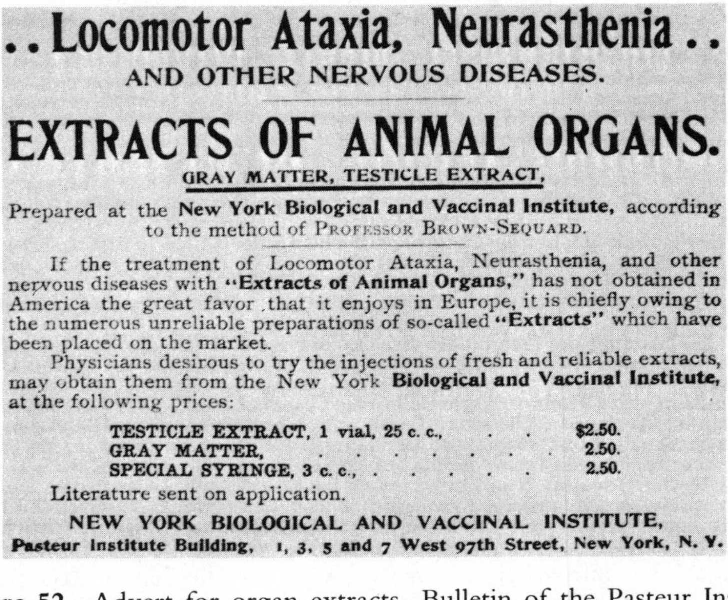

Figure 52 Advert for organ extracts, Bulletin of the Pasteur Institute, New York, 1897

at least during 1893–1898. This treatment of organotherapy was regretted as "an unhappy episode in the histories of both medicine and science"[3].

Borell refers to F. G. Young's citation of Herbert Evans: ". . . in this way 'Endocrinology' – suffered obstetric deformation at its very birth"[49], and she adds rightly:

> Rarely has it been pointed out that active principles of both, the thyroid and adrenal glands were discovered in the 1890s, when organotherapy was being heralded by many physicians as an exciting new field.[3]

THE PITUITARY GLAND: PIERRE MARIE AND ACROMEGALY, 1886

The pituitary gland did not remain entirely neglected. It has been seen in previous chapters (13 and 14) that it was not merely its function which puzzled natural scientists and physicians, but also its anatomy. As Rolleston remarked: "The pituitary is complex both in structure and function, and its anatomy is not exactly the same in man as in animals"[50]. In 1838, Martin Heinrich Rathke (1793–1860) described the evagination from the anterior end of the fore-gut (entoderm): 'Ueber die Entstehung der Glandula pituitaria'[51]. But F. M. Balfour (1851–1882) in 1874[52], and G. V. Mihalkovics (1844–1899) in 1875[53], found that Rathke's pouch came from the embryonic buccal cavity and was ectodermal. Although this view was generally accepted, later authors thought that it is both entodermal and ectodermal; T. Lups said in 1929 that the anterior portion (pars distalis) is ectodermal, but that it is impossible to decide whether the posterior portion is ectodermal or entodermal[54]. The most recent studies are those by Peter M. Daniel and Marjorie M. Pritchard, which cover 25 years of painstaking and meticulous work on the pituitary and hypothalamus, both in man and in animals. The pars anterior was described separately in 1724 by Giovanni Domenico Santorini (1681–1737), one of the most able dissectors of his day. He expressed some milky fluid from it; he called it "glandula pituitaria potior"[55].

The posterior lobe has been called neuro-hypophysis, the pars nervosa, the infundibular body[56]. The small pars tuberalis (from its close anatomical relation to the tuber cinereum) had been described previously as the "anterior process" of the pituitary in 1871 by W. Mueller[57]. The complicated blood supply was described as early as 1874, when H. Duret described a branch from the posterior communicating artery on each side, supplying the tuber cinereum and the pituitary[58].

The even more complicated venous drainage was first described by G. Popa and V. Fielding in 1930[59]. A remnant, named 'Accessory or Nasopharyngeal Pituitary' was described by the Ear, Nose, and Throat surgeon Gustave Killian (1860–1921)[60]. This occasional remnant, consisting mainly of chromophobe cells and situated in the submucosa of the naso-pharynx at the anterior part of the pharyngeal tonsil, can be of importance, if there are no symptoms of hypo-pituitarism after removal of the pituitary gland or – very rarely – in a case like the acromegaly described by the Viennese pathologist Jakob Erdheim (1874–1937)[61]. He later also described pituitary dwarfism.

The histology of the pituitary also progressed only slowly. Adolph H. Hannover (1814–1894) described two kinds of cells in the anterior lobe[62]. S. Lothringer in 1886[63], and A. Dostoiewsky in the same year[64] described (1) non-granular, neutrophil, clear, chromophobe cells and (2) granular chromophil cells. The latter were further subdivided in 1892 by Schoenemann into oxyphil, acidophil, eosinophil or α-cells, which stain with acid dyes, and into basophil, cyanophil or β-cells, which stain with basic dyes[65]. Vacuoles which may be present in chromophil cells may possibly contain their secretion. Hubert von Luschka (1820–1875) found "rests" of squamous epithelium in close relation to the pituitary[66] in 1860.

In 1898 L. Comte noticed an increase in the size of the pituitary during pregnancy, which diminished quickly after delivery[67] (see also p. 315). In man, radiological examination has shown enlargement of the sella turcica after castration. This has been reported in the Skopzes, a Russian religious sect in which many of the men are castrated, often by self-immolation (see p. 33). It has also been reported by Julius Tandler (1869–1936) and S. Gross[68]. The posterior lobe was regarded as an anterior extremity of the brain by Carl Ernst von Baer (1792–1876), of mammalian ovum fame, in 1828[50]. It is composed of the infundibular process, covered over by the extension of the pars intermedia. Concerning the progress in the knowledge of the function of the pituitary in the 19th century, one can do no better than quote Rolleston on the subject (p. 55):

> The advance of knowledge and the recent elaboration of detail in connexion with endocrine function and disease are best illustrated by the history of the pituitary. Until nearly the beginning of this century it was regarded as little more than a vestigial relic; now it has become the head stone of the corner. In a review of nerve physiology in 1889, it was stated that the pituitary has 'little, or perhaps no, use in the organism of the higher vertebrates' (T. W. Shore), and in the same year it was described as 'probably the rudiments of an archaic sense organ' (MacAlister)[50].

Sir Victor Horsley in 1886 succeeded in excising the pituitary from two dogs and keeping them alive for 5–6 months without adverse results[69]. Yet as late as 1908, Schaefer and Percy Theodore Herring (1872–1967) referred to the anterior lobe of the pituitary as not having any physiological effect[70]. (See also pp. 310 and 343.)

Diseases of the pituitary

Rolleston quotes Johann Jacob Wepfer (1620–1695) of Schaffhausen, who first described cerebral haemorrhage in post-mortem examinations[71], that he recorded a pituitary in 1681, twice the normal size[72]; and also Théophile Bonet (1620–1689), who also referred in his post-mortem material to enlargement of the pituitary[73], as did Raymond Vieussens (1641–1715) in 1705[74]. However, Rolleston stresses at the same time that Matthew Baillie (1761–1823) pronounced in 1797 that "this gland is very little liable to be affected by disease"[75].

The Italian Andrea Verga reported on the first post-mortem examination, describing a pituitary tumour, which had destroyed the sphenoid and pressed on the optic chiasma. Verga called the disease "Prosopectasia"[76] (1864) (see also p. 309, referring to case XXXV with notes on the autopsy by Marie, in Ref. 77). In 1877, Vincenzo Brigidi found a pituitary tumour during the post-mortem examination of the celebrated actor Ghirlenzoni, whose skeleton was preserved (see also p. 309, referring to case XXXI in the 'Essays on Acromegaly'[77]). Carl Benda (1857–1933), demonstrated in 1900 that the pituitary tumour in acromegaly is an eosinophil cell tumour[78]. This was confirmed in 1895 by Édouard Brissaud (1852–1909) (who later also described thyroid infantilism) and by Henri Meige (1866–1940), both of the Salpêtrière in Paris[79]. The neurologist Hermann Oppenheim (1858–1919), of Berlin, demonstrated in 1899 that the sella turcica appeared enlarged on the X-ray plate, after Heinrich Embden had presented the radiological appearances of the acromegalic hand a year before.

Rolleston quotes[80]:

In an elaborate monograph (1891) on the anatomy of the Irish giant Cornelius Magrath (1742–68), "A Research into the Connexion which exists between Giantism and Acromegaly", D. J. Cunningham, who had left Edinburgh and was for twenty years professor of anatomy at Trinity College, Dublin, showed that from the large size of their pituitary fossae (in Magrath's skull capable of very nearly holding "half of a small tangerine orange"). Magrath and Charles Byrne or O'Brien

(1761–1783) – another Irish giant (whose skeleton John Hunter obtained for his museum (now No. 3865–1) at great trouble and expense, it is said £500) – were acromegalics. [New observations on Charles Byrne (O'Brien) confirmed that he had suffered from a growth-hormone-producing adenoma[228].] In Magrath's case the pituitary tumour appeared to have invaded the right orbit and so might have caused exophthalmos; his other ocular derangements were discussed by Swanzy. Magrath when about 16 years of age and 6 feet 8¾ inches in height, was befriended by George Berkeley (1685–1753), the famous Bishop of Cloyne, . . . and it was widely believed in Ireland that Magrath's huge frame was the result of the Bishop's experiments in giant-rearing.

Regrettably, Rolleston does not tell us what Berkeley's (the philosopher's) experiments in giant-rearing were and, so far, I have been unable to find out the nature of such experiments. Moreover, Magrath was 16 years of age in 1758 (according to Rolleston), but Bishop Berkeley had died in 1753. Be it as it may, Rolleston seems correct in his assumption that the observations on Magrath must have "antedated that (case) observed by Saucerotte in 1772 and unearthed by Marie" (case XXXVIII in Ref. 77), which Nicolas Saucerotte (1741–1812) had presented to the Académie de Chirurgie in that year[81].

Thus, the knowledge of pituitary disease dates mainly from 1886, when Pierre Marie (1853–1940) published the first of his papers on acromegaly. He was a French neurologist (see Section II), Director of the Laboratory attached to the Salpêtrière, and Charcot's most able pupil. His "Thesis" was published under the title: 'Sur deux cas d'acromégalie. Hypertrophie singulière non congénitale des extremités supérieures, inférieures et céphalique'[82]. The paper aroused much interest and was translated into English. It was published in London in 1891 by the New Sydenham Society under the title *Essays on Acromegaly*, by Dr. Pierre Marie and Dr. José Dantas de Souza-Leite. de Souza-Leite was born in 1859 in Bahia, Brazil, and was Marie's pupil and collaborator[77]. The publication contained Pierre Marie's original paper and "A (doctoral) Thesis on Acromegaly" (Marie's Malady) by Dr. Souza-Leite, with a collection of a total of 38 other cases, mainly from the literature, with a further addition of another 10 patients, bringing the total to 48. In the original paper Marie gives a full and classic description of the clinical symptoms. In both patients, a woman of 37 and a woman of 54, Marie noted "a very intense thirst, with abundant urine"[77] (p. 13). In the original paper Marie says this about the cause of the condition: "On the question of etiology, we have nothing definite."[77] (p. 13). He concludes:

. . . and that, on the whole, we have yet as yet no certain data as to the nature of this malady . . . 1st. There exists a disease specially characterised by an hypertrophy of the hands, feet and face, which we propose to call Acromegaly. . . . 2nd. Acromegaly is quite distinct from myxoedema, and from Paget's disease (osteitis deformans), as well as from leontiasis ossea of Virchow.

When Souza-Leite published in 1890 his 'Thesis on Acromegaly (Marie's Malady)'[77] there were available to him the results of seven autopsies: of patient No. II by A. Broca[83] who found the sella turcica much enlarged, and several by Pierre Marie himself, one by M. Henrot, and others. Souza-Leite stresses (p. 61):

The most specific of these (pathological-anatomical) lesions which may be considered as essential, since it has not been found absent, is the considerable increase in size of the pituitary body. This gland is changed into an hypertrophical mass of which the size varies from that of a pigeon's egg to that of a hen's egg or even an apple.

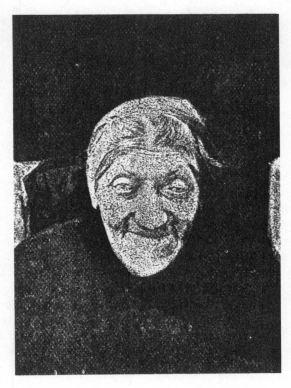

Figure 53 Case of acromegaly from *Essays on Acromegaly* by Pierre Marie and Souza-Leite, New Sydenham Society, London 1891

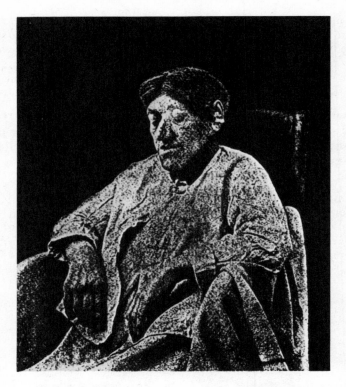

Figure 54   Case of acromegaly, as Figure 53

The greatly enlarged sella turcica, pressure on the optic nerve(s), are also a regular finding, explaining the ensuing neuro-retinitis and – eventually – blindness. "The sella turcica is increased in all its measurements – in length, width and depth"[77] (p. 64).

In spite of his excellent description and searching differential diagnosis, Souza-Leite ends the very short paragraph on treatment ("It is confined to the relief of the worst symptoms . . ." p. 80) as follows: "Knowing so little as to the etiology of the affection, it is impossible, at present, to formulate any very rational treatment." In chapter II, 'Etiology', he says: "In spite of recent researches, the knowledge of the causes, which produce Marie's disease, is still indefinite" (p. 34). He does, however, differentiate acromegaly from gigantism very definitely. He also differentiates acromegaly from hypertrophic pulmonary osteo-arthropathy (also described by Pierre Marie)[77] (p. 71).

Dr. Marie added to his observations by making the diagnosis of acromegaly in a number of patients described by authors, in some cases, long before his time. Nicolas Saucerotte (1741–1812) described to the Académie de Chirurgie à Paris in 1772 an "Accroissement singulier en grosseur des os d'un homme agé de 39 ans"[81], Noël having published the clinical details[84]. Unfortunately, the patient's (a Sieur Mirbeck) wife refused to allow an autopsy, but 3 years later the sternum, the left clavicle and a right rib were 'obtained' from the grave and now adorn the collection of the Musée Dupuytren (No. 435)[50]. Later, in 1908. F. Patry collected and published all the available information on this patient with illustration of the bones, in his 'Thèse de Paris', No. 153, 1907–1908[50]. Baron Jean Louis Marc Alibert (1768–1837), mainly interested in diseases of the skin, reported on a "scrofulous giant, aged 32, with diabetes"[85] which Pierre Marie was able to diagnose as acromegaly (case XXXVII, described in the original paper by Pierre Marie as case IV, where Alibert was quoted as saying that

> He was tormented with such an intense thirst, that he drank up to eighteen bottles of pure water every day; and his urine was proportionately abundant. Besides other symptoms there was want of sexual power.

Case VII of the original thesis of Marie, a man of 36, had been described by Dr. Henry Henrot of Rheims in 1877 and 1882 (with the post-mortem results) as a case of myxoedema[86]. Marie, however, recognized him as a patient with acromegaly. The pituitary was of the size of a hen's egg.

Of particular interest appears the account of Case XXVI of the collection, of a 30-year-old Russian musician, who was observed by Oscar Minkowski (1858–1931), later of pancreas extirpation fame. In his report 'Ueber einen Fall von Akromegalie' in 1887[87], he drew attention to the constant finding of pituitary enlargement in acromegaly, being the first to suspect a causal relation between the two conditions. In the 'collection', there were patients described by Samuel Wilks (No. XXIV), Erb (XX and XXI), Godlee (XXIII), Brigidi (XXXI), Lombroso (XXXVII), Verga (XXXV, with autopsy notes by Marie) and others. Additional cases contained No. XXXIX, XL, XLI and XLII, all by (Sir) Jonathan Hutchinson (1828–1913) reported mainly in the Archives of Surgery[87a, 87b].

Obviously, the condition in which people could become "so repulsive in appearance that he (Henrot's patient) attracted the attention of everyone who entered the hospital ward"[88], induced doctors, novelists and historians alike, to pin such a diagnosis – rightly or wrongly – on giants of the bible (see Chapter 5, pp. 34–35). The Piltdown skull, Hen Nekht, the giant pharaoh of Egypt (3000 BC) (see also Figure 4, head of Akhenaten), Gog and Magog, the Roman emperor Caius Julius Verus Maximinus Severus (AD 173–238), Henry IV of Castile (1425–1474), diagnosed by Maranon (see Section II), and many others. From paintings, it was found that in a battle scene between Centaurs and the Lapithae (Piero di Cosimo, 1441–1521, pinxit AD 1482), all the Lapithae and a few of the Centaurs show acromegalic faces. Max Sternberg of Vienna published a monograph 'Die Akromegalie', in 1897[89], based on 210 case reports with 47 necropsies. He also identified a life-size portrait in Schloss Ambras in Tyrol, of a giant at the court of Frederick II, Elector of the Palatinate, dated 1553[50]. The painters Thomas Rowlandson (1756–1827), H. W. Bunbury (1750–1811) and James Gillray (1757–1815), all utilized the features of acromegalics in some of their paintings. François Magendie's (1783–1855) description of two women (in 1839) belong in this group.

Last, but not least, attention has to be drawn to the remarkable autobiography of Leonard Portal Mark, MD (1855–1930), of St. Bartholomew's Hospital, London, where he was 'Pathological Draughtsman'. It was entitled: *Acromegaly, A Personal Experience*[90]. He was an acromegalic from the age of 24, but was 50 before he realized the nature of his illness, of which he kept a meticulous record all the time. In his book there is also an early X-ray (October 1911) of his enlarged sella turcica, reported on by Dr. A. Howard Pirie. At his wish, after his death a necropsy was performed on his body at St. Bartholomew's Hospital by Dr. Edward R. Cullinan (later Senior Physician to the hospital) on 5 September 1930, and reported in *St. Bartholomew's Hospital Journal* of November 1930 (pp. 22–23). In his life time, he had also been seen by Dr. Pierre Marie on a visit to London, who had confirmed the diagnosis. In a final chapter of his book, *Revery*, "After contemplating a Stone Figure of the Thirteenth Century carved on Reims Cathedral", he drew attention to several sculptures of acromegalics among the *ca.* 3000 figures adorning the Cathedral.

He reproduced one of a woman on a flying buttress, dating from the 13th century, but after the war (1914–1918), the figures mentioned by him could not be found. The summary of the postmortem report on Dr. Mark is as follows:

Acromegaly. Enlargement of the pituitary and thyroid glands. Advanced atheroma (with thrombosis of the common iliac and right popliteal arteries). Chronic interstitial nephritis (arterio-sclerotic type), hydronephrosis, pyonephrosis and renal calculi. Emphysema, chronic bronchitis and terminal confluent bronchopneumonia.

The skeletal system showed changes of acromegaly:

in a moderate degree. . . . The pituitary gland is slightly larger than

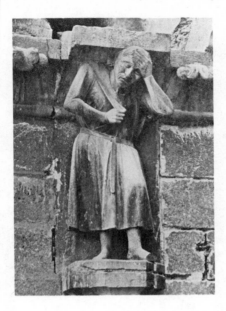

Figure 55 A 13th century figure on Reims cathedral

usual, especially in the downward direction. It has a soft consistency, but no other macroscopical abnormality. . . . The thyroid gland is enlarged. . . . The suprarenals and testes appear natural. . . . The thymus is not seen.

According to Rolleston[91], it was T. W. Chevalier in 1827 who gave the first good account of acromegaly in England: A woman of 29 had headache and impaired vision; on necropsy an "aneurysmal tumour" was found in the sella turcica, which did not communicate with the neighbouring vessels[92]. In spite of the fact that pituitary changes were usually seen to be associated with acromegaly, other remarkable explanations were suggested for years.

Rolleston, in a brief resumé, refers to them as follows[80]: "Trophoneurosis" (von Recklinghausen in 1890) and J. Dreschfeld (1845–1907) in 1894; "Acro-trophoneurosis" (Étienne Lancereaux, 1829–1910, in 1895). Lancereaux not only denied that there was a causal connection between the disease and the pituitary, but also that acromegaly was a morbid entity at all! (see also p. 306)[3].

Finally, another example of the 'forgotten men' has to be quoted. In 1884, a general practitioner of Glarus in Switzerland, Christian Friedrich Fritzsche (1851–1938) published, together with Theodor Albrecht Edwin Klebs (1834–1913) (see also Section II), who was then professor of pathology in Zürich, a paper 'Ein Beitrag zur Pathologie des Riesenwuchses' (=a contribution to the pathology of

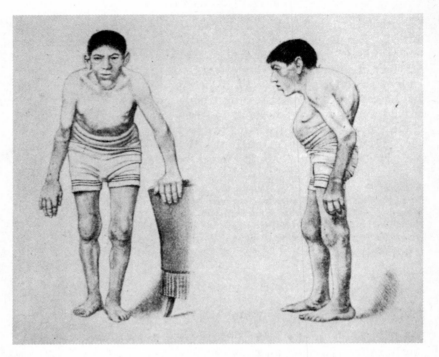

Figure 56 Fritzsche's patient [From Ciba Monograph No. 10, by kindness of Ciba–Geigy Ltd.]

gigantism)[94]. It was a full report on the history and the autopsy findings of a remarkable patient. He was an alpine cowherd, who first presented at the age of 36 with symptoms and signs which later developed into what was obviously a case of acromegaly. Fritzsche observed him for 8 years and presented him at a meeting of the 'Schweizer Naturforschende Gesellschaft' at Linthal. A few days later the patient died in hospital. Post-mortem examination by Klebs disclosed a persistent large thymus and a striking enlargement of the pituitary gland and of the sella turcica.

This early and accurate observation of acromegaly, published two years before Pierre Marie's treatise, remained hardly noticed; it was not even mentioned in the *Jahresbericht ueber die Leistungen und Fortschritte in der gesamten Medicin* (=Annual report on achievements and progress in all branches of medicine), which had a wide distribution at that time. Fritzsche had not given the disease a special name, and Klebs obviously failed to attribute any significance to the considerable enlargement of the sella turcica. He put the patient into the large group called 'general gigantism', although the Viennese anatomist Carl Langer (1819–1887) had written in his monograph on 'Wachsthum des menschlichen Skelettes mit Bezug auf den Riesen' (=Human skeletal growth in regard to gigantism), published in 1872, that enlargement of the sella is found only in those giants who exhibit a 'monstrous' lower jaw, thick lips and large nostrils. Yet Klebs actually referred to Langer's statement in his and Fritzsche's paper!

In 1885, two English observers, Walter Baugh Hadden (1856–1893) (who was translater of Charcot's 'Leçons sur les localizations des maladies du cerveau' in 1883) and (later Sir) Charles Alfred Ballance (1856–1936), presented to a meeting of the Clinical Society in London a patient with "hypertrophy of the subcutaneous tissue of the face, hands and feet", having the classic features of acromegaly[95], but in 1888 they redescribed it as acromegaly[80].

Like Pierre Marie and Souza-Leite, in his paper with Klebs Fritzsche had also collected descriptions of similar patients from the medical literature. It is only fair to state that Pierre Marie had no knowledge of the publication of Fritzsche and Klebs.

Pierre Marie was of the opinion (1896) that gigantism was an exaggeration of the normal and that acromegaly was abnormal. Maximilian Sternberg (in 1897) followed suit. However, E. Brissaud (1852–1909) and Henry Meige (1866–1940) maintained that gigantism is acromegaly during the period of growth, whereas acromegaly is gigantism in the adult[79]. Also in 1895, Woods Hutchinson (1862–1930) stressed that the pituitary was a growth centre for the whole body and that gigantism was, therefore, acromegaly in early or foetal life. P. E. Launois and P. Roy put it that hyperfunction of the pituitary will produce gigantism before the epiphyses are fused, and acromegaly after fusion[96]. This view, which still prevails today, was also supported by R. Massalongo (1857–1920) of Padua[97] ('Acromegaly represented abnormal delayed gigantism').

What's in a name? This question may well apply to the term 'acromegaly'. Pierre Marie preferred it to his original choice of 'acromacrie'. Souza-Leite called it "Maladie de Marie", based on the example of Paget's, Graves' or Addison's disease. Some authors accepted this term, but in 1890, Pierre Marie described hypertrophic pulmonary osteo-arthropathy, which was also sometimes called Marie's disease, which may have caused confusion. Of all other suggested names, such as 'macrosomia' (Lombroso in 1869, Taruffi in 1877 and Cushing in 1927; Cushing thought that the term 'acromegaly' referred to the extremities only); or 'prosopectasia' (A. Verga in 1864)[76], only acromegaly became firmly established; and there the matter will have to rest.

It will have been noted that the importance of polydipsia and polyuria was well recognized in diabetes mellitus (see Minkowski's pancreatectomized dog, p. 297), and in acromegaly (see Alibert's case, p. 309), but Avicenna had mentioned, as early as 1020 AD, an observation of 'multitudo urinae'. It is perhaps of importance to add an observation of Dr. Samuel Jones Gee (1839–1911), physician to St. Bartholomew's Hospital in London (of Gee's linctus) who published a two page note in *St. Bartholomew's Hospital Reports* in 1877 (pp. 79–80), entitled 'A Contribution to the History of Polydipsia'. In this paper he gave a brief account of eleven patients in a family of four generations, children and adults, who suffered "from polydipsia and polyuria (or diabetes insipidus)", stressing two points in the aetiology:

> I. First, the disease was inherited, an inheritance which was known to have afflicted the family for four generations.
> II. Secondly, the disease was congenital. Patient No. 8 cried for many hours after his birth and could not be comforted. His mother suspected that he might perchance be tormented with the family thirst, and begged her nurse to give him some water. At first the nurse refused; afterwards she gave water to the child, and straightaway his cries were stopped for the time. He died at six months of age, and of suffering from thirst.

J. P. M. Tizard, professor of Paediatrics at the University of Oxford, said, correctly, in his 'Samuel Gee Lecture 1972' to the Royal College of Physicians of London, that this meticulously careful observation, related in classic brevity, must have been the first description of nephrogenic diabetes insipidus[98] (see also p. 377).

MORE ABOUT THE PITUITARY

The pituitary had been regarded for too long as an organ without any known function. Richard Lower's and Thomas Willis's ideas (see Chapter 13) however brilliant they might have been, had not received any scientific experimental confirmation. This delayed the development of real knowledge of the gland until Pierre Marie noted the connection between acromegaly and, in many instances, the occurrence of a pituitary tumour. He did not realize, however, that a functional relationship existed between the structure of the tumour and with the substance some of the cells of the anterior pituitary produced and poured into the bloodstream. Minkowski did suspect a functional relationship when he reported on a patient with acromegaly a year later[99] – feeding of fresh or dried anterior (and posterior) lobe substance proved inconclusive (A. Schiff[100] and

J. Malcolm[101]). The most extensive such study was carried out by Emil Goetsch (1883–1963)[102], who was also a collaborator of Cushing. He fed rats from the time of weaning for 6–8 months on 0.05 g of acetone dried powder of whole pituitary glands, and claimed stimulation of growth and sexual development. This was, however, completely disclaimed by a later 3-year study by W. R. Sisson and E. N. Broyles[103]. Even Philip Edward Smith (1884–1970) started his brilliant career by the experimental feeding of fresh anterior pituitary substance to the hypophysectomized rats[104], as did Herbert McLean Evans (1882–1971)[105]. Although Evans' and Joseph Abraham Long's (b. 1879) rats enjoyed fresh anterior lobe substance as staple food and it proved to be of good food value, "the slightest traces of growth acceleration" could not be discovered. The same applied as regards the oestrus cycles[69].

For obvious technical reasons, satisfactory experimental hypophysectomy proved far more difficult than adrenalectomy. Brain damage and bleeding, especially in small animals, caused immediate or early death. That is why Julius von Michel's attempts failed in 1881[106]. It is also difficult to make certain that either all the pituitary tissue, or the whole anterior lobe, had been removed.

Sir Victor Horsley's successful experiment in removing the pituitary in two dogs in 1886 has already been mentioned[107]. The Bucharest physiologist Nicolas C. Paulesco (1869–1931) (about whom we shall have more to say), when telling the insulin story, introduced in 1907, in collaboration with the surgeon Balacesco, the subtemporal intracranial approach of hypophysectomy in dogs[108]. His 22 dogs and 12 cats died within 3 days after the operation, from which he concluded that the pituitary is essential to life. Separating the pituitary stalk produced the same result. Removal of the posterior lobe only had negative results. Paulesco summarized his experiments as follows:

> L'hypophysectomie totale est suivie, à bref delai, de la mort de l'animal. La durée moyenne de la survie, chez le chien, et de 24 heures. . . . En résumé, l'hypophyse est un organe indispensable à la vie, son absence étant rapidement mortelle. . . . Des diverses parties qui la constituent, la plus importante, au point de la vue fonctionnel, est la couche cortical du lobe épithelial.

> Total hypophysectomy is followed by the death of the animal, after a short delay. The average survival rate in the dog is 24 hours. . . . To sum up, the pituitary is an organ essential for life, its absence being rapidly fatal; of the various parts it consists of, the most important, from the functional point of view, is the cortical part of the epithelial lobe. [Translation V.C.M.]

Bernhard Aschner (1883–1960) and Harvey Williams Cushing (1869–1939) successfully used a modified Paulesco technique.

Cushing reported to the American Association for the Advancement of Science in Boston in 1910, on extensive studies carried out with Samuel James Crowe (1883–1955) and John Homans: 'Experimental hypophysectomy'[109], and on 'The functions of the pituitary body'[110], at the Hunterian Surgical Laboratories at Johns Hopkins. They had operated on over 100 dogs with a better survival rate, especially among the younger animals. Cushing confirmed Paulesco's findings, that apituitarism leads to death, preceded by listlessness, loss of appetite and weight, which Cushing defined as "cachexia hypophysiopriva". Removal of the posterior lobe, provided the anterior lobe remained intact, caused none of those symptoms. Paulesco[108], Crowe, Cushing and Homans[109,110] and, later, William Blair Bell (1871–1936)[111], all recorded that clamping of the pituitary stalk had the same effect as hypophysectomy, including atrophy of the ovaries and uterus. This was particularly important when partial hypophysectomy was carried out: if the animals survived for months, growth was reduced or stopped completely and – in puppies – sexual infantilism remained. Giulio Vassale (1862–1912) and Ercole Sacchi had reported, as early as 1892, that destruction of the pituitary gland caused disturbance of water and mineral metabolism[112], and (Sir) Henry Hallett Dale (1875–1968) reported on the oxytocic action of posterior pituitary extract injection in 1909[113].

It was, however, Bernhard Aschner (1883–1960) who deserves the greatest credit for his much improved technique of hypophysectomies, by the transbuccal approach, with minimal or little brain damage. He was critical of Paulesco's and Cushing's method, because it involved cerebral dislocation for the purpose of exposing parts "otherwise inaccessible", i.e. the dangling pituitary "could be exposed without cerebral injury or compression". Aschner maintained that the interference with the brain was still considerable. He worked out a buccal method via the sphenoid bone (which has no cavity in the dog), without levering the brain. He carried out more than 120 well planned and meticulously executed experiments, but, sadly, never received the recognition he deserved for his work. His dogs survived many months and experiments on puppies permitted X-ray studies of the cessation of growth of the long bones (confirmed by post-mortem examination) and control by litter mates. He also demonstrated the occurrence of genital hypoplasia in the animals[114].

In his historical review of the pituitary, Aschner mentioned Josef Engel, a pupil of Rokitansky, who recognized the pathological correlations of the pituitary, the thyroid and the pineal and described the occurrence of colloid, degeneration, and neoplasms in these

The Journal of the
American Medical Association

Published under the Auspices of the Board of Trustees

| VOLUME LIII | CHICAGO, ILLINOIS, JULY 24, 1909 | NUMBER 4 |

Address

THE HYPOPHYSIS CEREBRI

CLINICAL ASPECTS OF HYPERPITUITARISM AND OF HYPO-
PITUITARISM*

HARVEY CUSHING, M.D.

BALTIMORE

Few chapters in the history of medicine tell a more creditable story than that which relates our progress toward a better understanding of the thyroid and parathyroid glands. A combination of clinical, experimental and surgical experiences during the past twenty years has served to unveil many of the mysteries which formerly surrounded the function of these structures, whose normal activities prove to be so essential to the maintenance of physiologic equilibrium. Myxedema, cretinism, exophthalmic goiter, surgical myxedema (cachexia strumipriva) and tetany have come to be understandable maladies, definitely amenable to rational methods of treatment—and organotherapy, when glandular activity is subnormal, or partial surgical removal to correct functional over-activity, is a triumph of the experimental method in medicine, at the hands of Horsley, Kocher, Halsted, Gley, Vassale and Generale, Mac-Callum and a host of others.

Not the least memorable incident of the entire story was the recognition, first by the Italian investigators, of the important rôle played by the lesser glands—the parathyroid bodies—in occasioning the so-called acute cachexia thyreopriva with tetanoid symptoms; for without this knowledge the condition of myxedema must have remained obscure from inability to produce its experimental counterpart, and actual investigation of the parathyroids might have been long delayed.

No less satisfactory a tale is in the making as regards a hitherto even more obscure member of the family of ductless glands—the pituitary body—and it is my purpose on this occasion to recount briefly some of the steps already taken toward a better knowledge of the normal function and the part played in certain diseases by this peculiar and inaccessible structure—called "l'organe enigmatique" by Van Gehuchten. Our progress, such as it is, would have been much slower without the previous experiences with the cervical glands, for out of the confusion which long reigned in their case from lack of appreciation of the double glandular rôle a les-

* The Oration on Surgery, read in the Section on Surgery of the American Medical Association, at the Sixtieth Annual Session, held at Atlantic City, June, 1909.
* From an etymological point of view the terms *hyper-, hypo-, dys-,* and *a-pituitarism* are doubtless of badly mixed parentage, but there are certain obvious objections to such a combination as *hypohypophysism*, and I have therefore concluded to retain the Latin word with its Greek prefix. *Hyperpituitism*, etc., might possibly be less unwieldy.

son has been learned and applied to the pituitary body, for it likewise combines glandular structures of widely differing function.

Not only in view of the general awakening of interest in the subject, but owing to the fact that most of the recent work on the hypophysis has appeared in foreign languages, it has seemed to me that a simple review of our knowledge of the anatomy and physiology of the gland and some discussion necessarily of a more speculative character as to the part it plays in certain diseases would make an appropriate topic for this annual oration.

THE GLANDULAR STRUCTURE

Regarded by the ancients as an organ which discharged *pituita* or mucus into the nose, and by most scientists of the past century as a mere vestigial relic of prehistoric usefulness, our first insight into a possible functional activity of this gland came from the laboratories of the modern comparative anatomists and embryologists, with many of whom it has been a favorite object of research. As a knowledge of its structure, development and morphologic significance is essential to the proper understanding of matters relating to its function, it may not be out of place to briefly recall here some few of the more important facts:

Rathke, in 1838, described an invagination of mucous membrane, supposedly arising from the anterior end of the fore-gut—since known as Rathke's pouch—and correctly attributed to this origin the epithelial portion of the pituitary body, which before this time was thought to be wholly derived from the brain. It remained for Götte and Balfour and Mihalkovics, in 1874 and 1875, to show that the invagination described by Rathke was derived from the embryonic buccal cavity rather than from the primitive gut, and hence was of ectodermic rather than of entodermic origin.

This ectodermic and epithelial pouch of Rathke, therefore, projecting from the buccal cavity and pressing against the floor of the anterior cerebral vesicle, leads to a downward fold in its wall, which becomes the early infundibulum. The stalk of the epithelial pouch becomes cut off, leaving a closed sac—the hypophyseal sac—which embraces the thickening wall or infundibular body at the tip of the vesicular fold, and the combined epithelial and nervous structure represents the anlage of the adult hypophysis. As the primitive gland develops further the epithelium of the anterior or lower part of the closed sac representing the remains of Rathke's pouch becomes thickened, forming the anterior lobe of the pituitary body. A more or less definite cleft separates this portion of the gland from the so-called posterior lobe, composed of the upper portion of the primitive closed epithelial sac together with the infundibular body to which it has become intimately adherent and with which it remains functionally associated. It is the persistence of this cleft in the mammalian hypophysis which usually permits of an easy, gross anatomic or surgical separation of the two lobes.

Thus the neural portion of the gland (the infundibular body) becomes surrounded by an intimate epithelial investment pos-

Figure 57 Title page of "The hypophysis cerebri" by Harvey W. Cushing [By kind permission of the Royal Society of Medicine]

organs. He did not observe generalized trophic disturbances, but he knew of the genital organs being frequently affected as a consequence of pituitary changes; he regarded the pituitary as a secretory gland[114].

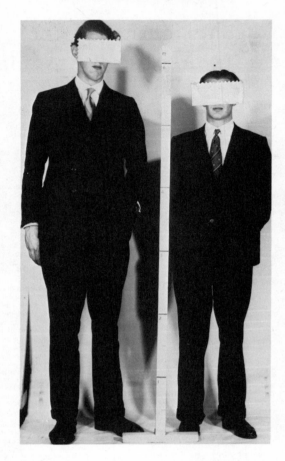

Figure 58   A case of gigantism (V. C. Medvei's patient)

Based on his own experimental work, Aschner is rightly critical of Pierre Marie's and Marinesco's theory that acromegaly is caused by a hypofunction of the pituitary[114]. He supported the view that the cause is a hyperfunction of the gland, in agreement with Benda, Max Sternberg and others[114]. It was Carl Benda (1857–1933) who demonstrated, in 1900, that the pituitary tumour of the anterior lobe in acromegaly consists of chromophil cells[115].

The whole epoch (between 1908 and 1912) was summarized by Cushing's address to the American Medical Association in June 1909, on 'The hypophysis cerebri'[116], in which he discussed the experimental findings in dogs, and the clinical symptoms in pathological conditions in man.

The address also contained the knowledge available on the Froehlich–Babinski–Cushing syndrome. On this occasion, Cushing introduced the new terms of "hyper- and hypo-pituitarism". However, it took another 13 years before one of his former students, Herbert McLean Evans, could postulate the specific growth-stimulating substance of the anterior pituitary. In the Summary of his address, Cushing said:

> Two conditions, one due to a pathological increased activity of the pars anterior of the hypophysis (hyperpituitarism), the other to a diminished activity of the same epithelial structure (hypopituitarism) seem capable of clinical differentiation.
>
> The former expresses itself chiefly as a process of overgrowth – gigantism, when originating in youth, acromegaly when originating in adult life. The latter expresses itself chiefly as an excessive, often a rapid, deposition of fat with persistence of infantile sexual characteristics when the process dates from youth, and a tendency toward a loss of the acquired signs of adolescence, when it first appears in adult life. . . . Experimental observations show not only that the anterior lobe of the hypophysis is a structure of such importance that a condition of apituitarism is incompatible with the long maintenance of life, but also that its partial removal leads to symptoms comparable to those which we regard as characteristic of lessened secretion (hypopituitarism) in man. . . . A tumour of the gland itself, or one arising in its neighbourhood and implicating the gland by pressure, is naturally the lesion to which one or the other of these condition has heretofore been attributed, though it is probable that over-secretion from simple hypertrophy, or undersecretion from atrophy, will be found to occur irrespective of tumour growth when examination of the pituitary body becomes a routine measure in the postmortem examination of all cases in which the conditions suggest one or the other of the symptoms-complex described. . . . When due to tumour, surgery is the treatment that these conditions demand, and at present, there are reasonably satisfactory ways of approaching the gland; but clinicians and surgeons must clearly distinguish between the local manifestations of the neoplasm due to the involvement of structures in its neighbourhood other than hypophysis, and those of a general character from disturbances of metabolism due to alterations of the hypophysis itself.

Two years after the report of Crowe, Cushing, and Homans[109,110], G. Ascoli and T. Legnani found another effect of hypophysectomy: atrophy of the adrenal cortex[117]. Craniopharyngiomas (Rathke's pouch tumours or hypophysial duct tumours) were clearly defined by the Viennese pathologist Jacob Erdheim (1874–1937) in 1904[118]; one of the first descriptions of these mostly squamous cell tumours was by the celebrated Jean Cruveilhier (1791–1874) as "tumeurs perlées" in 1829. As first professor of pathological anatomy in Paris, he described in his classic textbook[119] disseminated sclerosis and other conditions for the first time. Cushing later discussed the difficulties of surgical treatment of these tumours[120].

In June 1900, Joseph François Felix Babinski (1857–1932), a pupil of Charcot, reported to the Société de Neurologie in Paris on a girl of 17 as a 'Tumeur du corps pituitaire sans acromégalie et avec arrêt de développement des organes génitaux'[121]. The tumour occupied the sella turcica, was adherent to the pituitary gland and was probably a cranio-pharyngioma. The ovaries were very small. This presentation preceded the report on a boy of 14 by Alfred Froehlich (1871–1953) of Vienna, who wrote in 1901 on 'Ein Fall von Tumor der Hypophysis cerebri ohne Akromegalie'[122]. This is regarded as the classical description of dystrophia adiposo-genitalis, pituitary tumour, with obesity and sexual infantilism and drowsiness (Pickwick's fat boy): the boy was obese, had infantile testes, scanty pubic hair, dry skin, headache and vomiting.

In 1909, Harvey Williams Cushing (1869–1939) described 'Sexual infantilism with optic atrophy in cases of tumour affecting the hypophysis cerebri'[123]. But as Rolleston pointed out, in Britain, J. B. Story (1851–1926) from Dublin, showed a case of "optic atrophy in one eye and temporary hemianopia in the other", with drowsiness, headaches, increasing stoutness and irregular menstruation, to the Ophthalmological Society in 1887[124], and Edward Nettleship (1845–1913), suggested the presence of a pituitary tumour[124]. Post-mortem examination revealed a pituitary "of the size of a tangerine orange", of soft consistency. Microscopically, it was a round cell sarcoma.

Although Froehlich himself diagnosed a case of an obese woman, reported by Bernhard Mohr of Wuerzburg in 1840[125] (Mohr's Report appeared in the same number of the journal as Basedow's classic description of exophthalmic goitre) (see Figure 48), Babinski's description escaped him. In 1899, S. Pechkranz wrote on 'Sarcoma angiomatodes hypophyseos cerebri', describing a boy of 17 with genital hypoplasia[126]. Thus, the new syndrome of 'Dystrophia Adiposo-genitalis' was named after Froehlich and Babinski, with Cushing's name also sometimes added to it. It was not, however, the converse of acromegaly, as Philip Edward Smith (1884–1970) was able to show in one of his ingenious experiments. In this experiment, damage to the tuber cinereum of rats caused obesity and genital atrophy but no thyroid and adrenal cortical atrophy; but removal of the anterior pituitary caused arrest of growth in young animals and cachexia in adults (i.e. Simmond's disease), which is the converse of acromegaly[127]. In 1888, Sir Byrom Bramwell (1847–1931) (see Section II) had already suggested that the obesity, polyuria and glycosuria, occasionally observed in patients with pituitary

Originalartikel, Berichte aus Kliniken und Spitälern.

Aus der I. medicinischen Klinik des Herrn Hofrathes Prof. H. Nothnagel.

Ein Fall von Tumor der Hypophysis cerebri ohne Akromegalie.
Von Dr. Alfred Fröhlich.[*]

M. H.! Ich möchte mir erlauben, Ihnen einen Fall zu demonstriren, den ich in dem von Herrn Professor v. Frankl-Hochwart geleiteten Nerven-Ambulatorium der Klinik des Herrn Hofrathes Nothnagel zu beobachten Gelegenheit hatte und der mir in mancherlei Hinsicht Bemerkenswertes darzubieten scheint.

R. D., ein 14jähriger Knabe, steht seit November 1899 in unserer Beobachtung. Damals gab seine Mutter an, dass er zweimal wöchentlich, zuweilen in 14tägigen Intervallen von der Schule mit Kopfschmerz nachhause kam. Er musste sich zu Bett legen; zwei Stunden nachher Erbrechen, mitunter Erbrechen gleich beim Nachhausekommen. Dieser Zustand bestand seit April 1899. Kopfschmerz links, zuweilen beiderseits, meist im Vorderkopf. Er lernt gut, gutes Gedächtnis, keine Zeichen von Nervosität oder Hysterie. Keine früheren Erkrankungen, kein vorangegangenes Trauma. Sehen gut. Sonst keinerlei subjective Beschwerden.

Keine Blasen- und Mastdarmstörungen. Objectiv konnte keinerlei pathologischer Befund festgestellt werden. In der Krankengeschichte erscheint der Status, des negativen Befundes ungeachtet, ausführlich erhoben. Fundus normal. Der Augenhintergrund ist, wie die Mutter mittheilt, zu jener Zeit auch von Professor Königstein untersucht und normal befunden worden. Wir nahmen angesichts des negativen Befundes einen Zustand von Hemicranie an und ertheilten dementsprechende therapeutische Rathschläge. Dann verloren wir Pat. aus den Augen.

[*] Nach einer am 12. October 1901 in der Wanderversammlung des Vereines für Psychiatrie und Neurologie in Wien gehaltenen Demonstration.

Am 19. August 1901 erschien er wieder, diesmal mit einer Reihe ernster Beschwerden. Die Mutter giebt Folgendes an: Seit März 1899 begann Pat., der bis dahin ein mageres Kind war, rapid an Körpergewicht zuzunehmen. Jänner 1901 klagte er über Herabsetzung der Sehkraft am linken Auge, der aber keine weitere Beachtung geschenkt wurde. Juli 1901 begannen die Kopfschmerzen neuerdings aufzutreten und in der Folgezeit an Intensität zuzunehmen. Gleichzeitig klagte er über Mattigkeit. Oefters Erbrechen, besonders im Anschluss an Mahlzeiten. Weitere Abnahme der Sehkraft des linken Auges, dann Erblindung links. Später nahm auch die Sehkraft rechts ab.

Am 23. September 1901 konnte ich folgenden Befund erheben: Seit einigen Wochen subjectiv Besserung. Weniger Kopfschmerz, kein Schwindel. Seit 10 Tagen kein Brechreiz, Körpergewicht nimmt ab: 51 1/2 kg gegen 54 kg im Mai 1901. Appetit, Schlaf gut. Objectiv: Intelligenz. Sprache durchaus normal. Kopfbewegungen frei. Die linke Schläfengrube und nur diese auf Percussion schmerzempfindlich.

Keine Störungen des Geschmacks, Geruchs, sowie der Sensibilität im Gesichte. Gehör normal. Uebrige Hirnnerven normal. Motilität und Sensibilität an den Extremitäten und am Rumpfe durchaus normal. Sehnenreflexe, namentlich Kniereflexe lebhaft. Kein Fussclonus, kein Romberg'sches Phänomen. Sphincteren 0. Innere Organe normal. Urin frei von Zucker und Eiweiss.

Augenuntersuchung: Pupillen ca. 4 mm weit, gleich. Die linke Pupille reagirt auf Lichteinfall nicht, auf Accomodation sehr gut. Rechts prompte Reaction auf Licht und Accomodation. Bulbi frei beweglich, kein Nystagmus. Fundus: genuine Atrophia N. optici sin.; rechts normal. Links Amaurose, rechts 3/20 (Gläser bessern nicht); temporale Hemianopsie rechts.

Die Gesichtsfeldgrenzen des rechten Auges sind in der nasalen Hälfte ganz normal. Die sehende nasale Partie grenzt sich gegen die blinde temporale durch eine nahezu verticale Trennungslinie ab, welche aber nach aussen vom Centrum verläuft, dasselbe in einem sanft geschwungenen Bogen umgreifend. Die Papilla n. optici sin. ist schneeweiss, sehr scharf begrenzt; an den Gefässen keine Veränderungen.[*]

[*] Bei der letzten ophthalmoskopischen Untersuchung am 12. Nov. war die innere Hälfte der rechten Papille stark geröthet, opak und leicht geschwollen (Neuritis).

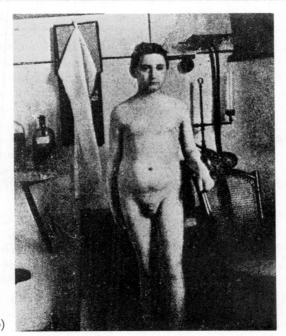

Figure 59 Froelich's report on dystrophia adiposogenitalis. (a) Frontispiece (by kind permission of the Institute for the History of Medicine, University of Vienna, Austria); (b) the patient [By kind permission of the Royal Society of Medicine, London]

321

tumours, were caused by the effect on the adjacent parts of the brain rather than by the actual changes within the pituitary[128]. The important connections, relations and pathways from the pituitary to the hypothalamus and the role of neuro-endocrine relations has taken over an ever-increasing part of the research in the field of endocrinology, especially in the last 20 years.

Today, it is often forgotten that the early efforts of surgical treatment of pituitary tumours often date from that period. In 1893 Richard Caton (1842–1926) and Frank Thomas Paul (1851–1941), in Liverpool, performed decompression in a married woman of 33 with acromegaly, to relieve cranial pressure[129]. However, it was really Herman Schloffer (1868–1937) of Innsbruck who first successfully operated on a pituitary tumour by the nasal route in 1906[130]: 'Erfolgreiche Operation eines Hypophysen-tumors auf nasalem Wege'[131], although it was Oskar Hirsch's endonasal method which later became better known (after 1911)[132].

Harvey Cushing (1869–1939) operated on his first patient with acromegaly in 1909. He removed about one third of the anterior lobe. The patient's condition was relieved and he "remained virtually symptom-free for some twenty years"[133]. Cushing remarked in a letter to his father that the pituitary "seems to be an important gland"[134]. It should be mentioned here that Froehlich's 15-year-old patient with the adiposo-genital dystrophy was successfully operated on by Anton von Eiselsberg (1860–1939), who removed a cystic tumour from the pituitary. The boy survived and was still alive and well 38 years later, when Froehlich had to leave Vienna after the Nazi occupation[135]. On Cushing's own patient, the 14-year-old girl with similar symptoms, where he made the diagnosis of a pituitary tumour, he attempted three exploratory operations, but could not find the tumour. The patient died and post-mortem examination revealed a large cystic tumour in the sella turcica which had almost destroyed the anterior lobe of the pituitary[135].

Von Eiselsberg's colleague, Julius von Hochenegg (1859–1940), carried out the first successful operation for acromegaly in Vienna on a woman on 14 February 1908, using Schloffer's technique. The initial mortality of 35% of these operations was gradually reduced to 10%, greatly aided by radiography making visible the enlargement of the sella turcica. It was first demonstrated by Herrmann Oppenheim (1858–1919) in 1899, at a meeting of the 'Berlin Society of Psychiatry and Nervous Diseases'.

The other important development was the observation by Julius Tandler (1869–1936) and S. Grosz of Vienna, that the human pituitary gland becomes enlarged in man and woman, following gonadectomy[136, 137]. This was followed in 1909 by the description of

Jacob Erdheim (1874–1937) and Emil Stumme of the changes of the pituitary gland during pregnancy, i.e. increase in size of the anterior lobe and the appearance of large, finely granular eosinophilic cells, which they called "pregnancy cells" and which are usually still present during lactation[138]. These cells have a certain similarity with the cells found in the anterior lobe adenomas of acromegalics; some enlargement of hands and face during pregnancy is not unknown. The enlargement in size of the pituitary during pregnancy was – as already mentioned – first described by L. Comte in 1898[67].

In fact, the study of interrelations between the pituitary and other endocrine glands became important. The influence of the pituitary on the gonads and vice-versa has already been mentioned, and we shall discuss the stimulating effect of the various pituitary hormones on the thyroid, etc. The influence of the other glands on the pituitary, however, was observed as early as 1886 to 1889 by N. Rogowitsch: 'Die Veraenderungen der Hypophyse nach Entfernung der Schilddruese'[139] (= The changes in the hypophysis after removal of the thyroid). He studied the result of thyroidectomy in rabbits, which, fortunately, possess a pair of extra-thyroidal parathyroids, and did not die, therefore, of the effect of the unintentional removal of those glands, as did dogs and cats, as Eugène Gley pointed out in 1891[140]. Thus, Rogowitsch found a definite enlargement of the pituitary and also a marked loss of eosinophils. The anterior lobe may contain colloid material, resembling that of the thyroid in appearance, but not its iodine content.

Bernhard Aschner noted in 1912, on the contrary, that in hypophysectomized puppies the thyroids appeared atrophic[114]. Ludwig Adler (1876–1958) reported in 1914[141], that if the pituitary body in large tadpoles is destroyed by cautery, in the few surviving animals metamorphosis does not occur if the anterior lobe is completely destroyed, and the thyroid appears atrophic. In contrast, J. F. Gudernatsch demonstrated in 1912, that metamorphosis can be induced in tadpoles by thyroid feeding[142]. A similar enlargement of the pituitary was also confirmed in myxoedema in 1892, by Wm. Hale White, and by R. Boyce and C. F. Beadles in 1893[143, 144]. Beadles reported it also in cretinism, but so did A. Nièpce as early as 1851[145], whereas A. Schoenemann reported it as usually completely atrophied[65]. In 1916, Philip Edward Smith (1884–1970) (see Section II)[146] and – independently of him – Bennett M. Allen[147] developed a method of incising Rathke's pouch in 4 mm tadpoles without damaging the brain. The surviving animals did not undergo metamorphosis and their thyroids became atrophic; but anterior lobe extracts were given, the thyroids recovered and metamorphosis occurred[148–150]. F. D. Thompson found that experimental parathyroidectomy caused an increased amount of 'colloid' in the pituitary[151].

It is sometimes forgotten that Oliver and Schaefer studied not only the pressor effect of adrenal extracts, but also those of the pituitary. Schaefer mentioned this briefly in his 'Address in physiology on internal secretions' to the British Medical Association on 2 August 1895[152] (see also p. 334). They also published a preliminary account 'On the physiological actions of extracts of the pituitary body and certain other glandular organs'[153]. Accordingly, extracts of fresh, whole pituitary glands, when given intravenously into mammals under anaesthesia, produce a rapid rise in blood pressure. But even fairly considerable doses will not produce the same rise as a small amount of suprarenal extract. Pituitary extract causes a slower pressure rate, but it is maintained longer. The vasoconstrictor action of such extracts in frogs with their nervous system destroyed has proved that the action was peripheral. This pressure raising action of pituitary extracts was confirmed by a number of research workers between 1895 and 1898, but William Henry Howell (1860–1945) proved that the pressor principle was in the infundibular body (=the posterior lobe)[154]. Howell also noted that the prolonged rise in blood pressure was more marked when the dog was not only anaesthetized, but had the vagal nerves cut, or was atropinized. He also described the phenomenon of 'tachyphylaxia', i.e. that successive injections may have less effect or even none, depending on the time interval and the dosage used. These observations were confirmed by Schaefer and Swale Vincent[155, 156], who also confirmed a further observation of Howell, that their pituitary extracts may have a depressor effect and lower the blood pressure. The cause for this phenomenon could be (a) reduction of myocardial bloodflow through constriction of the coronary arteries[157]; or (b) crude extracts may contain histamine or histamine-like substances[158].

The diuretic and anti-diuretic activity of the pituitary will be discussed later, but the former had already been noted by Schaefer and his co-workers and reported in 1901[159, 160]. It was also confirmed by the studies of R. G. Hoskins and W. Means[161].

Meanwhile, Morris Simmonds (1855–1925) of Hamburg gave what was thought to be the first clinical account of the result of atrophy of the anterior lobe in man[162], in his patient combined with septic puerperal infarction of the anterior lobe. The name of Simmonds' disease was introduced in 1922 by L. Lichtwitz[163]. Simmonds thought that the arteries of the anterior lobe are endarteries, which would explain the risks in the case of puerperal sepsis, syphilis, tuberculosis, but there were patients where the anterior lobe was destroyed by a cyst or a tumour (see also Chapter 18). Later it was found that L. K. Glinski had published a case-history of *post-partum* necrosis of the anterior lobe of the pituitary a year before Simmonds (in 1913), but – unfortunately – in the Polish language, which was, therefore, overlooked[164].

DISCOVERY OF A SPECIFIC PHYSIOLOGICAL RESPONSE TO ADRENAL EXTRACT[6]

Sir Henry Dale has told the story in his charmingly written essays 'Accident and Opportunism in Medical Research', how the vaso-pressor effects of adrenal extract were discovered "in circumstances which, if not entirely accidental, had at least something of that character"[165].

George Oliver (1841–1915) was a physician in Harrogate from 1876 to 1908. His practice in a Spa being seasonal, he spent the winter months mainly in London (see Section II). Oliver was aware of the claims of Brown-Séquard and interested in the role of organ extracts. These were partly his reasons for wishing to examine the effect of an extract of the adrenal gland, as many other physicians were in-terested in the therapeutic potential of extracts of all sorts of organs. Oliver's visit to Schaefer in the autumn of 1893 has now become part of the best known medical anecdotage. The clinician Oliver was playing about with various organ extracts, one of which, he thought, had certain effects. He decided to consult Edward Albert Schaefer, then Professor of Physiology at University College in London, the brilliant, very busy and somewhat intolerant academic, who resented any unnecessary intrusion upon his time and did not believe for a moment that Oliver could have possibly found anything of impor-tance. He conceded to try and use Oliver's extract which the latter had on his person, towards the end of one of his (Schaefer's) experiments, mainly to demonstrate to Oliver that his intrusion presented a nuisance. He was completely taken aback when Oliver proved his point, particularly as glycerine extracts of several organs had been available to Schaefer, and he was equally dubious of the effect of all of them. The effect of Oliver's adrenal extract on the blood pressure of the experimental animal was convincing. It led to a close co-operation between them in the ensuing winter months and resulted in Oliver and Schaefer presenting their first report on 10 March 1894: 'On the physiological action of extract of the suprarenal capsules' to the Physiological Society[166, 167]. The account of their first meeting reads much more amusingly in Sir Henry Dale's version[165] than in the somewhat stilted account of Sir Edward Schaefer[168].

Schaefer's description of his meeting with Oliver:

In the autumn of 1893 there called upon me in my laboratory at University College a gentleman who was personally unknown to me, but with whom I had a common bond of interest – seeing that we had both been pupils of Sharpey, whose chair at that time I had the honour to occupy. I found that my visitor was Dr. George Oliver, already distinguished not only as a specialist in his particular branch of medical practice, but also for his clinical application of physiological methods. Dr. Oliver was desirous of discussing with me the results which he had been obtaining from the exibition by the mouth of extracts of certain animal tissues, and the effects which these had in his hands produced upon the blood vessels of man, as investigated by two instruments which he had devised – one of them the haemodynamometer, intended to read variations in blood pressure, and the other, the arteriometer, for measuring with exactness the lumen of the radial or any other superficial artery. Dr. Oliver ascertained, or believed he had ascertained, by the use of these instruments, that glycerine extracts of some organs produce decrease in calibre of the arteries and increase of pulse tension, of others the reverse effect[168].

Sir Henry Dale's account of the same event:

He (Oliver) went up to London to tell Professor Schaefer what he thought he had observed, and found him engaged in an experiment in which the blood pressure of a dog was being recorded; found him, not unnaturally, incredulous about Oliver's story and very impatient at the interruption. But Oliver was in no hurry, and urged only that a dose of his suprarenal extract, which he produced from his pocket, should be injected into a vein when Schaefer's own experiment was finished. And so, just to convince Oliver that it was all nonsense, Schaefer gave the injection, and then stood amazed to see the mercury mounting in the arterial manometer till the recording float was lifted almost out of the distal limb[165] (p. 454).

Borell remarks:

"It is interesting that Oliver was using glycerine extracts, as Murray had done, and that, like many of his countrymen, he administered extracts by mouth. One wonders what other extracts had been tested by Oliver. One cannot help but suspect that these were far more numerous than Schaefer deigned to mention in 1908, fifteen years after their first encounter[6].

Borell makes a further, fundamental observation which leads to the discussion of an important development in the history of endocrinology in one of the next chapters. She says:

In the meeting of the clinician Oliver and the physiologist Schaefer, one can observe a tension between two visions of what constitutes an adequate demonstration of a new phenomenon. Oliver had observed an effect in a human subject. . . . Schaefer questioned that effect. It is this confrontation and complementation which constitutes the 'accidental' circumstances which Dale related[165]. . . . The tension between these two approaches contributes a major theme in the history of endocrinology. The 'crisis' of medical endocrinology which emerged in the 1920s effected a re-evaluation of the relative merits of medical and physiological research for the progress of this field[6].

Schaefer continued in his Oliver–Sharpey Lectures of 1908:

Although the conclusions were interesting, it was easy to see that results which were obtained under mechanical conditions, which were somewhat complex and not easy of interpretation, could not be expected to decide an important physiological question of this nature, and that it was essential, in order to obtain exact knowledge of the actions, if any, of such extracts, to conduct the investigations with the employment of all means at the disposal of the modern physiologist. With the suggestion that we should undertake such an investigation, Dr. Oliver promptly agreed, and it was then and there arranged to devote that winter to a thorough examination of the physiological effects of such extracts.

The result of this conjunction of effort, brought about by the fortunate chance foreseen by old Montesquieu (see p. 179), speedily showed that, whilst many of the extracts which had been dealt with clinically by Oliver were inert or, at any rate, not specific in their action, the suprarenal capsules, and to a lesser extent the pituitary body, yielded to glycerine, to water and to saline solutions principles which have an extraordinary effect upon the tone of the heart and arteries, transcending that of any known drug.

George Oliver, as stated by Schaefer above, was also the inventor of the arteriometer, which measured the diameter of the radial artery, and which he allegedly tried out on his own son[169].

In the course of their continued collaboration, Oliver and Schaefer investigated the effect of a clear watery extract "obtained from Paris (in a sealed tube) and furnished to us by the kindness of Dr. Hale White"[170]. William Hale White (1857–1949) was physician, and lecturer on Materia Medica at Guy's Hospital. He had worked on a very popular subject at that time. As outlined previously, since the work of Mering and Minkowski, Laguesse and of Opie, the attempt to treat diabetes mellitus by feeding the patient with raw pancreas or giving injections of pancreatic juice had been attempted many times, although no one seemed to be able to cure or even improve the condition by these means. Hale White's report on his experiments appeared in the *British Medical Journal* on 4 March 1893[30,31]. He fed two patients on raw pancreas and he also gave them subcutaneous injections of "liquor pancreaticus" (pancreatic extracts). Both patients liked eating the raw, fresh sheep's pancreas, finely chopped and flavoured with pepper and salt, but the first developed an (obviously allergic) rash and sore throat, "of the same nature as that due to shell fish, or that brought about in myxoedematous patients treated with thyroid gland"[30,31]. Later 5 minims of Benger's liquor pancreaticus were injected night and morning in both cases for *ca.* 8 days. A steady diet was maintained and weight and urine carefully monitored. Hale White's summary was as follows:

> The general conclusions at which we may arrive, if we may judge from two cases only, are that it is very doubtful whether feeding on fresh pancreas or the subcutaneous injection of liquor pancreaticus is of any benefit in diabetes mellitus. Neither appear to have any influence on the quantity of the urine, its specific gravity, or the urea; perhaps they decrease the amount of sugar passed and very slightly increase the weight and feeling of strength. Patients like raw pancreas, but one great disadvantage is that it may cause severe erythema with fever and a slight sore throat. . . .

> I hope the publication of these two cases will lead others to try the treatment, so that we may soon have sufficient cases to form a just estimate of it.

White seems to have obtained his Benger's liquor pancreaticus from a laboratory in Paris. In this context, it may be of further interest to note that very recent experiments seem to show that whole pancreas transplants reversed the metabolic defects of diabetes in animals. Moreover, the classical complications of diabetes were diminished, if not prevented, in grafted animals. These experiments are the work of a team under the direction of Dr. Marshall J. Orloff, Professor of Surgery at the University College of San Diego, California[171].

To return to the experiments with adrenal extracts: in 1895, Oliver and Schaefer gave a concise summary of the results of their work 'The physiological effects of extracts of the suprarenal capsules'[172].

It appears to be established as the result of these investigations that, like the thyroid gland, the suprarenal capsules are to be regarded although ductless, as strictly secreting glands. The material which they form and which is found, at least in its fully active condition, only in the medulla of the gland, produces striking physiological effects, on the muscular tissue generally and especially upon the heart and arteries. Its action is to increase the tone of all muscular tissue, and this result is produced mainly if not entirely by direct action. On the other hand, the removal of the suprarenal capsules produces extreme weakness of the heart and muscular system generally, and great want of tone in the vascular system. A similar result is known to be characteristic of advanced disease of these organs (Addison's disease). It may fairly be concluded, therefore, that one of the main functions, if not the main function, of the suprarenal capsules is to produce a material which is added in some way or another to the blood, and the effect of which is to assist by its direct action upon the various kinds of muscular tissue in maintaining that amount of tonic contraction which appears to be essential to the physiological activity of the tissue. Any further conclusion than this we cannot legitimately draw from our experiments, and we do not propose at this time to discuss such other conclusions as it may be possible to arrive at from the results of ablation experiments. . . .

Following Oliver and Schaefer's work, John Jacob Abel (1857–1938), of Cleveland, Ohio, Professor of Pharmacology at Johns Hopkins University in Baltimore (see Chapter 20) and Albert Cornelius Crawford (1869–1921) of Baltimore, Maryland, Abel's assistant at the Johns Hopkins, obtained the active principle of the adrenal gland as a monobenzoyl derivative. Abel called this "epinephrine". This was the first isolation of an endocrine secretion as a chemically-pure substance. They reported it in 1897 under the heading 'On the blood-pressure raising constituent of the suprarenal capsule'[173]. Two other achievements of the greatest importance were – many years later – Abel's production of crystalline insulin (1925–1928), and the study and evaluation of the oxytocic-pressure-diuretic principle of the infundibulum of the pituitary gland (see Chapter 20).

It is one of the ironies of all scientific progress that when discoveries are 'in the air', research workers in different places may make the same important discovery, independently. If there is, in addition, a language problem, communication may become difficult or completely lacking. This became apparent particularly in the case of the discovery of insulin, as we shall see in Chapter 19. It also applied, however, in the case of the discovery of the pressor effect of the medullary hormone, which seems to have been discovered independently by Oliver and Schaefer and by N. Cybulski and Ladislaus Szymonowicz. Cybulski was Professor and Director of the Institute for Physiology and Histology of the Jagellonian University at Cracow, which at that time belonged to Austria, but the official languages were Polish and German. Dr. Szymonowicz was one of his assistants, who became 'Private-Docent' (=Associate Professor) by presenting a paper, in Polish, on the results of his experimental study on the function of the adrenal gland, suggested by Cybulski and published in September 1895. Oliver and Schaefer had presented their first report 'On the physiological action of extract of the suprarenal capsules' to the Physiological Society on 19 March 1894, having met in the autumn of 1893 for the first time. Szymonowicz then reported the main results of his experiments in German on 'Die Function der Nebenniere'[174]. He dates there his first (extirpation) experiment on a dog on 10 May 1894, carrying out another seven similar experiments until 21 December 1894. On 17 December 1894, he began his experiments to study the result of an injection of adrenal gland extracts into 11 dogs and one big cat. In two other dogs (making thus a total of 13), he removed the adrenals before injecting the extracts: the last experiment was recorded on 20 September 1895.

As he was travelling abroad for several months in January 1895, his chief, Professor Cybulski, carried out a number of similar experiments in dogs, rabbits and cats, finding that watery, glycerin and alcohol extracts had the same effect.

The Summary of Cybulski and Szymonowicz's conclusions was as follows:

(1) The adrenal is an organ essential for life, a gland with internal secretion.
(2) Especially the medulla produces a substance and introduces it into the blood, which controls the function of the vasomotor nerve-centres, the vagus nerve, and of the accelerating nerves, also of the respiratory centre and – most likely – of the centres responsible for muscular tonus, and which keeps all of them in a condition of tonic tension[174]. [Translation from the German: V.C.M.]

And Professor Cybulski added:

All nerve impulses and chemical stimuli are – as it were – accidental and could not maintain the action of the above mentioned centres; in order to be independent of casual stimuli, the organism possesses, within its own economy, a gland, which provides the blood continually with a substance which maintains the functions of these centres. We have been used to regard the nervous system as the most important factor in the organism; we encounter here a new factor, without which the action of the nervous system itself would become impossible. We

find here, therefore, as rarely elsewhere, the strictly reciprocal dependence of the functions of the organism of itself and the mutual influence
of various organs. We may thus reduce the importance of the nervous
system, but do we not approach – by so doing – a more exact
understanding of the real conditions within the organism? [Translation
from the German: V.C.M.][175]

Szymonowicz next relates that they received a letter from Professor Schaefer in London, dated 3 June 1895, containing the two
reports of the experiments by Oliver and Schaefer, along similar
lines and with similar results. One report, dated 10 March 1894,
was ahead of that by Cybulski and Szymonowicz, "the second,
16 March, later than ours" (the exact meaning of that statement,
concerning the second date, is not quite clear: V.C.M.). Thus,
Szymonowicz concluded, their work was carried out quite independently of that of Oliver and Schaefer, and it gave them great
satisfaction, that they achieved the same important results[174]. In their
interesting list of references, they quote (apart from Oliver and
Schaefer), 11 papers by Jaques Emile Abelous (1864–1940) and Jean
Paul Langlois (1862–1923) (and some of their collaborators) on 'Note
sur les fonctions des capsules surrénales chez les grenouilles'[176]
(= note on the functions of the suprarenal capsules in frogs), also,
ergographic studies in Addison's disease and diuresis "after injection
of extract"[177]. There was also a report mentioned from Antoine de
Martini: 'Sur un cas d'absence congéniale des capsules surrénales'[178]
(an unreliable report: V.C.M.), without any signs of Addison's
disease. The pigmentation in Addison's disease was regarded by
Szymonowicz as being of nervous effect, i.e. caused by changes in
the nervous and sympathetic ganglia![174]

Biedl removed inter-renal (=cortical) tissue in some fishes, where
chromaffin tissue was placed separately. Although this was not easy
to carry out, it tended to show that the inter-renal organs had the task
of preventing adrenal insufficiency[179]. T. D. Wheeler and S. Vincent
removed one adrenal and half of the other, in dogs, then cauterized
the medullary tissue in the remaining fragment. The remaining
cortical fraction, if not damaged, sufficed to maintain good health[180].
Frank A. Hartman and Katherine A. Brownell, in their monograph
on *The Adrenal Gland*[181], suggested that the period of the experimental investigations after Addison's description in 1855 should
be called Addisonian epoch. They called the period from the
discovery of the pressor effect of epinephrine in 1894, and the
investigation of that problem, the epinephrine period. The third
period, they thought, concerns the investigation of the function of
the cortex and they marked the beginning of that period by the
publication of Wheeler and Vincent's paper.

Bernardo Alberto Houssay (1887–1971) of Buenos Aires, and J. T. Lewis made similar experiments to Biedl's (with elasmobranchs), as did Wheeler and Vincent (with dogs), using a much more sophisticated technique. They came to the conclusion that "dogs survive extirpation of all chromophil tissue . . . in the adrenals when the remaining cortex is in a good state"[182]. As Robert Gaunt has pointed out[183], the results of the adrenal extirpation experiments in rats vary because survival times after adrenalectomy are influenced by the following factors: (1) hereditary strain differences (partly due to accessories), (2) the age of the animals, (3) the sodium and potassium content of the diet, (4) environmental conditions, (5) presence or absence of temporary life sustaining therapy, enabling some adjustment (development of accessories), and (6) avoidance of an early stress-induced death from shock. Julius Moses Rogoff (1883–1966) and George Neil Stewart (1860–1930) of Case Western Reserve University, were particularly critical of sloppy operation techniques, and were pioneers of meticulous observations of experimental adrenal insufficiency, especially in dogs[184, 185]. In 1922 Frank A. Hartman, the joint author of the monograph *The Adrenal Gland*[181], then of Buffalo, later of Ohio University, wrote cautiously that "from all the evidence available, we may conclude that of the two tissues the cortex is more important"[186].

In the meantime, the first clinical report on phaeochromocytoma should be recorded. This was in 1886, by Felix Fraenkel, who was at the time of the observation at the medical school of the University of Freiburg im Breisgau and presented it as his doctoral thesis. In the winter of 1883 the patient, a girl of 18, suddenly developed the symptoms of classic attacks of phaeochromocytoma. In addition, she had signs of retinitis and albuminuria, and an enlarged thyroid. She went rapidly downhill and died within 10 days of admission, having had several attacks of paroxysmal hypertension. The post-mortem examination revealed a growth the size of a fist, which had destroyed the left adrenal, and a similar growth the size of a walnut in the right adrenal. Microscopic examination indicated that the two tumours were identical and that the one on the right might have originated in the adrenal medulla, although the pathologist assumed that the tumour was an angiosarcoma. The kidneys did not present evidence of chronic nephritis but there were pathological changes in the aorta, major and minor arteries, and the heart showed enlargement. It is interesting to note that throughout the time of observation as an in-patient, the blood pressure was never taken. From the extravasation of blood in various organs it was concluded that they might have occurred during sudden rises of blood pressure. In the discussion, the role of the adrenals was considered. After nearly 30 years, the causal connection between Addison's disease and the adrenals was still regarded as not proven, but Gotschau's studies in Basle are quoted as proof that the suprarenals are glands. Remarkably, the title of the thesis is: 'A case of bilateral, completely latent tumour of the adrenals with concurrent nephritis, with changes in the circulatory system and retinitis[187] (Translation: V.C.M.). This in spite of the admission that the microscopical examination of the kidneys showed only some changes in the arteries, but no evidence of chronic nephritis.

The work of Oliver and Schaefer also marked a turning point in another respect: as already indicated. Murray, Oliver and Hale White were clinicians. The participation of Schaefer, one of the leading English physiologists, meant that the investigation of organ extracts was now accepted as a serious pre-occupation of physiological research; but the research proceeded from a different angle. The clinicians attempted to prove that an organ extract may contain a potent drug because it cured or prevented a specific disease. Physiologists, like Schaefer, were trying to find physiological responses to the hypothetical drugs in organ extracts, which could be measured, studied and their actions repeated under set circumstances. Thus they were beginning to approach Edward A. Doisy's set of four criteria (see p. 6):

1. Recognition of the gland; 2. Methods of detecting internal secretion; 3. Preparation of extracts leading to a purified hormone; 4. The isolation of the pure hormone, determination of its structure and, finally, its synthesis.

This new era was heralded in by Schaefer's Address to the British Medical Association in Physiology in London on 2 August 1895, entitled 'On Internal Secretions'[152].

ON INTERNAL SECRETIONS

Schaefer's address is so important for the history of endocrinology that the first part must be quoted in full.

My definite subject – the subject of internal secretions – is one of far-reaching interest, although its full importance has only lately come to be recognised. A secreting organ is one which separates certain materials from the blood and pours them out again, sometimes after effecting change of some sort in them, usually upon external surfaces, or at least upon surfaces which are connected with the exterior. These are the secretions which are most commonly known under that name.

on preserving health you may have every reason to hope that you will pass through it successfully—and, I trust, satisfactorily—and may return to this country in health and vigour and with large experience with the prospect of doing useful work at home—it may be in this great school. I will not detain you longer than to say that in bidding you farewell I wish you every prosperity and success, and trust that your highest aspirations may be realised.

Address in Physiology

ON

INTERNAL SECRETIONS.

Delivered at the Annual Meeting of the British Medical Association at London, Aug. 2nd, 1895.[1]

BY EDWARD A. SCHÄFER, F.R.S.,

JODRELL PROFESSOR OF PHYSIOLOGY IN UNIVERSITY COLLEGE, LONDON.

MR. PRESIDENT AND GENTLEMEN,—My definite subject —the subject of internal secretions is one of far-reaching interest, although its full importance has only lately come to be recognised. A secreting organ is one which separates certain materials from the blood and pours them out again, sometimes after effecting change of some sort in them, usually upon external surfaces, or at least upon surfaces which are connected with the exterior. These are the secretions which are most commonly known under that name. On the other hand, some secreted materials are not poured out upon an external surface at all, but are returned to the blood. These may be termed internal secretions, and they may be and are of no less importance than the better known and more fully studied ordinary or external secretions. The name of gland is one which is usually applied to a secreting organ; and to those which have been believed to furnish only internal secretions the name "ductless glands" has been applied. It is not, however, the ductless glands alone which possess the property of furnishing internal secretions, for it is clear, according to our definition, that this will apply to any organ of the body. Every part of the body does, in fact, take up materials from the blood, and does transform these into other materials. Having thus transformed them they are ultimately returned into the circulating fluid, and in that sense every tissue and organ of the body furnishes an internal secretion. Moreover, certain important glands which are provided with ducts possess not only the faculty of yielding an external secretion, but have equally important, if not even more important, functions in connexion with internal secretion. Thus both the liver and the pancreas are as essential to life, by virtue of the internal secretions which they furnish to the blood, as they are by their better known external secretions. The evidence of this is complete. The entire removal of either of these organs causes death, and this is due to the removal of the influence which they exert on the metabolism of the body by the loss of their internal secretions, not necessarily to the loss of their external secretions; for in the case of the liver it is well known that the bile may be diverted by a fistulous opening without any serious interference with the vital functions, and the same is the case for pancreatic juice. The kidney is another instance. It might, indeed, at first appear that a similar statement will not apply so well here; but it has been shown by the researches of Dr. Rose Bradford that the kidney is not a real exception to the rule laid down, for enough of the kidney substance may be left to carry on the excretory products of the body, and yet the removal of the remainder of the organ may cause such disorganisation of the nitrogenous metabolism of the body as to lead speedily to wasting and death. The same result is not obtained with all glands. The salivary glands may be entirely removed without any marked symptom supervening. And this is also well known to be the case with the mammary glands. On the other hand, removal of the generative glands leads to marked alterations

[1] Professor Schäfer intended to illustrate his address by lantern slides, but the hall being unsuitable for this he gave his audience a good idea of his meaning by tracing the curves with his finger.

in the development of other parts of the body. In the last-mentioned case the changes are without doubt produced through the nervous system, and are not connected with the internal secretion of the glands; and with respect to the salivary and mammary glands we may assume that, although they yield an internal secretion of some sort to the blood, it is of the same nature as that yielded by other organs, and that such other organs may act vicariously for those removed. This is, however, inapplicable to the liver, the kidney, or the pancreas; removal of which or restriction of their internal secretions is inevitably followed by a fatal result.

I do not propose to dwell further upon the internal secretions of the liver and kidney, and for contrary reasons—namely, that in the one case the subject has become too large for the limits of a short address; and in the other because the subject is one with regard to which we have at present too little information. But before leaving the liver I would point out that it affords an excellent illustration of the fact that internal secretions may, like ordinary or external secretions, either serve some useful purposes in the body, or may be formed only to be got rid of (excretions). The formation of glycogen and sugar is an example of a useful internal secretion—that of urea—of what would be termed in the ordinary sense an excretion, although it is not actually got rid of by the liver, but is produced by that organ only to be got rid of by the kidney. The internal secretion of the pancreas may detain us somewhat longer. Among the racemose secreting glands the pancreas offers a peculiarity of structure which in the first instance it may be well to note. For we meet here, besides the secreting alveoli and ducts, a peculiar epithelium-like tissue which occurs in isolated patches throughout the organ and which is characterised by its extreme vascularity. These islands of epitheloid tissue are quite characteristic of pancreas. We know of no other externally secreting gland which contains them.

Now it was formerly believed that the sole function of the pancreas was to yield pancreatic juice, and this, it must be confessed, is in itself a sufficiently important function, seeing that this fluid contains ferments which act on all the principal organic constituents of the food. Before 1889 it had indeed been remarked that cases of glycosuria occurring in the human subject were frequently associated with disease of some kind of the pancreas. Frerichs found that 20 per cent. of the total number of cases of diabetes which came under his notice were accompanied by obvious changes in the pancreas. This observation led to experimental inquiry. Claude Bernard had long previously attempted to entirely remove the pancreas, but all his attempts were unsuccessful, in so far that the animals speedily succumbed. In 1889, however, the operation was successfully performed by Von Mering and Minkowski. They found that all cases in which the entire pancreas was removed the operation was followed within the space of a very few hours by the appearance of sugar in the urine, and this to a great extent—as much as 5 to 10 per cent. being found even in fasting animals. Accompanying the condition of glycosuria there is also produced polyuria; and these conditions occur even under a purely flesh diet, and are accompanied, as might be supposed, by a rapid wasting, and followed within the space of fifteen days or less by death. This result is not due to the loss of the pancreatic secretion, for, as we have already seen, the pancreatic juice may be diverted by a fistula, and the animal may remain in perfect health. Nor is it due to the loss of the secreting structure; for it has been found possible to destroy the secreting structure of the organ without the supervention of diabetes. This was done successfully by Schiff in 1872. Schiff's method, which was a repetition of experiments by Bernhard, was the injection of paraffin into the duct of Wirsung. In Bernhard's original experiments all the dogs operated on speedily died; but this was probably due to accidental causes, and not to the actual destruction of the pancreatic tissue; for in Schiff's experiments the dogs survived and remained in perfect health. The fact that removal of the pancreas is followed by glycosuria was not at that time known, and the appearance of sugar in the urine was not therefore looked for by Schiff. But there can be no doubt of the absence of any severe form of diabetes, because the animals underwent no wasting.

Quite recently the experiment has been repeated by Thiroloix, who found that, although the gland was reduced by the process of atrophy supervening on the injection to a mere rudiment, symptoms of diabetes do not occur as when the whole gland is removed. It is now well known that if a

Figure 60 Schaefer's address in physiology

On the other hand, some secreted materials are not poured out upon an external surface at all, but are returned to the blood. These may be termed internal secretions, and they may be and are of no less importance than the better known and more fully studied ordinary or external secretions. The name of gland is one which is usually applied to a secreting organ; and to those which have been believed to furnish only internal secretions the name 'ductless glands' has been applied. It is not, however, the ductless glands alone which possess the property of furnishing internal secretions, for it is clear, according to our definition, that this will apply to any organ of the body. Every part of the body does, in fact, take up materials from the blood, and does transform these into other materials. Having thus transformed them they are ultimately returned into the circulating fluid, and in that sense every tissue and organ of the body furnishes an internal secretion. Moreover, certain important glands which are provided with ducts possess not only the faculty of yielding an external secretion, but have equally important, if not even more important, functions in connexion with internal secretion. Thus both the liver and the pancreas are as essential to life, by virtue of their internal secretions which they furnish to the blood, as they are by their better known external secretions. The evidence of this is complete. The entire removal of either of these organs causes death, and this is due to the removal of the influence which they exert on the metabolism of the body by the loss of their internal secretions, not necessarily to the loss of their external secretions; for in the case of the liver it is well known that the bile may be diverted by a fistulous opening without any serious interference with the vital functions, and the same is the case for pancreatic juice. The kidney is another instance. It might, indeed, at first appear that a similar statement will not apply so well here; but it has been shown by the researches of Dr. Rose Bradford that the kidney is not a real exception to the rule laid down, for enough of the kidney substance may be left to carry on the excretory products of the body, and yet the removal of the remainder of the organ may cause such disorganisation of the nitrogenous metabolism of the body as to lead speedily to wasting and death. The same result is not obtained with all glands. The salivary glands may be entirely removed without any marked symptom supervening. And this is also well known to be the case with the mammary glands. On the other hand, removal of the generative glands leads to marked alterations in the development of other parts of the body. In the last-mentioned case the changes are without doubt produced through the nervous system, and are not connected with the internal secretion of the glands; and with respect to the salivary and mammary glands we may assume that, although they yield an internal secretion of some sort to the blood, it is of the same nature as that yielded by other organs, and that such other organs may act vicariously for those removed. This is, however, inapplicable to the liver, the kidney, or the pancreas; removal of which or restriction of their internal secretions is inevitably followed by a fatal result.

Schaefer then discussed the experimental evidence that diabetes mellitus will not supervene if the islands of epithelioid cells are not destroyed, but all the other cells of the pancreas are. He then gave a resumé of the physiological investigations of the thyroid gland and an account of the symptoms following thyroidectomy. Next he considered, surprisingly briefly, the pituitary body, quoting experiments which demonstrated that this gland supplied an internal secretion which caused contraction of the heart's arteries (see also pp. 304, 305 and 343). He then described in detail the role of the supra-renal bodies, referring to Addison's disease, as well as to the experiments of Brown-Séquard and others; finally, he discussed at length the results of his work with Oliver during the last 2 years, concerning the experiments with extracts of the adrenal medulla. He concluded:

> The general results to which we are led from a consideration of these facts, and others to which I had no time so much as to allude, point strongly in favour of a theory of internal secretions, and it is obvious that such internal secretions may be of no less importance than the better recognized functions of the external secreting glands. These internal secretions have to be definitely reckoned with by the physician, while at the same time the therapeutist will be able to avail himself of the active principles which they contain and in certain cases to use extracts of internally secreting glands in place of the hitherto more commonly employed vegetable medicaments. That the subject has a vast future there can be no doubt, for, in spite of the advances which have been made in elucidating it during the last few years, a great number of points still remain obscure. Nevertheless, the way which the physiologist has attempted to show may be followed by the practitioner, and the result of these physiological experiments may now be utilised for the diagnosis and treatment of disease.

The following comments seem appropriate. It was 2 years after the first communication with Oliver on their work on adrenal extract that Schaefer decided to make 'internal secretion' a recognized term in physiology and, therefore, in medicine. Thus, this term, presented by Claude Bernard on 9 January 1855 had come of age 40 years later. Secondly, and this seems even more important, Schaefer extended the meaning of internal secretion far beyond the field of ductless glands, and made it applicable to every organ of the body; this is a fact which seems to have been occasionally overlooked by some observers during the first quarter of the 20th century. His discussion on the role of the liver and the kidneys in particular, as organs with an internal as well as an external secretion, deserves our full attention. The role of the pancreas and especially of the epithelial islet cells are presented in an almost prophetic manner, considering that he knew of von Mering and Minkowski's and of Schiff's experiments, but Opie's work was not carried out until 1900 and Ssobolew's until 1902! He quotes Schiff's ingenious method (in 1872), repeating Claude Bernard's earlier experiments, without the risk of the major operation which killed the dogs. Schiff injected paraffin into the duct of Wirsung: the dogs survived and remained perfectly healthy, without any wasting.

It is also remarkable that Schaefer, who proved himself to be such a lucid analyst and forecaster, refused to recognize the endocrine function of the gonads, in spite of the fact that the work of John Hunter, Berthold, von Baer, von Koelliker and others was available. In particular, Schaefer knew of the main works of Brown-Séquard and d'Arsonval. Was he perhaps so antagonistic to Brown-Séquard's flamboyant personality and methods as to be almost allergic to his work? Or was it an Englishman's subconscious dislike of focussing the limelight on sex? Perhaps his contemporary, Sigmund Freud (1856–1939) would have had something to say about that! (Joseph Breuer's, 1842–1925, and Sigmund Freud's first book on hysteria with the revelation of the 'unconscious mind' was published in 1895[188].) Be it as it may, the fact that a man of Schaefer's stature publicly entered the field of the scientific study of endocrinology, gave an enormous stimulus to the subject. As Borell succinctly puts it[189]:

> He was then forty-five years old, Jodrell Professor of Physiology at University College, a Fellow of the Royal Society, and an active member of the Physiological Society. With his sanction, internal secretion became a problem of increasing importance to British physiologists.

Borell also notes that it was

> significant that he did not comment on the numerous clinical studies which had been made with testicular and ovarian extracts. It is curious that he did not suggest the possibility of further study of sex glands' physiology by means of experimental grafts. He simply dismissed the idea that the sex glands produced internal secretion.

Moreover, Schaefer was quite prepared to argue that the theory was untenable that the effects of removal of the thyroid were caused by damage to the neighbouring nervous structures in the neck. "But this, as in the similar theory propounded to account for the effects of the extirpation of the pancreas, is absolutely negatived by the results of thyroid grafting"[190]. Yet, in the same address, Schaefer had pronounced that on removal of the generative glands, the marked alterations in the development of other parts were produced "without doubt" through the nervous system and are not connected with the internal secretion of the glands, in ignorance of, or deliberately

337

ignoring John Hunter's and Berthold's transplant experiments. On the other hand, we must remember that in 1867 Obolensky had recorded that the testicle atrophied on cutting the spermatic nerve[191] and Steinach thought in 1894 that sensory nerve impulses in the maturing testis caused the sexual activity of male frogs in the breeding season[192]. We have also seen that Nussbaum thought – as late as 1905 – that secretions from the transplanted testicle acted via the central nervous system[193].

Virchow and Pflueger assumed that the mechanism of the menstrual cycle is based on reflexes[194].

The reproduction of Schaefer's address in *The Lancet* was also noteworthy. A number of major topics were presented by the editors as short extracts only; for example: "Professor Schaefer here considered the various theories which have been put forward as to the function of the pancreas as an internally secreting organ, and went on to say. . ."[195]. Miss Borell rightly poses the question, what had changed? "Why did Schaefer raise the notion of internal secretion to the status of a theory?"[6]. There was no difference from the views propounded by Brown-Séquard and d'Arsonval in 1891. Yet, there was. Formerly, mainly the clinicians observed the effect of deficiency of certain organs due to disease (Addison, Murray, Brown-Séquard) and the treatment of such deficiencies by means of organ extracts; similarly, the surgeons noted the results of extirpation of certain organs and the prevention of dangerous or fatal sequels by organ transplants and injections of extracts. But now the physiologists had stepped in. They studied the effects of organ extracts scientifically in controlled experiments in their laboratories, which were measurable by well established scientific methods and could be compared with the effects of well-known drugs. Moreover, very soon the physiological chemist would succeed in isolating the active substance of organ extracts and then synthetize them and produce them in crystalline form. Thus, the characteristics of potency, pharmacological effects and side effects of all tissue extracts could be assessed and measured, to the great benefit of the study of animal and human physiology and of diagnostic and curative medicine. Borell summed it up: "This was rational, scientific medicine"[6]. She was, indeed, so impressed with Schaefer's contribution, that she added another paper to the subject: 'Setting the standards for a new science: Edward Schäfer and endocrinology'[196], in which she considered "Schaefer's role in the emergence of the new field of endocrinology" and emphasized his contributions to the establishment of scientific medicine in Britain. This became even more important when he had to be not only a leader of the new development but also to act as its critic, to keep some control of an over-enthusiastic application of the new science.

Borell points out that "Sir Edward Sharpey-Schaefer (as he called himself after the war of 1914–18), later emphasized the changed perception of the central problem of his profession by calling this the 'New Physiology'"[197]. According to Schaefer's argument 'The Old Physiology',

> was based, as we have seen, on *nervous regulation*; the New Physiology is based on *chemical regulation*[197]. . . . The changes of physiology which have resulted from this knowledge constitute *not merely an advance in degree but an alteration in character*. The doctrine of internal secretion forms a new departure. We must in future explain physiological changes in terms of chemical regulation as well as of nervous regulation[198].

This last sentence appears almost – perhaps subconsciously – prophetic, to the present writer. The perspective of the 'newest' physiology is certainly one of neuro-chemical transmission and some of the modern terms like 'neuro-endocrinology' appear, perhaps, less new, if one reads again those addresses given 40 to 50 years ago.

The 'Birth of Endocrinology' was a long drawn-out procedure: it was another 15 years before its physiological and biochemical fundaments became established. Moreover, with the rapidly increasing body of knowledge, the fast expanding field changes from the mechanism of the regulation of metabolism to that of the mechanism of cellular communication by means of chemical messengers[6]. Far beyond that, the newly developing science of genetics entered the field and expanded it even further. Thus, the clinicians and physiologists were soon joined by the embryologists, biochemists, and even physicists (e.g. Erwin Schroedinger's lectures on 'What is Life'[199]), philosophers and sociologists (on problems of fertility and contraception), not to forget the psychiatrists and neurologists. Even the historians attempted to explain the events of history due to endocrine causes: Louis XVI's alleged hypothyroidism, Napoleon's Froehlich's disease affecting his paternity, and even the outcome of the Battle of Waterloo, and many other events (we have already discussed the role of the eunuchs in ancient Egypt, in the Imperial Service of ancient China, in the Civil Service of the Byzantine and later of the Ottoman empires).

HORMONES

In the decade following Schaefer's address of August 1895, there first occurred new developments brought about by the work of (Sir) William Maddock Bayliss (1860–1924) and Ernest Henry Starling

(1866–1927) (see Section II), both friends, associates and followers of Schaefer and his collaborators at the Department of Physiology at University College in London. When Schaefer (1850–1935) moved to Edinburgh in 1899 (where he remained until 1933), he was succeeded by Starling. One of Starling's closest collaborators, Bayliss, referred to him as "My Fellow-Worker", but they were also brothers-in-law.

Bayliss and Starling were investigating the manner by which the pancreas was excited to activity, when they became aware that the chemical agent concerned, to which they had given the name 'secretin', was one of a class of substances of which others had been known. They found that a crude extract of duodenal mucosa injected into the blood stream of an experimental animal excited pancreatic secretion[200, 201]. The main characteristic of this group of substances was that they were produced in one organ, then carried by the blood to another organ, on which their effect became manifest. Their first experiment was carried out on 16 January 1902. In 1927, (Sir) Charles Martin, described the scene[227]:

> I happened to be present at their discovery. In an anaesthetized dog a loop of jejunum was tied at both ends and the nerves supplying it dissected out and divided so that it was connected with the rest of the body only by its blood vessels. On the introduction of some weak HCl into the duodenum, secretion from the pancreas occurred and continued for some minutes. After this had subsided a few cubic centimetres of acid were introduced into the denervated loop of duodenum. To our surprise a similarly marked secretion was produced. I remember Starling saying 'Then it must be a chemical reflex'. Rapidly cutting off a further piece of jejunum he rubbed its mucous membrane with sand and weak HCl, filtered and injected it into the jugular vein of the animal. After a few moments the pancreas responded by a much greater secretion than had occurred before. It was a great afternoon.

Such substances, which include adrenaline and other internal secretions, serve as chemical messengers, by means of which the activity of certain organs is co-ordinated with that of others. This co-ordinating system via the blood exists alongside that of the nervous system; there is also a direct link between the two systems forming the base of a neuro-humoral or neuro-endocrine system throughout the body. The already existing term of 'internal secretion' did not sufficiently cover their nature and function as 'messengers' or 'guide-messengers'. Nor did it permit the wider view, that such functions are not limited to 'glands', be it glands with both external and internal secretion, or to glands with internal secretion only, but to all organs of the body, to every tissue and, in fact, every cell. This

340

was merely to confirm de Bordeu's hypothesis of 1775, re-stated by Brown-Séquard in 1891; moreover, phylogenetically, chemical control occurs earlier than nervous control in the animal kingdom, but reflex action was recognized long before the concept of internal secretion was understood. René Descartes (1596–1650) recognized it in man in 1649 (Des passions de l'âme, see also p. 130), Robert Boyle (1627–1691) in a decapitated viper, Johann Bohn (1640–1718) of Leipzig, in a decapitated frog[202]. Bohn showed that the nerves do not contain a 'nerve juice'. Georg Prochaska (1749–1820) of Prag and Vienna, assumed that reflexes operate directly through the ganglia and anastomosing nerve filaments by means of direct and psychic stimuli of the 'ascending nerves' to be reflected (reflectendae) from the 'sensorium commune' (see also p. 213). It was rediscovered by Marshall Hall (1790–1857)[203] who invented the term 'reflex action'. Independently, Johannes Mueller (1807–1858) of Berlin regarded the discovery of reflex action as an "epoch-making advance".

Pavlov had regarded the secretion of pancreatic juice as a reflex from the duodenal mucous membrane (Ivan Petrovitch Pavlov, 1849–1936[204]), until Bayliss and Starling proved that duodenal mucosa 'secretin' specifically stimulates the pancreas. Later Dale and George Howard Parker (1864–?)[205, 206] concluded that the control of the vegetative parts of the body in the animal kingdom may be nervous or humoral, which mechanisms may be alternative or combined. Z. M. Bacq of Belgium, who worked with Sir Henry Dale and with Walter Bradford Cannon (1871–1945), wrote Les Transmissions Chimiques de l'Influx Nerveux[207], which was translated into English in 1975 on the occasion of the Sir Henry Dale centenary, under the title of Chemical Transmission of Nerve Impulses – A Historical Sketch; this will be discussed in a later chapter.

After the discovery of 'secretin' and in the course of extensive discussion on the nature of these newly discovered substances, (Sir) William B. Hardy (1864–1934) of Cambridge suggested the name 'hormone', which was first used by Starling in his Croonian Lectures at the Royal College of Physicians of London, On the Chemical Correlation of the Functions of the Body, in June 1905 (see also p. 7), and subsequently in two addresses given in Germany. It has now been universally accepted, but it is occasionally forgotten that the definition of 'hormone' was meant to transcend the definition of secretion from a 'blood-gland' (see Wilhelm Falta)[208] from the onset. Although 'secretin' had proved very important in the progress of scientific thought about hormones, Bayliss and Starling did not succeed in isolating it. We know now that it is a polypeptide of moderate molecular weight, the isolation of which was not possible until very recently. In his Croonian Lectures, Starling said:

These chemical messengers . . . or 'hormones' (from ὁρμάω = I excite or arouse), as we may call them, have to be carried from the organ where they are produced to the organ which they affect, by means of the blood stream, and the continually recurring physiological needs of the organism must determine their repeated production and circulation through the body.

In this context it is important, however, to quote Hermann Zondek's (1887–1979), of Berlin and Jerusalem, observation, when discussing hormones:

One of the peculiarities of the hormones is the *minute quantity* needed to cause marked *generalized effects*. How minute these amounts are may be inferred from animal experiments. Thus millionfold and even higher dilutions of thyroxine notably accelerate the metamorphosis of tadpoles, and even 1 in 5,000 millions of thyroxine causes some acceleration of their metamorphosis and inhibition of growth (Romeis). The human body, too, undoubtedly produces very important cellular processes by means of minute quantities of hormones. . . . The fact indicates that the hormone acts as a catalyst. *It is an organic catalyst*; together with the other regulative forces acting upon the cell surface, *it directs the cell's function, regulates its intensity, and links up the functional activities of different organs, thus ensuring a harmonious functional performance*. The importance of the last-named function, i.e., the power of the hormones to act upon *many regions of the body* should be specially stressed; it is manifested in the action of thyroxine, pituitrin and probably insulin. In contrast with other catalysts, e.g., the ferments, the catalytic action of the hormones seems to depend upon the *intact condition of cellular* structure. They appear to influence especially the physical forces acting on the cell, viz., permeability, adsorption, absorption, etc. We therefore regard the hormone as a *physical catalyst*[209].

As Borell says, the rejuvenation studies of first Brown-Séquard in the 1890s, and later of Eugen Steinach (1861–1944) by ligation of the vas deferens[210] in the 1910s, and later still by Serge Voronoff (1866–1951) by testicular transplants[211] in the 1920s had surprisingly little visible impact on the direction of British endocrinology.

Under the leadership of Schaefer and his younger colleagues, Bayliss, J. N. Langley, J. S. Haldane, C. S. Sherrington, F. G. Hopkins and Benjamin Moore, the co-ordination of physiological events by means of chemical messengers or hormones, that is, the active principles of the internal secretions, became a problem of fundamental concern to physiologists, and the rational control of physiological events remained the goal of scientific medicine. From 1904, no less an organization than the British Association for the

Advancement of Science began to provide research grants for the study of internal secretions. The chairman of the Committee on the Ductless Glands was Schaefer; the secretary, his former student and assistant Swale Vincent (1868–1933). Over one-quarter of all British Association funds allocated for research in physiology during the years 1904–1920 were granted for such studies[196]. It has to be noted, however, that Schaefer's approach remained so conservative that – as late as 1908 – he maintained that the anterior lobe of the pituitary had no physiological effect[70]. Borell continues: "As such, Schaefer was able to remain an advocate for endocrinology during what Hans Lisser has called the years of drought" (see p. 379). Accordingly, in Britain, social problems bordering on endocrine knowledge, such as eugenics, birth control, and sexual behaviour did not influence the progress of endocrinology until the end of the 1920s. As to the role of Swale Vincent, his controversy with Starling and the crisis in endocrinology in Britain in the early 1920s, we shall discuss the position in Chapter 18.

Meanwhile, the study of endocrinology progressed elsewhere too. We have already discussed Ssobolew's fundamental experiment on the islands of Langerhans[212], and Naunyn's monograph (see p. 297) on diabetes. Jôkicki Takamine (1834–1922) isolated adrenaline as "The blood-pressure-raising principle of the suprarenal glands" in 1901[213]. Independently of Takamine – who had previously worked in Abel's laboratory – Thomas Bell Aldrich (1861–?) succeeded in isolating adrenaline in a crystalline form ($C_9H_{13}NO_3$) (=laevomethylamine–ethanol–catechol)[214]. Adrenaline was thus the first hormone to be isolated, fulfilling one of Doisy's essential criteria of hormone investigation: preparation of active extracts, isolation, synthesis. Synthesis was achieved by Friedrich Stolz in 1904[215]. The granules in the cells of the adrenal medulla were, after Henle's (1809–1885) and P. Manasse's staining experiments, later called 'chromaffin', 'chromophil', or 'phaeochrome' cells, because they stained with chromaffine salts[216].

Eugène Gley (1857–1930) (see Section II) re-discovered the parathyroids[217]. Only later did he come across Sandstroem's first description. Gley's path of research was, however, not smooth then, nor later. He removed the two parathyroids then known in animals, without any fatal effect; he then removed the thyroid without causing death. He observed that after thyroidectomy the 'parathyroids' became hypertrophic and showed histological changes, their tissue resembling the thyroid. Accordingly, he drew the conclusion that the parathyroids were potential thyroid tissue. He was opposed by Giulio Vassale (1862–1912) and Francesco Generali ('Sugli effeti dell estirpazione delle ghiandole paratiroide')[218, 219], who showed that removal of the parathyroids is followed by tetany, whereas removal of the thyroid is followed by myxoedema. Moreover, Walter Edmunds (1850–1930) showed that after thyroidectomy the parathyroid did not become thyroid tissue[220], an idea which was later abandoned also by Gley and his collaborators. Later, D. A. Welsh[221], William Stewart Halsted[222] (1852–1922), and Artur Biedl (1869–1933)[223] carried out experimental parathyroidectomy. They proved that the complete removal of all parathyroid tissue led to severe tetany with fatal outcome. Kohn in 1899 and 1900 established the anatomical independence of the parathyroids, which he called 'Epithelkoerperchen', a name which is still popular in German-speaking countries[224, 225]. But Swale Vincent and W. A. Jolly found in 1905 that accessory parathyroid tissue is common in some animals, often embedded in the thymus, which modifies attempted parathyroidectomy and prevents 'tetania parathyreopriva'[226].

REFERENCES

1. Brown-Séquard, C. É.: Expérience démontrant la puissance dynamogénique chez l'homme d'un liquide extrait de testicules d'animaux. Arch. Physiol. Norm. Pathol. **5**, sér. 1, 651–658, 1889.
2. Brown-Séquard, C. É.: Arch. Physiol. Norm. Pathol. **5e**, sér. **1**, 739–746, 1889.
3. Borell, Merriley: Brown-Séquard's organotherapy and its appearance in America at the end of the nineteenth century. Bull. Hist. Med. **50** (3), 309–320, 1976.
4. Brown-Séquard, C. É.: C. R. Hebd. sèance. Mêm. Biol. **9**, sér. **1**, 415–419, 1889.
5. Annotation: Br. Med. J. **1**, 1416, 1889.
6. Borell, M.: Organotherapy, British physiology and discovery of internal secretions. J. Hist. Biol. **9**, (2), 236–268, 1976.
7. Br. Med. J. **1**, 451–454, 1889.
8. As 6: p. 238.
9. Waterhouse, W. D.: Report of the Clinical Evening of the Harveian Society, 7th Jan. 1891. Br. Med. J. **1**, 229, 1892.
10. Murray, George R.: Note on the treatment of myxoedema by hypodermic injections of an extract of the thyroid gland of a sheep. Br. Med. J. **2**, 796–797, 1891.
11. Brown-Séquard, C. É. and d'Arsonval, Arsène: De l'injection des extraits liquides provenant des glandes et des tissues de L'organisme comme méthode thérapeutique. C.R. Soc. Biol. 9 sér., **3**, 248–250, 1891.
12. Eiselsberg, Anton von: Ueber erfolgreiche Einheilung der Katzenschilddruese in die Bauchdecke u. Auftreten von Tetanie nach deren Exstirpation. Wien. Klin. Wochenschr. **5**, 81–85, 1892.
13. Bircher, H.: Samml. Klin. Vortraege, Leipzig (Chir. No. 110), 3393, 1900.
14. Fenwick, H. and Collins, W. J.: Lancet **1**, 1003, 1891.

15. Wright, J. A.: Lancet **1**, 609, 1892.
16. MacPherson, J.: Edin. Med. J. **37**, 1021, 1891–1892.
17. Kocher, Albert: Br. Med. J. **2**, 560, 1923.
18. Murray, G. R.: Br. Med. J. **2**, 797, 1891.
19. Murray, G. R.: Br. Med. J. **1**, 359, 1920.
20. Murray, G. R.: Br. Med. J. **2**, 136, 1934.
21. Fenwick, H.: Lancet **2**, 941, 1892.
22. Mackenzie, Hector: Br. Med. J. **2**, 940, 1892.
23. Fox, E. L.: Br. Med. J. **2**, 941, 1892.
24. Howitz, F.: Br. Med. J. **1**, 266, 1893.
25. Gley, Eugène: Note préliminaire sur les effets physiologiques du suc de diverses glandes et en particulier du suc extraits de la glande thyroide. C.R. Soc. Biol. 9 sér., **3**, 250–251, 1891.
26. The treatment of myxoedema. Br. Med. J. **2**, 965, 1892.
27. Charcot, Jean Martin: Myxoedème, cachexie pachydermique en état crétinoide. Gaz. Hôp. No. 10, 1891.
28. Harley, V.: Br. Med. J. **2**, 452–454, 1892.
29. Murray, G. R.: Br. Med. J. **2**, 449, 1892.
30. White, W. H.: The treatment of diabetes mellitus by means of pancreatic juice. Br. Med. J. **1**, 63–64, 1893.
31. White, Wm. Hale: Br. Med. J. **1**, 452–453, 1893.
32. Mering, Joseph von: Ueber d. experimentellien Diabetes. Verh. Congr. Inn. Med. **5**, 185–189, 1886.
33. Frerichs, F. Th.: Ueber d. Diabetes. Berlin, 1884.
34. Mering, J. von and Minkowski, O.: Arch. Exp. Pathol. Pharmakol. **26**, 371–387, 1890.
35. Naunyn, B.: Der Diabetes Mellitus. Wien, A. Hoelder, 1898.
36. Cited from Young, F. G.: Ideas about Animal Hormones, p. 137, in The Chemistry of Life (ed. Needham, J.) London, 1970.
37. Opie, E. L.: J. Exp. Med. **5**, 397; 527–540, 1900/1901.
38. Ssobolew, Leonid Wassilyevitch: Die Bedeutung der Langerhans'-schen Inseln. Virchows Arch. Pathol. Anat. **168**, 91–128, 1902.
39. MacCallum, William George: On the relation of the Islands of Langerhans to glycosuria. Johns Hopkins. Hosp. Bull. **20**, 265–268, 1909.
40. Rondelet, G.: Methodus curandorum omnium morborum corporis humani in tres libros distincta. Lugd, apud G. Ronillium, 1576.
41. Lusk, G.: Metabolism in Diabetes. Harvey Lecture (1908–09) pp. 69–96, 1910.
42. Brown-Séquard, C. É.: On a new therapeutic method consisting in the use of organic liquids extracted from glands and other organs. Br. Med. J. **2**, 1145–1147; 1212–1214, 1893.
43. Ibid.: p. 1213.
44. Leading Article: Animal extracts as therapeutic agents. Br. Med. J. **1**, 1279, 1893.
45. Brown-Séquard, C. É.: C.R. Soc. Biol. **9**, sér. **3**, 535–536; 722–725, 1891.
46. Brown-Séquard, C. É.: Arch. Physiol. Norm. Pathol. **5**, sér. **1**, 730–746, 1889.
47. Dunbar, Newall (ed.): Boston, J. G. Cupples Co., 1889.
48. Delhoume, Léon: De Claude Bernard à d'Arsonval, p. 350. Paris, J. B. Baillière, 1939.
49. Evans, Herbert: Present position of our knowledge of anterior pituitary function. J. Am. Med. Assoc. **101**, 425–432, 1933.
50. Rolleston, Sir H. D.: The Endocrine Organs in Health and Disease with an Historical Review, p. 44, p. 80 etc. London, Oxford University Press, 1936.

51. Rathke, M. H.: Arch. Anat. Physiol. Wiss. Med., Berlin 482–485, 1838.
52. Balfour, F. M.: Q. J. Microsc. Sci. Lond. **14**, 362, 1874.
53. Mihalkovics, G. V.: Anarch. Mikrosk. Anat., Bonn **11**, 389, 1875.
54. Lups, T.: Anat. Anz., Jena **67**, 161, 1929.
55. Santorini, G. D.: Observationes Anatomicae, p. 70. Venetis, apud J. B. Recurti, 1724.
56. Howell, Wm. H.: J. Exp. Med. **3**, 245, New York, 1898.
57. Mueller, W.: Jenaische Z. Med. Naturwiss. **6**, 354, 1871.
58. Duret, H.: Arch. Physiol. norm. pathol., Paris et **16**, 73, 1874.
59. Popa, G. and Fielding, V.: J. Anat. **65**, 88, Cambridge, 1930.
60. Killian, G.: Morphol. Jahrb. **14**, 718, 1888.
61. Erdheim, Jakob: Beitr. Pathol. Anat. Allg. Pathol. **46**, 233, 1909.
62. Hannover, A. H.: Recherches Microscopiques sur le Système Nerveux, p. 26, 1844.
63. Lothringer, S.: Arch. Mikrosk. Anat., Bonn **23**, 257, 1886.
64. Dostoiewsky, A.: Arch. Mikrosk. Anat., Bonn **26**, 592, 1885/6.
65. Schoenemann, A.: Virchow's Arch. **129**, 310, 1892.
66. Luschka, H. von: Der Hirnanhang u.d. Steissdruese d. Menschen, Berlin, 1860.
67. Comte, L.: Beitr. Pathol. Anat. Allg. Pathol. **23**, 90, 1898.
68. Tandler, J. and Gross, S.: Arch. Entw. Mech. **54**, 157, 1934.
69. Evans, H. M. and Long, J. A.: Anat. Record. **21**, 62, 1921.
70. Schaefer, E. A. and Herring, P. Th.: Philos. Trans. R. Soc. Lond. B., **199**, 1, 1908.
71. Wepfer, J. J.: Observationes anatomicae, ex cadaveribus eorum, quos sustulit apoplexia. Schaffhusii, J. C. Suteri, 1658.
72. Wepfer, J. J.: Observations anatomicae ex Cadaveribus. Amsterdam, 1681.
73. Bonet, Th.: Sepulchretum, sive anatomia ex cadaveribus morbo donatis. Genevae, L. Chouet, 1679.
74. Vieussens, R.: Novum Vasorum Corp. Hum. Systema, p. 242, Amsteradami, 1705.
75. Baillie, M.: The Morbid Anatomy of Some of the Most Important Parts of the Human Body, 2nd ed., p. 451, London, 1797.
76. Verga, A.: Caso Singolare di Prosopectasia. Rendic. 1st di Lombardia, Vol. **1**, p. 111, Milano, 1864.
77. Marie, P. and de Souza-Leite, J. D.: Essays on Acromegaly. London, New Sydenham Society, 1891.
78. Benda, C.: Beitraege zur normalen und pathologischen Histologie der menshlichen Hypophysis Cerebri (=Contributions to the normal and pathological histology of the human pituitary); Berl. Klin. Wschr. **37**, 1205–1210, 1900.
79. Brissaud, E. and Meige, H.: Rev. Sci., Paris, 4 ser, **3**, 575, 1895.
80. As 50: pp. 83–84, 86–87.
81. Saucerotte, Nicolas: Mélanges Chir. **1**, 407–411, 1801.
82. Marie, Pierre: Sur deux cas d'acromégalie. Hypertrophie singulière non congénitale des extrémités supérieures, inférieures et céphaliques. Rev. Méd. **6**, 297–333, 1886.
83. Broca, A.: Arch. Gén. Méd. ii, 663, 1888.
84. Noël,: J. Méd., Chir. Pharmacol. **1**, 225, 1779.
85. Alibert, Baron J. L. M.: Précis théorique et Pratique des Maladies de la Peau, Vol. III, p. 317, Paris, 1822.
86. Henrot, Henri: Notes de Clinique Méd. Rheims, p. 57, 1877.
87. Minkowski, O.: Berl. Klin. Wochenschr. **24**, 371–374, 1887.

87a. Hutchinson, J.: A case of acromegaly. Arch. of Surgery, II, 141–148; 1889–90.
87b. Hutchinson, J.: Three cases of acromegaly, illustrating the stage of premonitory symptoms. Arch. of Surgery, II, 296–298, 1890–91.
88. As 50: p. 81.
89. Sternberg, Max: Spez. Path. Therapie (Nothnagel), Vol. viii, Wien, 1897.
90. Mark, L. P.: Acromegaly. A Personal Experience. London, 1912.
91. As 50: p. 83.
92. Chevalier, T. W.: Lond. Med. Physical. J. **58,** 498, 1827.
93. Lancereaux, É.: Semaine Méd., Paris **15,** 61, 1894.
94. Fritzsche, Ch. F. and Klebs, Th. A. E.: Ein Beitrag zur Pathologie d. Riesenwuchses, Leipzig, 1884.
95. Abderhalden, R.: The Development of Clinical Endocrinology. CIBA Monograph No. 10, pp. 333–358, Bombay, 1951. (Translation by V.C.M.)
96. Launois, P. E. and Roy, P.: Bull, Mém. Soc. Méd. hôp. Paris 3 sét, **20,** 543, 1903.
97. Massalongo, R.: Riforma Med., Napoli, VIII, 74, 1892.
98. Tizard, J. P. M.: J. R. Coll. Physicians, London, **7,** 193–206, 1973.
99. Minkowski, O.: Klin. Wochenschr. **24,** 371–374, 1887.
100. Schiff, A.: Wien. Klin. Wochenschr. **10,** 277–285, 1897.
101. Malcolm, J.: J. Physiol. **30,** 270–280, 1904.
102. Goetsch, Emil: The influence of pituitary feeding upon growth and sexual development. Bull. Johns Hopkins. Hosp. **27,** 29–50, 1916.
103. Sisson, W. R. and Broyles, E. N.: Bull. Johns Hopkins Hosp. **32,** 22–30, 1921.
104. Smith, P. E.: Am. J. Physiol. **81,** 20–26, 1927.
105. Evans, H. M.: in Glandular Physiology and Therapy, p. 59, Chicago, Am. Med. Assoc., 1935.
106. Koenig,: Berlin Kiln Wochenschr. **37,** 1040, 1900.
107. Horsley, Sir Victor: Functional nervous disorders due to loss of thyroid gland and pituitary body. Lancet **2,** 5, 1886.
108. Paulesco, N. C.: L'hypophyse du cerveau. J. Physiol. Path. Gen. **9,** 441–456, 1907.
109. Crowe, J., Cushing, H. W. and Homans, J.: Experimental hypophysectomy. Bull. Johns Hopkins Hosp. **21,** 127–169, 1910.
110. Cushing, H. W.: The functions of the pituitary body. Am. J. Med. Sci. **139,** 473–484; 1910
111. Bell, Wm. B.: Experimental operations on the pituitary. Q. J. Exp. Physiol. **11,** 77–126, 1917.
112. Vassale, G. and Sacchi, E.: Sulla Distruzione della Ghiandola Pituitaria, Riv. Sper. Freniat. **18,** 525–561, 1892.
113. Dale, Sir Henry H.: The action of extracts of the pituitary body. Biochem. J. **4,** 427–447, 1909.
114. Aschner, Bernhard: Ueber die Funktion der Hypophyse. Pfleuger's Arch. Ges. Physiol. **146,** 1–146, 1912.
115. Benda, Carl: Beitraege zur normalen u. pathol. Histologie d. menschlichen Hypophysis cerebri. Berlin Klin Wochenschr. **37,** 1205–1210, 1900.
116. Cushing, H. W.: The Hypophysis Cerebri. J. Am. Med. Assoc. **53,** 250–255, 1909.
117. Ascoli, G. and Legnani, T.: Die Folgen d. Exstirpation d. Hypophyse. Muenchn. med. Wochenschr. **59,** 518–521, 1912.
118. Erdheim, J.: Sitzungsber. Kais. Akad. Wiss., Mathem. Naturwiss. Kl., Wien **113,** 537, 1904.

119. Cruveilhier, Jean: Anatomie pathologique du corps humain. Tom. 1, livre 2, p. 2, Paris, J. B. Baillière, 1829–42.
120. Cushing, H. W.: The Pituitary Body and its Disorders. p. 173, 1912.
121. Babinski, J. F. F.: Rev. Neurol., Paris **8**, 531, 1900.
122. Froehlich, A.: Wien. Klin. Wochenschr. **15**, 883–886; 906–908; 1901.
123. Cushing, Harvey W.: J. Nerv. and Ment. Dis., Chicago **33**, p. 704, 1906.
124. Story, J. B.: Br. Med. J. **1**, 1334, 1887.
125. Mohr, B.: Wochenschr. Ges. Heilk. **6**, 565–571, 1840.
126. Pechkranz, S.: Neurol. Centralbl., Leipzig **18**, 203, 1899.
127. Simmonds, M.: Zwergwuchs bei Atrophie d. Hypophysen Vorderlappens. Munch. med. Wochenschr. **45**, 487–488, 1919.
128. Bramwell, Sir Byrom: Intracranial Tumours, p. 164, London, 1888.
129. Caton, R. and Paul, F. T.: Notes on a case of acromegaly treated by operation. Br. Med. J. **2**, 1421–1423, 1893.
130. Schloffer, H.: Zur Frage d. Operationen an der Hypophyse. Beitr. Klin. Chir. **50**, 767–815, 1906.
131. Schloffer, H.: Erfolgreiche Operation eines hypophysen-tumors auf nasalem Wege. Wien. Klin. Wochenschr. **20**, 621–624, 670–671, 1075–1078, 1907.
132. Hirsch, Oscar: Berl. Klin. Wochenschr. **48**, 1933–35, 1911.
133. Cushing, H. W.: Partial hypophysectomy for acromegaly with remarks on the function of the hypophysis. Ann. Surg. **50**, 1003–1017, 1909.
134. Fulton, J. F.: Harvey Cushing, p. 288. Thomas, Springfield Ill. 1946.
135. Ibid.
136. Tandler, J. and Grosz, S.: Ueber den Einfluss der kastration auf den Organismus. Wien. Klin. Wochenschr. **20**, 1596–1597; 1907.
137. Tandler, J. and Grosz, S.: Untersuchungen an Skopzen, Wien. Klin. Wochenschr. **21**, 277–288, 1908.
138. Erdheim, J. and Stumme, E.: Ueber die Schwangerschaftsveraenderung der Hypophyse. Beitr. Pathol. Anat. Allgem. Pathol. **46**, 1–136, 1909.
139. Rogowitsch, N.: Die Veraenderungen der Hypophyse nach Entfernung der Schilddruese. Beitr. Pathol. Anat. Allgem. **4**, 137, 1889.
140. Gley, E.: Sur les fonctions de la glande thyroide chez le lapin et chez le chien. C.R. Soc. Biol., Paris **43**, 843–847; 1891.
141. Adler Ludwig: Metamorphosenstudien an Batrachierlarven. 1. Exstirpation endokriner Druesen: A. Exstirpation der Hypophyse. Arch. Entwicklungsmech. Organ. **39**, 21–45, 1914.
142. Gudernatsch, J. F.: Arch. Entwicklungsmech. Organ. **35**, 457–483, 1912.
143. White, Hale Wm.: Trans. Clin. Soc. Med., London **18**, 159, 1886.
144. Boyce, R. and Beadles, C. P.: J. Pathol. Bacteriol. Edinburgh **1**, 223, 1893.
145. Nièpce, A.: Goitre et Crétinisme. Paris, 1851.
146. Smith, P. E.: The effect of hypophysectomy in the early embryo upon growth and development of the frog. Anat. Record. **11**, 57–64, 1916.
147. Allen, Bennett M.: The result of extirpation of the anterior lobe of the hypophysis and of the thyroid of Rana Pipiens larvae. Science **44**, 755–757, 1916.
148. Smith, P. E. and Smith, I. P.: The effect of intraperitoneal injection of fresh anterior lobe substance in hypophysectomised tadpoles. Anat. Record. **23**, 38–39, 1922.
149. Smith, P. E. and Smith, I. P.: The repair and activation of the thyroid in the hypophysectomised tadpole by the parenteral administration of fresh anterior lobe of the bovine hypophysis. J. Med. Res. **43**, 267–283, 1922.
150. Allen, B. M.: The relation of the pituitary and thyroid glands of Bufo and Rana to iodine and metamorphosis. Biol. Bull. **36**, 405–417, 1919.

151. Thompson, F. D.: Phil. Trans. R. Soc. London B., **201,** 91, 1910.
152. Schaefer, E.: Address in Physiology: On Internal Secretion. Lancet **2,** 321–324, 1895.
153. Oliver, G. and Schaefer, E.: On the physiological actions of extracts of the pituitary body and certain other glandular organs. J. Physiol. London **18,** 277–279, 1895.
154. Howell, Wm. H.: The physiological effects of the hypophysis cerebri and infundibular body, J. Exp. Med. **3,** 245–258, 1898.
155. Schaefer, E. A. and Vincent, Swale: The physiological effects of extract of pituitary injected intravenously. J. Physiol. London **24,** XIX–XXI, 1899.
156. Ibid: **25,** 87–97, 1899.
157. De Bonis, V. and Susanna, V.: Ueber die Wirkung des Hypophysen-extraktes auf isolierte Blutgefaesse. Zentralbl. Physiol. **23,** 169–175, 1909.
158. Abel, J. J. and Nagayama, T.: J. Pharmacol. Exp. Ther. **15,** 347–399, 1920.
159. Magnus, R. and Schaefer, E. A.: The action of the pituitary extract upon the kidney. J. Physiol. London **27,** IX–X, 1901.
160. Schaefer, E. A. and Herring, P. T.: Phil. Trans. R. Soc., B., **199,** 1–29, 1908.
161. Hoskins, R. G. and Means, W.: The relation of vascular conditions to pituitrin diuresis. J. Pharmacol. Exp. Ther. **4,** 435–441, 1913.
162. Simmonds, Morris: Ueber Hypophysisschwund mit toedlichem Ausgang. Dtsch. Med. Wochenschr. **40,** 322–323, 1914; and Virchow's Arch. Pathol. Anat. **217,** 226–239, 1914.
163. Lichtwitz, L.: Klin. Wochenschr. **1,** 1877, 1922.
164. Glinski, C. K.: Z. Kazuistyki Zmian anatomo-patologicznych w przysada Mózgowej. Przogl. Lek. **4,** 13–14, 1913.
165. Dale, Sir Henry: Br. Med. J. **2,** 451–455, 1948.
166. Oliver, G. and Schaefer, E. A.: Proc. Physiol. Soc., **9,** 1, 1894.
167. Oliver, G. and Schaefer, E. A.: J. Physiol. **16,** i–v, 1894; and **17,** pp. ix–xiv, 1895.
168. Schaefer, E. A.: "Oliver-Sharpey Lectures on the present condition of our knowledge regarding the functions of the suprarenal capsules. Br. Med. J. **2,** 1281, 1908.
169. Bishop, Peter M. F.: The development of British endocrinology. Br. Med. J. **1,** 867, 1955.
170. As 167: p. 1.
171. Orloff, Marshall J.: Diabetes Outlook **13** (7), 2, 1978.
172. Oliver, G. and Schaefer, E. A.: J. Physiol. London **18,** 230–276, 1895.
173. Abel, J. J. and Crawford, A. C.: Johns Hopkins Hosp. Bull. **8,** 151–157, 1897.
174. Szymonowicz, L.: Die Function der Nebenniere. Pflueger's Arch. Ges. Physiol. **64,** 97–164, 1896.
175. As 174: pp. 148–149.
176. Abelous, J. E. and Langlois, J. P.: Note sur les fonctions des capsules surrénales chez les grenouilles. C.R. Soc. Biol., Paris **43,** 793–798, 1891.
177. Abelous, J. E. and Langlois, J. P.: C.R. Soc. Biol. 623, 1892.
178. Martini, Antoine de: Sur un cas d'absence congèniale des capsules surrénales. C.R. Acad. Sci. **43,** 1052–1053, 1856. (An unreliable report – V.C.M.)
179. Biedl. A.: Innere Sekretion. Berlin, Wien, Urban & Schwarzenberg, 1910.
180. Wheeler, T. D. and Vincent, S.: The question as to the relative importance to life of cortex and medulla of the adrenal bodies. Trans. R. Soc. Can. **11,** 125–127, 1917.
181. Hartman, F. A. and Brownell, K. A.: The Adrenal Gland. p. 17. London, H. Kimpton, 1949.

182. Houssay, B. A. and Lewis, J. T.: The relative importance to life of cortex and medulla of the adrenal glands. Am. J. Physiol. **64**, 513–521, 1923.
183. Gaunt, Robert: History of the adrenal cortex, in Handbook of Physiology, Section 7, Endocrinology, Vol. III, Chap. 1, p. 3, 1975.
184. Rogoff, J. M. and Stewart, G. N.: Am. J. Physiol. **84**, 649–659, 1928.
185. Ibid.: **86**, 20–24, 1928.
186. Hartman, F. A.: The general physiology and experimental pathology of the suprarenal glands, in Endocrinology and Metabolism (Ed. Barker, L. F.) Vol. II, p. 119, New York, Appleton, 1922.
187. Fraenkel, F.: Ein Fall von doppelseitigem, voellig latent Verlaufenen Nebennierentumor und gleichzeitiger Nephritis mit Veraenderungen am Circulations – apparat und Nephritis. Virchow's Arch. Pathol. Anat. **103**, 244–263, 1886.
188. Breuder, J. and Freud, S.: Studien ueber Hysterie. Leipzig, Deuticke, 1895.
189. As 6: p. 260.
190. As 152: p. 322.
191. Obolensky, J.: Die Durchschneidung d. Nervus spermaticus u. deren Einfluss auf d. Hoden. Centralbl. Med. Wiss. 497–500, 1867.
192. Steinach, E.: Untersuchungen z. vergleichenden Physiologie d. maennlichen Geschlechtsorgane insbesondere d. accessor. Geschlechtsdruesen. Arch. Ges. Physiol. **56**, 329, 1894.
193. Jørgensen, C. Barker: John Hunter, A. A. Berthold and the origins of endocrinology. Acta. Hist. Scient. Nat. Med., Odense, U.P. **24**, 329, 1971.
194. Ibid.: p. 330.
195. As 152: p. 322.
196. Borell, Merriley: Setting the standards for a new science: Edward Schaefer and endocrinology. Med. Hist. **22**, 282–290, 1978.
197. Sharpey-Schafer, Sir E. A.: in Endocrine Physiology, Irish J. Med. Sci. 6th series, No. 69, pp. 483–505, 484, 1931.
198. Ibid.: p. 505.
199. Schroedinger, E.: What is Life? Cambridge University Press, Cambridge, 1945.
200. Bayliss, W. M. and Starling, E. H.: On the causation of the so-called 'peripheral reflex secretion' of the pancreas. Proc. R. Soc. London **69**, 352–353, 1901/2.
201. Bayliss, W. M. and Starling, E. H.: The mechanism of pancreatic secretion. J. Physiol. **28**, 325–353, 1902.
202. Bohn, J.: Circulus anatomico-physiologicus. Lipsiae, J. F. Gleditsch, 1686.
203. Hall, Marshall: On the reflex function of the medulla oblongata and medulla spinalis. Phil. Trans. **123**, 635–665, 1833.
204. Pavlov, I. P.: Lectures on Conditioned Reflexes, New York, 1928–41.
205. Dale, H. H. and Parker, G. H.: The Elementary Nervous System. Philadelphia, Lippincott, 1919.
206. Dale, H. H. and Parker, G. H.: Humoral Agents in Nervous Activity. Cambridge, 1932.
207. Bacq, Z. M.: Les Transmissions Chimiques de l'Influx Nerveux. Paris, Gauthier-Villars, 1974. (Trans. Chemical Transmission of Nerve Impulses – A Historical Sketch. Pergamon Press, Oxford, 1975.)
208. Falta, W.: The Diseases of the Bloodglands, p. 3, Berlin, Julius Springer, 1913.
209. Zondek, H.: The Diseases of the Endocrine Glands, 4th (2nd English) Edition. London, p. 6, Edward Arnold, 1944.

210. Steinach, E.: Verjuengung durch experimentelle Neubelebung der Alternden Pubertaetsdruese. Berlin, Springer, 1920.
211. Voronoff, S.: Greffes Testiculaires. Paris, O. Doin, 1923.
212. As 38.
213. Takamine, J.: Ther. Gaz. **17,** 221–224, 1901 and Am. J. Pharmacol. **73,** 523–531, 1901.
214. Aldrich, Thos. B.: Am. J. Physiol. **5,** 457–461, 1901.
215. Stolz, Friedrich: Ber. Dtsche. Chem. Ges. **37,** 4149–4154, 1904.
216. Manasse, P.: Virchow's Arch. **135,** 263, 1894.
217. Gley, Eugène: Sur les fonctions du corps thyroide. C.R. Soc. Biol., Paris **43,** 841–847, 1891.
218. Vassale, G. and Generali, F.: Riv. Patol. Nerv. Ment. **1,** 95–99, 1896.
219. Vassale, G. and Generali, F.: Arch. Ital. Biol. xxv, 459, 1895.
220. Edmunds, Walter: Proc. Physiol. Soc., p. xxx; J. Physiol. **18,** 1895.
221. Welsh, D. A.: J. Pathol. Bacteriol. **5,** 20, 1898.
222. Halsted, Wm. S.: Auto- and isotransplantation in dogs of the parathyroid glands. J. Exp. Med. **11,** 175–194, 1909.
223. Biedl, Artur: Zur Aetiologie d. parathyreogenen Tetanie. Ztrbl. Physiol. Pathol. Stoffwechs. No. **11,** 1911.
224. Kohn, A.: Arch. Mikrosk. Anat. Bonn. **49,** 366, 1895.
225. Kohn, A.: Die Epithelkoerperchen. Erg. Anat. Entwick. 1899, 1900.
226. Vincent, Swale and Jolly, W. A.: J. Physiol. **32,** 65, 1905.
227. Martin, C. J.: Obituary. Ernest Henry Starling. Br. Med. J., **1,** 900–905, 1927.
228. Landott, A. M. and Zachmann, M.: The Irish giant: New observations concerning the nature of his ailment. Lancet **1,** 1311–1312, 1980.

CHAPTER SEVENTEEN

THE BIRTH OF ENDOCRINOLOGY – PART III

CONTRACEPTION

WHAT of contraception in the 19th century? Where there existed a need or, indeed, a desire for control of conception, there was a lack of effective prevention; in fact the effectiveness of methods of contraception did not meet expectations. This is proved by the existence of abortion and infanticide in early cultures. Such knowledge of control of conception as existed was certainly not widely diffused and was "the possession essentially of the upper, more privileged classes"[1].

In the 19th century, however, in Western countries, such as England, Germany, and France, contraceptive practices began to become popular and spread rapidly. Industrialization, urban life, greater freedom for women and loss of authority of the churches were greatly responsible for this. It seems that contraceptive practices have been more widespread in Western societies since the beginning of the 19th century than in any major culture before. In 1838, Friedrich Adolph Wilde, a German gynaecologist, published a treatise[2] which stressed the prevention of conception by discussing the indications for contraception and the magical (ineffective) measures – the condom, coitus interruptus, the sponge and the rubber cap. He remarked that the condom would tear easily and that withdrawal was also ineffective. He, therefore, recommended a rubber cervical cap specially moulded to fit each individual woman. This was a fore-runner of the type later used in Dr. Marie Stopes' clinic. Wilde rejected the idea that prevention of conception was immoral, but maintained that it might be more justifiable than a dangerous Caesarean section. Continence, which was usually recommended by physicians of his time as a safe method, may produce great difficulties in maintaining a happily balanced marriage. The cap should be made of rubber ("ein Pessarium aus Resina elastica") without an opening. It shoud be constantly worn by women, who are endangered by pregnancy, and only removed during the period.

One of Wilde's contemporaries, C. A. Weinhold, a German Malthusian, developed some sound ideas on overpopulation but – unfortunately – propagated the cruel method of infibulation, a bizarre male method which was known in ancient Rome.

A modified and simplified cervical cap was eventually used in the United States, where it was made and sold in a few sizes. It was later displaced by the 'diaphragm' of Dr. Wilhelm Peter Johann Mensinga, who wrote in 1891 *Ein Beitrag zum Mechanismus der Conception (Empfaengnis)* (=A contribution to the mechanism of conception)[3]. It was not a cervical cap, but fitted longitudinally into the vagina, the front end under the pubic bone, the distal end in the posterior fornix. Although invented by Mensinga, it was often referred to as the 'Dutch cap', because Dr. Ruttgers and his colleagues in Holland popularized it. Mensinga, originally of Flensburg, on the Danish Border, later became Professor of Anatomy in Breslau. He recommended the use of the diaphragm by discussing the medical indications for contraception at some length. It was first introduced in the early 1880s and its use soon spread to Holland. It was several years before it arrived in England, and it was hardly known in the United States until 1920.

In English, the main writers on contraception between 1823 and 1830 were Francis Place, Richard Carlile, Robert Dale Owen, and Dr. Charles Knowlton. They all considered its social implications – underlying the 19th-century thought on contraception were the social and economic desirability. Francis Place (1771–1854), an English workman who became a friend of Thomas Wakley, the founder and first editor of *The Lancet*, published in 1822 his 'Illustrations and Proofs of the Principle of Population'. This was "the first treatise on population in English to propose contraceptive measures as a substitute for Malthus' 'moral restraint'"[1]. Incidentally, Malthus' "moral restraint" did not imply restriction of intercourse in marriage, but postponement of marriage until the couple were able to support expected offspring. Place followed this with the dissemination of handbills on contraception in working-class districts. The later drafts of these handbills refer only to the use of the sponge and – as an alternative – a tampon of lint, fine wool, cotton, flax or whatever may be at hand. Curiously, no legal procedure was taken against Place's handbills. Place himself said that he had "taken pains

TO
THE MARRIED OF BOTH SEXES
IN
Genteel Life.
⚬●●●⚬

AMONG the many sufferings of married women, as mothers, there are two cases which command the utmost sympathy and commiseration.

The first arises from constitutional peculiarities, or weaknesses.

The second from mal-conformation of the bones of the Pelvis.

Besides these two cases, there is a third case applicable to both sexes: namely, the consequences of having more children than the income of the parents enables them to maintain and educate in a desirable manner.

The first named case produces miscarriages, and brings on a state of existence scarcely endurable. It has caused thousands of respectable women to linger on in pain and apprehension, till at length, death has put an end to their almost inconceivable sufferings.

The second case is always attended with immediate risk of life. Pregnancy never terminates without intense suffering, seldom without the death of the child, frequently with the death of the mother, and sometimes with the death of both mother and child.

The third case is by far the most common, and the most open to general observation. In the middle ranks, the most virtuous and praiseworthy efforts are perpetually made to keep up the respectability of the family; but a continual increase of children gradually yet certainly renders every effort to prevent degradation unavailing, it paralizes by rendering hopeless all exertion, and the family sinks into poverty and despair. Thus is engendered and perpetuated a hideous mass of misery.

The knowledge of what awaits them deters vast numbers of young men from marrying and causes them to spend the best portion of their lives in a state of debauchery, utterly incompatible with the honourable and honest feelings which should be the characteristic of young men. The treachery, duplicity, and hypocrisy, they use towards their friends and the unfortunate victims of their seductions, while they devote a large number of females to the most dreadful of all states which human beings can endure extinguishes in them to a very great extent, all manly, upright notions; and qualifies them to as great an extent, for the commission of acts which but for these vile practices they would abhor, and thus to an enormous extent is the whole community injured.

Marriage in early life, is the only truly happy state, and if the evil consequences of too large a family did not deter them, all men would marry while young, and thus would many lamentable evils be removed from society.

A simple, effectual, and safe means of accomplishing these desirable results has long been known, and to a considerable extent practised in some places. But until lately has been but little known in this country. Accoucheurs of the first respectability and surgeons of great eminence have in some peculiar cases recommended it. Within the last two years, a more extensive knowledge of the process has prevailed and its practice has been more extensively adopted. It is now made public for the benefit of every body. A piece of soft sponge about the size of a small ball attached to a very narrow ribbon, and slightly moistened (when convenient) is introduced previous to sexual intercourse, and is afterwards withdrawn, and thus by an easy, simple, cleanly and not indelicate method, no ways injurious to health, not only may much unhappiness and many miseries be prevented, but benefits to an incalculable amount be conferred on society.

Figure 61 Place's handbill

in my inquiry on this subject . . . amongst surgical and medical (as well as) amongst intelligent elderly women . . . ".

Richard Carlile, one of Place's most ardent pupils, followed in 1826 with the publication of *Every Woman's Book; or, What is Love?*[5] Although, according to Himes, there was no obvious effect of these propaganda measures on the English birthrate, it was certainly part of the new type of thought on population problems[4].

In the United States this new thought on birth control was represented by Robert Dale Owen and Charles Knowlton. In 1830 Owen published the *Moral Physiology*, the first small book to be published in America on birth control. At the time of Owen's death

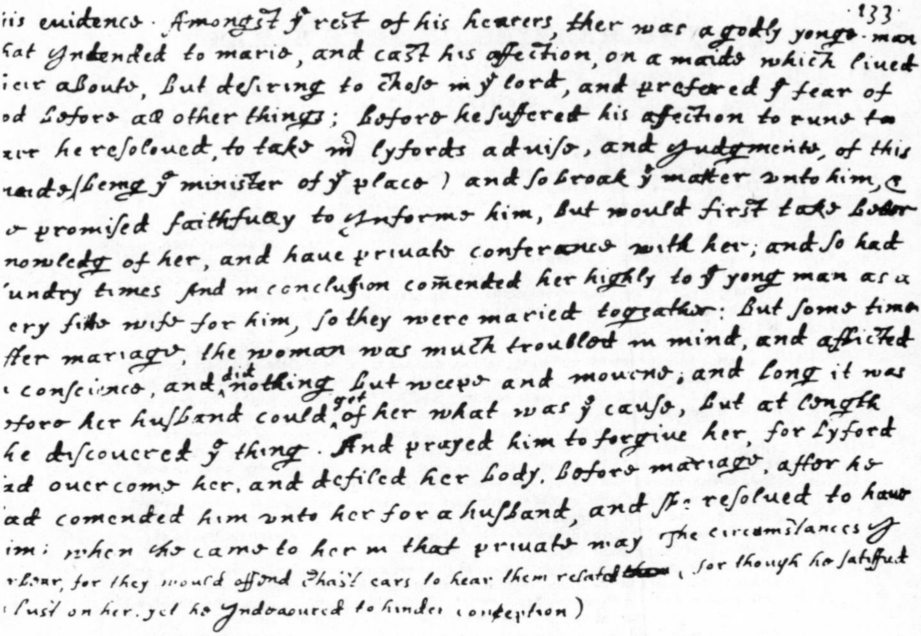

133

his euidence. Amongst y rest of his hearers, ther was a godly yonge man
sat yntended to marie, and cast his afection, on a maide which liued
icir abouts, but desiring to those m y lord, and prefered y fear of
od before all other things; before he suffered his afection to runs to
xce he resolued, to take m Lyfords aduise, and judgments, of this
mids (being y minister of y place) and so break y mater vnto him, e
o promised faithfuly to informe him, but would first take better
nowledg of her, and haue priuate conferance with her; and so had
undry times and in conclusion comended her highly to y yong man as a
ery fitte wife for him, so they were maried togeather: But some time
fter mariage, the woman was much troulled in mind, and afflicted
i conscience, and did nothing but weepe and mourne; and long it was
ifore her husband could got of her what was y cause, but at length
he discouered y thing. And prayed him to forgiue her, for Lyford
ad ouercome her, and defiled her body, before mariage, affter he
ad comended him vnto her for a husband, and [He] resolued to haue
im: when she came to her in that priuate way. The circumstances y
vliar, for they would offend chaist cars to hear them related, for though he satisfied
lust on her, yet he yndeauoured to hinder conception)

Figure 62 Governor Bradford's MS

in 1877, 75 000 copies had been sold in England and America. The main method recommended by him was coitus interruptus. Himes produced interesting documentary evidence from Governor Bradford's manuscript ['(History) of Plimmoth Plantation (Colony)'; Date 1630–1650; Source: Original Manuscript on Deposit in State House Library, Boston, Mass.] that the Puritan forefathers were acquainted with coitus interruptus[1].

Dr. Charles Knowlton's (1800–1850) treatise was first published anonymously in New York in 1832: *By a Physician, The Fruits of Philosophy, or the private companion of young married people*. Later editions had additions by other authors. His book was the most complete on the subject, at his time and place. The main method he recommended was douching, solutions of alum and of astringent vegetables, white oak bark, green tea, etc. As a general rule, "a solution of saleratus (sodium bicarbonate), is the best and most convenient thing to use". In his opinion, these methods were cheap, harmless, caused no sterility and meant no sacrifice during intercourse; above all, control remained in the hands of the woman, where it ought to be. *Fruits of Philosophy* went through numerous editions until 1877, in the United States and in England, until

Charles Bradlaugh and Mrs. Annie Besant succeeded in winning a test case (1877–1879) and vindicated the right of publication. A trial of the elderly Free-thought publisher, Edward Truelove of London, for re-issuing Owen's *Moral Physiology* was less successful. He was sentenced to 4 months in prison. However, the circulation of the *Fruits of Philosophy*, which was *ca*. 1000 copies per year before the trial, increased to 185 000 during the next 3½ years (to August, 1881)! At the same time, French and Dutch editions were printed. Next, the Knowlton pamphlet was replaced by Mrs. Besant's *Law of Population; its Consequences and its Bearing upon the Human Conduct and Morals*[6]. In the one hundred and ten thousandth copy of the *Law of Population* she modified her advice on technique, recommending as most reliable the soluble pessary, the cervical cap and the sponge soaked in a solution of 20 grains of quinine in water, and a douche of quinine in the morning before removing the cap.

In 1854, Dr. George Drysdale published the *Elements of Social Science*, "a radical treatise on sex education, critical of the institution of marriage, warmly advocating the principles of Malthusianism and of classical political economy"[7]. At the time he wrote the book, the full title of which was: *The Elements of Social Science; or physical, sexual and natural religion. An exposition of the true cause and only cure of the three primary social evils: poverty, prostitution and celibacy*, he was a student of medicine. He mentioned five techniques: the sponge; its combination with a douche of tepid water; the 'sterile period' (2 days before the period and 8 days after); withdrawal, which he regarded as physically injurious; and the sheath, which he thought unaesthetic and which "dulled enjoyment".

INFERTILITY AND THE MENSTRUAL CYCLE

The study of infertility, especially in women, received new impetus. It had become obvious that the problem must be approached on a more scientific basis. The recommendation of Boerhave's pupil, (Baron) Gerard L. B. van Swieten (1700–1772) to Maria Theresa might have been based on sound practical experience, when she at first did not become pregnant after her marriage to Francis of Lorraine (later Emperor Francis of Germany): "Ceterum censeo vulvam Sanctissimae Majestatis ante coitum esse titillandam", because she produced afterwards sixteen children, but it took nearly another hundred years, before a major step forward was made.

James Marion Sims (1813–1883), the surgeon and gynaecologist who dominated the American scene from the middle of the century onwards, published in 1866 his *Clinical Notes on Uterine Surgery, with*

Special Reference to the Management of the Sterile Condition[8]. In it, he not only described the duck-bill speculum which he invented[9], but also gave a remarkably accurate description of the fertile period in relation to the menstrual cycle[10]. Sims wrote the book in Paris, where he lived at the time in voluntary exile, because of the Civil War. The book is based on his answers to the question: "What are the conditions essential to Conception?"

(1) It occurs only during menstrual life.
(2) Menstruation should be such as to show a healthy state of the uterine cavity.
(3) The os and cervix uteri should be sufficiently open to permit the free exit of the menstrual flow, and also admit the ingress of the spermatozoa.
(4) The cervix should be of proper form, shape, size and density.
(5) The uterus should be in normal position, i.e. neither ante-verted, nor retro-verted to any great degree.
(6) The vagina should be capable of receiving and retaining the spermatic fluid.
(7) Semen, with living spermatozoa, should be deposited in the vagina at the proper time.

The secretions of the cervix and vagina should not poison or kill the spermatozoa. It took 50 years before his account was re-discovered and really understood. He stressed that Section 7, mentioned above, involved three considerations: first, the nature and properties of the semen, secondly, its passage to the cavity of the uterus, and third, the proper time for this[11]. He continued

A short time ago, it was generally supposed that sterility was a thing that belonged almost wholly to the opposite sex. Mr. Curling [Thomas Blizzard Curling, 1811–1888, FRS, Surgeon to the London Hospital, *Observations on Sterility in Man* with cases[12]. See also Curling's observation on cretinism, p. 246] has recently brought this subject prominently before the profession, and has established very conclusively that sterility in the male does positively exist, and that it may depend upon – 1st. Congenital malposition of the testes. 2nd. Chronic inflammation of these glands; and 3rd. Stricture. In the first and second, the testes fail to produce spermatozoa; in the third, the semen regurgitates into the bladder.

Sims clearly differentiates between impotence and sterility. He made particular use of the vaginal speculum for regular gynaecological examinations, which was eventually accepted by the profession, in spite of some bitter opposition from both America and Britain. This was an instrument Soranus had used (see also p. 61) so many hundreds of years ago. In a later address in 1868, to the New York County Medical Society, on 'The Microscope as an Aid in the Diagnosis and Treatment of Sterility', Sims stressed the importance of demonstrating live spermatozoa in the semen. He complained that he was misrepresented, maligned and positively abused, "both here and abroad", for his insistence on semen studies, and cited the *Medical Times Gazette*, which charged that "this dabbling in the vagina with speculum and syringe was incompatible with decency and self-respect"[13].

In the 'Notes . . .', Sims also recorded a successful artificial insemination in the case of a woman of 28, who had been married for 9 years without becoming pregnant. She was the only one of about half a dozen patients where he had attempted uterine injection, because operation (of incising the os and cervix, which Sims regarded the correct treatment) was refused. He carried out a total of 27 such injections with originally three or four drops of seminal fluid, eventually reduced to half a drop, which proved successful. These injections in her case extended over a period of nearly 12 months, on eight occasions, 2–7 days after her periods had finished. In 1868, Girault mentioned ten cases of artificial insemination and Sims mentions that Professor George Harley, of University College, London, "informs me that he has repeatedly performed the experiment of injecting the semen into the cavity of the uterus, but with no result". In 1877, a Papal Encyclical condemned artificial insemination as abominable[13]. (See also John Hunter's successful artificial insemination, recorded by Everard Home in 1799: this book, p. 205.)

Of other causes of female sterility, Murray, who had been first to treat thyroid deficiency with thyroid extract in 1891, knew that such an extract was an old, though controversial standby in the treatment of infertility (George Redmayne Murray, 1865–1939).

Far more important proved to be the observations of Emil Noeggerath (1827–1895) in his book *Die latente Gonorrhoe im weiblichen Geschlecht* (=The latent gonorrhoea in the female sex)[14], especially after Albert Ludwig Sigmund Neisser had discovered the gonococcus in 1879[15].

In 1865, Thomas Addis Emmet (1828–1919), a disciple of Sims, reported 'On the treatment of dysmenorrhoea and sterility, resulting from anteflexion of the uterus'[16]. About that time, tuberculosis of the female pelvic organs was also noted as a cause of sterility[13]. After the discovery and, initially, somewhat indiscriminate use of X-rays by Wilhelm Conrad Roentgen (1845–1923) in 1895, the sterilizing effect of these rays applied to human ovaries and testicles was recorded by Davis and Varrier in 1903. It was also known that fertility was impaired in young women suffering from diabetes mellitus. The discovery of insulin, in 1921, altered this outlook from very poor to fairly optimistic. Finally, Isadore Clinton Rubin's (1883–1958) carbon-dioxide insufflation test to determine and treat tubal patency was another milestone in the analysis and treatment of female sterility[17,18] (these articles deal with intra-uterine inflation with oxygen and production of an artificial pneumo-peritoneum).

The discovery of the role of the hormones produced by the ovary (pp. 396–401) had a great influence on the understanding of some aspects of sterility in women, but especially on that of the menstrual cycle. This phenomenon had aroused the interest of physicians and naturalists since antiquity. The connection with the calendar, or rather with the phases of the moon (hence the names of 'menses', 'Regeln', 'monthly periods', 'caramenia', etc.) seemed obvious. Less clear appeared the purpose of the bleeding. Because of its occasionally putrifying appearance, the smell, the pain, it had been assumed since Hippocrates that the period was a form of detoxication of the blood-poisoning women encountered. This view was also carried by Aristotle, Galen, Pliny and the other scientists who succeeded them[19]. This was also underlined by the fact that women priestesses of antiquity were often regarded as unclean during their menstrual periods and were not allowed to carry out their religious functions. As to the place of the menstruating woman in the Old Testament, she was definitely unclean, both as regards preparation of certain food and of sexual activity (see also Chapter 5). C. F. W. Ludwig (1816–1895) still used in 1861 the term "monatliche Reinigung", or monthly purging, for menstruation[24].

There was no real progress in the knowledge of the menstrual period during the 17th, 18th and 19th centuries, in spite of the great scientific discoveries, because anatomical and physiological observations remained static until the end of the 19th century. Hans Georg Mueller-Hess (born 1914) mentions that, in 1657, Lambert Velthuysen (1622–1685) postulated "a fermenting menses-inducing force derived from the 'semen-like' fluid which comes from the female testes into the blood circulation"[20]. But that assumption was not based on observation, or on experiment. The first clinical experiment was Percival Pott's (1713–1788) report in 1775 of the removal of both ovaries in a young woman for correction of 'ovarian herniae', which was followed by shrinkage of her breasts and cessation of her menses[21]. Whereas Pott did not comment on the significance of this observation, John B. Davidge (1768–1829), an American student in Edinburgh, learned of Pott's case and put it into his doctor's thesis in 1794[22], which he reprinted in 1814 with an English translation (from the Latin)[23]. He concluded from Pott's observation, that "menstruation is attributable to a peculiar condition of the ovaries serving as a source of excitement to the vessels of the womb. . . ." Until 1872, this was the only scientific account of the effect of bilateral oophorectomy on the periods. Simmer stresses that "there is no evidence that in 1861 Eduard Friedrich Wilhelm Pflueger (1829–1910) demonstrated that menstruation did not take place in women whose ovaries have been removed", as Bullough and Voght maintained (see Note 36 in Ref. 24).

According to Nardone[19], Negrier in 1840 and Rivelli in 1893 laid a scientific foundation for connecting the menstrual period with ovulation, showing that a follicle bursts every month, and that women born without ovaries have no periods; furthermore, that there is no ovulation before menarche nor after the menopause, and that there is no period nor ovulation during pregnancy and often none during lactation. Girwood showed in 1842, based on a number of autopsies, that the number of follicular scars corresponded to the total number of periods the deceased woman had had during her lifetime[19]. Fritz Hitschmann (1870–1926) and Ludwig Adler (1876–1958) gave, in 1908, the first description of the histological cyclical changes in the endometrium, as part of the normal process closely connected with the ovarian hormones[25]. The regulation of menstruation was further confirmed by the work of Schroeder and Meyer in 1913–1914[19]. German (first Great) War data indicated that human fertility was highest in the week after menstruation (a fact not unknown to Sims[10]) falling gradually to virtual sterility in the week preceding menstruation (Fraenkel and Robert Schroeder)[26].

In 1917, Charles Rupert Stockard (1879–1939) and George Nicholas Papanicolaou (1883–1962) presented their classic study of the histological changes in the vagina. They noted that at the beginning of the menstrual cycle, even the lower part of the vaginal epithelium of rodents becomes cornified and this could be recognized by the microscopical examination of vaginal smears[27]. The final breakthrough in the understanding of the menstrual cycle, beginning with the isolation of oestrin by Edgar Allen (1892–1943) and Edward Doisy (b. 1893) came in 1923 and will be discussed in Chapter 20.

Halban, in 1905, as Corner put it[28]: ". . . by cogitation in his armchair, not (this time) by experiment . . .", suggested the placenta to be a source, together with the ovary, of a hormone acting on the mammary gland. In his Croonian Lectures in 1905, Starling (see p. 342) mentioned some experiments he had made in conjunction with Dr. Janet E. Lane-Claypon (1877–1967), in which they had produced hypertrophy of the mammary glands in virgin rabbits, and in some cases actual secretion of milk, by the daily subcutaneous injection of the filtered watery extract of young rabbit foetuses. In his Harveian Oration on *The Wisdom of the Body* in 1923, he withdrew the result of those experiments as inconclusive because of a "weak point . . . that the ovaries had not been previously extirpated"[29].

From 1912 onwards, several research workers in Austria, France and in the United States found that the secret of the ovarian hormone lay in extraction with lipid solvents. Henri Iscovesco was a gynaecologist in Paris; he had a Roumanian name, but presumably trained in France. In July 1912, he reported to the Société de Biologie that one of his liquid extracts, prepared from sows' ovaries, contained a potent substance, which – when injected into young rabbits – caused growth of the uterus[30]. Clinical application seemed to give good results in dysmenorrhoea, amenorrhoea and in some types of hypogonadism[31]. In Vienna, another assistant at Schauta's clinic, Otfried O. Fellner, independently made lipid extracts from sows' ovaries and from human placentas; he reported on their action on the uterus of young female rabbits and guinea pigs[32]. The third observer was another young Viennese gynaecologist, Edmund Hermann, who began his studies in about 1911 and published his results in 1915. He used extracts made from the general ovarian tissue, from the corpus luteum and from the placenta, but – unfortunately – "he did not clearly distinguish between the effects of his extracts and therefore some of his pictures show what we now recognise as progesterone effects"[28].

Hermann's illustrations[33], however, gave Corner and Willard Allen ". . . one of our best leads when we first attempted to isolate the corpus luteum hormone"[28].

The fourth research worker was Robert T. Frank of New York, who started his studies *ca.* 1904.

In 1915, he collaborated with Jacob Rosenbloom, and they reported on physiologically active substances in the placenta and corpus luteum with which they could prevent castrate atrophy in rabbits[34]. When published, their paper carried references to Iscovesco and to Hermann, but as Corner remarks, it was submitted in July 1914, well before Hermann's paper had appeared. Corner stresses, however, that at the beginning of 1923, before Allen and Doisy's first paper appeared (see also Chapter 20), "the literature of ovarian endocrinology was in a very confused state"[28].

In a review written in that year Corner said, ". . . we should probably have to wait a long time for the identification of these (follicle and corpus luteum) hormones and their exact sources". In a paper published under the auspices of the American Medical Association in 1924, A. J. Carlson, a physiologist in Chicago, was even more sceptical: "Until it has been conclusively shown in spayed females that these extracts (of the German, French and Austrian investigators) prevent the atrophy of the uterus and maintain oestrus periods typical for the species, it seems clear that experimental ovarian organo-therapy has not been placed on a scientific basis"[35]. This was almost identical with the views of Swale Vincent and of A. J. Clark in Britain and of Eugène Gley in France, which will be discussed in Chapter 18.

Although there had been a great deal of concern about the nature of the spermatozoa (von Koelliker), testicular transplant studies (A. A. Berthold), and experiments with testicular extracts (Brown-Séquard, d'Arsonval and others), studies of the histology of the male gonads were only few. Franz Leydig (1821–1908) described the interstitial cells of the testis in 1850[36]. Conrad Eckhard (1822–1915) carried out important studies on the erector mechanism of the penis in the dog[37].

The importance of the discussion on fertility and reproduction within the framework of the field of endocrinology can be gauged by the fact that Dr. Borell, whose careful researches on the historical development of modern endocrinology have already been mentioned, has recently prepared a major study, entitled: 'The Origins of Modern Research on Fertility and Reproduction: Physiology and the Discovery of Hormones 1889–1930'[38]. In her preface, she says: "Although by the mid-nineteenth century, physicians had developed a physiological model to explain and guide sexual activity, laboratory investigators did not begin to comment until the first decades of the twentieth." She comments on the "Lack of systematic study of reproductive physiology before 1900"; but, eventually, even Schaefer and his laboratory, especially Francis Hugh Adam Marshall (1878–1949) and William Adam Jolly (1873–1945) made up for the neglect of this important subject. Before discussing their work, however, we shall have to fill in a few facts, to serve as background and to lead up to Marshall and Jolly's investigations.

MORE REPRODUCTIVE PHYSIOLOGY

We have already recorded Carl Ernst von Baer's discovery of the mammalian ovum (p. 276). In his Sir Henry Dale Lecture for 1964: *The Early History of the Oestrogenic Hormones*, George W. Corner pointed out that the castration of sows has not fundamentally changed in its technique since the days of Aristotle[39]. "The term 'sow-gelder' appears in English in 1515 and repeatedly thereafter, for example in Burton's *Anatomy of Melancholy* and Butler's *Hudibras*", and all this without giving useful hints for the investigation of ovarian function. Nor did physicians "profit by the second clue – so long known to farmers and camel drivers – that to remove the ovaries stops the oestrus cycle". Nor did castrate atrophy of the uterus appear in the medical literature until Albert Puech, a French physician, wrote in 1873 about the spaying of sows[40]: "It is worthy of note, that following the operation, which is commonly done during the first two months of life, the uterus ceases to grow, and its volume remains stationary".

At that time antiseptic surgical operations for removal of the human ovaries had become frequent; in 1872, Robert Battey of Atlanta, Georgia, had made oophorectomy popular for dysmenorrhoea and various neuroses! (Battey's operation). In Germany, Alfred Hegar of Freiburg-im Breisgau (1830–1914), became particularly interested in it and also personally carried out spaying of sows for experimental purposes. His drawing of one of these experiments, showing complete aplasia of the (sow) uterus in his book *Die Castration der Frauen*[41] is the first illustration of castrate atrophy ever published. Ferdinand A. Kehrer (1837–1914), of Giessen, took up the same study, by spaying a few young rabbits and reporting on the results in 1879[42]. After that 20 years elapsed before anyone resumed that particular line of study.

We now return to Brown-Séquard again. In a second note on his report on the effect of subcutaneous injections of testicular extract in 1889, he expressed the view that the ovaries of animals must produce an extract which has the same effect on women as the testicular extracts have on men[43]. This he followed with a report in 1890, that a midwife known to him in Paris had given herself a liquid made from pigs' ovaries, with beneficial effect. Just before this, a Marseilles surgeon, Villeneuve, used Brown-Séquard's method on two women. One of them was not benefited; "The other, who suffered with hysterical seizures following oophorectomy, was cured"[44]. In a further report, in 1890, Brown-Séquard announced that an American woman doctor, Dr. Augusta Brown (a graduate of Paris, unrelated to him) had given more than a dozen old women filtered juice of guinea-pigs' ovaries with good effect in cases of hysteria, in various uterine affections, and in debility due to age[45]. This was confirmed in a report by H. R. Andrews in 1904[46], who reported on 46 such women patients but – he said – "without much success".

We must now turn to the results of the very exhaustive studies on the development of endocrinology in the field of gynaecology and obstetrics carried out by Hans H. Simmer in the past decade. In two major papers he discussed 'The First Experiments to Demonstrate an Endocrine Function of the Corpus Luteum'. The first of these is also dedicated to the 100th birthday of Ludwig Fraenkel (1870–

1951)[47]. The second part is subtitled: 'Ludwig Fraenkel versus Vilhelm Magnus'[48].

In 1865, Otto Spiegelberg (1830–1881), obstetrician and gynaecologist at Breslau, restated that the corpus luteum caused rupture of the follicle. Although both Vesalius (1514–1564) and Volcher Coiter (1534–1576) have been credited with the first description of the corpus luteum, it was Marcello Malpighi (1678–1694) who introduced the term in 1681, in his letter to Spon[49].

The leading German anatomist of that time was Wilhelm Waldeyer (full name: Heinrich Wilhelm Gottfried Waldeyer-Hartz), (1836–1921) of Hehlen, who was a pupil of Henle and Professor in Breslau and later in Berlin. Among his important contributions was research on the ovaries, on which he published a monograph: *Eierstock und Ei*[50] (=Ovary and ovum). Waldeyer stressed that the corpus luteum started to develop before ovulation, "to cover, as Pflueger has pointed out, the loss of substance associated with the evacuation of the Graafian follicle". To Waldeyer and Pflueger the corpus luteum represented an evolutionary process. Others, supported by Robert Heinrich Johannes Sobotta (1869–1945), later professor of Anatomy in Bonn, and John Goodrich Clark (1867–1927), believed that the corpus luteum restored ovarian circulation as well as the lost tension, making ovulation possible again.

Eduard Friedrich Wilhelm Pflueger, 1829–1910, a pupil of Johannes Mueller and du Bois Reymond, succeeded Helmholtz as Professor of Physiology in Bonn and founded in 1868 the famous *Pflueger's Archiv fuer die gesamte Physiologie*. He loved scientific controversy and argument. He had written a monograph: 'Ueber die Eierstoecke der Saeugethiere und des Menschen' (='On the ovaries of the mammalia and of man'.)

Sobotta, for many years Prosector at the Institute of Comparative Anatomy, Embryology and Histology at Wuerzburg, made an extensive study of the impregnation of the ovum in the mouse and its early development, and numerous publications on the subject bore witness of his work from 1893 to 1898. Although he had at one time been a pupil of Waldeyer, and later of von Koelliker, he prepared the ground for a new hypothesis of the corpus luteum as an endocrine gland. He introduced the principle of serial study (he looked at some 1500 mouse corpora lutea in all stages of development). He felt, however, that the final answer to the many questions raised by his researches would need physiological experimentation. To his own work he added some careful studies of rabbit corpora lutea in 1897[51]. The paper on the rabbit corpora lutea showed a fully developed corpus luteum graviditatis. His meticulous drawings influenced John Beard (1858–1924) in 1897 to assume that the corpus luteum had the function of suppressing ovulation[52]. It also made Auguste Prénant (1861–1927) specify this as an endocrine function in 1898[53].

As we shall see, Beard's and Prénant's ideas became of importance later, in the search for hormonal contraception (see p. 373).

Gustav Born, Professor and head of the Embryological Division of the Anatomical Institute of the University of Breslau, was much impressed by Sobotta's work, on which he based his new hypothesis on the function of the corpus luteum. Unfortunately he was by then suffering from angina of effort and in July 1900 he died without having published his hypothesis. He had, however, persuaded his pupil Ludwig Fraenkel (1870–1951: see also Section II), then in practice as a gynaecologist in Breslau, to carry out some experiments, to prove his hypothesis. He had also discussed it with Vilhelm Magnus (1871–1929), an American-born Norwegian doctor who happened to be at Born's Institute at the time, studying histology and experimental embryology. In May 1900, while Born was still alive, Ludwig Fraenkel started to carry out some experiments on the rabbit, assisted by Franz Cohn (1880–?), then a medical student. At that time, Fraenkel was quite familiar with the anatomy and histology of the female rabbit's sexual organs, although – like his contemporaries – he was not aware that in the rabbit ovulation does not occur spontaneously, but some 10 hours after coitus as a result of that stimulus. This fact was first recognized by Walter Heape in 1905[54]. In spite of this, Fraenkel's experimental plans and his interpretation of results were not influenced by it.

After Born's death, Cohn participated in a total of 39 experiments until the end of 1901. After that, Fraenkel was assisted by Lili Conrat (Mrs. Fraenkel, née Lili Conrat, since 1900). In 1903 he carried out 75 more experiments and between 1904 and 1910, 277 more. All those experiments, assisted by Conrat, were carried out in his private hospital, in a small laboratory where they studied and operated on 400 pregnant rabbits. When he reported to the Deutsche Gesellschaft fuer Gynaekologie in Giessen on 3 May 1901, he and Cohn had already performed 19 valid experiments. The gist of these complicated experiments was to prove that the ovary has two functions: to develop and release eggs and to permit implantation of the eggs into the uterus. "Most likely this new function is confined to the corpus luteum[55]." Fraenkel stressed that although the original hypothesis was entirely Born's achievement, the experimental approach was his own. On 1 July 1901, Fraenkel, for the first time, destroyed a corpus luteum by electrocautery. "By this method I could prove the exclusive dependence of the egg-insertion on the corpus luteum". All his experiments were carried out under careful anaesthesia, under aseptic conditions. The technique used was as careful as that employed by him on his own patients.

In the meantime, Vilhelm Magnus had returned from Breslau to Christiania (Oslo), where he was resident in Neurology. Probably between April and early August 1901, he carried out experiments almost identical to those which Fraenkel and Cohn had been doing in 1900 (bilateral oophorectomies) as well as cauterizations of the corpora lutea, using electrocautery on the advice of the physiologist Torup (Sophus Carl Fredrik Torup, 1861–1937). He reported his findings in a lecture to the Medical Society of Christiania, entitled: 'The importance of the ovaries for pregnancy, with special regard to the corpus luteum'. He concluded that a nervous influence initiated by the ovary, on to the uterus, was not possible. He called the internal secretion from the corpus luteum 'differentierinsstoffe' (='differentiating substances'). Because the uterus did not atrophy after destruction of the corpora lutea, he further concluded that the "ovarian stroma also had an endocrine secretion, the function of which was to maintain the uterus". Magnus posed a number of pertinent questions, to which he was unable to find answers. Yet, after presentation of his work on 11 September 1901 "never again was he to return to his subject"[56]. Thus it came about that in 1902, two identical reviews appeared within the German literature. In *Frommel's Jahresberichten* a review of Magnus' paper was followed by a discussion of the first two papers of Fraenkel.

From these reviews it became obvious that the authors had not only arrived at similar conclusions. Fraenkel's work, it was said, indicated the importance of the corpus luteum for nidation. Magnus' experiments additionally demonstrated a continuous, though limited, influence of the corpus luteum after nidation[57].

The controversy is difficult to adjudicate. Neither Fraenkel nor Magnus mentioned one another in their first publications of 1901. Magnus was still in Breslau when Fraenkel and Cohn began their first experiments, which they discussed with Born. Magnus himself reported discussing Born's hypothesis with the latter. Magnus' paper was published in Norwegian, which Fraenkel could not read, nor is it likely that Norwegian medical journals would be available in Breslau, unless sent there specially by Magnus. It is not known if there existed a correspondence between the two, but there is no evidence to suggest it. The fact remains, however, that Magnus seemed to have used electrocautery independently and successfully, to remove the corpora lutea. He also studied the time factor before Fraenkel did, namely that the corpus luteum protected pregnancy until about the 15th to the 20th day. In contrast to Fraenkel, Magnus did not observe any atrophy of the uterus after removal of the corpora lutea, hence he thought that the 'ovarian stroma' by its own internal secretion, maintains the uterus. In other words, he correctly predicted the existence of two ovarian hormones.

In the meantime, discussions at meetings in Germany, including in Vienna in 1903, extended the experimental findings on to clinical experience in the human. Moreover, some new, bright young people appeared in the field of gynaecological endocrinology and they must now be considered. It should be mentioned, however, that Starling, in the fourth of his Croonian Lectures of 29 June 1905 (in the first of which he had introduced the new term of chemical messengers or 'hormones'), discussed Fraenkel's experiments in detail. These, he said, "have been confirmed by Marshall and Jolly, who conclude that the ovary is an organ providing an internal secretion which is elaborated by the follicular epithelial cells or by the interstitial cells of the stroma". Fraenkel was also "deeply gratified" when the chemists Slotta (his son-in-law) and Ruschig (a student of Slotta) and his own pupil and assistant Fels, isolated pure progesterone, the hormone which is mainly responsible for the action of the corpus luteum[58]. Fraenkel never lost interest in the corpus luteum, which he also studied in the rat, dog, cat, sheep and snakes. We have already referred to his study of the corpus luteum in an armadillo when discussing de Graaf's work on *De Mulierum Generationi* . . . (in Chapter 13.

In 1896, Emil Knauer (1867–1935), a 29-year-old assistant to Rudolf Chrobak, chief of one of the gynaecological clinics in Vienna, carried out a few experimental transplantations of fragments of rabbit ovaries into the same individuals at new sites. When such grafts survived, they prevented the castrate atrophy which oophorectomy would cause without re-grafting. The nervous connections had been severed by the transplantation. It followed that there must exist an ovarian internal secretion. Knauer reported his results in a paper entitled: 'Einige Versuche ueber Ovariantransplantation bei Kaninchen'[59], in ignorance of Arnold Berthold's parallel experiments with testicular transplants in 1849 (see p. 217). (Incidentally, these had been attempted again by Heinrich Lode in 1891.) Knauer's final report was published as a monograph in 1900[60]. His work won him recognition in the form of a professorial title in Vienna and – in 1903 – of a call to the chair of Obstetrics and Gynaecology in Graz, where he remained until 1934, long enough to see the use in his clinic of the hormone he had so obviously foretold. Knauer was able to show that autotransplants of ovarian tissue were often successful and homoeotransplants at least occasionally so. At that time, however, he had not yet referred to "internal secretion" of the ovaries.

When Knauer discussed his experiments at a meeting of the Vienna *Gesellschaft der Aerzte* on 1 December 1899, Josef Halban (1870–1937), a young trainee of Professor Friedrich Schauta (1849–1919), at the other clinic for Gynaecology and Obstetrics in Vienna, spoke during the discussion. He reported on his own experiments of transplanting ovarian tissue into castrated newborn guinea-pigs, with the result that there was normal development of the uterus and the salpinges. Halban's conclusions from the result of Knauer's and his own experiments were that the transplants, deprived of their nerve supply, were connected with the host body solely by means of newly formed blood vessels; from which it followed that the ovaries must produce a substance which is taken into the circulation and is capable of having specific effect on the uterus and the rest of the genital organs; furthermore, that the presence of this substance in the body is absolutely necessary for the maintenance and for the development of the sexual organs and the mammary glands.

Remarkably, during the same period, a young New York surgeon, Robert Tuttle Morris (1857–1945), became a pioneer in human ovarian transplants. He achieved great reputation as a general surgeon – he became Professor of Surgery at the New York Post-graduate Medical School – and was regarded (and remembered) as a distinguished writer, a brilliant and witty speaker, as a man "with a singular degree of 'serenity, urbanity, and dignity of mind', as a surgeon with 'poetry in the dexterity of his hands', as a researcher of continuous and restless curiosity and persistent skepticism, and finally as an unorthodox and entertaining teacher"[61]. Moreover, he survived into the modern phase of medicine. However, one of his most outstanding achievements seems to have been overlooked and forgotten. Fielding H. Garrison found him worthy to be included in his *Introduction to the History of Medicine*[62], but merely to remark, en passant, "Other prominent American surgeons of the Listerian period are . . ." followed by sixteen names; in fourteenth position: "Robert T. Morris of Seymour, Connecticut, author of many technical improvements and original ideas". It is true that Morris, in his younger years, toured famous hospitals in Europe and visited (Lord) Lister at King's College Hospital in London. Special credit is due to Professor Hans H. Simmer for having rescued from oblivion one of Morris' outstanding feats, his successful transplants of human ovarian tissue, which he began early in 1895[61]. It was, incidentally, also the year, Simmer records, in which the first oophorectomy for breast cancer was carried out, with "an explanation as an endocrine ablation"[63].

Unfortunately, Morris' first report was a short record in a monograph *Lectures on Appendicits and Notes on Other Subjects*[64] (under notes on other subjects) to which he later referred in a short letter to the Editor of the *New York Medical Journal* on 16 September 1895, to report successful ovarian transplants in two patients. One of those patients menstruated for the first time 2 months after a homotransplant into her womb; the second woman, who had received a tubal autotransplant, had become pregnant a month after the operation. Morris called auto – and homotransplants – to use the terminology of today – 'homo- and heterotransplants', respectively. The technique used was also ingenious. After removal of a pea-sized segment from a normal ovary, he inserted it either into a slit into the fundus uteri, reached via the pouch of Douglas, or into the tube. Later, he also implanted ovarian tissue transabdominally into the peritoneum of the broad ligament at some point near the ovarian site, and this was the approach which proved most successful. Morris undertook ovarian transplants in order to prevent unnecessary hysterectomy with inflammatory disease of the appendages, especially in women before the menopause. Furthermore, he knew of the results of transplants of thyroid tissue in man; in fact, he referred in his report of 1895 to "the well-known fact that transplanted portions of other organs continue in their function"[64]. "It is not improbable", he continued, "that menstruation and normal sexual impulse may continue in women who carry an ovarian graft . . .". He decided to treat in this manner a group of women who had lost their adnexa because of disease; secondly, a group who had rudimentary adnexa and an infantile uterus. By 1901, Morris had recorded 12 transplant operations. For six of those, he had a longer term follow-up. Of them, three had received autotransplants and menstruated for several years afterwards; one even conceived, but aborted in 1895; but that pregnancy was based only on the patient's information. Surprisingly, three other patients with homotransplants also had their menses restored. Morris regarded as his major achievement in these patients the avoidance of premature menopause; four of those six patients were also relieved of their dysmenorrhoea. Side effects occurred in the form of (suspected) pelvic thrombophlebitis in one patient, cystic degeneration of the transplant from a cystic ovary, and in another instance a suspected extrauterine pregnancy, but the diagnosis was not proved, because the patient disappeared. Whether the patient who had her 'cirrhotic' ovaries removed in February 1902, and a transplant grafted from another 33-year-old patient, really became pregnant (in 1905 with a $7\frac{1}{2}$ lb baby-girl being born in 1906), because of the ovarian graft or whether some ovarian tissue had been left (the patient produced later another two living children) is very difficult to prove.

Thus Morris anticipated Martin-Théodore Tuffier's (b. 1857) ovarian transplants[65] by 10 years; yet Garrison named Tuffier ". . . a pioneer in pyelography and ovarian transplantation . . ."[66]. Emil Knauer might have known of Morris' work, as the letter to the *New York Medical Journal* of September, 1895, was reviewed in the *Oesterreich-Ungarischen Centralblatt der Medizinischen Wissenschaften* in 1896, but this was a month after Knauer's first paper. However, Knauer did refer to that review and to the second edition of Morris' monograph[60], although he himself never attempted ovarian transplants in the human. In 1910, William Estes (1855–1940) modified Morris' technique by implanting ovarian grafts into the 'horns' of the uterus from which the tubes had first been excised[67,68]. Estes gave proper credit to Morris, but Morris' original work was eventually forgotten.

A further problem Halban (see also Section II) tackled, was Pflueger's hypothesis of 1865, that the menstrual period is due to the stimulus to the ovarian nerves which the maturing follicle causes, and that the ovulation, followed by genital hyperaemia and uterine bleeding, is caused by reflex action of the nerves. A meticulous and excellent discussion of Pflueger's nerve reflex theory of menstruation as a "product of analogy, teleology and neurophysiology" is given in a recent paper by H. H. Simmer in honour of Professor Erna Lesky's 65th birthday (1977)[24]. Halban decided to test Pflueger's hypothesis by some more simple but carefully planned transplant experiments. Halban obtained permission for his next experiments to use four baboons from the Vienna Zoo, because they are one of the few mammals who have menstrual periods like humans. On two of them he managed to disprove Pflueger's reflex theory of the periods by means of producing amenorrhoea after castration, but restoring the periods after ovarian transplant. His observation on one of the animals was that the periods did not start again, although the uterus appeared normal in every respect anatomically and histologically. He was so confident in the correctness of his planning his experiments and of the faultless technique of their execution, that he concluded, correctly, that in internal secretion the production and presence of hormones is not sufficient; the target organ must also be able to react and respond to the stimulus.

Halban could later confirm Ludwig Fraenkel's observation that in the human female, ovulation occurs between two menstrual periods. Fraenkel had also postulated that the corpus luteum is responsible through its internal secretion for causing the uterine bleeding of

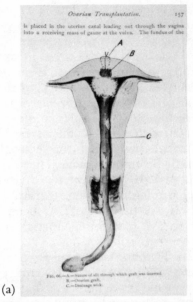

(a)

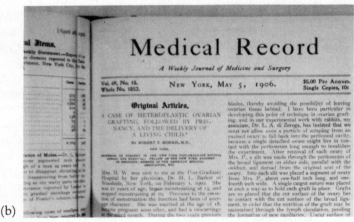

(b)

Figure 63 (a) Figure 2 of Simmers on Morris's technique. (b) Frontispiece of Morris' article in *Medical Record*

menstruation. Halban, later supported by his assistant Robert Koehler, disproved this view. Halban had already criticized Fraenkel's interpretation of some observations after extirpation of corpora lutea at a meeting of the Vienna Society for Obstetrics and Gynaecology on 15 December 1903. About 10 years later, Halban and Koehler removed and transplanted corpora lutea in patients who had to undergo gynaecological operations for other reasons. The post-operative observation gave direct proof that it was not the hormone production of the corpus luteum which released the menstruation but – on the contrary – the cessation of the internal secretion of the corpus luteum is responsible for the menstrual bleeding. These investigations were based on the Beard–Prénant hypothesis and Loeb's experiments to show that the corpus luteum may suppress ovulation (see p. 366). This remarkable piece of Halban's work is hardly known, nor is the attached clinical study 'Blutungen nach Eingriffen am Follikelapparate'[69] (=uterine bleeding after intervention at the level of the follicular arrangement). H. H. Simmer recorded this especially in his address on the occasion of Halban's centenary of birth in 1970[70].

In England, as we have already said, it was notably F. H. A. Marshall (1878–1949) (see Section II) and Wm. A. Jolly (1873–1945), who followed the line of investigations in reproductive physiology. They were able to confirm the results of Knauer's and Halban's experiments. George W. Corner, who knew Marshall personally (he met him first in the winter of 1923–1924), said this about him:

> . . . (he) did a great service to ovarian endocrinology by submitting it to detailed investigation as a branch of general biology, not merely as a special interest to gynaecologists. . . . Marshall had the great advantage of knowing the female cycle by observation of domestic animals, the ewe, ferret, and bitch, rather than of women, whose cycles, marked by menstruation instead of oestrus, were still imperfectly understood by the puzzled clinicians[71]. (See also p. 363.)
> Marshall's real contribution throughout his career was to sort out the confused observations of his predecessors, place them in order, and retest them by experiment[71].

His 'Contributions to the physiology of mammalian reproduction', written together with Jolly, has remained a classic even after a lapse of over 70 years[72]. In their general conclusions they say:

> The ovary is an organ providing an internal secretion which is elaborated by the follicular epithelial cells or by the interstitial cells of the stroma. This secretion circulating in the blood induces menstruation and heat. After ovulation, which takes place during oestrus, the corpus luteum is formed, and this organ provides a further secretion, whose function is essential for the changes taking place during the attachment and development of the embryo in the first stages of pregnancy.

After Marshall and Jolly had shown that ovarian grafts prevented uterine atrophy, Schaefer felt obliged to review his former ideas on the gonads being governed by nervous influences. He now said:

> The only rational explanation of the results of these experiments is contained in the assumption that the grafted organ produces, besides

ova, which may be regarded as the main function of the tissue, also an internal secretion which by virtue of the hormones which it contains, and which pass with it into the blood, can materially influence the development and structure of distant parts[73].

Dr. Borell remarks:

The influence of extracts of the ovaries and testes on the growth of young animals had not yet been studied by the physiologists. Clearly, the previous mode of appraisal of the effects of these extracts, that is the measurement of cardiovascular events, was not satisfactory. Growth and development were much more difficult processes to monitor and measure than those sudden and striking phenomena evoked either by adrenalin or even the recently discovered intestinal hormone, secretin. Histological studies of castrated animals would be imperative. The ignorance of physiologists regarding the reproductive process became glaringly apparent. At the same time, the nervous energy theory of sexuality together with its normative associations began to lose its force. . . . Several lines of research appeared to be promising[74].

One was, obviously, the study of the results of (male and female) castration. Secondly, the role of the ovary in the cycle of oestrus (ovulation and menstruation) had to be elucidated, and the events occurring during pregnancy (see also Chapter 18). Marshall was obviously the man for the job of systematic study of a number of those problems. In all fairness, it must be said that Schaefer recognized this, supported Marshall and encouraged him to sum up the result of his work in his book, *The Physiology of Reproduction*[75], a comprehensive study which appeared in the same year (1910) as Artur Biedl's book, *Innere Sekretion*[76] the first complete textbook on the physiology, pathology and therapy of internal secretion. Marshall's study was comprehensive as it "provided the first analysis of all data relating to the reproductive process, including breeding seasons, cyclical changes in the reproductive organs, gametogenesis, fertilisation, pregnancy, lactation and fertility, as well as discussion of internal secretory activity within the gonads"[77]. Thus "Marshall cut across rather more disparate lines of study uniting agricultural, morphological and physiological investigations under the common theme of reproductive physiology"[77].

Some progress had been made in anatomical observation of the ovary: Charles Philippe Robin (1821–1885) in 1857 suggested the name of 'ovariule' (=scar of the ovary) for the corpus luteum[78]. The corpus luteum of 'menstruation' was called 'false' corpus luteum, in contrast to the large 'true' corpus luteum of pregnancy[79]. It was described as a gland with internal secretion in 1898 by Born and A. Prénant (1861–1927) independently (see also p. 366)[80].

The epoopheron or parovarium, which corresponds to the epididymis, was described in 1802 by J. C. Rosenmueller (1771–1820) ('Organ of Rosenmueller')[81]. Marshall said in the introduction to his book that ". . . no attempt has yet been made to supply those interested in the reproductive processes with a comprehensive treatise dealing with this branch of knowledge". Accordingly, he consulted ". . . works on zoology and anatomy, obstetrics and gynaecology, physiology and agriculture, anthropology and statistics" in order to bring together those observations which have a "bearing on the problems of reproduction".

So it happened that, after 1910, no one seriously questioned the existence of gonadal hormones; only the best method of their study, definition, isolation, assay and possible synthesis were still subject to contention. In addition, as we have already seen from our discussion of the problems of contraception, they also became important as problems of social relevance.

NEW SYNDROMES

In 1886, Sir Jonathan Hutchinson (1828–1913) reported on 'Congenital absence of hair and mammary glands, with an atrophic condition of the skin and its appendages in a boy'[82]. He was a boy of 17 who died of senile decay, whose mother had been almost completely bald from alopecia areata from the age of six. The name 'micromegaly' was suggested, as the condition seemed to be the opposite of acromegaly. Hastings Gilford (1861–1941) wrote 'On a condition of mixed premature and immature development' in 1897; in a further, more complete description in *The Practitioner*[83], he called the condition 'progeria'. (=προγηρος = prematurely old). Post-mortem on one patient by Gilford: "The pituitary appeared to be normal, but was not further examined, the thyroid was normal, the thymus persistent and fibrous; the microscopic appearance of the adrenals was like that in the fibrous organs of the aged." Similar cases were described, independently, by others. Later, abortive cases of Simmonds' disease were described, which appeared to be the same as progeria (Hutchinson-Gilford syndrome) but occurred in adults[84].

John J. Mackenzie, in 1922 Professor of Pathology and Bacteriology at the University of Toronto, wrote in his contribution 'The pathological anatomy and histology of the suprarenal glands' in *Endocrinology and Metabolism*:

An interesting relationship between suprarenal pathology and general growth is seen in the condition described by Gilford as 'progeria' and by Variot and Prionneau as 'nanisme type senile'. Three cases have been described [the one by Hutchinson a year before had obviously escaped him – V.C.M.], two by Gilford and one by the French authors. In each case growth ceased before the fifth year of life, the hair of the head, eyebrows, eyelashes and trunk was almost entirely absent, the genital organs were hypoplastic and at the end there was extreme feebleness. In Gilford's case the autopsy showed fibrous atrophy of the suprarenals. The French case showed fibrous changes not only in the suprarenals but also in the spleen, lymph glands, pancreas, thyroid and hypophysis. . . . It is quite possible that the senile type of nanism is a manifestation of pluriglandular disease rather than simple involvement of the suprarenals, as the authors seemed to think[85].

Wilhelm Falta (1875–1950) of Vienna felt, however, that there were features in the case of at least three patients which make the diagnosis of a *primary* generalized sclerosis of the 'bloodglands' difficult to support. Firstly, intelligence was fairly well developed, which makes a primary major affection of the thyroid unlikely; secondly, he thought that the premature ossification of the long bones indicated a generalized sclerosing process, independently of the 'bloodglands'. He assumed, therefore, that 'progeria' might be a condition of generalized progressive sclerosis of many organs of the body, including the endocrine glands, sometimes perhaps following some generalized infection[86].

Between 1866 and 1910 a number of clinical syndromes were described, which became household words in endocrine literature, the underlying pathology of which have indicated the extension of the concept of the field of endocrinology to the brain itself and the close link with the field of genetics. A syndrome of a complex nature, which we have mentioned several times before, and which also received attention during that period, was diabetes insipidus. Whether Thomas Willis (1621–1675) actually distinguished diabetes mellitus from insipidus, is doubtful (see p. 141). Johann Peter Frank (1745–1821) first defined diabetes insipidus (see p. 174) and separated it from diabetes mellitus; he called it diabetes insipidus or spurius, a diabetes without glycosuria.

Robert Willis (1799–1878) gave in his book *Urinary Diseases and their Treatment*[87] an account of several forms of diabetes insipidus, according to the associated excretion of urea. William Prout (1785–1850), in *An Inquiry into the Nature and Treatment of Diabetes and Calculus*[88], described excess of urea, divided into those with and without polyuria. Experimental polyuria was produced by Claude Bernard (1813–1878) (see also p. 709) in 1849, by injury to the floor of the fourth ventricle[89], a little anterior to the 'glycosuric' centre. In 1870 C. Eckhard found that injury to certain other parts of the brain may also cause polyuria[90]. In 1901 Rudolf Magnus (1872–1927), and Schaefer (1850–1935) demonstrated that intravenous injection of pituitary extract can be followed by a severe degree of diuresis[91], and in 1908, Schaefer and Percy Theodor Herring (1872–1967) showed that there was a diuretic principle in the posterior pituitary[92]. In 1906, there was published the paper by Joseph Jules Dejerine (1849–1917) and Gustave Roussy (1874–1948) on 'Le syndrome thalamique'[93], studies of the result of localized thalamic injury, later to be followed by J. Camus and Roussy's studies on polyuria caused by injury to the floor of the third ventricle[94]. Reference has already been made to Dr. Samuel Jones Gee's (1839–1911) *Contribution to the History of Polydipsia* in 1877, perhaps the first description of familial nephrogenic diabetes insipidus (see p. 314).

A congenital and familial condition of mental deficiency, excessive obesity and hypogenitalism with retinitis pigmentosa, polydactyly and syndactyly became popular after the description by G. Bardet in Paris in 1920[95], which was followed by one by Artur Biedl (1869–1933) in 1922[96,97]. It was then discovered that the first complete description of such a condition had been given by John Zachariah Laurence (1829–1870) and Robert Charles Moon (1844–1914) in 1866[98], in the short-lived *Ophthalmic Review* (1864–1867), of which one of the editors was Laurence.

Laurence was the founder of the South London Ophthalmic (now the Royal Eye) Hospital in 1857. Earlier descriptions of similar patients date back to 1864, when Hoering of Erlangen reported one[99]. It is now called the Laurence–Moon–Biedl–Bardet syndrome and it is a complex congenital disorder; although the mode of inheritance appears to be autosomal recessive, the polydactyly has been regarded as dominant (Julius Bauer, 1887–1979)[100]. The epiblastic and mesoblastic changes are perhaps recessive and due to mutations of two genes in the same chromosome[101]. In some cases there are also other bone anomalies, such as oxycephalus, present[102,103]. The strong involvement of the endocrine system is striking.

We cannot, however, close this long and tangled tale of the 'Birth of Endocrinology' without mentioning a few authors who added contributions to the development of genetics and heredity (see also pp. 272–276). It should also be recalled that it was perhaps the *Philosophie Zoologique* of Jean Baptiste Pierre Antoine de Monet Lamarck (1744–1829) (see Section II), published in 1809 which had a great influence on further ideas[104]. Being one of the great comparative anatomists he propounded the theory of evolution by inheritance of acquired characteristics as a result of the use (or disuse) of organs in response to external stimuli (see also Chapter 23: *Somatic*

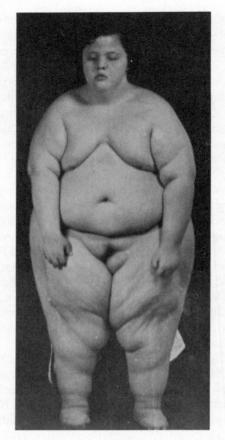

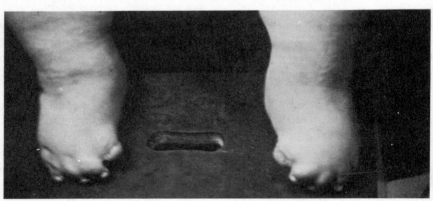

Figure 64   (Apert–)Laurence–Moon–Biedl–Bardet syndrome

*Selection and Adaptive Evolution: On the Inheritance of Acquired Charac-
teristics,* by E. J. Steele).

Joseph Adams (1756–1818) pioneered in medical genetics when he
published, in 1814, *A Treatise on the Supposed Hereditary Properties of
Diseases*[105] (see Chapter 15).

Of the many important contributions in this field, we wish to
mention only one other, at this stage: Edmund Beecher Wilson
(1856–1939) studied the influence of the reproductive chromosome
on heredity[106].

Between 1910 and 1925 the highlights of progress in endocrine
research were the production of crystalline thyroid hormone (1914–
1915), and the isolation of insulin in 1921. It was also the period
which contained the Great War, 1914–1918. Just before its outbreak,
there appeared in 1912 the first English textbook on *Internal Secretion
and the Ductless Glands* by Swale Vincent (1868–1933) (see Section II),
one of Schaefer's pupils. Like Marshall's *The Physiology of Reproduction,* Swale Vincent's book also acknowledged Schaefer's influence
on its production, and carried a warm recommendation by Schaefer
in the form of an introduction. Schaefer himself made a contribution
to the subject, by publishing a modified version of his Lane Medical
Lectures at Leland Stanford Jr. University in San Francisco (in 1913)
under the title: *An Introduction to the Study of Endocrine Glands and
Internal Secretions* in 1914, which he revised and enlarged two years
later, to be published as *The Endocrine Organs.* But otherwise, Hans
Lisser's words applied (see also p. 343) that after Brown-Séquard's
work was decried in 1895, "a drought descended upon the field of
clinical endocrinology which persisted with but a few scattered
refreshing contributions for almost 30 years"[107].

REFERENCES

1. Himes, N. E.: Medical History of Contraception. pp. 210 ff. Gamut Press,
    New York, 1936.
2. Wilde, F. A.: Das weibliche Gebaerunvermoegen. Eine medizinisch juri-
    dische Abhandlung zum Gebrauch fuer praktische Geburtshilfe, Aerzte
    und Juristen, Berlin, 1838. (=The inability of a woman to give birth. A
    medico-legal treatise for the use of practical obstetrics, for doctors and
    lawyers.)
3. Mensinga, W. P. J.: Ein Beitrag zum Mechanismus der Conception
    (Empfaengnis). Leipzig, Ernst Fiedler, 1891.
4. As 1: p. 223.
5. Carlile, R.: Every Woman's Book or What is Love? London, R. Carlile, 1825.
6. Besant, A.: Law of Population; its Consequences and its Bearing upon the
    Human Conduct and Morals. London, 1879.
7. As 1: p. 233.

8. Sims, J. M.: Clinical Notes on Uterine Surgery, with Special Reference to the Management of the Sterile Condition. London, Robert Hardwicke, 1866.
9. Ibid.: pp. 16–18.
10. As 8: pp. 381–387.
11. As 8: p. 361.
12. Curling, T. B.: Observations on Sterility in Man, with Cases. Reprinted from the British and Foreign Medico-Chirurgical Reviews, April 1874.
13. Johnston, R. D.: The History of Human Infertility. Fertil. Steril. **14**, 266 ff., 1963.
14. Noeggerath, E.: Die latente Gonorrhoe im weiblichen Geschlecht. Bonn, M. Cohen, 1872.
15. Neisser, L. S.: Ueber einen der Gonorrhoea eigentuemlichen Micrococcus. Zbl. Med. Wiss. **17**, 497–500, 1879.
16. Emmet, Thos. A.: New York Med. J. **1**, 205–219, 1865.
17. Rubin, I. C.: J. Am. Med. Assoc. **74**, 1017, 1920.
18. Rubin, I. C.: J. Am. Med. Assoc. **75**, 661–667, 1920.
19. Nardone, G. E.: Evoluzione del concetto di meccanismo della menstruazione. Pag. Stor. Med., 7 s, anno 14, no. 1, Roma, 1970.
20. Mueller-Hess, H. G.: Die Lehre von der Menstruation vom Beginn der Neuzeit bis zur Begruendung der Zellenlehre. Dissertation. Med. Fakultaet Berlin, pp. 50–54, 1938.
21. Pott, P.: An ovarian hernia, in The Chirurgical Works, pp. 791–792, London, 1775.
22. Davidge, J. B.: Dissertatio physiologica de causis catameniorum. Birmingham, T. Pearson, 1794.
23. Davidge, J. B.: Menstruous action, in Physical Sketches and or Outlines of Correctives, Applied to Certain Modern Errours in Physick, pp. 31–56. Baltimore, Warner & Robinson, 1814.
24. Simmer, H. H.: Pflueger's nerve reflex theory of menstruation: the product of analogy, teleology and neurophysiology. Clio Medica **12**, 57–90, 1977.
25. Hitschmann, F. and Adler, L.: Der Bau d. Uterusschleimhaut des geschlechtsreifen Weibes, mit besonderer Beruecksichtigung d. Menstruation. Mschr. Geb. Gynaekol. **27**, 1–82, 1908.
26. Garrison, F. H.: An Introduction to the History of Medicine. 4th ed. Repr., p. 684. Philadelphia, W. B. Saunders, 1929.
27. Stockard, Ch. R. and Papanicolaou, G. N.: The existence of a typical oestrus cycle in the guinea-pig; with a study of its histological and physiological changes. Am. J. Anat. **22**, 225–283, 1917.
28. Corner, George W.: J. Endocrinol **31**, (2), Proc. Soc. Endocrinol. pp. iii–xxxii, 1964/5.
29. Starling, E. H. The Wisdom of the Body. The Harveian Oration, delivered to the R. Coll. Physicians London. London, Lewis & Co., 1923.
30. Iscovesco, H.: Les lipoides de l'ovaire. C.R. Soc. Biol., Paris **63**, 16–18, 1912.
31. Iscovesco, H.: Lipoides homo-stimulants de l'ovaire et du corps jaune. Rev. Gynécol. **22**, 161–198, 1914.
32. Fellner, O. O.: Arch. Gynaekol. **100**, 641–719, 1913.
33. Hermann, E.: Ueber eine wirksame Substanz im Eierstocke und in der Placenta. Mschr. Geburtsh. Gynaekol. **41**, 1–50, 1915.
34. Frank, R. T. and Rosenbloom, J.: Surg. Gynaecol. Obstet. **21**, 646–649, 1915.
35. Carlson, A. J.: Physiology of the mammalian ovaries. J. Am. Med. Assoc. **83**, 1920–1923, 1924.
36. Leydig, Franz: Zur Anatomie d. maennlichen Geschlechtsorgane u. Analdruesen d. Saeugethiere. Z. Wiss. Zool. **2**, 1–57, 1850.

37. Eckhard, C.: Untersuchungen ueber die Erection des Penis beim Hunde. Beitr. Anat. Physiol. **3,** 123–170, 1863.
38. Borell, Merriley: The Origins of Modern Research on Fertility and Reproduction: Physiology and the Discovery of Hormones 1889–1930. Prepared for Workshop on Historical Perspectives on the Scientific Study of Fertility. Am. Acad. Arts Sciences, Boston, MA, 9–10 December 1977. Revised for Scientific Workshop, 5–6 May 1978.
39. Aristotle: Historia Animalium, Vol. IV, translated by D'Arcy W. Thompson, p. 632, lines 15 ff. in the English edition of the Works of Aristotle, by J. H. Smith and W. O. Ross, Oxford, 1910.
40. Puech, A.: Les Ovaires, de leur Anomalies. Paris, 1873.
41. Hegar, A.: Die Castration der Frauen. Leipzig, 1878.
42. Kehrer, Ferdinand A.: Beitr. Klin. Exp. Beb. Gynaekol., Giessen **2,** Heft 2, 1879.
43. Brown-Séquard, C. E.: C.R. Soc. Biol., Paris **41** (new series, vol. **1**), 420–422, 1889.
44. Villeneuve: Quelques faits pour servir à l'histoire des injections sous-cutanées de suc de tissue testiculaire et ovarien. Marseille-med. (Aug.), 458–468, 1889.
45. Brown-Séquard, C. E.: Remarques sur les effets produits sur la femme par des injections souscutanées d'un liquide retiré d'ovaire d'animaux. Arch. Physiol. Norm. Pathol. Ser. 5, **2,** 456–457, 1890.
46. Andrews, H. R.: The internal secretion of the ovary. J. Obstet. Gynaecol. **5,** 448–465, 1904.
47. Simmer, Hans H.: "Ludwig Fraenkel" Sudhoffs Arch. **55,** Heft 4, 392–417, 1971.
48. Simmer, Hans H.: Ludwig Fraenkel versus Vilhelm Magnus, Sudhoffs Arch. **56,** Heft 1, 76–99, 1972.
49. Malphighi, Marcello: Praeclarissimo et Eruditissimo Viro D. Jacobo Sponio, Medicinae Doctori et Lugdunensi Anatomico Accuratissimo. Phil. Trans. R. Soc. London **14,** 630, 1685.
50. Waldeyer, W.: Eierstock und Ei. Leipzig, W. Engelmann, 1870.
51. Sobotta, Johannes: Anat. Hefte **8,** 469, 1897.
52. Beard, J.: The Span of Gestation and the Cause of Birth, Jena, Fischer, 1897.
53. Prénant, A.: Sur la valeur morphologique sur l'action physiologique et thérapeutique possible du corps jaune. Rev. Med. Est. **30,** 385, 1898.
54. Heape, Walter: Proc. R. Soc. London B. **76,** 260, 1905.
55. As 47: p. 410.
56. As 48: p. 77.
57. As 48: p. 78.
58. Slotta, Karl H., Rushig, H. and Fels, W.: Reindarstellung der Hormone aus dem Corpus Luteum. Ber. Dtsch. Chem. Ges. **67,** 1270, 1934.
59. Knauer, Emil: Einige Versuche ueber Ovariantransplantation bei Kaninchen, Zbl. Gynaekol. **20,** 524–528, 1896.
60. Knauer, Emil: Die Ovarientransplantation. Exp. Stud. Arch. Gynaekol. **60,** 322–376, 1900.
61. Simmer, H. H.: Robert Tuttle Morris (1857–1945): A pioneer in ovarian transplants. Obstet. Gynecol. **35,** 314–328, 1970.
62. As 26: p. 601.
63. Simmer, H. H. Oophorectomy for breast cancer patients: Its proposal, first performance, and first explanation as an endocrine ablation. Clio medica. Cit. in Ref. 61.
64. Morris, R. T.: Lectures on Appendicitis and Notes on Other Subjects. New York, G. R. Putnam's Sons, 1895.

65. Tuffier, M-T.: Étude chirurgicale sur 230 greffes ovariennes. Acad. Méd. Bull. Ser. 3, **86**, 99, 1921.
66. As 26: p. 728.
67. Estes, W. L. J.: A method of implanting ovarian tissue in order to maintain ovarian function. Penn. Med. J. **13**, 610, 1910.
68. Estes, W. L. J.: Further results with ovarian implantation. J. Am. Med. Assoc. **83**, 674, 1924.
69. Halban, J. and Koehler, R.: Wien. Klin. Wochenschr. **38**, 612, 1925.
70. Simmer, H. H.: Wien. Med. Wochenschr. **121**, 549–552, 1971.
71. As 28.
72. Marshall, F. H. A. and Jolly, Wm. A.: Contributions to the physiology of mammalian reproduction. Phil. Trans. R. Soc. London **198**, 99–141, 1906.
73. Schaefer, A. E.: The hormones which are contained in animal extracts: their physiological effects. Pharm. J. **79**, 670–674, 1907.
74. As 38: p. 19.
75. Marshall, F. H. A.: The Physiology of Reproduction. London, Longmans, Green, 1910.
76. Biedl, A.: Innere Sekretion. Berlin und Wien, 1910.
77. As 38: p. 20.
78. Robin, C. P.: Compt. rend. Soc. biol. Paris, III., p. 139, 1857.
79. Clark, J. G.: Johns Hopkins Hosp. Reps., Baltimore, IX., 593, 1900.
80. Pratt, J. P.: Bibliography of the corpus luteum. Arch. Pathol. Chicago, XIX, 380, 1935.
81. Rosenmueller, J. C.: De Ovariis Embryonum et Foetorum Humanorum. Leipzig, 1802.
82. Hutchinson, Sir Jonathan: Congenital absence of hair and mammary glands, with an atrophic condition of the skin and its appendages in a boy. Med.-Chir. Trans. **69**, 473–477, 1886.
83. Gilford, H.: On a condition of mixed premature and immature development. Med.-Chir. Trans. **80**, 17–45, 1897.
84. Gilford, H.: Practitioner, **73**, 188–217, 1904.
85. Mackenzie, John J.: The pathological anatomy and histology of suprarenal glands, in Endocrinology and Metabolism. (Ed. Barker, L. F.) Vol. II, p. 273, New York, Appleton, 1922.
86. Falta, W.: Die Erkrankungen der Blutdruesen, p. 305. Wien, Springer, 1913.
87. Willis, R.: Urinary Diseases and their Treatment. London, 1838.
88. Prout, W.: An Inquiry into the Nature and Treatment of Diabetes and Calculus, 3rd ed., p. 92. London, 1840.
89. Bernard, Claude: C.R. Soc. Biol. (Paris) **1**, 60, 1850.
90. Eckhard, C.: Beitr. Anat. Physiol., Giessen **5**, 147, 1870.
91. Magnus, R. and Schaefer, E. A.: Proc. Physiol. Soc., p. ix, in J. Physiol. **27**, 1901.
92. Schaefer, E. A. and Herring, P. Th.: Phil. Trans. London Ser. B. **199**, 1, 1908.
93. Dejerine, J. J. and Roussy, G.: Rev. Neurol. **14**, 521–532, 1906.
94. Camus, J. and Roussy, G.: C.R. Soc. Biol. Paris, **75**, 628, 1913.
95. Bardet, G.: Thèse de Paris. No. 470, 1920.
96. Biedl, Artur: Geschwisterpaar mit adiposo-genitaler Dystrophie. Dtsch. Med. Wochenschr. **48**, 1630, 1922.
97. Raab, W.: Wien. Arch. Inn. Med. **7**, 443–530, 1924.
98. Laurence, J. Z. and Moon, R. C.: Four cases of 'retinitis pigmentosa', occurring in the same family, and accompanied by general imperfections of development. Ophthal. Rev. **2**, 32–41, 1866.

99. Hoering: Klin. Monatsbl. Augenh., Erlangen **2**, 233, 1864.
100. Bauer, Julius: Innere Sekretion. Berlin, Springer, 1927.
101. Rieger and Trauner, Z. Augenh., Berlin **118**, 235, 1929.
102. Medvei, V. C.: Personal observations.
103. Pool, F. L.: Wien Arch. Inn. Med. **31**, 187–200, 1937.
104. Lamarck, J. B. P. A. de M.: Philosophie Zoologique. Paris, Baillière, 1809.
105. Adams, J.: A Treatise on the Supposed Hereditary Properties of Diseases. London, J. Callow, 1814.
106. Wilson, E. B.: The Cell in Development and Inheritance. New York, Macmillan, 1896.
107. Lisser, Hans: The Endocrine Society: the first forty years (1917–1957). Endocrinology **80**, 5–28 (p. 7), 1967.

CHAPTER EIGHTEEN

THE TROUBLED AND EXCITING YEARS OF THE FIRST FOUR DECADES OF THE 20th CENTURY – PART I

In 1918 The Great War was over, but the scars were to remain for a long time, especially in Europe. Although Anglo–American links were strengthened, the scientific communications with Europe and within Europe had been interrupted. Their restitution took several years, and the economic and political upheavals on the continent of Europe made a return to the pre-war level of zest and high standard of research and teaching difficult. Personal friendships across the frontiers had been severed; the feeling of bitterness and animosity had not escaped the scientific field. Sir Edward Schaefer, an upright and kindhearted man, found it necessary to change his name by adding that of his teacher and predecessor in the chair of physiology, Sharpey, to his own, in order to dissociate himself clearly from the war-oriented direction which Central-European science had taken. The autumn issue of the *Journal of the History of Biology* for 1976 is largely taken up with the development of Endocrinology during that period, and in "A brief introduction" of that "special section of endocrinology", Professor Diane Long Hall and Dr. Thomas F. Glick discuss the interesting papers presented, which "indicate the extent to which the history of this complex field may be used to throw light on the intellectual and social history of the twentieth century"[1].

THE PERIOD OF THE DROUGHT AND OF THE CRISIS

On the Continent Artur Biedl's and Wilhelm Falta's textbooks, published before the war, were leading the field; in Britain, Sharpey-

Schafer and his pupils: Bayliss, Starling, Swale Vincent, F. H. A. Marshall and W. A. Jolly, were in the forefront of the 'New Physiology'. In France, Arsène d'Arsonval (1851–1940), former assistant and successor to Brown-Séquard, was still active, and, especially, so was Eugène Gley, of whom we shall talk in greater detail. In the United States, there was the well established figure of Harvey Cushing; the other dominant emerging figure was Herbert McLean Evans, to whom we shall devote our full attention. There was the experimental work of Bennett M. Allen and Philip E. Smith, and the pioneering chemical studies of Edward C. Kendall.

In 1915, Walter B. Cannon published from the Harvard Physiological Laboratory: *Bodily Changes in Pain, Hunger, Fear and Rage: An Account of Researches into the Function of Emotional Excitement*[2]. Professor Ian Stevenson wrote in the Foreword to the Torchbook Edition of Cannon's book in 1963:

> I wonder whether any modern textbook treating the physiological subject by Cannon would also include discussion of such topics as a mediaeval combat of knights or the sensations felt by a man trying to kill himself by starvation. . . . This correlating of social stimuli and physical responses made Cannon one of the founders of psychosomatic medicine.

Cannon stressed particularly the interrelation of nervous and hormonal responses with emotional derangement. He demonstrated the role of adrenal secretion in emotional excitement and pain, and studied the physical basis of fear, rage, hunger and thirst. He also postulated that emotional expression results from action of subcortical centres in the optic thalamus. Later, he summarized his views in a book, *The Wisdom of the Body*[3], in which he discussed the sympathetic and adrenal mechanism. Ernest H. Starling, in his Harveian Oration of 1923 'The Wisdom of the Body'[4], referred to Cannon's work as follows:

> As Cannon has pointed out, this secretion (the internal secretion of the medulla of the supra-renal bodies) is poured into the blood during conditions of stress, anger, or fear, and acts as a potent reinforcement to the energies of the body. It increases the tone of the bloodvessels, as well as the power of the heart's contraction, while it mobilises the sugar bound up in the liver, so that the muscles may be supplied with the most readily available source of energy in the struggle to which these emotional states are the essential precursors or concomitants[5].

Cannon's observations on the physiology of emotion followed his studies on *The Mechanical Factors of Digestion*[6]. He also succeeded in producing hyperthyroidism experimentally[7], the occurrence of which, following excessive emotional stress, he also discussed in his researches on emotion.

In Canada, the figures of Macleod, Banting and Best were looming in the background, two of whom were to emerge triumphantly on the field of Nobel Prize winners, leaving another claimant to fame, Paulesco in Roumania, rightly or wrongly, to disappear in the shadows of oblivion.

For the moment, however, we shall consider the position in Britain.

The position in Britain

In spite of the apparently steady development of the 'New physiology', the initiative which had been given by Sharpey-Schafer, and which was continued by his collaborators, pupils and successors, a rift gradually appeared between the views of two of the most prominent representatives, namely Swale Vincent and Ernest Henry Starling. We have seen in Chapter 16 that it was particularly Schaefer's Address in Physiology to the British Medical Association on 2 August 1895, which made "Internal Secretion" a respectable, scientifically based, field of medicine. Ernest H. Starling followed this 10 years later, when he introduced in his Croonian Lectures on the 'Chemical Correlation of the Functions of the Body', in June 1905, the newly coined term 'hormone', i.e. chemical messenger (see p. 341). This had a broader definition than that originally given for 'internal secretion' by Schaefer and followed by Swale Vincent in his textbook on *Internal Secretion and the Ductless Glands* in 1912. Eventually, in 1923, Starling summed up the position again, as he saw it, in The Harveian Oration, given to the Royal College of Physicians in London, entitled: 'The Wisdom of the Body'[4], with the motto:

> Who hath put wisdom in the inward parts?
> Or who hath given understanding to the heart?

The first part of his oration dealt with the discussion of the progress of knowledge concerning the circulation and the action of the heart since Harvey; the second part with 'The chemical integration of the body'. At that time, not only Cannon's work was known, but also that of Kendall on the chemistry of the thyroid and several of the pituitary hormones, David Marine's work on goitre prevention and Banting and Best's discovery of insulin. Starling – as was to be expected from this romantic figure among the many brilliant scientists of his generation – took a broad, enthusiastic and optimistic view of the development in the field of hormones during the last 18 years and of the future. It was, therefore, somewhat surprising when Swale Vincent, now Professor of Physiology at the Middlesex Hospital in London, gave a major lecture at about the same time, on 'The Present Position of Organotherapy' to the Royal Society of Medicine (on 9 January 1923)[8], which was very similar in tenor to his Arris and Gale Lecture on 'A Critical Examination of Current Views on Internal Secretion', delivered to the Royal College of Surgeons of England in the previous year[9], Swale Vincent's analysis and definition was – to say the least – different from Starling's. Moreover, he spoke of a 'crisis in the field of endocrinology' which threatened its existence as a respectable scientific medical specialty. Swale Vincent had, at that time, worked in endocrinology for 25 years, and had made important contributions to the physiology of the adrenals, thyroid, parathyroids, pituitary, and of the islets of Langerhans. He was very slightly younger than Starling and he had also been a student, assistant and colleague of Sharpey-Schafer. His attitude was so strange that Professor Diane Long Hall felt sufficiently puzzled to devote a paper to the study of the situation: 'The critic and the advocate: contrasting British views on the state of endocrinology in the early 1920s'[10].

T. Swale Vincent (1868–1933) (see Section II) developed, under the influence of Schaefer, a histological and metabolic approach to endocrine research. One of his former students, J. W. Cramer, called him a man "with a highly critical mind, ... which enabled him to clear the new science of endocrinology from many pseudo-scientific weeds"[11]. In this respect, he was a man of "firm principles and ideals", and quite "uncompromising".

Starling said in the last chapter of his Harveian Oration 'The Therapeutics of Hormones'[4]:

> There seem to be three possible methods by which we medical men can interpose our art in the hormonic workings of the body: (1) In the first place we may find what is the effective stimulus to the production of the hormone, and by supplying this, increase its production by the responsible cells ... (2) Where a disordered condition is due to diminished production of some specific hormone, we may extract the hormone from the corresponding gland or tissue in animals. It is characteristic of these hormones that, so far as we know, they are identical throughout all the classes of vertebrates, and it is possible that they may be found far back in the invertebrate world ... (3) The ideal but not, I venture to assert, the unattainable method will be to control, by promotion or suppression, the growth of the cells themselves, whose function it is to form these specific hormones ... (p. 26)

Starling had said before in his Oration:

> Each specific hormone is manufactured by a group of cells and turned into the blood, in which it travels to all parts of the body, but excites definite reactions in one or a limited number of distant organs. The production and action of these substances are continually going on in the normal animal. (p. 22)

He also gave this definition of a hormone:

> The typical hormone, however, is a drug-like body of definite chemical composition, which in a few cases is actually known, so that the substance has been synthesised outside the body. It is more or less diffusible, and may even withstand without alteration the temperature of boiling water. It is generally easily oxidisable in a neutral or alkaline medium, so that after its production does not remain long in the blood; it delivers its message and is then destroyed. (pp. 21–22)

Finally, and most importantly Starling stated:

> These hormones may apparently be formed by any kind of tissue. In many cases a gland which has, in the evolutionary history of the race, poured its secretion by a duct into the alimentary canal or on to the exterior, loses its duct and becomes a ductless gland, the secretion being now transferred either immediately or through the lymphatics into the blood stream. In either case these chemical messengers may be formed from masses of cells which have at no time had a glandular structure, and may be modified nervous tissue, germinal tissue, or some part of the mesoblast.

Not so Vincent; he attacked such physiological and therapeutic generalizations. In his view the field had been clearly defined by William Carpenter, and after him by Claude Bernard, in the middle of the 19th century. In 1852, William B. Carpenter (1813–1885) said:

> The vascular glands (spleen, thymus, thyroid, adrenals) ... exactly correspond with ordinary glands in all that part of their structure by which they withdraw or eliminate certain matters from the blood; and they differ only in being unprovided with excretory ducts for the discharge of the products of their operation. These products, instead of being carried out of the body, are destined to be restored to the circulating current apparently in a state of more complete adaptiveness to the wants of the nutritive function[12].

According to Vincent, therefore, the correct basis for good endocrinology is the definition within the limits laid down by the above pioneers and by the progress achieved by the exact science of anatomy, histology and physiology. It involves the agreement among the research workers "that the act of secretion can only be carried out by certain kinds of tissue – namely those which consist of highly specialised epithelial cells". He thus repeats the definition given in his own textbook, i.e. "the process consists in the preparation and setting free of certain substances of physiological utility . . . by certain cells of a glandular type; the substances set free are not passed out on to a free surface but into the blood stream"[9].

Accordingly, Long Hall remarks:

> the only discoveries worthy of a place in a textbook of endocrinology are thyroxine and adrenalin. Both have been found in the gland, both have been chemically identified, and both have clear metabolic effects[10].

Those were also the standards of Sharpey-Schafer and of Eugène Gley in Paris, another of the puritans of endocrine physiology. Vincent does not accept 'adrenin' as a hormone because (a) it has a "drug-like", non-specific action on the neuro-muscular and cardiovascular system, and (b) because its advocates have overstated their case. This meant that Vincent rejected Walter B. Cannon's 'Emergency Theory' of the action of adrenin (as he preferred to call adrenalin). Cannon concluded:

> . . . since the adrenal glands are innervated by autonomous fibres of the mid-division, and since adrenal secretion stimulates the same activities that are stimulated nervously by this division, it is possible that disturbances in the realm of the sympathetic, although initiated by nervous discharges, are automatically augmented and prolonged through chemical effects of the adrenal secretion[13].

Vincent regarded Cannon (and, no doubt, Starling too) a "tutored romantic", who was more dangerous to the future of the field of endocrinology than the "untutored" ones and the commercial druggists[10]. Vincent did not – at that time – accept the reality of insulin (officially discovered by Banting and Best), "simply on the grounds of insufficient evidence"[10]. He also rejected the gonadal hormones, discovered after 1923. He did accept 'secretin' discovered by Bayliss and Starling in the pancreas, as a hormone, the stimulant to intestinal function. Vincent was as critical as some of his other colleagues – like the Professor of Pharmacology at University College, London, A. J. Clark.

There were only three classes of people interested in endocrinology:

(1) Scientific investigators with critical minds, who analyse accumulated evidence with dispassionate interest.

(2) Persons engaged in attempting to cure disease whose optimism and eagerness to help, sway their deficient critical sense until they seize at any straw which seems to point towards

390

success. There is often a love of romance in these people which makes them delight in spinning a misty intellectual mesh which completely obscures any possible facts. This is a large and sincere class, including a mass of general practitioners, most dispensing chemists, a number of consultants, not a few journalists, many medical men.

(3) Persons who have realized the commercial possibilities in exploiting the human weakness characteristic of the last-named class. Some of the firms placing 'endocrine' preparations on the market, belong to this class. "The result is that endocrine therapy is coming to bear a suspicious resemblance to mediaeval magic; the savage believes that eating the heart of his enemy will confer on him the virtues of this enemy, and the more enthusiastic vendors of endocrine remedies suggest that the consumption of extracts of practically any organ will cure diseases of that organ"[14].

Professor Clark began his address, a British Medical Association Lecture on the 'Experimental Basis of Endocrine Therapy'[14], as follows:

The laboratory worker and the clinician naturally regard therapeutic measures from a slightly different angle, since the former is concerned chiefly to know what facts can be considered as fully proved, and the latter wishes to know what measures offer a fair chance of benefiting patients. The history of therapeutics teaches us, however, with no uncertain voice, that once speculation and imagination get free from the restraint of rigidly controlled observation there is no limit to the distance which they may wander from the paths of truth. Complex systems of treatment based on inaccurate deductions have repeatedly been built up, and have been almost universally accepted and followed until some advance of knowledge, or even some change in fashion, has sufficed to upset the whole system, and the treatment has been universally discarded and often has come to be regarded not only as useless but actually harmful.

When considering any system of treatment it is very necessary to distinguish clearly between that part of it which is definitely proved and that part which is based merely on plausible deductions, and in no case is this attitude more essential than when considering the recent developments of endocrine therapy.

Vincent made his position abundantly clear. He strictly defined the study of the internal secretions of ductless glands. From his definition it followed that unless the internal secretion of a gland was identified, its hormone isolated, its metabolic action proved, an effective extract could not be obtained; useless extracts should not be prepared nor prescribed. Although he had made valuable contributions to the field of endocrinology himself and wished the 'New Physiology' to develop successfully, his standards became so high, his criteria so strict, his views so rigid, that he produced some critical and even angry reaction. Leonard Williams, who had written the foreword to the English translation of Artur Biedl's textbook in 1913, wrote in a letter to the *Lancet*:

> Moreover, Professor Swale Vincent, by his valuable contributions to endocrinology, has done his bit in stimulating that very enthusiasm which he is now so tireless in rebuking. It is a pity that he should be tiresome as well as tireless[15].

Clark, in his above-mentioned address[14], accepted the three criteria, laid down by Gley, that must be fulfilled before it can be assumed that an organ produces an internal secretion:

(1) The histological condition. The organ must contain secretory cells in intimate relation with the blood vessels and without any duct for external secretion.

(2) The chemical condition. A specific chemical substance must be identified both in the organ and also either the venous blood or lymph coming from the organ.

(3) The physiological condition. The venous blood or lymph coming from the organ must produce the pharmacological actions produced by the specific substance.

We shall see later that Gley's strict, though logical, requirements caused difficulties in establishing endocrinology as a special field in Spain.

Applied to endocrinology, Clark considered therapy to rest on a solid scientific foundation when the following criteria existed:

(a) The destruction of the gland causes a characteristic syndrome.

(b) Administration of extracts of the gland relieves this syndrome.

(c) Some chemical or pharmacological test exists by which the activity of the extract can be recognised and, if possible, be measured[14].

He then discussed the nine glands in which the first condition was fulfilled, although he stressed that "Recent work makes it doubtful if the destruction of the suprarenal medulla produces any very definite effects ..."!

On mentioning the islet tissue of the pancreas, Clark said, interestingly; "but the difficulty of extracting the active principle from the pancreas has only recently been overcome by the work of Banting and Macleod". The address was reported in the *British Medical Journal* of 14 July 1923, the year that Banting and Macleod received the Nobel Prize (for detailed discussion see the section on 'The Story of Insulin' in Chapter 19). The names of Best or of Collip were not mentioned by Professor Clark and that of Paulesco was obviously unknown to him.

After describing the contemporary atmosphere in Britain and the background, polarized around the personalities of Starling and Vincent, Professor Diane Long Hall came to the conclusion that

> The 'crisis' to which Starling was responding in his lecture lay, I believe, not in the science, but in the push for medical reform. Historians have used contemporary sources on those changes, the most famous being the accounts by Abraham Flexner, who published in 1910 an effective call for the reform of American and Canadian medicine on scientific lines. Flexner was also anxious to introduce such reforms into Britain, which he visited in 1910, and revisited in 1922[10].

Starling's extreme advocacy of medical science was effective because he was a respected and persuasive leader in the medical profession. Medical education was made more scientific, and biological science became less medical. Likewise, Vincent's critical voice was heard, and acted upon in medical circles. As the Editors of the *British Medical Journal* remarked in 1937:

> Indiscriminate endocrine therapy brought about the inevitable reaction, and clinical endocrinology came to be looked upon with suspicion. The intense work carried out over the past decade has gone far to remove the disfavour into which endocrinology had fallen, and it is now becoming possible to put the matter into some kind of perspective. Solid achievements have been made. Possibilities are daily becoming probabilities[16].

'Crisis' in Spain

A 'Crisis' in endocrinology was not restricted to Britain. Thomas Glick of the Department of History, Boston University, devoted a study: 'On the Diffusion of a New Specialty; Marañon and the "Crisis" of Endocrinology in Spain'[17], which was originally presented as a 'Model for the Study of Medicine in Different Social and Cultural Contexts', (Harvard University, April 1974). Glick found that barriers to scientific communication were at the core of structural deficiencies which have impeded the growth of science in modern Spain. There, physiologists carried out animal experiments to obtain the exact physiological action of hormones; 'endocrinologists' concentrated on organotherapeutic procedures in the human subject.

In Spain, all research on the endocrine glands at that time seemed to be directed to the service of clinical medicine. The 'Institutionalization' of endocrinology as a medical specialty was the work of Gregorio Marañon (1887–1960) alone (see Section II). 'Institutionalization' is, according to Nicholas C. Mullins[18], the fourth stage in his model describing the formation of a new scientific specialty.

Marañon explained the theory of internal secretions to his colleagues and to the general public; he carried out much publicized organotherapy and stressed the effects of internal secretion on human behaviour, presenting the 'Don Juan personality' as a 'hypergonadal' individual. Marañon spoke of a 'pre-endocrine era' before the 19th century; of a period of "latency" from Berthold, Bernard and Brown-Séquard to 1900, and of a period of "explosive growth" from 1900 to 1910. He regarded Biedl's formulation in 1910 of the doctrine of internal secretion as the basis of his own statement to the Spanish public in 1915. Next, there followed a "hyperbolic" period of excessive overpopularization and overvaluation of the endocrine field between 1910 and 1919, causing a movement or reaction; this started with a course of lectures: 'Quatre Leçons sur les Sécrétions Internes' at the Societad de Biologia in Barcelona, given in 1919 by Professor Eugène Gley of Paris, the Swale Vincent of France[19].

The reaction movement went on to 1922, when Marañon noted a general 'crisis' in the field, which he helped to resolve; he thought the final and 'classical' period would follow, when endocrinology would no longer be subject to attack from the physiologists. The 'crisis' had been caused by Gley's attack on the significance, uncritically given to the importance of internal secretion by the clinicians who called themselves 'endocrinologists'. Gley described the "incomplete experiments, adventurous hypotheses, vain theories and even errors"[19] of the over-zealous clinicians. In 1924, Swale Vincent quoted Gley's criticism of Marañon's "uncritical use of the method of organic extracts" as an example of excesses of the clinicians[20]. At that time many people in Spain carried out adrenaline research, which was sharply criticized by Gley and his Spanish supporters. Juan Negrin, Professor of Physiology in Madrid, criticized George Neil Stewart's (1860–1930) and Julius Moses Rogoff's (1883–1966) technique of experimentally inducing glycosuria in rabbits[21]. Stewart and Rogoff, on their part, were engaged in the controversy with Walter B. Cannon's 'Energy Theory' of adrenal action (see pp. 507–509). Another physiologist who supported Gley was Augusto Pi Suñer of Barcelona, who also felt that the concept of internal secretion had been applied too generally, without clear definitions. According to him, hormone action (or general chemical action) is only one component of human physiology, no more important than any other[17]. No wonder that Marañon felt himself threatened in his organotherapeutic orientation. He defended the thyroid as a gland of internal secretion, which – according to Gley – did not fulfil two of his (Gley's) three necessary criteria of such a gland[22] (see p. 392). Moreover, surgeons like Léon Cardenal of Madrid performed a series of Steinach's rejuvenation operation by ligating the vas, and reported success in a number of patients. The whole episode was reminiscent of the controversy Brown-Séquard's method had created. In February 1926, Marañon and Cardenal carried out a series of much publicized clinical experiments: an adrenal transplant on a patient with Addison's disease, a pituitary transplant on another patient; finally, Cardenal carried out a testicular transplant in a case of impotence and on a eunuchoid young man, according to the method of Serge Voronoff (1866–1951)[23]. This brought about a sharp attack by José Madinaveitia in the daily newspaper *El Sol* (Las operaciones de injertos glandulares en la Facultad de Medicina. *El Sol*, 1 March 1926). Marañon's reply was the creation of a Department of Medical Endocrinology (in 1925), with himself as Director, by re-organizing the Institute of Medical Pathology in Madrid. This he carried out with great courage, in virtual isolation from his colleagues. His first and most important step was to insert himself into an international network of communication. He linked up with Ehrlich's group in Frankfurt. At home, he collected researchers, usually people who had studied abroad. By 1935, his pupils, friends and followers were able to publish a bibliography of all his own work or of work inspired by him directly. By that time, he had 158 collaborators, most of them his pupils. All but nine were Spaniards, seven of the nine being Latin Americans. There was no doubt that endocrinology had emerged as a specialty under the leadership of Gregorio Marañon, a clinician. The present writer, sitting next to Marañon at a dinner in the early 1950s, complimented him on his achievements; one of Marañon's pupils had worked with him in the 1930s. Marañon's sole remark was: "Yes, he has done well; he is one of our most promising clinical endocrinologists" (Dr. José Monguio).

In Spain, therefore, the 'Diffusion of a New Speciality' occurred differently from in Britain or Austria, due to the different background of the development of science; and that is what Glick endeavoured to demonstrate, together with the practical application of Nicholas C. Mullins' proposition of a four-stage model describing the formation of new scientific specialties.

REPRODUCTIVE PHYSIOLOGY

Miss Borell remarked in her paper on 'Edward Schaefer and endocrinology'[24] that the years from 1890 to 1930 have been referred to as the "heroic age of reproductive endocrinology". We must now briefly survey the end of that period, during which occurred the isolation of the gonadal and related pituitary hormones.

Oestrin

It became clear that the ovaries were necessary for the development of the accessory organs of procreation, for the cyclical changes of oestrus (proved by the Viennese Ludwig Adler (1876–1958) in 1912[25]) and for the maintenance of the early phase of pregnancy. F. H. A. Marshall and W. Jolly[26] (and later others) removed the ovaries in the later stages of pregnancy, both experimentally and clinically, without causing abortion or preventing the onset of labour. A. Kohn[27] and A. Brachet[28] came to the conclusion that the ovary is originally hermaphrodite, the cortex being feminine and the medulla masculine. This view is supported by the occasional finding of an ovo-testis.

In 1923/24, Edgar Allen (1892–1943) and Edward Adelbert Doisy (b. 1893) published two papers which signified the beginning of a new era in the study of the endocrinology of female reproduction. Those were: 'An ovarian hormone'[29] which meant the isolation of 'oestrin', the active principle of the ovarian hormone (see also Ref. 30) and 'The induction of a sexually mature condition in immature females by injection of the ovarian follicular hormone'[31]. Allen and Doisy summarized:

(1) That no hormone can be said to be capable of taking the place of the ovary unless tested on *ovariotomized* animals (many of the earlier workers used 'virgin' animals).

(2) That the criteria for oestrus which were used by some of the earlier workers had little meaning.

(3) That an oestrus-producing extract can be made from liquor folliculi.

(4) That *no* oestrus-producing extract can be made from the corpora lutea.

(5) This means that the oestrus-producing hormone is produced by the maturing follicle.

Robert Courrier, using guinea pigs, worked with the liquor folliculi and produced oestrus-like effects in ovariotomized guinea pigs. When injected during pregnancy, the active principle passed through the placenta and produced hyperaemia of the uterus of female foetuses[32,33]. Allen and Doisy proved the existence of a hormone in the fluid of the ovarian follicles of pigs. It was cholesterol-free, unsaponifiable substance, soluble in most lipid solvents, but not in water. They also succeeded in measuring its potency in physiological terms by establishing the Allen-Doisy rat unit. The hormone was present in the follicles, in the whole ovary, and in the placenta. It prevented castrate atrophy in the rat, which meant that it was most likely the same as that found by Iscovesco, Hermann, and the others. As to the name, Rolleston[34] quotes as "Synonyms and Derivatives": oestrin, folliculin (Courrier), oestrone, theelin (crystalline oestrone), menformon (Laqueur), thelykinin (Loewe) and pregynon.

Particularly interesting for the historian is the origin of the collaboration of the two men, Allen and Doisy, which Corner has related with great gusto[35].

Allen was fortunate; he was "an outgoing enthusiast. Heavily built, with a large head on broad shoulders, he was a partial albino with white hair, blue eyes and pink skin"[35]. Doisy was "slender and dark, was a quieter and more reflective man, but always mentally alert"[35].

Neither of them was a medical man, nor had they much previous knowledge of the oestrous cycle. Doisy (see Section II) was a Harvard-trained biochemist, who had done work on colorimetric methods of the determination of phosphorus in the urine and in blood (in 1920). Allen was a zoologist. He learned about the ovarian cycle when working for his Ph.D. thesis. He had also come across Stockard and Papanicolaou's paper of 1917 on the oestrous cycle of the guinea pig (see p. 361), when he was still a student. The second paper of importance he noted, was based on the previous one: it was Joseph Abraham Long (b. 1879) and Herbert McLean Evans' (1882–1971) work on 'the oestrus cycle in the rat and its associated phenomena'[36]. Using the Long-Evans method, Edgar Allen, then an instructor in anatomy at Washington University, was struck by the recurrent presence of large follicles at the time of oestrus, which – he began to suspect – might contain an oestrogenic hormone. With the new Long-Evans method to hand, he collected follicle fluid from pigs' ovaries and injected them into spayed mice. Within hours, the characteristic cytological changes of the oestrous phase of the cycle were present.

Corner tells Doisy's side of the story. He and Allen had become friendly when forming a successful faculty baseball team. It came about that Doisy gave Allen regular lifts from the latter's home to the Medical School. Doisy was working on the purification of insulin, and managed in a dramatic incident, in September 1922, to supply insulin to save the life of a baby who was in a diabetic coma. While talking about his work to Allen in the car, in March 1923, Doisy suddenly told him about his work on the ripening of the follicles, and his ideas. They decided to study the problem together, but before Doisy had finished the preparation of the first extract, Allen had already carried out the crucial experiment mentioned above.

Marshall had – 17 years before – also suspected that the follicles might produce an effective hormone, but had no practical method available to prove it. Doisy, however, proceeded to purify the follicular fluid successfully. Their co-operation lasted until 1927. One of their last important papers was that on 'The menstrual cycle of the monkey, *Macacus rhesus*: observations on normal animals, the effects of removal of the ovaries and the effects of injection of ovarian and placental extracts into the spayed animals'[37], in which it was shown that uterine bleeding is produced as a withdrawal effect, when oestrogen stops acting on the endometrium.

Only after Allen and Doisy had established the nature of oestrin did they find out, from a search of the previous literature, that Iscovesco, Fellner, Hermann and others had attained a similar method of partial purification of the hormone (see p. 362 of the previous chapter), although Doisy managed to carry it a stage further.

This seems to me particularly interesting. As Professor (Sir) Alan Sterling Parkes said at the beginning of his Sir Henry Dale Lecture for 1965 on 'The Rise of Reproductive Endocrinology'[38]:

> . . . I enjoyed Corner's [Dale Lecture of 1964] greatly; much in it was new to me because forty years ago, when I should have read the early literature, I took the view, like most young men and Henry Ford, that history was bunk. I have since learned by experience, as did Allen and Doisy, that those who ignore the past are likely to find themselves re-living it.

These sentiments still exist, however, even today. There are quite a few of our young – and not so young – leading lights in endocrinology whose knowledge of the past of their own special field is considerably less than one would expect. One of the most remarkable men in this respect was the celebrated Fuller Albright (1900–1969) of the Massachusetts General Hospital. When he wrote the Introduction to the section on 'Diseases of the Ductless Glands' in the sixth edition of Cecil's *Textbook of Medicine*[39], he refused to give the derivation of the word 'hormone', which had been coined by Starling; similarly, he would not mention the experiments of Claude Bernard, leading to the term 'internal secretion'; he did not refer to castration, animal or human, a milestone in the early history of endocrinology, nor to Hunter's or Berthold's experimental transplant studies. He refused to list even the names of people who first described endocrine syndromes, from Addison to the more modern ones. He decided to discuss instead, what *is* endocrinology and what it is *not*. Endocrinology *is*, according to Albright (and correctly in our opinion) an indivisible part of internal medicine. It is *not* the fat boy, with slightly delayed sexual development, or the otherwise normal tall girl. Theodore B. Schwartz, of the Rush-Presbyterian-St. Luke's Medical Center, relates in his 'Foreword' to Will G. Ryan's book: *Endocrine Disorders: a Pathophysiological Approach*[40] another of Albright's anecdotes: He 'concluded a presentation with a projected slide which stated: "I have told you more than I know".' As he regarded any form of medical history as bunk, perhaps he was more right than he thought.

Parkes continued in his Dale Lecture of 1965:

Corner is a distinguished historian of science, I am not a historian of any kind. As an eye-witness, however, even at the risk of being anecdotal and parochial, I want to take this chance of putting some flesh on the bare bones of history[28].

Allen and Doisy missed, however, the importance of the special endocrine function of the corpus luteum. They also missed the fact that the general ovarian tissue is a major source of the hormone, as Alan S. Parkes of the (British) National Institute of Medical Research in Hampstead demonstrated in 1926[41,42]. As to the selection of a name for the newly purified hormone 'theelin' (from the Greek 'thelys' = $\theta\eta\lambda\acute{\upsilon}\varsigma$), the fact that the pure crystalline compound was protected by a university-held patent, precluded general use of this designation. Courrier's 'folliculin' was regarded as too narrowly significant, because of the high yield in the placenta. Parkes and Bellerby in 1926[42] hit upon the happy idea of calling it 'oestrin', which proved also a manageable stem, from which a number of new words could be derived, which were needed for the rapidly expanding subject.

As it happened, it was the chemists who developed the field. S. Loewe and F. Lange described in 1926 that oestrogenic hormones are present in human urine[43]. Next came Selmar Aschheim's observation, that a much larger quantity is found in the urine during pregnancy[44], to be followed by the Aschheim–Zondek (Bernhard

Zondek 1891–1966) test for pregnancy from the urine[45]. Until then, Allen and Doisy were handicapped by the limited quantities of their raw material that were available. This discovery guaranteed rapid progress, and the isolation of the oestrus-producing substance in crystalline form was achieved in 1929, not only by Doisy, Thayer and Veler in St. Louis[46], but also by Adolf Friedrich Johann Butenandt (b. 1903)[47] of Goettingen. In 1930, Ernst Laqueur (1880–1947) and his team in Amsterdam isolated a similar active material, which Laqueur called "Menformon"[48].

Doisy and Butenandt independently reached the conclusion that the formula of the pure cystalline hormone 'Oestrone' or 'Theelin' was $C_{18}H_{22}O_2$, a hydroxyketone. A further impetus to this line of research was given by B. Zondek's discovery that the urine of pregnant mares was a rich source of oestrin substances. Thus 100 000 to 500 000 mouse units per litre of mare's urine became a source of commercial utilization. The use of placenta extracts and of urinary products for treatment of sexual disorders in mediaeval China has already been discussed (Chapter 11). Even more remarkable were the discoveries that small quantities of oestrone were present in the urine of human males[49], also the demonstration by E. A. Haeussler that the testes of stallions contain 500 times more oestrone than ovaries of sexually mature mares[50].

In 1930, Guy Frederic Marrian (1904–1981), then of University College, London (see Postscript), announced that he had found other oestrogenic substances in the urine of pregnant women[51]. Marrian, who worked virtually single-handed under difficult conditions, was first disbelieved but, eventually, fully vindicated. It was confirmed that apart from oestrone, there was present in pregnancy urine 'oestriol' as a separate entity. Marrian's further observation that more active substance could be obtained from stale and decomposed urine than from fresh was later explained by the fact that oestrogen was excreted in conjugated form and had to be hydrolysed before becoming biologically active again.

A further important step was taken when, in July 1932, the first meeting of the International Conference on the Standardization of Sex Hormones took place in London. Doisy, Laqueur, Marrian, Parkes, Butenandt, Marshall, Collip, Dodds, Girard and Schoeller, under the chairmanship of Sir Henry Dale, agreed on a standard preparation for urinary hydroxyketone. A nice touch occurred when discussing the scarcity of material, Doisy and Butenandt – hesitantly – offered a contribution of 500 mg each. When the unknown Girard asked diffidently if 20 grams would be any good, he was met with disbelief, especially when he actually produced the crystalline substance from his waistcoat pocket! It turned out to be, however, the true bill, the happy result "of the application to mare's urine of a new ketone reagent"[38].

At that meeting, the terminology was extended: to oestrin were added oestrone, oestriol and oestradiol. A minute amount of oestradiol was isolated by Doisy and his team from sows' ovaries in 1936. The slight similarity of the nucleus of the oestrogens to that of some synthetic carcinogenic substances posed another problem, which has not been resolved yet. More happily, (Sir) Edward Charles Dodds (1899–1973) of the Middlesex Hospital in London, and his co-workers, found in 1938 that certain synthetic compounds, primarily detected as impurities of anol and without a steroid nucleus, had oestrogenic activity. This was the introduction of stilboestrol, the first synthetic 'oestrogen'[52], to be followed soon by that of dynoestrol[53]. Both these clinically effective preparations could be produced by the kilogram, but the problem of their carcinogenic effect also raised its ugly head.

Progesterone

We have seen in the previous chapter (p. 362) that Edmund Hermann of Vienna published the results of his studies in 1915. Extracts had been made from general ovarian tissue, from the corpus luteum and from the placenta, with results similar to those of other research workers. Henry Iscovesco in France and Robert T. Frank in New York. Corner remarked that in 1923, the literature on the subject was still in "a very confused state". Ludwig Fraenkel's work has also been discussed in detail (see pp. 366–368). Allen and Doisy's discoveries made it clear, however, that Hermann must have used a mixed extract. The situation which Corner and his team (especially Willard Myron Allen, b. 1904) had to face, was made more complex by the fact that relatively large amounts were needed for the specific biological test, which was also time-consuming as it was based on maintaining pregnancy in adult rabbits after mating. Corner and Willard Allen attempted to use progestational proliferation in immature rabbits, but after some time it became clear that such response could be achieved only if the immature rabbit uterus was first primed with oestrogen. By December 1928, they submitted their second and third papers on the 'Physiology of the corpus luteum'. In their Summary they said: "It appears, therefore, that the extracts of corpus luteum contain a special hormone which has for one of its functions the preparation of the uterus for reception of the embryos by inducing progestational proliferation of the endometrium"[54].

In the summary of the third paper the final sentence reads[55]:

The evidence is now complete that in the rabbit the corpus luteum is an organ of internal secretion which has for one of its functions the production of a special state of the uterine mucosa (progestational proliferation) and that in turn the function of the proliferated endometrium is to nourish or protect the free blastocysts and to make possible their implantation.

It is surprising that it took another 5 years before Willard M. Allen and Oscar Paul Wintersteiner (b. 1898) could report the isolation of cystalline 'progestin', almost coincidentally with Adolf F. J. Butenandt and Ulrich Westphal (b. 1910); moreover, with Max Hartmann (b. 1884) and Albert Wettstein of Switzerland; and, finally, with Karl H. Slotta (b. 1895) and his team. The isolation procedure needed enormous quantities of the raw material. Butenandt used the corpora lutea of 50 000 pigs to obtain a few milligrams of the hormone! In the same year (1934), Butenandt [and also Karl H. Slotta, who was Ludwig Fraenkel's son-in-law (see p. 368[56])], determined the chemical structure of the corpus luteum hormone. Butenandt had already, in 1931, isolated the male sex hormone (androsterone) in crystalline form[57].

Thus, at the Second International Conference on Standardization of Sex Hormones in 1935, at the London School of Hygiene, with Sir Henry Dale as Chairman, a standard of crystalline material could be established for the hormone of the corpus luteum. Professor Alan S. Parkes told amusingly how the name 'progesterone' was born[59]. At the Second International Conference, Willard Allen and George Corner presented as the name for their crystalline substance, 'Progestin'; Butenandt came forward with 'Luteosterone', and a lengthy (and boring) discussion seemed to loom ahead. 'Progesterone' had been thought of by Willard Allen, but he was not enthusiastic about it. Parkes and Marrian, however, thought it a good name; at the pre-conference party, given by Sir Heny Dale, they tried it on Butenandt and others, successfully.

The name progesterone may thus be said to have been born, if not conceived, in a place of refreshment near the Imperial Hotel in Russell Square, where Willard Allen was staying[59].

In the meantime, Professor Solly Zuckerman (b. 1904), now Lord Zuckerman, had shown that the extra-ovarian features of anovular cycles could be stimulated in castrated animals by sequential changes in oestrogen dosage and those of normal cycles by changes in the appropriate levels of oestrogen and progesterone, thus solving the major mystery of the menstrual cycle. Similarly, Professor Robert Courrier in Algiers studied the behaviour of oestrogen and progesterone during pregnancy in various species[60]. Parkes assumed[61] that the corpora lutea of pregnancy, pseudo-pregnancy and lactation have four functions: (1) The inhibition of ovulation and of the oestrous changes in the accessory organs: (2) the sensitization of the uterus for the implantation of the fertilized ova ('progestational proliferation'); (3) the development of the mammary glands from the condition they are in oestrus to that at the end of the luteal phase.

The role of the two ovarian hormones at the time of the climacteric was described by Bernhard Zondek (1891–1966) as[62] (1) an excessive secretion of oestrin (the poly-oestrone phase); (2) followed by a decline of oestrin secretion (the oligo-oestrone phase) and (3) by an increase of secretion of pituitary gonadotrophic hormone (the poly-gonadotrophic phase), often to remain permanently in the urine.

Marañon regarded the climacteric as a pluriglandular disorder of ovarian and pituitary insufficiency, hyperthyroid tendency and hyperadrenalism[63]. Bernard Zondek's poly-oestrone phase may last weeks or months. In the oligo-oestrone phase, the precipitate decline of the hormone is typical; it is characterized by the signs of vasomotor instability. After the ovaries stop functioning, in the third stage, the considerable increase in urinary gonadotrophin may remain a permanent feature. The three stages may merge imperceptibly into one another.

Androgens

The connection of the testicles with procreation and the effects of castration in animals as well as in man, belong – as we have seen in previous chapters – to the oldest experiences of an endocrine nature. Added to it were the more recent studies by de Graaf, Leeuwenhoek, Spallanzani, von Koelliker and others, including embryological investigations. Last, but by no means least, one must remember John Hunter's and Berthold's testicular transplant experiments and Brown-Séquard's organotherapy. Microscopically, it was known after Franz Leydig's (1821–1908) description of the cells named after him that there are two main cell groups of importance in the testicle (see also Chapter 17, and Ref. 36 therein).

Enrico Sertoli (1842–1910), Italian histologist, described the tall epithelial cells in the tubules of the testes, named after him; to their ends become attached the spermatids until they change into mature spermatozoa; they are also called sustentacular cells. Then there is the vascular connective tissue, whereas the Leydig cells described in 1850[64], also called interstitial cells, form the basis of the interstitial tissue, also called the 'interstitial gland' of the testis, or – according to Eugen Steinach (1861–1951) – the 'puberty gland'[65]. It was soon reported by various observers that in man and animals with cryptorchidism, in whom there is no spermatogenesis but the interstitial cells are intact, the secondary sex characteristics do develop and function normally. If the Leydig cells have been damaged or disappear, signs of castration become evident. Botin and Ancel studied ligation of the vasa deferentia in rabbits: after a few months, the germinative part of the testicles, including the spermatogonia, spermatocytes, spermatids and spermatozoa disappear, only a thin layer of Sertoli cells remaining. The interstitial cells, however, show considerable proliferation; the secondary sex characteristics show no change. A. Loewi and Hermann Zondek destroyed the germinative tissue by adequate doses of X-rays (checked histologically)[66]. During the entire experiment, metabolism remained at a normal level, even though one testicle was removed for histological examination. Only after removal of the second testicle appeared the signs of castration, with a drop in metabolism of 15–20%, after only a few days. Steinach's rejuvenation operation, i.e. ligation of the vas deferens in man, was based on the above experiments[65]. It was much argued whether the results justified the attempt. The re-awakening of libido in old people is not necessarily entirely desirable. Other signs, such as growth of hair in the original natural colour instead of white, increase in body weight, and improved working efficiency appeared transient and perhaps also auto-suggestive. Yet, A. Loewi and H. Zondek came to the conclusion that Steinach's operation did result in genuine rejuvenation[66], after carefully studying a number of men between the ages of 57 and 66, who had been suffering from various complaints of old-age and sexual deficiency and had undergone the operation. Its effects, however, last only a number of weeks or months.

Next, it was Serge Voronoff (1866–1951), working in Algiers, who reported his experimental rejuvenation by means of testicular implants (originally in 1919)[23]. He grafted sections of chimpanzee's or baboon's testicles into the scarified tunica vaginalis (in farm animals and humans). He attracted much publicity and in 1927 an international deputation visited him in Algiers, including F. H. A. Marshall from Cambridge, F. A. E. Crew from Edinburgh, W. C. Miller and others. According to A. S. Parkes, their report to the Ministry of Agriculture "was very cautious"[38].

It is surprising, therefore, that the isolation of the male hormone and the production of active testicular extracts was so long delayed.

This was not only due to technical problems, but also to the idea that (male) ageing was mainly due to the gradual running down of the testicular function and that all that was needed to restore it was to graft testicular tissue or to inject whole-testicle extracts. The idea that the interstitial cells produce a hormone concerned with the development of the secondary sex characteristics and the sexual instincts, was mooted by S. G. Shattock in 1897[67], and before him by F. Reinke in 1896[68]. Rolleston quotes Victor Robinson as reading "a vague foreshadowing of endocrinology into a passage of Aretaeus: 'for it is the semen, when possessed of vitality, which makes us to be men, hot, well braced in limbs, well voiced, spirited, strong to think and act' "[69].

Lemuel Clyde McGee (b. 1904) in the United States prepared perhaps the first active extract, from the lipoid fraction of bull testicles in 1927[70]. In his report he gave a preliminary description of the capon–comb test, which was given in greater detail in a paper by Carl Richard Moore (1892–1955), T. F. Gallagher and F. C. Koch in 1929: 'The effects of extracts of testis in correcting the castrated condition in the fowl and in the mammal'[71]. They had obtained a potent testicular extract containing androsterone. Moore's group (including McGee) developed the capon–comb test (comb growth in capons) for the essay of the male hormone. When Ernst Laqueur (1880–1947) and his team in Amsterdam eventually isolated a crystalline hormone from the testicle in 1935, they gave it – as A. S. Parkes put it[38] – "the dreadful name 'testosterone' ". In the meantime, it had been found that male urine contained the active principle, and in 1931 Butenandt[57] (see also p. 402) isolated a crystalline substance from 25 000 litres of male urine, which he called 'androsterone' and for which he was to share the Nobel Prize in 1939 with Leopold Ruzicka, who managed to synthetize androsterone by preparing isomerides from cholesterol in 1934[58] (see also p. 790). Laqueur's team observed that highly purified testicular extract lost its biological activity, whereas the admixture of fatty acids or esterification increased the effectiveness of synthetic androgens by delaying absorption at the site of injection. This brought A. S. Parkes to the development of solid pellets of steroid hormones, which – implanted subcutaneously or intramuscularly – gave improved and prolonged biological action[38]. One little-known result of this work is related by Parkes with great gusto: his presentation by (Sir) E. Charles Dodds (1899–1973) at a dinner at the Catalyst Club with a record of an old popular ballad, which had been signed by Dodds, (Lord) Zuckerman, Robert Robinson, and others. The title of the ballad was: "If I should plant a tiny seed of love (In the Garden of your Heart)" by MacDonald and Tate!

Parkes and Zuckerman could also show that prolonged injection of androsterone into an immature male mandrill would produce the rainbow colours of the fully grown male[38]. In the further progress of the research on the steroid sex hormones a new discovery was made: namely, that the clear delineation and separation of maleness and femaleness does not hold good!

Ambivalence of sexuality

In 1928, Brouha and Simmonet demonstrated that testicular extracts could cause vaginal cornification[38]. We have already mentioned that Bernhard Zondek, and also E. A. Haeussler, found in 1934 that the testicles of stallions are the richest source of oestrone[50]. B. Zondek also found that stallion urine has a high oestrone content, whereas the urine of the non-pregnant mare or of a gelding has a low one. Similarly, extracts from blood and urine from men produced vaginal cornification. Finally, it was shown that oestrone and probably oestriol were present in men's urine[38].

Vice-versa, androgenic active substances were found in women's urine in similar amounts as those in men's; and – in 1938 – R. K. Callow and Callow demonstrated that the two main androgens, androsterone and di-hydro-epi-androsterone, were identical. Similarly, the chemical structural formulae of progesterone and testosterone are very similar. Finally, studies on gonadectomized men and women showed that much of the androgen and oestrogen in the urine was not of gonadal origin and that the adrenal cortex was the source of the extragonadal production[38]. Although this helped to explain the features of the adreno-genital syndrome, it put an end to the expectation that the excretion of the sex steroids could be used to measure hyper- or hypo-function of the gonads. A. S. Parkes put it wittily:

> The present wonder, therefore, is not that intersexual conditions occur, but that the balance of endocrine factors usually comes down on one side or the other to produce a recognisable male or female – perhaps in these days, I should say, a more or less recognisable male or female[38].

The gonadotrophins of the anterior pituitary

The idea that the functions of the sex glands might be influenced and controlled by some extragonadal factor, most likely the anterior lobe of the pituitary, had been 'in the air' since the beginning of the 20th century. We mentioned in Chapter 16 (see also p. 304). Ref. 67, and p. 323, Ref. 138) that Le Comte in 1898 noted the increase in size of the pituitary during pregnancy, and that Erdheim and Stumme described the pregnancy cells. Aschner's, Cushing's, and others' observations and experiments (see Chapter 16) confirmed that anterior hypopituitarism led to genital hypoplasia. During the course of two lectures in 1926, Bernhard Zondek and Selmar Aschheim (b. 1878) reported that they had succeeded in producing precocious sexual maturity in mice by transplantation of the anterior lobe of the pituitary. Herbert McLean Evans (1882–1971), with Joseph Abraham Long (b. 1879), had already studied the effect of continued intraperitoneal injections of an anterior pituitary extract on growth, maturity and oestrous cycle of the rat in 1921[72] and found an acceleration in the growth rate of their laboratory animals. Evans later (in 1924) described that such injections of bovine extract inhibited the oestrous cycle and caused marked luteinization of the follicles[73]. Philip E. Smith (1884–1970), however, was able, in the course of his experiments, to induce precocious sexual maturity in rats and mice by pituitary homeo-transplants, on which observation he reported in detail with his co-worker Earl Theron Engle (1896–1957) under the heading: 'Experimental evidence regarding the role of the anterior pituitary in the development and regulation of the genital system'[74]. Macerated pituitary tissue implants made the immature mouse ovary increase up to twenty times in weight. As a first step leading up to these results, Philip E. Smith described his successful method of hypophysectomy on the 25-day juvenile rat, whom he could keep alive for many months, and which resulted in "an almost complete inhibition of growth in the young animal and a progressive loss of weight in the adult"[75]. The adult animals became prematurely senile, with atrophy of the gonads, thyroid, parathyroids and adrenal cortex; in short, they developed a syndrome which in the human was described by M. Simmonds (see Chapter 16) as a consequence of atrophy of the anterior lobe.

As already mentioned, B. Zondek and S. Aschheim achieved the same results in their experiments, independently, on which they reported in detail in 1927[76,77]. Zondek and Aschheim had also found that the urine of pregnant females contained a substance with the same action as the gonadotrophic principle in the anterior pituitary, which forms the basis of the Aschheim–Zondek pregnancy test, published in 1928[45]. The identity of the pituitary and the urinary principle have, however, been contested. The objection that the animal's own pituitary might have been stimulated by the treatment was invalidated by Smith's further experiments in which injections of macerated tissue preparations fully restored sexual function in hypophysectomized rats.

Zondek and Aschheim called the substance they had found gonadotrophin or prolan. Moreover, they believed that there are two distinct hormones, Prolan A and Prolan B. They said that Prolan A governs follicle maturation and Prolan B controls luteinization. They put forward the following argument[76]:

Anterior Pituitary Reaction I: Test for Prolan A:	Maturation of follicle and ovum; Production of oestrone: oestral reaction
Anterior Pituitary Reaction II: Test for Prolan A + B:	"Blood Points", i.e. haemorrhages in enlarged follicles.
Anterior Pituitary Reaction III: Test for Prolan B:	Luteinization, i.e. formation of true corpora lutea with enclosed ova (atretic corpora lutea)

This was strongly criticized by James Bertram Collip (1895–1965) of Montreal, who would not accept the prolan of B. Zondek or the existence of two prolans in the placenta[78,79]; nor did E. C. Dodds accept that the existence of two prolans had been proved[80]. Fevold, F. L. Hisaw and S. L. Leonard[81], and also M. Hill and A. S. Parkes put forward evidence for two distinct hormones influencing the ovarian cycle[82]. Harry Fevold and Hisaw of Wisconsin described a method of separating the follicle-stimulating and the luteinizing hormone[83].

Today, we talk of FSH = Follicle Stimulating Hormone and LH = Luteinizing Hormone; in the male, it is the ICSH = Interstitial Cell Stimulating Hormone. These terms developed following the work of Herbert McLean Evans and his group (e.g. Evans, H. M., Korpi, K., Pencharz, R. I. and Wonder, D. H.[84]), who also distinguished an 'Antagonistic Factor' and a 'Synergistic Factor'; but it is possible that the LH, ICSH and the antagonistic factor are identical.

It seemed that the hormone in pregnancy is produced in the chorionic villi of the placenta. It was, therefore, called 'chorionic' gonadotrophin in contrast to the 'pituitary' gonadotrophins. The extrahypophysial origin of the chorionic gonadotrophin in early-pregnancy urine was confirmed mainly by J. B. Collip and his team in 1930. B. Zondek himself carefully worked out the quantitative differences of the action of pituitary and chorionic gonadotrophic hormone[62]. He also found that the effect of pituitary gonadotrophic hormone is greatly increased by delayed absorption at the site of injection, by addition, e.g. of zinc sulphate, tannic acid, etc.[62]. H. M. Evans and M. E. Simpson showed[85,86] that the gonadotrophic hormone is produced by the basophil cells of the anterior lobe. This was confirmed by B. Zondek and W. Berblinger[87], and by H. M. Teel and Harvey Cushing[88]; but – according to E. J. Kraus[89] – the acidophil cells also participate. Hermann Zondek stresses the important fact that the

> gonadotrophic hormone is the *superior and sexually undifferentiated sex hormone*; both, in the male and female sexual organs gonadotrophic effects are induced by implanting the anterior lobe of either sex[90].
> Factor A (FSH) stimulates the follicles in the female and the Sertoli cells in the male; factor B (LH) stimulates the corpus luteum in the female and Leydig's interstitial tissue in the male.

Fee and A. S. Parkes could show in acute experiments in 1928 that hypophysectomy of the female rabbit within 45 minutes of mating prevented ovulation[38], but their somewhat crude method of partial decerebration was criticized by Philip E. Smith, who achieved the same result by his usual meticulous surgical technique.

Another problem mentioned by A. S. Parkes was created by the fact that the main sources of pituitary material differed considerably in their actions. Herbert McLean Evans, in his growth experiments, mainly used horse pituitary, which contains mostly FSH, whereas the ox pituitary mainly contains LH[38].

A further gonadotrophic hormone, not identical with either the pituitary or the placental ones, was discovered in the blood of pregnant mares by Harold Harrison Cole (b. 1897) and George H. Hart (b. 1883) in 1930, and also by B. Zondek in the same year[38].

The last discovery and also the existence of gonadotrophins in human pregnancy urine and in the placenta proved a rich source of gonadotrophic hormone which now became readily available for clinical and experimental use, considering that, for example, Laqueur and his associates obtained only 10 mg of male hormone from 100 kg of bull testicle in 1935! On the other hand, A. S. Parkes pointed out that for clinical use only human pituitary gonadotrophic hormone proved effective.

In 1928, P. Stricker and F. Grueter made the observation that lactation could be produced in ovariectomized pseudo-pregnant rabbits by administration of anterior pituitary extracts (lactogenic hormone)[91]. In fact, Walter Lee Gaines (b. 1881) had demonstrated the action of the pituitary in lactation as early as 1915[92].

Remarkably, the French research workers did not follow up their results and the 'prolactin' story was taken up elsewhere. We discussed John Hunter's interest in the phenomenon of 'pigeon's milk' (see p. 197), which, much later, was found to be controlled by the lactogenic hormone, now called 'prolactin'. Oscar Riddle (1877–1968) took over from Stricker and Grueter. Oscar Riddle, R. W. Bates and S. W. Dykshorn published the result of their research on 'the preparation, identification and assay of prolactin – a hormone of the anterior pituitary'[93]. Joseph Halban, in 1905, believed that lactation was controlled by active principles of the chorionic villi of the placenta[94]. Ernest H. Starling and Janet E. Lane-Claypon, in 1906, thought it was regulated by those of the embryo[95], and others had different ideas again. George Corner supported Riddle's findings. The latter's team had, moreover, demonstrated that the prolactin fraction was distinct from the other growth-stimulating principles of the anterior pituitary. The pigeon's crop-gland reaction, introduced by them, became the standard test for the assay of prolactin. John Hunter would have been pleased!

According to A. S. Parkes, the discovery of prolactin in fish pituitaries "prompted the thought that in the course of evolution organisms find new uses for old substances, and even that 'the by-product of today is the hormone of tomorrow' "[38]. The main actions of prolactin are: (a) production of milk in mammals, and activation of the pigeon's crop-gland; (b) inhibition of menstruation in women, delayed oestrus in mammals, atrophy of the gonads in pigeons (anti-gonadal activity); (c) induction of maternal instinct [nest-building; care and protection of the young, even of the strange young (cuckoo-in-the-nest)]; (d) loss of flight-reaction in pigeons; (e) unknown action of it in fishes. To all this we have to add some newer pathological syndromes for hyper-prolactinaemia, often linked with amenorrhoea in mammals.

The existence of a second, 'mammotrophic' hormone to 'prepare' the mammary gland for lactation, could not be conclusively proved, especially as the necessary growth of the mammary gland can be caused by oestrone, which produces proliferation of the excretory ducts and pigmentation of the nipple and enlargement of the Montgomery tubercles. Progesterone causes proliferation of the alveoli. This stimulation occurs in a modest manner during each menstrual period and more definitely during pregnancy. The high level of oestrone and progesterone in the blood paves the way for the secretion of prolactin in the pituitary. The sudden withdrawal of oestrone and progesterone from the body at birth is the final stimulus for high level production of prolactin in the pituitary. Experimental proof for the existence of prolactin was given by the fact that hypophysectomy immediately stops lactation; this was done by H. Allen and P. Wiles[96] in 1932, and also by Hans Selye, James B. Collip and D. L. Thomson[97].

This feverish research activity needed solutions for the difficult problems of standardization arising from it. In 1938, the third Conference on the Standardization of Sex-Hormones took place in Geneva, again with Sir Henry Dale in the chair[75]. The large number of participants included this time Herbert McLean Evans, Oscar Riddle, and others concerned with the new discoveries. Agreement was reached on new standards for chorionic gonadotrophin, mare serum gonadotrophin and for prolactin, but *not* for the pituitary gonadotrophins, which had to wait until long after the war to arrive at a solution[38].

Philip E. Smith summed up the position concerning the anterior lobe hormones in 1935:

> . . . it is evident that no less than six and possibly eight hormones have been extracted from the anterior pituitary. That this small gland, which in man averages less than 0.5 grams in weight, secretes this number of hormones as separate entities throughout the entire secretory process, taxes the imagination[98].

If he could have only foreseen the position existing in 1979, I am certain he would have added "and the mind boggles"!

Hermann Zondek answered the question

> how in an organ as small as the pituitary, so many different hormones can be elaborated? Probably these various substances are but *modifications derived from a chemically uniform basic substance by comparatively insignificant molecular changes*[99].

This idea was also shared by Julius Bauer (1887–1979) in Vienna in 1937[100].

Hermann Zondek devoted a whole chapter (IV) of his textbook to 'The Relations between the Different Hormonal Glands'[101] and a further chapter (VIII) to 'The Autonomic Nervous System and its Relations to the Hormonal System'[102].

NEURO–ENDOCRINOLOGY

The inter-hormonal relationships, the inter-glandular relationships, the development of the role of the feed-back phenomenon, the discovery of the 'endocrine orchestra' conducted by the pituitary led, inevitably, to the idea of yet higher placed control by the hypothalamus and, eventually, by the cerebral cortex itself. Thus, students and explorers of the endocrine expanse found themselves back in the field of neuro-endocrinology, so new and yet so old. A. S. Parkes put it eloquently:

> . . . neural factors were known to be involved in ovulation in the rabbit and pseudo-pregnancy in mice and rats. . . . Further information was provided in the 1930s by Marshall and others who showed that pharmacological agents which stimulated the central nervous system might cause ovulation in the rabbit.

In his 'Croonian Lectures' to the Royal College of Physicians of London in 1936: 'Sexual Periodicity and the Causes which Determine it'[103], Francis H. A. Marshall, then at Cambridge, mentioned W. Heap, who had put forward in 1905 the theory that some substance is found in the body in small amounts that is responsible for growth and reproduction, pointing out that, broadly speaking, reproduction begins when growth ceases or, at least, slows down[104].'' In that lecture, Marshall came to the following conclusions[103]:

> . . . Speaking generally, there is an internal rhythm of reproduction depending primarily upon the alteration of periods of rest and activity; in correlation with this rhythm, hormones are periodically elaborated by the gonads and act upon the accessory organs and secondary sexual characters. But in the higher animals, the internal rhythm is brought into relation with seasonal changes and other external environmental phenomena, these not merely conditioning the metabolic processes (as they do also in all or most of the lower animals, as well as in plants), but, in part at any rate, acting extraceptively through the nervous system and probably through the hypothalamus upon the anterior pituitary and thence upon the testis and the ovary. . . . The primary periodicity is a function of the gonad, the anterior pituitary acting as a regulator, and the internal rhythm is adjusted to the environment, by the latter acting on the pituitary, partly or entirely, through the intermediation of the nervous system.

Prophetic words, these! – To continue Parkes' assessment:

> Moreover, it was evident that some reciprocating mechanism must exist, whereby the gonads were protected from overstimulation by excessive amounts of pituitary gonadotrophin. This mechanism was found to depend on the fact that the presence of excessive amounts of gonadal hormones, provided exogenously or produced by overstimulated secretion, and thus on gonad activity. This 'feedback mechanism' was exploited in various ways in the 1930s and is now, of course, the cornerstone of oral contraception. . . . Historically, neuroendocrine effects in reproduction, currently receiving a great deal of attention, provide a happy marriage between the early views that neural effects dominated the reproductive processes and the later ones, developed in the period under review, that endocrine effects were all-important[38].

The last three projects A. S. Parkes and his group (Idwal Row-lands, C. W. Emmens and R. K. Callow) worked on, between January 1932 and 1940, at the Medical Research Council's Institute at Hampstead (under Sir Henry Dale) were: (1) the study, in animals, of anti-gonadotrophic principles (mainly Idwal Rowlands); (2) the study of the relations, or lack of them, between gonadal condition and steroid excretion (mainly Emmens and Callow); (3) the stock-piling and biological evaluation of desiccated pituitary powder and its extracts of (a) human pituitary glands, which were individually recorded, and (b) of dried horse pituitary glands, now hard to come by[38].

But to return to the history of neuro-endocrinology. We have already referred to Dr. Geoffrey Wingfield Harris, FRS, whose early death on 29 November 1971 was a great loss to British physiology and to international neuro-endocrinology. He was from 1962 Dr. Lee's Professor of Anatomy and Head of the Department of Human Anatomy in Oxford; his special work was carried out at his Neuro-endocrinology Research Unit, where he furthered the de-velopment and application of highly sensitive assays for pituitary and steroid hormones in human and animal studies. His death occurred only 6 months after being awarded the Dale Medal of the Society of Endocrinology and after giving the Sir Henry Dale Lecture for 1971 (on 27 May 1971) on 'Humours and Hormones' (see p. 65). He called it 'Humours' because he referred to Galen, Conrad Victor Schneider (1614–1680) of Wittenberg and to Richard Lower (1631–1691) concerning the idea "that neurosecretory material . . . pass down the nerve fibres, through the infundibulum to the posterior pituitary . . .". We have also mentioned that H. H. Simmer felt that Thomas Willis and Richard Lower were wrongly credited with the suggestion of pituitary hormones, the key to such claim being the translation of one of Willis's sentences from the Latin (see Chapter 13). Be it as it may, it is obvious that the idea of chemical (or humoral) transmission to the nervous system is older than many people, even research workers in that field, realize. F. J. Gall in 1818[105] and J. Vimont[106] mentioned that unilateral castration causes atrophy of the contralateral hemisphere of the cerebellum:

Toutes les fois qu'on a enlevé un seul testicule à un animal, de quelque espèce qu'il soit, le lobe du cervelet, du côté opposé, s'atrophie visiblement, ou est altéré dans sa substance, d'une manière quelconque; . . . J'ai fait châtrer, unilatéralement, plusieurs lapins, les uns du côté droit, les autres du côté gauche. Les ayant fait tuer six a huit mois après, j'ai trouvé sans exception, le lobe du cervelet, du coté opposé à celui où la castration avait été opérée, plus petit, et la bosse occipitale plus aplatie que l'autre[107].

Vimont wrote:

> Chez quatre autres lapins que je fait nourrir pendant dix-huit mois, j'ai trouvé après la mort une diminution apparente du lobe cérébelleux opposé[108].

Similarly, reports that gonadal hypoplasia could be observed in men with agenesis of the olfactory lobes was ignored when first recorded by A. Maestre de San Juan in Spain in 1856[109] and F. Weidenreich in 1914[110]; but when more such reports appeared, T. Mirsalis in 1929[111], T. Kanai in 1940[112], G. Gauthier in 1960[113], etc., the condition had to be reconsidered and was confirmed by experimental studies (E. Scharrer and B. Scharrer[114]). The late G. W. Harris was one of the few research workers who studied neuro-endocrine development in the foetus[115]. In 1890 R. Zander noted the connection between the adrenals and other organs, especially the brain[116], referring to observations on the absence of the adrenal cortex in anencephali recorded by Morgagni in 1733, Soemmering in 1792, and Meckel in 1802.

More recently, in 1951, Emile Moeri has discussed the situation: 'Les surrénales chez le foetus, le nouveau-né, le nourrisson et l'enfant'[117]. Scharrer and Scharrer emphasize that A. A. Berthold, in his celebrated and overlooked experiment of the testicular transplant in 1849, "implicated the nervous system as a target organ, but this thought was not pursued until Steinach's experiments in 1912 received widespread attention"[114]. They also comment on the remarkable fact that Brown-Séquard, who was both a neurologist and a pioneer in endocrine research with a lively and fertile imagination, "never seems to have become interested in possible connections between the nervous system and the endocrine glands"[114].

In 1913, G. Peritz summed up the state of affairs at that time in his contribution to the *Handbuch der Biochemie*, 'Nervensystem und innere Sekretion'[119], mainly posing questions to which, even now, many of the answers are missing. F. H. Lewy declared in his 60-page account on the diseases of the endocrine glands – obviously written for the benefit of the neurologists in 1929[120], that "die vegetativen Kerne im Zentralnervensystem and Hypophysenhinterlappen ein einziges zusammengehoeriges System bilden" (= the vegetative nuclei in the central nervous system form with the posterior lobe of the pituitary a single, consecutive system). However, the concept of the chemical transmission of nerve impulses faced great difficulties between 1910 and 1950 before it became accepted. Three of its main pioneers, Sir Henry Dale, Walter B. Cannon and Otto Loewi of Graz (Nobel Prize winner), are all now deceased. It is fortunate, therefore, that two of the eye witnesses have written a memoir of that period:

Wilhelm Feldberg on 'The early history of synaptic and neuro-muscular transmission by acetylcholine: reminiscences of an eye witness'[121], and Z. M. Bacq of Liège (Belgium): "Les transmissions chimiques de l'influx nerveux" in 1974. An English translation of this work was published in 1975 for the celebration of the Sir Henry Dale centenary: *Chemical Transmission of Nerve Impulses*[122].

Feldberg stresses that for the true beginning of his narrative ". . . we must go back to Dale's early publication in 1914 on 'The action of certain esters and ethers of choline', in which he made the fundamental distinction between two types of action of acetylcholine, a muscarine and a nicotine action . . ." that was the true beginning of the story of acetylcholine in synaptic and neuromuscular transmission.

In 1937, Dale penned a note for the *Proceedings of the Physiological Society* on 'Du Bois–Reymond and chemical transmission', illustrating that 60 years previously, in 1877, Raymond had clearly suggested a chemical transmission from motor nerve endings to striated muscle[123]. "Then there was the brilliant anticipation of this mode of action", Feldberg continues: "by T. R. Elliott, who had been the first to conceive the idea of chemical transmission in the autonomic nervous system". In 1914, Elliott said:

> I have tried in vain to discover an active principle in the muscle plates of striped muscles. And Professor Herring was also disappointed when he examined for this purpose the electric organs of the skate which are exaggerated motor end plates . . .

The prediction came true, when Feldberg and Fessard published a paper in 1942 'On the cholinergic nature of the nerves to the electric organ of *Torpedo*[121] (p. 68).

Bacq, in his historical sketch, said:

> The concept of a neuro-endocrine system, as W. B. Cannon defined it in the 1920s, is still valid. The most striking example is the series of catecholamines, of which some (adrenaline, noradrenaline) are real hormones secreted into the blood by the adrenal medulla during emotional shock, physical exercise, cold, or when the blood sugar concentration drops below the point tolerable to nerve cells. These same hormones are also the chemical mediators or transmitters, the indispensable substances for the transmission of excitation in one class of nerve fibres which innervate the heart, smooth muscles and glands[122] . . . until 1930–35 physiologists believed that it was the difference in the electric potential itself, the eddy current, which passed from the endings of the axon to the membrane of the effector cell and brought about the transmission. Today we know that, with rare exceptions, transmission of the nerve impulse is effected in all tissues

(smooth muscles, glands, striated muscles, heart and nerve cells) through molecules which are stored in the presynaptic nerve endings. The electric events are naturally linked to the release of these transmitters and we therefore speak in a general way of 'electro-chemical events' that occur at the synapses. The neurone can, therefore, be looked upon as a kind of electrical device which transmits quanta of very active molecules from its axon terminals whenever a nerve impulse reaches them.

In pursuing the tale, Bacq quotes 'The forerunners', E. Du Bois Reymond[123] (see p. 415).

Von bekannten Naturprocessen, welche nun noch die Erregung vermitteln koennten, kommen, soviel ich sehe, nur zwei in Frage. Entweder muesste an der Grenze der kontraktilen Substanz eine reizende Sekretion, in Gestalt etwa einer duennen Schicht von Ammoniak oder Milchsaeure oder einem anderen, den Muskel heftig erregenden Stoff stattfinden. Oder die Wirkung muesste elektrisch sein.

= Of the known processes of nature, which could transmit the excitation, there could be only two, I can perceive. There would have to be at the border of the contractile substance either a stimulating secretion, in form, e.g. of a thin layer of ammonia or lactic acid or of another substance which excites the muscle vehemently. Or the effects would have to be electric.

At this point, the flash of intuition of Schiefferdecker must be registered. It was reported in 1905 in a comparatively obscure record of a little-known German Society for Biology and Medicine in Bonn[118]. He described his theory of the secretion of endocrine substances by neurons or between a neuron and an effector cell in muscle or gland. These ideas were based on Tigerstedt's "automatic irritability" theory, where the irritation is caused by metabolic products of internal secretion, and on Schiefferdecker's own observations.

Apart from mentioning T. R. Elliott, Bacq referred to Howell, an American physiologist, who in 1906 showed that small changes in the cation concentration of saline solutions used for studying isolated organs produced effects similar to those which occur on nerve stimulation[122] (p. 12). He next recalled O. Loewi's fundamental experiment to prove the existence of the 'Vagusstoff', giving Loewi's own version of how he got the idea for his experiment. He briefly discussed Feldberg's work (who is still an active research worker) and commented: "Without Feldberg the research on chemical transmission of nerve impulses might well have taken a very different course"[123] (p. 23). Bacq discussed further not only the questions of cholinergic and adrenergic transmission (W. B. Cannon's main work; Bacq arrived at Harvard in 1929 to work at Cannon's laboratory for more than a year), but also the opposition to the theory of chemical transmission, the leaders of which were Leon Ascher of Basel, several French physiologists, especially Malmëjac (then in Algiers) and J. C. Eccles, who later emigrated to Australia and New Zealand, but continued his controversy with Dale's school of thought. Eccles "tried to refute the solid arguments provided by G. L. Brown, Dale, Feldberg and myself [Z. M. Bacq] from 1935–1938 . . ."[122] (pp. 57–63). It was only in 1944 that Eccles began to admit an error of misinterpretation, particularly after meeting Karl Popper, the Austrian philosopher, in New Zealand. Afterwards Eccles placed himself firmly behind Sir Henry Dale's interpretation. In 1963, he became a Nobel Prize winner.

Bacq also presents an interesting account of 'Working in Sir Henry Dale's Department' and a few thumbnail sketches of the personalities of the outstanding scientists he had come across during his wandering years. Finally, he describes several international symposia on the subject of chemical transmission, which helped to clarify the situation considerably, e.g. one in Philadelphia on 10 and 11 September 1953, another at Bethesda in October 1958, and the Third International Catecholamine Symposium at Strasbourg in June 1973[122] (p. 94). Among his personality portraits, which include Dale, Feldberg, Eccles, Otto Loewi, Walter Bradford Cannon, the one of (Sir) John Henry Gaddum FRS (1900–1965), must be mentioned especially. Gaddum was also one of Dale's men. In 1934 he went to Cairo for a year. In 1942, he succeeded A. J. Clark (see pp. 390–393) as Professor of Pharmacology at the University of Edinburgh.

> With the help of Marthe Vogt, Gaddum made his Institute in Edinburgh one of the great centres for pharmacological research. He ended his career as Director of the Institute of Animal Physiology at Babraham (near Cambridge) where he continued his work with Marthe Vogt, mainly on the central nervous system[122] (p. 103).

Specific examples of close connections between endocrine and nervous mechanisms can be found in the literature with increasing frequency from 1920, and especially from 1930 onwards (C. von Monakow, 1919[124], R. G. Hoskins, 1934[125] and 1941[126], L. Roizin, 1936[127], C. R. Stockard, 1938[128]. As early as 1919, Carl Caskey Speidel reported on 'Gland-cells of internal secretion in the spinal cord of skates'[129]. Seymour Reichlin, of the Tufts University School of Medicine in Boston, believes that the first clue of the pituitary–thyroid axis arose in the 1840s, from autopsy studies of cretins who were found to have enlarged pituitary glands[130]. In the 1920s, but mainly from 1928 to 1940, there is the considerable contribution to the subject by Ernst and Berta Scharrer (and other co-workers), originally from Germany, later from the United States. Their work went on into the 1970s, witness of which are some 40 papers and their very important book on *Neuroendocrinology*[114] in 1963, written from the Albert Einstein College of Medicine in New York. The importance of their studies is enhanced when one realizes that their painstaking work covers insects, invertebrates, vertebrates and man. We shall have to devote more space to the discussion of the impact of their work. The most important collection and analysis of the then available data, however, was the publication of Gustave Roussy and Michel Mosinger's great volume (of 1106 pages!) in 1946; *Traité de Neuro-endocrinologie: Le Système Neuro-endocrinien; Le Complexe Hypothalamo-Hypophysaire; La Neuro-ergonologie et son Evolution Récente*[131]. In the Introduction the authors write:

> Les sciences médicales, comme les sciences biologiques d'ailleurs, ont pris une orientation nouvelle au cours de ces dernières années. Après une étape longue de plus de deux siècles, durant laquelle les disciplines morphologiques, physiologiques et cliniques ont établi leur assises sur des bases essentiellement analytiques, la médecine s'engage aujourd'hui sur des voies nouvelles. Elle tente de rapprocher ce qu'elle avait, peut-être, trop longtemps séparé. Elle cherche à aborder de plus en plus, en un esprit de synthèse et dans une vue d'ensemble, l'étude des vastes problèmes relatifs au mécanismes régulateurs de la vie normale des tissus et des organes, ainsi que leurs dérèglements au cours des processus morbides.
>
> Il en est ainsi de la Neurologie et de l'Endocrinologie. Ces disciplines tendent aujourd'hui à se rapprocher l'une de l'autre à tel point que l'étude des régulations nerveuses et celle des régulations hormonales se confondent de plus en plus en une science de synthèse: la Neuro-endocrinologie . . .

(After mentioning Pierre, Cushing and Biedl, they continue:) . . .

> Puis Aschner, J. Camus et G. Roussy[132] ont démontré, par des expériences devenues classiques, la possibilité de provoquer ces syndromes par des lésions nerveuses. Or, les corrélations anatomiques et fonctionelles entre l'hypothalamus – noeud vital du système neuro-végétatif – et l'hypophyse, gland directrice de toutes les manifestations de la vie organique, se sont révélées par la suite extrémement étroites, en même temps que d'une grande complexité.

= The medical sciences, like the other biological sciences, have taken a new direction in the course of the last ten years. After a long phase of more than two centuries, during which the morphological, physiological and clinical disciplines had established their standards, mainly on an analytical basis, medicine to-day is running along new tracks. It attempts to bring together what was perhaps separated for too long. It seeks to tackle more and more, in a spirit of synthesis and a general overview, the exercise of the large problems concerning the regulatory mechanism of the normal life of tissues and organs, and their disorders in the course of pathological processes.

This is also the case in neurology and endocrinology. These disciplines tend to-day to run closer together to the point where the actions of the nervous regulations and of the hormonal ones become more and more intermingled in a science of synthesis: Neuro-Endocrinology. . . . After Aschner, J. Camus and G. Roussy have demonstrated by experiments which now have become classic, the possibility of provoking these syndromes by nervous lesions. The anatomical and functional correlations between the hypothalamus, the vital junction of the neurovegetative system, and the pituitary, which is the governing gland of all manifestations of organic life, have been revealed to be extremely close and, at the same time, of great complexity. [Translation: V.C.M.]

Ernst and Berta Scharrer placed the sentence "Il en est ainsi de la Neurologie et de l'Endocrinologie . . ." at the beginning of their book as motto. In their multiple studies the Scharrers and their group noted large cells filled with secretory droplets in the hypothalamus of teleost fishes. Some of them were multinuclear and surrounded by capillaries. This observation was published in 1928[133]. They continued their studies in other fish, because "there is so great a variety . . . that every species must be studied and described separately"[134]. The varied appearances which would be observed in the cells of a single species were tentatively interpreted as a series of stages in a cycle of formation and discharge of inclusions of cells, leading to the concept of neurosecretion; and after 1937 similar observations could be made in the nervous system of insects[135]. Other vertebrate studies were carried out on reptiles, birds and mammals (including man), where it was found that in the cells of the supraoptic and paraventricular nucleus, the secretory granules displace the Nissl staining material to the periphery (and the cell nucleus), giving an appearance of chromatolysis[136]. This secretory material was, in both fish and man, traced along the axons leading to the neurohypophysis[137].

At the beginning of the 1950s, after many discussions and studies, evidence was eventually accumulating to prove that posterior lobe hormones of the pituitary originated from two large-celled hypothalamic nuclei. David Bodian, in 1951, described the posterior lobe of the opossum, which permits a particularly clear histological study. The nerve terminals were found surrounded by discharged neurosecretory substances, enveloping them "in sleeve-like fashion"[138]. At this point, it is important to note that since 1913 J. Camus and G. Roussy had insisted on the predominance of the hypothalamus[132]. In 1933 G. Roussy and M. Mosinger recorded three phases of opinion[139]: (1) The hypophyseal, when the pituitary was in the focus of attention of such research workers as, for example, Biedl, Cushing and Marañon. (2) The phase of the tuber

419

cinereum, when the function of the pituitary was overshadowed by the tuber cinereum, based on the work of Bernhard Aschner[140] in 1912, and Camus and Roussy in 1913[131], and confirmed by Bernardo Alberto Houssay (1887–1971)[141] in Los Angeles, and others. The nuclei in the hypothalamus were thought to control the metabolic functions. (3) Phase III, according to which the control of the hypothalamus over the pituitary and the other endocrine glands has been recognized as the central neuro-humoral mechanism[139].

To complete the picture, one has to add the concept of feedback mechanism which emerged towards the end of the 1940s when R. G. Hoskins introduced it into the field of endocrinology[142], following a suggestion of Norbert Wiener that the engineers' idea of feedback control should be applied to biological systems[143]. In 1956, C. von Euler and B. Holmgren injected minute quantities of thyroxine into the anterior lobe of the pituitary, causing a reduction in radio-iodine release from the thyroid[144].

Whereas the neurologists were hesitant to join the endocrinologists in the exploration of the new field of neuro-endocrinology, the psychiatrists appeared more receptive. J. H. W. van Ophuisen, writing in 1951 on endocrinological orientation to psychiatric disorders[145] records that Sigmund Freud himself believed that many of the disturbances which he tried to understand from a psychological angle might become amenable to treatment by hormones. Scharrer and Scharrer remark critically on a fashionable trend which existed for a time "to treat the mentally ill with irradiation and surgical removal of endocrine organs or administration of hormones, although the causal relationships between psychiatric disorders and endocrine function were but little understood"[146]. They add:

> The fact that M. Bleuler could accumulate a bibliography of 2700 references, published between Laignel-Lavastine's first papers on 'Psychiatrie Endocrinienne'[147,148] in 1908 and his own *Endokrinologische Psychiatrie*[149] in 1954, does not mean that the area had been successfully explored. Quite the contrary; as Bleuler points out, the endocrine disturbances, if any, in cases of neuro- and psychopathic conditions and the psychological symptoms in patients suffering from endocrine malfunctions are of an unpredictable multitude, and no generally applicable conclusions have yet been reached beyond what Bleuler designates as the 'endocrine psychosyndrome'[146].

That term denotes the fact that endocrine disorders are frequently accompanied by hyperexcitability as in hyperthyroidism, depression as in Cushing's syndrome, or diminished response as in hypothyroidism. In fact, M. Besser *et al.* could show a few years ago that in some cases of depression, the blood cortisol level is raised, reminiscent of Cushing's syndrome[150].

Max Reiss (d. 1970), when still working in Bristol, showed particular interest in the subject; in fact, he was the leading spirit of the short-lived Psycho-endocrine Society in England in the 1950s (of which the present writer was also an 'endocrine' member). He came, however, to the conclusion that it is not only doubtful that further accumulation of casuistic material will help to elucidate relationships between the functioning of the endocrine system and abnormal behaviour, but that clinical studies are unsuitable for research in this field[151]. J. Lhermitte (in the same year) was more optimistic[152]:

> ... qui peut, en effet, douter aujourd'hui que le système endocrinien, source des hormones, exerce une importance de premier plan dans la régulation de la vie psychique ...

> = who can, in fact, doubt to-day, that the endocrine system, the source of the hormones, exerts an influence of the greatest importance on the regulation of mental life. [translation: V.C.M.]

In fact a conference was held on neuro-endocrinology in May 1956, at Columbia University's Arden House on the Hudson. The twelve papers presented and discussed were in fact mainly on psychiatric subjects and the proceedings were edited by Dr. Hudson Hoagland of the Worcester Foundation for Experimental Biology at Shrewsbury, Massachusetts and published under the title: *Hormones, Brain Function and Behaviour*[153].

THYROXIN(E)

We have seen (see p. 257) that Adolf Oswald made considerable efforts between 1897 and 1925 to obtain an accurate determination of iodine in connection with the thyroid. It meant determination of iodine in the thyroid itself and in food, water, soil, etc. The problem was to achieve destruction of organic matter without incurring loss of iodine. One of the methods was to carry it out in the presence of an excess of alkali. There were, however, several possible sources of error in the simple experiments made previously. Oswald made good progress and identified the protein of the colloid as 'thyreoglobulin' (later known as thyroglobulin of Robert Hutchison). Surprisingly, Oswald, who had succeeded in isolating di-iodotyrosine from artificially iodinated proteins[154], failed to isolate it from thyroglobulin by the tryptic digestion of thyroglobulin itself or of the peptic digestion product. Others (A. Nuernberg in 1907 and 1909) also failed to isolate di-iodotyrosine from a thyroglobulin hydrolysate. Thus – as Rosalind Pitt-Rivers says in her excellent recent summary on 'Thyroid hormones; historical aspects'[155]: "No significant developments in the field occurred until Kendall's isolation of thyroxine." Edward Calvin Kendall (1886–1972) was given the task of isolating the active principle of the thyroid gland in 1910, on joining the firm of Parke, Davis & Co. He left them a year later, going first to St. Luke's Hospital in New York and joining the Mayo Clinic in Rochester, Minnesota, another three years later. After some initial experiments in a different direction, Kendall soon tackled the problems of hydrolysis, based on a modification of a method used by A. Hunter of alkaline hydrolysis. (Sir) Charles Robert Harington described the details of Kendall's technique in 1933 (in the Appendix of his book: *The Thyroid Gland: its Chemistry and Physiology*[156], and commented:

> This method leaves little to be desired in simplicity and accuracy so far as the determination of iodine in the thyroid gland is concerned; it is also generally applicable to the determination of organic compounds, so long as these are not volatile.
>
> The determination of the traces of iodine which may be present in samples of water, food, etc., presents a more difficult analytical problem. . . .

Apparently, Th. von Fellenberg eventually succeeded in obtaining a method: 'Die Bestimmung kleinster Jodmengen in organischen Materialen' (The determination of minimal amounts of iodine in organic substances)[157] which appeared tricky but satisfactory. Be it as it may, by the end of 1914, Kendall realized that the physiological activity of the thyroid was linked with the acid–insoluble portion of the products of alkaline hydrolysis of the gland substance (which also explained the failure of Adolf Oswald to achieve an active product in his earlier experiment, when the hydrolysis liquid was neutralized with sulphuric acid[158,159]. On 25 December 1914, Kendall had achieved the crystals which he first called 'iodine-A' and which turned out to be active in dogs and in hypothyroid patients, causing increase in pulse rate and the basic metabolic rate and producing thyrotoxic symptoms when given in excess. In 1917, by which time he had accumulated 7 grams of crystals, Kendall gave a detailed account of the physical, chemical and physiological characteristics of the new compound[160]. In it he called the crystals 'thyroxin', which is a contraction of thyroxindole; this had to be changed to 'thyroxine', to conform with established chemical nomenclature.

Pitt–Rivers quotes Kendall's remark:

> Any reference to iodine in the hormone is purposely omitted from the name of the substance, because the work we have done concerning the physiologic action removes the attention from iodine[155].

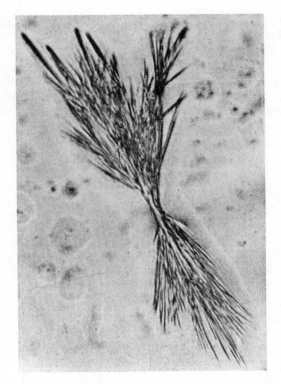

Figure 65   Thyroxine crystals – C. Kendall

Pitt-Rivers continues:

> This emphasis on the importance of the *structure* of thyroxine for biological action rather than its iodine content seems to be prophetic: We now know that the thyroxine molecule may have all the iodine atoms replaced by other substitutents and still retain its physiological activity[161].

Two important observations of that period must be mentioned. First, that the actual amount of thyroxine isolated was so small that it took three tons of pigs' thyroids to obtain 33 grams of pure thyroxine[162,163]. Secondly, that there was noticed a long latent period, which meant that 48 hours might pass before any effect would be observed after intravenous injection of pure thyroxine into man. Furthermore, the duration of the eventual effect is prolonged and may last two weeks, reaching a peak after eight days. (Henry Stanley Plummer, 1874–1937, and William Meredith Boothby, 1880–1953: 'Specific dynamic action of thyroxine'[164].)

When thyroxine was put on the market by Squibb and Son, New York, Kendall later related that the price of $350.00 per gram did not cover the actual cost of production (quoted after Pitt-Rivers[155]). Until Harington devised an improved method of isolation in 1926, and Harington and George Barger (1878–1939) established the constitution and synthesis of thyroxine in 1927[165], minute amounts of the substance were available only for biological tests.

(SIR) CHARLES ROBERT HARINGTON, PHD, FRS (1897–1972)

Harington became Lecturer in Pathological Chemistry at the University College Hospital Medical School, London, in 1922 (see also Section II). Before taking up his appointment, he spent a year in America, working mainly with D. D. Van Slyke, who had worked on the blood urea clearance test at the Rockefeller Institute, and with Henry Drysdale Dakin (1880–1952). Dakin had made extensive studies on oxidation and reduction processes in the body (1908–1912) and later became interested in antiseptic substances ('Dakin's solution' for the treatment of infected wounds, 1915), in his laboratory at Scarborough on Hudson. It was the latter who persuaded Harington to investigate the structural formula for thyroxine, which Kendall had proposed. After his return to London, and after a year's frustration, Harington embarked with F. H. Carr of British Drug Houses on a new trail, the project being supported financially by the medical school. His final solution to the problem was achieved by a two-stage hydrolysis, to begin with dilute and then with concentrated baryta. At the end of the day, Harington obtained a much increased, 25-fold yield of thyroxine from desiccated thyroid at a cost reduced from £70.00 to £6.10 per gram[166], Pitt-Rivers relates that H. D. Dakin

> had come to the same conclusion as Harington, regarding the constitution of thyroxine. When he heard that Harington had submitted a paper on the same subject to the *Biochemical Journal*, he generously withdrew a manuscript he had submitted to the *Journal of Biological Chemistry*.

In 1940, Harington and Pitt-Rivers improved on that method[167].

Harington and Barger next elucidated the constitution of thyroxine[165]. They then succeeded in obtaining the synthesis of thyroxine, the synthetic substance having properties identical to the natural compound and both having indistinguishable biological properties[168].

It was mentioned in Chapter 15 that E. Drechsel isolated 'gorgonin' (see also p. 257) or iodo–gorgonic acid, from the axial skeleton of the coral[169]; H. L. Wheeler and G. S. Jamieson demonstrated this substance to be 3:5-di-iodotyrosine[170] which, however, is devoid of thyroid activity. Rosalind Pitt-Rivers regards it rightly as "remarkable that more than 30 years were to pass after its first isolation, before Harington and S. S. Randall obtained it in a poor yield by stepwise baryta hydrolysis of desiccated thyroid"[155] (p. 409).

Another problem which exercised the minds of the leading research workers in this line of studies then, and for many years to come, was the nature of the hormone in the blood. Kendall, in 1929, came to the conclusion that the thyroid secretion was, in fact, thyroglobulin (cit. after Pitt-Rivers[155]). Pitt-Rivers quotes him:

> In regard to the chemical nature of the vehicle by which thyroxine is carried, the experimental results have been uniform. They indicate that active thyroxine leaves the gland in combination with the protein molecule.

Harington[171] and – later – W. T. Salter[172], agreed in their assumption that circulating thyroxine was bound in peptide linkage; moreover, Harington thought that the peptide contained di-iodotyrosine as well. Pitt-Rivers stresses that V. Trevorrow (1939) and others, who reviewed the situation up to 1975 (J. Robbins in *Thyroid Hormone Metabolism*[173]) confirmed that thyroxine, added to plasma proteins, behaved as regards dialysis, protein precipitants, and ethanol extraction identically to natural hormone, and this applied to experiments with ^{131}I labelled hormone[174].

Biological assay and standards were attempted as soon as sufficient thyroxine was at hand; that is from the 1920s onward.

The main methods used were:

(1) The results when feeding tadpoles on various mammalian tissues and organs, which J. F. Gudernatsch had observed in 1912[175–177]. Gudernatsch found that thyroid had a specific effect in accelerating differentiation (metamorphosis) in amphibian larvae (of *Rana temporaria, Rana esculenta, Bufo vulgaris* and *Triton alpestris*). B. M. Zavadovsky and E. V. Zavadovsky, in 1926, used a modification: 'Application of the axolotl metamorphosis reaction to the quantitative assay of thyroid gland hormones'[178]. The axolotl was found most useful for the study of a number of biological problems by the Viennese zoologist B. Hatschek at the turn of the century.

The main difficulty in the quantitative application of this test had been to establish the best criterion to determine the time of the effect. For that reason the Zavadovskys adopted the completion of the metamorphosis as the end-point of their axolotl based test.

(2) Effects of growth retardation and organ hypertrophy in laboratory animals (e.g. white rats) as studied by A T. Cameron and J. Carmichael[179] and also by Percy Theodore Herring (1872–1967)[180]. They studied the changes (hypertrophy) in the adrenals and the adrenaline content of those glands, respectively, as a compensatory attempt to inhibit the activity of the thyroid, while B. Romeis investigated the effect of thyroxine on the body-weight and liver glycogen content of white mice[181].

(3) Adolf Magnus-Levy (1865–1955)[182] observed the basal metabolic rate in man under the influence of thyroid and in diverse pathological conditions as early as 1895. Henry Stanley Plummer (1874–1937) and William Meredith Boothby (1880–1953) found a quarter of a century later, in a study on 69 myxoedematous patients, that 1 mg thyroxine produced, in the adult human being, an increase of the metabolic rate of 2.8%, with the highest point of rise usually occurring on the 8th day after administration of a single massive dose of thyroxine[164]. J. R. Mørch designed an ingenious method for the 'Standardization of thyroid preparations': under constant conditions of temperature, diet, etc. mice responded to continuous administration of thyroid with an increase of carbon dioxide production, achieving its maximum after three weeks. Thus all that was needed was to determine the basic CO_2 production at the beginning of the experiment and after three weeks[183].

(4) Finally, there was the unusual test devised by Reid Hunt (1870–1948): 'The acetonitril test for thyroid and of some alterations in metabolism'[184], in 1923, which he had, however, first described in 1905. It worked only in white mice, kept on a uniform diet – given thyroid, they became highly resistant to the toxic effect of aceto-nitrile, i.e. to the liberation of hydrocyanic acid, in contrast to rats and guinea pigs. Harington remarked[185]: ". . . the most serious objection to the test is the theoretical one of its complete lack of relation to any known physiological property of thyroid". Gudernatsch observed[186]: ". . . the thyroid-fed tadpoles possessed far less resistance against noxious influences than the others, as if the thyroid food had weakened their systems". Harington handed the final word on the subject to H. Paal, who found that

thyroidectomy, ". . . so far from reducing the resistance of mice towards acetonitrile, actually increases it by 80%, although it must be stated that the protective action of a given dose of thyroxine is less in a thyroidectomised than in a normal mouse"[187]. But Pitt-Rivers observed[155] (p. 410) that it soon became apparent that the physiological activity of thyroid material "could not be entirely accounted for by its thyroxine content". In fact, Reid Hunt in 1923[184] found that thyroxine had only one third of the activity of thyroid, and other workers obtained similar results. Professor George Barger (1878–1939) in Edinburgh suggested, therefore, in a review in 1928[188]: "Perhaps the [thyroid] gland is able to synthesize a substance which is more active than thyroxine, but which is lost or converted to inactive iodine containing compounds [during isolation]."

E. C. Kendall and D. G. Simonsen published in the same year an important paper on the 'seasonal variations in iodine and thyroxine contents of the thyroid gland'[189], referring back to the results Atherton Seidell (b. 1878) and F. Fenger reported sixteen years before on 'Seasonal variation in the iodine content of the thyroid gland (in sheep, pigs and oxen)'[190], the conclusions of which paper (dating from 1912!) they confirmed. The iodine content was highest in the autumn and lowest in the spring. The reduction in winter-iodine is accompanied by an increase in the size of the thyroid, which should be considered with the seasonal variations in the incidence of goitre. It was stated:

> The increase is basal metabolism which is produced by desiccated thyroid cannot be due only to the influence of the thyroxine which can be isolated in thyroxine form . . . it is necessary to assume that there is a substance present in the thyroid gland which is not thyroxine but which has the same action qualitatively as thyroxine, quantitatively it is more active than thyroxine.

Harington did not accept this view until 1952, when tri-iodothyronine was discovered by Jack Gross (b. 1921) and Rosalind Venetia Pitt-Rivers (b. 1907)[191]. Although in his Oliver-Sharpey Lectures in 1935, Harington admitted that there existed an unexplained discrepancy between the action of the whole thyroid and its equivalent as thyroxine[192], he said in a review in the same year: ". . . all the knowledge we possess of the chemical features responsible for the type of physiological activity exhibited by thyroxine indicates the intrinsic unlikelihood of the existence of a second unstable active principle"[193].

How did Harington explain the observed discrepancy? He thought that there existed a peptide of thyroxine, more active than thyroxine itself, which was destroyed during isolation. In spite of the veneration in which Pitt-Rivers rightly held Harington, she and Gross had the last laugh in 1952! Plummer and Boothby[194] based their success in the use of pre-operative iodine for the prevention of post-operative deaths in hyperthyroidism, on Paul Julius Moebius' (1853–1907) hypothesis of the production of an abnormal hormone produced in hyperthyroid glands[195], which Plummer thought to be a thyroxine not completely iodized.

> This incompletely built up thyroxine, as it leaves the gland, can enter into catabolic reaction faster than the normal, stable molecule and raise the metabolic rate more rapidly. If, therefore, we can change the character of the molecule, we can change the basal metabolism.

Pitt-Rivers recalls that Dr. James Howard Means, on the first day of her visit to the Massachusetts General Hospital in the autumn of 1953, asked her: "Do you think that triiodothyronine is Plummer's abnormal hormone in Graves' disease?"[155] (p. 412) Kendall believed persistently that the thyroid did contain another compound more active than thyroxine. His reasons were based on the observation that (1) some samples of desiccated thyroid with pronounced activity "do not contain any thyroxine that can be separated in crystalline form"; (2) that in exophthalmic goitre there is an increase in the acid-soluble content of the glands[196]; (3) that "all of the iodine-containing compounds insoluble in concentrated baryta solution are not thyroxine", and that re-treatment of mother liquor after thyroxine crystallization gives barium-insoluble salts of iodine containing compounds which "are stable in strong alkali but which cannot be crystallized from an alcoholic solution as thyroxine"[197]. "The properties described in (2) and (3)", Pitt-Rivers remarks, "would apply to triiodothyronine, which is much more acid soluble than thyroxine, and which would not crystallize under the conditions referred to in (3)." With a certain smug but justifiable satisfaction Pitt-Rivers concludes[155] (p. 412). "If Kendall had biologically tested his second crop of barium-insoluble salts, it is likely that the discovery of triidothyronine would have been anticipated by more than 20 years."

REFERENCES

1. Long Hall, Diana and Glick, T. F.: Endocrinology: a brief introduction. J. Hist. Biol. **9**, 229–233, 1976.
2. Cannon, Walter B.: Bodily Changes in Pain, Hunger, Fear and Rage. An Account of Researches into the Function of Emotional Excitement. 2nd, rev.

ed., 1929. Reprinted: New York, Evanston, and London, Harper Torch-books, 1963.

3. Cannon, Walter B.: The Wisdom of the Body. New York, Norton, 1932.
4. Starling, Ernest H.: The Wisdom of the Body. The Harveian Oration delivered to the R. Coll. Physicians, London, 1923. London, H. K. Lewis, 1923.
5. Ibid.: pp. 24–25.
6. Cannon, Walter B.: The Mechanical Factors of Digestion. London, E. Arnold, 1911.
7. Cannon, Walter B.: Am. J. Physiol. **36,** 363–364, 1915.
8. Vincent, T. Swale: The present position of organotherapy. Lancet **1,** 130–132, 1923.
9. Vincent, T. Swale: A critical examination of current views on internal secretion. The Arris and Gale Lecture. Lancet **2,** 315-320, 1922.
10. Long Hall, Diana: The critic and the advocate: contrasting British views on the state of endocrinology in the early 1920s. J. Hist. Biol. **9,** 269–285, 1976.
11. Cramer, J. W.: Professor T. Swale Vincent. Nature (London), 128–129, 1934.
12. Carpenter, William B.: Cyclopaedia of Anatomy and Physiology (ed. Todd, B. R.), Vol. IV, p. 440, London, 1852.
13. As 2: p. 36.
14. Clark, A. J.: Experimental basis of endocrine therapy. Br. Med. J. ɪɪ, 50–53, 1923.
15. Williams, Leonard: Letter to the Lancet. Lancet **1,** 255–256, 1923.
16. Editors of the Br. Med. J.: The endocrines in theory and practice. Articles republished from Br. Med. J. London, H. K. Lewis, 1937.
17. Glick, Thomas F.: On the diffusion of a new specialty: Marañon and the 'Crisis' of endocrinology in Spain. J. Hist. Biol. **9,** 287–300, 1976.
18. Mullins, Nicholas C.: The development of a scientific specialty. Minerva **10,** 51–82, 1972.
19. Gley, Eugène: Quatre Leçons sur les Sécrétions Internes (to the Societad de Biologia in Barcelona, 1919). Paris, 1920.
20. Vincent, T. Swale: An Introduction to the Study of Secretion, p. 152. New York and London, 1924.
21. Negrin, Juan: El papel de loss adresses en las glucosurias de origen bulbar. Libro en Honor de D. S. Ramon Y Cajal, Vol. II, pp. 383–384, Madrid, 1922.
22. Marañon, G.: Obras Completas, Vol. II, p. 22, Madrid, 1921.
23. Voronoff, Serge: Greffes, Testiculaires. Paris, O. Doin, 1923.
24. Borell, Merriley: Setting the standards for a new science: Edward Schaefer and endocrinology. Med. Hist. **22,** 282–290, 1978.
25. Hitschmann, Fritz, Adler, Ludwig: Der Bau d. Uterusschleimhaut d. geschlechtsreifen Weibes mit besonderer Beruecksichtigung d. Menstruation. Mschr. Geburtsch. Gynaekol. **27,** 1–82, 1928.
26. Marshall, F. H. A., Jolly, W.: Phil. Trans. R. Soc. B. **198,** 1905.
27. Kohn, A.: Arch. Entwicklungsmechan Organ. Leipzig, **47,** 47, 1920.
28. Brachet, A.: Traité d'Embryologie des Vertébrés. Paris, 1921.
29. Allen, Edgar, Doisy, E. A.: An ovarian hormone. J. Am. Med. Assoc. **81,** 819–821, 1923.
30. Allen, Edgar, Doisy, E. A.: The extraction and some properties of an ovarian hormone. J. Biol. Chem. **61,** 7–11–27, 1924.
31. Allen, Edgar, Doisy, E. A.: The induction of a sexually mature condition in immature females by injection of the ovarian follicular hormone. Am. J. Physiol. **69,** 577–588, 1924.

32. Courrier, Robert: C.R. Soc. Biol. **90,** 45, 1924.
33. Courrier, R.: C. R. Acad. Sci., Paris **178,** 2197, 1924.
34. Rolleston, Sir H. D.: The Endocrine Organs in Health and Disease with an Historical Review. p. 403, London, Oxford University Press, 1936.
35. Corner, George W.: The Early History of Oestrogenic Hormones. The Sir Henry Dale Lecture for 1964. Proc. Soc. Endocrin., J. Endocrinol. **31,** III–XVII, 1965.
36. Long, Jos. A., Evans, H. M.: The oestrus cycle in the rat and its associated phenomena. Memoirs Univ. California, No. 6, Berkeley, Univ. California Press, 1922.
37. Allen, Edgar, Doisy, E. A.: The menstrual cycle of the monkey, *Macacus rhesus*: observations on normal animals, the effects of removal of the ovaries and the effects of injection of ovarian and placental extracts into the spayed animals. Contr. Embryol. Carnegie Inst. **19,** 1–44, 1927.
38. Parkes, Alan S.: The rise of reproductive endocrinology 1926–1940. The Sir Henry Dale Lecture for 1965. J. Endocrinol. **34,** No. 3, Proc. Soc. Endocrinol. XX–XXXII, 1965.
39. Albright, Fuller: Introduction to the Diseases of the Ductless Glands, in A Textbook of Medicine (eds. Cecil, Russell L. and Loeb, Robert F.). 6th ed. Philadelphia, London, W. B. Saunders, 1943.
40. Ryan, Will G.: Endocrine Disorders: A Pathophysiological Approach. Chicago, Year Book Med. Publishers, 1975.
41. Parkes, Alan S.: On the occurrence of the oestrus cycle after X-ray sterilisation. Part I: Proc. R. Soc. B. **100,** 172–199, 1926. Part II: Proc. R. Soc. B. **101,** 71–95, 1927; Part III: Proc. R. Soc. B. **101,** 421–449, 1927.
42. Parkes, A. S., Bellerby, C. W.: The distribution in the ovary of the oestrus-producing hormone. J. Physiol. London **61,** 562–575, 1926.
43. Loewe, S., Lange, F.: Der Gehalt des Frauenharnes an brunsterzeugenden Stoffen in Abhaengigkeit vom ovariellen Zyklus. Klin. Wochenschr. **5,** 1038–1039, 1926.
44. Aschheim, Selmar: Weitere Untersuchungen ueber Hormone und Schwangerschaft. Das Vorkommen der Hormone im Harn der Schwangeren. Arch. Gynaekol. **132,** 179–183, 1927.
45. Aschheim, S., Zondek, B.: Schwangerschaftsdiagnose aus dem Harn (durch Hormonnachweis). Klin. Wochenschr. **7,** 8–9; 1404–1411; 1453–1457, 1928.
46. Doisy, E. A., Thayer, S., Veler, C. D. J. Biol. Chem. **136,** 499, 1930.
47. Butenandt, A. F. J.: Dtsch. Med. Wochenschr. **55,** 217, 1929.
48. Laqueur, Ernst, Hart, P. C., De Jongh, S. E., Wissenbeck, J. A.: Dtsch. Med. Wochenschr. **52,** 4; 1247; **52,** 1331, 1926.
49. Zondek, B., von Euler (Cit. by Rolleston, pp. 406 and 408, see Ref. 34).
50. Haeussler, E. A.: Helv. Chim. Acta **17,** 531, 1934.
51. Marrian, G. F.: The chemistry of oestrin. I. Preparation from urine and separation from an unidentified solid alcohol. Biochem. J. **23,** 1090–1098, 1929; The chemistry of oestrin: III. An improved method of the preparation and the isolation of active crystalline material. Biochem. J. **24,** 435–445, 1930.
52. Dodds, E. Ch., Goldberg, L., Lawson, W., Robinson, R.: Nature (London) **141,** 247–248, 1938.
53. Dodds, E. C. *et al.*: Nature (London) **142,** 34, 1938.
54. Corner, G. W., Allen, Willard Myron: Physiology of the corpus luteum (II) Production of a special reaction: progestational proliferation, by extracts of the corpus luteum. Am. J. Physiol. **88,** 326–339, 1929.
55. Corner, G. W., Allen, Willard Myron: Normal growth and implantation of

embryos after very early ablation of the ovaries, under the influence of extracts of the corpus luteum. Am. J. Physiol. **88,** 340–346, 1929.

56. Slotta, K. H., Rushig, H., Fells, W.: Reindarstellung der Hormone aus dem Corpus Luteum. Ber. Dtsch. Chem. Ges. **67,** 1270, 1934.
57. Butenandt, F. J.: Z. Angew. Chem. **44,** 905–908, 1931.
58. Ruzicka, L.: Ueber die Synthese des Testikelhormons (Androsteron) und Stereo-isomerer desselben durch Abbau hydrierter Sterine. Helv. Chim. Acta **17,** 1395–1406, 1934.
59. Parkes, Alan S.: Br. Med. J. II, 71, 1962.
60. Courrier, R., Potvin, R.: C.R. Soc. Biol., Paris **94,** 878, 1926.
61. Parkes, Alan S.: Internal Secretions of the Ovary. p. 175, London, 1929.
62. Zondek, B.: Cit. after H. Zondek: The Diseases of the Endocrine Glands, 2nd ed, p. 411. London, E. Arnold, 1944.
63. Marañon, G.: L'Àge Critique. p. 2, Paris, 1934.
64. Bovin, P., Ancel, P.: C.R. Acad. Sci., Paris **138,** 110, 1904.
65. Steinach, Eugen: Verjuengung durch experimentelle Neubelebung d. alternden Pubertaetsdruese. Berlin, J. Springer, 1920.
66. Loewi, A., Zondek, H.: Dtsche Med. Wochenschr. **47,** 349, 1921.
67. Shattock, S. G.: Br. Med. J. I, 460, 1897.
68. Reinke, F.: Arch. Mikrosk. Anat., Bonn. **47,** 34; 1896.
69. Robinson, Victor: Cit. after Rolleston: As Ref. 34, p. 390.
70. McGee, L. C.: The effect of the injection of a lipoid fraction of bull testicle in capons. Proc. Inst. Med. Chicago. **6,** 242–254, 1927.
71. Moore, C. R., Gallagher, T. F., Koch, F. C.: The effects of extracts of testis in correcting the castrated condition in the fowl and in the mammal. Endocrinology **13,** 367–374, 1929.
72. Evans, H. M., Long, J. A.: Anat. Rec. **21,** 62–63, 1921.
73. Evans, H. M.: Harvey Lect., New York **19,** 212, 1924.
74. Smith, P. E., Engle, E. Th.: Experimental evidence regarding the role of the anterior pituitary in the development and regulation of the genital system. Am. J. Anat. **40,** 159–217, 1927.
75. As 38: p. xxix.
76. Zondek, B., Aschheim, S.: Das Hormon des Hypophysenvorderlappens. Klin. Wochenschr. **6,** 348–352, 1927.
77. Zondek, B.: Ibid. **7,** 831–835, 1928.
78. Collip, J. B.: Lancet **1,** 1208, 1933.
79. Collip, J. B.: Lancet **2,** 347, 1933.
80. Dodds, E. C.: Lancet **1,** 931, 1934.
81. Fevold, H. L., Hisaw, F. L., Leonard, S. L.: Am. J. Physiol., Boston **97,** 291, 1931.
82. Hill, M., Parkes, A. S.: Proc. R. Soc. Lond. B **97,** 291, 1931.
83. Fevold, H. L., Hisaw, F. L.; Am. J. Physiol., Boston **109,** 655, 1934.
84. Evans, H. M., Korpi, K., Pencharz, R. I., Wonder, D. H.: Univ. California Publ. (Anat.) I, 255; 1936.
85. Evans, H. M., Simpson, M. E.: J. Am. Med. Assoc. **91,** 1337, 1928.
86. Evans, H. M., Simpson, M. E.: Am. J. Physiol. **89,** 371, 379, 1929.
87. Zondek, B., Berblinger, W.: Klin. Wochenschr. **10,** 1061, 1931.
88. Teel, H. M., Cushing, H.: Endokrinologie, Leipzig **6,** 401, 1930.
89. Kraus, E. J.: Klin. Wochenschr. XI, 471, 1933.
90. As 62: p. 49.
91. Stricker, P., Grueter, F.: Action du lobe antérieur de l'hypophyse sur la montée laiteuse. C.R. Soc. Biol. Paris **99,** 1978–1980, 1929.
92. Gaines, Walter L.: Am. J. Physiol. **38,** 285–312, 1915.

93. Riddle, O., Bates, R. W., Dykshorn, S. W.: The preparation, identification and assay of prolactin – a hormone of the anterior pituitary. Am. J. Physiol. **105,** 191–216, 1933.

94. Halban, J.: Arch. Gynaekol, Berlin **75,** 353, 1905.

95. Starling, E. H., Lane-Claypon, Janet E.: Proc. R. Soc. London B., **77,** 505, 1906.

96. Allan, H., Wiles, P.: J. Physiol., London **75,** 23; 1932.

97. Selye, H., Collip, J. B., Thomson, D. L.: Proc. Soc. Exp. Biol. Med. NY, xxxi, 588, 1933.

98. Smith, P. E.: General physiology of the anterior hypophysis. J. Am. Med. Assoc. **104,** 548–553, 1935.

99. As 62: p. 55.

100. Bauer, Julius: Personal communication, Vienna, 1937.

101. As 62: pp. 20–24.

102. As 62: pp. 106–109.

103. Marshall, F. H. A.: Sexual periodicity and the causes which determine it. Croonian Lectures, R. Coll. Physicians London, 1936. Phil. Trans. R. Soc. London B. **226,** 423–456, 1936.

104. Heape, W.: Proc. R. Soc. London B. **76,** 260, 1905.

105. Gall, F. J.: Anatomie et Physiologie du Système Nerveux en Générale et du Cerveau en Particulier. Vol. III, pp. 108–131. Paris, Librairie Greque-Latine-Allemande, 1818.

106. Vimont, J.: Traité de Phrénologie Humaine et Comparée. 2nd ed. Brussels, Établissement Encyclographique (with Atlas), 1835.

107. As 105: pp. 112, 113.

108. As 106: p. 321.

109. Maestre de San Juan, A.: Falta total de los nervios olfactorios con anosmia en un individuo en qui en existia una atrofia de los testiculos y membro viril; observacion recogida por el Dr. M. de San Juan. p. 211, Madrid, El Siglo Medico, 1856.

110. Weidenreich, F.: Ueber Partiellen Riechlappendefekt und Eunuchoidismus beim Menschen. Z. Morphol. Anthropol. **18,** 157–190, 1914.

111. Mirsalis, T.: Ein neuer Fall von Arhinencephalie. Anat. Anz. **67,** 353–360, 1929.

112. Kanai, T.: Ueber d. kombinierte Vorkommen des partiellen Riechlappen defektes mit dem Eunuchoidismus. Okajima Folia Anat. J. **19,** 199–213, 1940.

113. Gauthier, G.: La dysplasie olfacto-génitale. (Agénésie des lobes olfactifs avec absence de développement gonadique à la puberté). Acta Neuro-veget (Vienna) **21,** 345–394, 1960.

114. Scharrer, Ernst, Scharrer, Berta: Neuroendocrinology. New York and London, Columbia U.P., 1963.

115. Harris, G. W.: The relationship between endocrine activity and the development of the nervous system. In Biochemistry of the Developing Nervous System (ed. Waelsch, H.), pp. 431–442. New York, Academic Press, 1955.

116. Zander, R.: Ueber functionelle und genetische Beziehungen der Nebennieren zu anderen Organen, speciell zum Grosshirn. Beitr. Pathol. Anat. **7,** 439–534, 1890.

117. Moeri, E.: Les surrénales chez le foetus, le nouveau-né, le nourisson et l'enfant. Acta Endocrinol., Copenhagen **8,** 259–311, 1951.

118. Schiefferdecker: Ueber die Neuronen u. die innere Sekretion. Sitzgsber. Niederrhein. Ges. Naturu. Heilkde, Bonn, 46–54: 1905.

119. Peritz, G.: Nervensystem und innere Sekretion, in Handbuch d. Biochemie

des Menschen u. der Tiere (ed. Oppenheimer, C.). Ergaenzungsband, pp. 496–536. Jena, G. Fischer, 1913.

120. Lewy, F. H.: Die Erkrankungen d. endokrinen Druesen, Fortschr. Neurol. Psychiatr. Grenzg. **1**, 347–408, 1929.

121. Feldberg, Wilhelm: The early history of synaptic and neuromuscular transmission by acetylcholine: reminiscences of an eye witness. In The Pursuit of Nature. Informal Essays on the History of Physiology. pp. 65–83, Cambridge, C.U.P., 1977.

122. Bacq, Z. M.: Chemical Transmission of Nerve Impulses. A Historical Sketch. Oxford, New York, Toronto, Pergamon Press, 1975.

123. Du Bois Reymond, E.: Gesammelte Abhandlungen d. allgemeinen Muskel- und Nervenphysiologie **2**, 700, 1877.

124. Monakow, C. von: Psychiatrie und Biologie. Schweiz. Arch. Neurol. Psychiatr. **4**, 13–235, 1919.

125. Hoskins, R. G.: Endocrinology, in The Problem of Mental Disorder, pp. 234–240. New York, McGraw-Hill, 1934.

126. Hoskins, R. G.: Endocrinology. New York, Norton, 1941.

127. Roizin, L.: Sensorial Organs as Originators of Neuro-Endocrine-vegetative Reflexes in the Diencephalo-pituitary Region. Thesis, Univ. Milan (in Italian). Published also in Ras. Neurol. Vegetat. **1**, 348–383, 1936.

128. Stockard, C. R.: The interactions of the endocrine glands and the nervous system. Diplomate **10**, 44–51, 1938.

129. Speidel, C. C.: Gland-cells of internal secretion in the spinal cord of skates. Carnegie Inst. Wash. Publ. No. 13, 1–31, 1919.

130. Reichlin, S.: Med. Clin. N. Am. **62**, 305–312, 1978.

131. Roussy, G., Mosinger, M.: Traité de Neuro-endocrinologie: Le Système Neuro-endocrinien; Le Complexe Hypothalamo-Hypophysaire; La Neuro-ergonologie et son Évolution Récente. Paris, Masson & Cie, 1946.

132. Camus, J., Roussy, G.: C.R. Soc. Biol., Paris **75**, 628, 1913.

133. Scharrer, E.: Die Lichtempfindlichkeit blinder Elritzen. (Untersuchungen ueber das Zwischenhirn d. Fische. I.) T/Z. Vergl. Physiol. **7**, 1–38; 1928.

134. Scharrer, E., Scharrer, B.: Secretory cells within the hypothalamus. Res. Publ. Assoc. Nerv. Ment. Dis. **20**, 170–194, 1940.

135. Scharrer, Berta: Histophysiological studies on the corpus allatum of *Leucophaeae maderae*. V. Ultrastructure of sites of origin and release of a distinctive cellular product. Z. Zellforsch., Mikrosk. Anat. **120**, 1–16, 1971.

136. LeGros Clark, W. E. *et al.*: Morphological aspects of the hypothalamus. In The Hypothalamus, Morphological, Functional, Clinical, Surgical Aspects. pp. 1–68, Edinburgh, 1938.

137. Gaupp, R., Scharrer, E.: Die Zwischenhirnsekretion bei Mensch und Tier. Z. Ges. Neurol. Psychol. **153**, 327–355, 1935.

138. Bodian, D.: Nerve-endings, neurosecretory substance and lobular organisation of the neurohypophysis. Bull. Johns Hopkins Hosp. **89**, 354–376, 1951.

139. Roussy, G., Mosinger, M: C.R. Soc. Biol. Paris **112**, 775, 1933.

140. Aschner, Bernhard: Arch. Gynaekol. Berlin **97**, 200, 1912.

141. Houssay, B. A.: Endocrinology, Los Angeles **18**, 409, 1934.

142. Hoskins, R. G.: The thyroid-pituitary apparatus as a servo (feed-back) mechanism. J. Clin. Endocrinol. **9**, 1429–1431, 1949.

143. Wiener, N.: Cybernetics. New York, 1948.

144. von Euler, C., Holmgren, B.: The thyroid 'receptor' of the thyroid–pituitary system. J. Physiol. **131**, 125–136, 1956.

145. Van Ophuisen, J. H. W.: A new phase in clinical psychiatry. Part I and

Introduction. Endocrinologic orientation to psychiatric disorders. J. Clin. Exp. Psychopathol. **12**, 1–4, 1951.

146. As 114: p. 5.
147. Laignel-Lavastine, M.: Les troubles psychiques par perturbations des glandes à secrétion interne, in Congrès des Médecins Aliénistes et Neurologistes de France et des Pays de Langue Française, xviii session, Dijon, pp. 1–188. Paris, Masson & Cie, 1908.
148. Laignel-Lavastine, M.: Sécrétions internes et psychoses. Presse Méd. Année 1908 (No. 62), p. 491.
149. Bleuler, M.: Endokrinologische Psychiatrie, 1954. cit. from Scharrer, E., Scharrer, B.: Neuroendocrinology. New York and London, Columbia U.P. p. 5., 1963.
150. Butler, P. W. P., Besser, G. M.: Pituitary–adrenal function in severe depressive illness. Lancet **1**, 1234–1236, 1968.
151. Reiss, Max: Application of endocrinological research methods in psychiatry. J. Endocrinol. **7**, 235–241, 1950/51.
152. Lhermitte, J.: Le Cerveau et la Pensée. Paris, Bloud et Gay, 1951.
153. Hoagland, H.: (ed.) Hormones, Brain Function and Behavior. Proceedings of a Conference on Neuroendocrinology (1956) New York, Academic Press, 1957.
154. Oswald, A.: Neue Beitraege zur Kenntnis d. Bindung des Jods im Thyreo-globulin nebst einigen Bemerkungen ueber das Jodothyrin. I. Arch. Exp. Pathol. Pharmacol. **60**, 115–130, 1909.
155. Pitt-Rivers, Rosalind: The thyroid hormones; historical aspects. In Hormonal Proteins and Peptides. Vol. VI., pp. 399–422. New York, Academic Press, 1978.
156. Harington, C. R.: The Thyroid Gland: Its Chemistry and Physiology. p. 192. London, O.U.P., 1933.
157. Fellenberg, Th. von: Die Bestimmung kleinster Jodmengen in organischen Materialen. Biochem. Z. **224**, 170, 1930.
158. Kendall, E. C.: J. Am. Med. Assoc. **64**, 2042–2043, 1915.
159. Kendall, E. C.: A method for the decomposition of the proteins of the thyroid with a description of certain constituents. J. Biol. Chem. **20**, 501, 1915.
160. Kendall, E. C.: Collected Papers, Mayo Clinic, Mayo Foundation, **9**, 309–336, 1917.
161. Compston, N., Pitt-Rivers, R.: Lancet, **1**, 22–23, 1956.
162. Kendall, E. C.: Thyroxine. New York, Chem. Catalog Co., 1929.
163. Kendall, E. C.: J. Biol. Chem. **39**, 125, 1919.
164. Plummer, H. S., Boothby, W. M.: Specific dynamic action of thyroxine. Am. J. Physiol. **55**, 295, 1921.
165. Harington, C. R., Barger, G.: Chemistry of thyroxine. III. Constitution and synthesis of thyroxine. Biochem. J. **21**, 169–183, 1927.
166. Barger, G.: Pharmcol. J. **119**, 609–614, 1927.
167. Harington, C. R., Pitt-Rivers, R.: J. Chem. Soc. 1101–1103, 1940.
168. As 156: pp. 107–111, 93–96.
169. Drechsel, E.: Beitraege zur Chemie einiger Seethiere. Z. Biol. **33**, 85–107, 1895/96.
170. Wheeler, H. L., Jamieson, G. S.: Synthesis of iodogorgonic acid. Am. Chem. J. **33**, 365–372, 1905.
171. Harington, C. R.: Lancet **1**, 1199–1204; 1261–1266, 1935.
172. Salter, W. T.: Physiol. Rev. **20**, 345–376, 1940.
173. Robbins, J.: In Thyroid Hormone Metabolism (ed. Harland, W. S. and Orr, J. S.) pp. 1–22. New York. Academic Press, 1975.

174. Leblond, C. P., Gross, J.: J. Clin. Endocrinol. Metab. **9**, 149–157, 1949.
175. Gudernatsch, J. F.: Feeding experiments on tadpoles: I. The influence of specific organs given as food, on growth and differentiation. Arch. Entw. Mech. Org. **35**, 457–483, 1912.
176. Gudernatsch, J. F.: Feeding experiments on tadpoles: II. A further contribution to the knowledge of organs with internal secretion. Am. J. Anat. **15**, 431, 1913/14.
177. Gudernatsch, J. F.: Anat. Rec. **11**, 357–359, 1917.
178. Zavadovsky, B. M., Zavadovsky, E. V.: Application of the axolotl metamorphosis reaction to the quantitative assay of thyroid gland hormones. Endocrinology **10**, 550–559, 1926.
179. Cameron, A. T., Carmichael, J.: Contributions to the bio-chemistry of iodine: III. J. Biol. Chem. **45**, 69–100, 1920/21.
180. Herring, P. T.: Q. J. Exp. Physiol. **12**, 115, 1917.
181. Romeis, B.: Biochem. Z. **135**, 85–106, 1903.
182. Magnus-Levy, A.: Berlin Klin. Wochenschr. **32**, 650–652, 1895.
183. Mørch, J. R.: Standardization of thyroid preparations. J. Physiol. **67**, 221–241, 1929.
184. Hunt, Reid: The acetonitril test for thyroid and of some alterations in metabolism. Am. J. Physiol. **63**, 257–299, 1923.
185. As 156: p. 139.
186. As 175: p. 477.
187. Paal, H.: Schilddruesenfunktion u. die Reaktion nach Reid Hunt. Arch. Exp. Pathol., Pharmacol. **148**, 232, 1929/30.
188. Barger, G.: Ergebn. Physiol., Biol. Chem. Exp. Pharmakol. **27**, 780–831, 1928.
189. Kendall, E. C., Simonsen, D. G.: Seasonal variations in iodine and thyroxine contents of the thyroid gland. J. Biol. Chem. **80**, 357–377, 1928.
190. Seidell, A., Fenger, F.: Seasonal variations in the iodine content of the thyroid gland (in sheep, pig and oxen). J. Biol. Chem. **13**, 517–526, 1912.
191. Gross, J., Pitt-Rivers, R. V.: Triiodothyronine. I. Isolation from thyroid gland and synthesis. Biochem. J. **53**, 645–651, 1953.
192. Harington, C. R.: Lancet **1**, 1199–1204, 1261–1266, 1935.
193. Harington, C. R.: Ergebn. Physiol. Biol. Chem., Exp. Pathol. **37**, 210–244, 1935.
194. Plummer, S. H., Boothby, W. M.: The value of iodine in exophthalmic goitre. J. Iowa Med. Soc. **14**, 66–73, 1924.
195. Moebius, P. J.: Arch. Psychol. **17**, 301–321, 1886.
196. Kendall, E. C.: Am. J. Med. Sci. **151**, 79–91, 1916.
197. Kendall, E. C.: ACS, **47**, 63, 1929.

CHAPTER NINETEEN

THE FIRST FOUR DECADES OF THE 20TH CENTURY – PART II

INTERLUDE: CONTRACEPTION IN THE 1920s AND 1930s

MISS Borell says in her paper 'Origins of modern research on fertility and reproduction: physiologists and the discovery of hormones, 1889–1930'[1] under the heading 'Enlarging the scope of scientific concern' (p. 23):

> . . . from the teens and twenties (of the present century) the emerging science of reproductive endocrinology was observed to be applicable to the resolution of a variety of topical and controversial issues, prominent among them the debates surrounding family limitation. After the Great War (1914–1918), voluntary parenthood began to have increasing appeal among the middle classes. Physicians and physiologists were asked to participate in the evaluation of safe and effective means for birth control.

Just over a hundred years ago the Malthusian League was founded in England, in the wake of the Bradlaugh–Besant trial (1877–79). Charles Bradlaugh, a lawyer, and Annie Besant, both of the Freethought Movement, challenged the Establishment by starting the Freethought Publishing Company for the purpose of publishing Dr. Charles Knowlton's pamphlets (see also p. 356) and forcing – courageously – a legal test case, which they succeeded in winning.

The Malthusian League, which – according to Norman E. Himes[2] – was really a 'Neo-Malthusian' League, was disbanded with a celebration dinner in 1927, because they felt they had fulfilled their aims. Their moving spirit was Dr. Charles Henry Drysdale, supported by his wife, Dr. Alice Drysdale–Vickery, who was an

English feminist (she was a witness in the Bradlaugh–Besant trial). A medical branch of the League was soon formed, and in August 1881, an International Medical Congress was held in London, where the Medical Branch of the League had called a meeting of British and foreign physicians to discuss 'Malthusianism and parental prudence'. About 40 medical practitioners attended, with Dr. Drysdale in the chair. That conference was apparently a forerunner of the International Conference in Zurich of 1931, although the first real First International Medical Congress had taken place in 1879 under the secretaryship of Dr. Guye of Amsterdam. A long time had passed since the use of the tampon was mentioned in the Papyrus Ebers (see also p. 23), and the plugging of the vagina, which was used in ancient China and India, to the time when Casanova used the gold ball of 18 mm in diameter. (He used it for 15 years and later described it in his 'Memoirs'.) Between the two conferences in 1879 and 1931, there was another development: advisory clinics on contraception had begun, especially after 1918. Many of them, including that of Dr. Marie Stopes, still advocated the use of the barrier method. This had been popular in Japan in antiquity, when oiled silk paper called 'misugami' was rolled into a ball and placed high up into the vagina[3]. Until recently, Hungarian peasant women made discs from melted bees' wax, placed it into the vagina and forced it into shape. Bees' wax does not melt at human body temperature. In 1916, a report was published in London by the National Council of Public Morals in connection with the investigations of the National Birth-rate Commission. The latter was established in 1913. It had 60 members, experts in 'religion, science, statistics, economics and education', who produced their report under the title: 'The Declining Birth Rate, its Causes and its Effects'. The parent organization, the National Council of Public Morals, was a voluntary organization supported by charitable contributions.

In July 1923, *The Practitioner*, one of the most read monthly medical magazines in Britain, published a 'Special Issue on Contraception'[4]. In it was presented the following concluding paragraph of a paper on 'Birth control and economy', by Mr. Henry Corby, Professor of Gynaecology and Obstetrics at the University College of Cork, in the South of Ireland:

> Now to sum up; contracepts undoubtedly tend to produce ill-health in both husband and wife, and the resulting nervous irritability tends to banish the harmony and love that should subsist between them. The children that are permitted to come into existence lose all the gaieties and joys of childlife. If the advocates of these self-limiting practices are successful in making them at all widespread, the land will be cumbered by a weakly degenerated race of neurasthenics and hypochondriacs, not

a small percentage of whom will drift into lunatic asylums where, poor creatures, they will be in the midst of their fellow masturbators. Nature is a stern goddess, who relentlessly punishes those who set at naught her beneficent ordinances. (pp. 62–73)

In due fairness, it must be stated, however, that another contributor to the same issue of *The Practitioner* was Dr. Norman Haire, who by that date had analysed 1400 cases of contraceptive techniques.

One may wish to contrast the sentiments expressed by Corby with the title of a seven-page handout for women, presented by the Health Education Board, obtained by the author in February 1979 at the Out-Patients' Department of a teaching hospital in London. It reads:

THE PRACTITIONER

JULY

1923

Contraception.

THE subject of Birth Control, with which this Special Number deals, is one which has occupied the thoughts of political economists for about two centuries. The facts and problems which the question presented were, however, first clearly stated by the Rev. Thomas Malthus, an intellectual and philosophical divine, who in 1803 published a learned treatise entitled *The Principles of Population*, in which he showed that, although the population of these islands increased in geometrical ratio, the means of subsistence never increased beyond arithmetical ratio. And he went on to argue that unless some effective means of birth control were practised, results economically and politically disastrous must surely ensue. The opinions expressed in this little work evoked a storm of hostile criticism, but as the facts could not be gainsaid, the matter was gradually transferred from a noisy and nebulous religious atmosphere to one of solemn and slumberous scientific calm. In this academic peace it was allowed to rest until, in the late seventies, Charles Bradlaugh and Annie Besant started a platform and pamphlet campaign

1   A

Figure 66 Contraception number of *The Practitioner*, July 1923 [by kind permission of the Royal Society of Medicine, London]

"Have as many children as you want". Underneath there is a colour photograph of a family with nine children and a caption: "We wanted two children". Beneath is a picture of a pregnant woman, complaining: "I did not want any children". On page two, there are three paragraphs, headed:

(1) Contraception isn't just stopping babies. (". . . But a baby every year – which is possible for healthy women – is rarely the right way to build up a healthy and happy family . . .");

(2) There is nothing new about contraception ("3000 years ago the Ancient Egyptians concocted weird contraceptive creams from crocodile dung and honey . . .");

(3) Some methods that don't work (". . . or wearing charms . . .").

Next follows a description of "How to get pregnant". This is followed by "How to stop getting pregnant"; "The Pill"; "The IUD"; "The Sheath"; "The Cap"; "Foaming tablets, creams, films, aerosol foams or spermicide jellies"; "The Safe Period" (Rhythm Method); to the latter is added: "The Staff of the Catholic Marriage Advisory Council are especially skilled in giving advice on the use of this method". Next follow paragraphs on "Withdrawal", "Douching", "Combined Methods"; "Sterilization". All these sections are illustrated with simple, coloured, explanatory sketches. The last page is devoted to: "How to get help":

(1) Your Family Doctor (Free contraceptive services are available to women from most family doctors. Your local Family Practitioner Committee or Main Post Office will have a list of doctors who will provide this service . . .);

(2) Your local family planning clinic (. . . run by the National Health Service and contraceptives prescribed and dispensed by them are free too . . .) Whether you are married or single, man or woman, young or old, you can go to a clinic for private or confidential help . . .);

(3) If you need to know more: The Health Education Department of your local Health Authority may be able to help . . . (address given).

I understand that unmarried girls of 16 can get advice and help at such clinics or from their family doctors without knowledge or consent of their parents, although some family doctors draw the line at such requests. What a change in fifty-five years!

Dr. Borell mentions that Professor Corby modified 19th century arguments against contraception "to include scientific evidence that the testes produce some important chemical substances".

440

Corby's conclusion was that – unless male and female secretions mix – there will occur pathological congestion of the testicles. As the use of condoms prevented such mixture and intercourse in such a manner would amount to mere masturbation, disease would inevitably follow[5].

Be it as it may, the National Council of Public Morals, eventually, felt obliged to set up a Medical Committee to report on the 'Medical Aspects of Contraception', in 1927. This Committee was chaired by Mr. Charles Gibbs and had thirteen other members, Among them, Sir Arthur Newsholme (Vice-Chairman), C. J. Bond, A. K. Chalmers, Mrs. Agnes Dunnett, J. S. Fairbairn, Letitia D. Fairfield, A. E. Giles, Professor Leonard Erskine Hill, Frances Ivers, Professor F. H. A. Marshall and Sir James Marchant. This was a formidable array of well known personalities, among whom Professor Hill and F. H. A. Marshall promised a strong expert medical contribution, not to overlook Sir Arthur Newsholme (1857–1943), as a leading authority on public health and preventive medicine. J. S. Fairbairn had published, in 1923, a paper on 'Birth control – medical advice'[6]; Dr. Fairfield had written on 'The State and birth control' in *Medical Views on Birth Control* edited by Marchant and introduced by Sir Thomas (later Lord) Arthur Horder, to which Sir Arthur Newsholme, Professor Hill and A. E. Giles had also contributed[7,8]. Giles also wrote in *The Lancet* on 'The *need* for medical teaching on birth control'[9].

Sir James Marchant himself edited the report of the Medical Committee: 'Medical Aspects of Birth Control'[10]. This report was addressed to ". . . those medical men and women upon whom responsibility lies for giving advice on this most difficult subject". The report was praised by reviewers like Dr. Sidney Webb as "the most candid, the most outspoken and most impartial statement that this country has yet had . . ."[11].

The Medical Committee defined as 'Health': The relevant biological (physiological and psychological) factors which affect normal life[12]. Among the problems to be considered were "The medical reasons for exercise of contraceptive control". . . . "The effect on health of sexual abstinence, partial or complete, in married life" . . . "the reliability . . . of the so-called 'safe period' . . ."; "the effects of the use of various contraceptives on (I) the subsequent fertility and (II) the health of the persons concerned"[12]. Borell remarks that on the first two questions only clinicians could give an opinion, whereas the last two could be evaluated by experimental investigation only[13].

The Committee came to the conclusion that at that time neither suitable clinical nor statistical data existed to obtain any answers. Because of this fact, "the Medical Committee must necessarily fall

441

back on the knowledge and experience of witnesses and of others who have prescribed or used contraceptives"[14]. There was a change in attitude since Brown-Séquard: (1) Sexual exertion was no longer regarded dangerous to health or morality. (2) Abstinence in marriage was no longer accepted as a realistic method of birth control, ". . . in view of the fact that for many married people it is impossible to avoid sexual excitement, the non-gratification of the physiological act may lead to psychological ills, and if the normal sexual impulse be not satisfied – irregular sexual practices may follow"[14]. Although even the most certain of the contraceptive methods, like the sheath, sometimes produced neurasthenic symptoms, coitus interruptus was much more likely to cause such conditions in both persons involved[14]. In fine, sexual satisfaction was essential to the emotional and physical health of both partners[14] and a "reliable method of birth control was a necessity which should be made available to couples who needed it for medical reasons or excessive child bearing or poverty"[14]. Maintenance of sexual activity in marriage was essential to the stability of the family.

Dr. Gertrude Sturges of New York, Executive Secretary of the Committee on Maternal Health of New York City (founded to "study the questions of sterility, fertility, including contraception and sterilization from a medical and public health point of view") took part in the (British) Medical Committee's deliberations. Her own committee in New York was supported privately and by a grant from the Bureau of Social Hygiene, and the subcommittee on research had as one of its members Dr. Robert T. Frank, Head of the Department of Gynaecology of the Mount Sinai Hospital, whom we have encountered in his studies (partly with Jacob Rosenbloom) on hormones in the placenta and corpus luteum between 1904 and 1915 (see Chapter 17, p. 362). The American Committee also attempted to find definitions "of medical indications for contraception and sterilization", "clinical study of contraceptive methods" and "biological research" in support of their problems[15]. The subcommittee on research were already studying "the time of ovulation", "the period and conditions of receptivity in the female", and "spermatoxin"[16]. Dr. Robert Latou Dickinson, the American gynaecologist and obstetrician in the forefront of the reformers of sexual activity, birth control and contraception, since the early 1920s (who published the daring book on *Human Sex Anatomy: A Topographical Atlas*[17], in 1933) wrote[18]:

In March, 1923, The Committee on Maternal Health (of New York) began work on questions of human fertility and sterility. It was self-constituted as no scientific organization could be found that was willing to include a study of birth control.

Dr. Sturges gave evidence that "we are trying to secure clinical evidence of experience with the various mechanical methods. Our biologists may meanwhile discover a better method"[19]. The Chairman of the Medical Committee of the British Commission called her evidence "the only initial attempt towards a scientific investigation"[19].

It was interesting to note that Dr. Marie C. Stopes (1880–1958) (see also Section II) was not a member of the Committee. She had been writing on the remedy of overpopulation, on birth control, and on its methods, since the 1910s, an especially important book of hers being *Contraception (Birth Control): Its Theory, History and Practice. A Manual for the Medical and Legal Profession*[20], which reached a number of editions and was translated into several European languages. She also set up a Mothers' Clinic for Constructive Birth Control in London, on the work of which she reported in 1925: *The First Five Thousand (being) the First Report of the First Birth Control Clinic in the British Empire*[21]. By that time, there were a great number of writers on birth control in England. Dr. Helena Wright who – at 93 years of age – is still actively engaged in writing and lecturing on the subject today, was one of the six founders of the National Birth Control Association in 1930, the name of which was later changed to the Family Planning Association. Her husband, Dr. H. Wright, Julian Huxley, Lord Dawson of Penn, the Royal Physician, C. J. Bond, Dr. Norman Haire, and Dean Inge are just a few names of those who expressed their views on the subject.

Of the mid-19th century American writers, there should be mentioned J. Soule, MD who published a 72-page pamphlet in Cincinnati, Ohio, in about 1856: *Science of Reproduction and Reproductive Control*, discussing contraceptive technique in the few pages of the last (4th) part of it. Russell Thacher Trall (1812–1877) published his *Sexual Physiology* in 1866, which went through several editions over 20 years. Dr. Stopes thought him particularly important. John Humphrey Noyes (1811–1886) introduced a special method of contraception, practised by the community founded by him near Oneida, New York: Male Continence (or Karezza) (or 'coitus reservatus') which consists of normal entry, followed by movements, but avoiding the approaching climax; detumescence takes place intravaginally until normal conditions are achieved (in contrast to coitus interruptus where ejaculation follows). Thus nervous harmful effects are avoided[22]. Noyes, who was a congregational minister, established the Oneida community in 1847 as a Communal Society, which held all things to be of joint ownership. However, Noyes had to recant his system of complex marriage ('The Oneida Community Experiment') in 1880; he died six years later, a frightened and feeble old man, "in exile" in Canada, away from his community.

It was Dr. Alice Stockham who popularized 'Karezza' in her books (e.g. 'Karezza, parenthood and tokology'[23], and 'Karezza. Ethics of Marriage'[24] etc.). As a writer she had a romantic and somewhat mystic style. An example may suffice:

> Karezza gives a free motherhood, whether in a Government controlled by men or women. Karezza is a mutual relation and removes all vestiges of the old idea of man's domination over women.

In general, important medical leaders such as Dr. John B. Reynolds, in 1890 President of the American Gynaecological Society, displayed a strong reactionary attitude to birth control. This changed somewhat at the beginning of the 20th century, especially after the First World War.

Dr. Abraham Jacobi (1830–1919), an ex-president of the American Medical Association, wrote on medical aspects of birth control between 1906 and 1917[25]; he also advocated an examination and a medical certificate that men and women contemplating marriage are free from venereal and serious transmissible disease, which recommendation has been adopted in a number of the states of the U.S.A.

Dr. William Allen Pusey was another former president of the American Medical Association, who discussed contraception and eugenics in his 1924 presidential address on the 'Social Problems of Medicine'[26] and also participated in the Sixth International Neo-Malthusian and Birth Control Conference in New York in 1926[2].

Thomas Robert Malthus (1766–1834) published his celebrated 'An essay on the principle of population, as it affects the future improvement of society' in London in 1798. He argued the thesis that populations increase in geometrical ratio, but that subsistence increases only in arithmetical ratio. Hence checks on population increase are essential if one wishes to avoid the creation of misery and want. In his opinion, only certain naturally occurring events, such as disease, epidemics, vice and war, would prevent a population explosion. In later editions of his book he suggested "moral restraint" to restrain an undesirable growth of the population. By this he meant that marriage should be postponed until a much later age and that during marriage, strict sexual abstinence should help to regulate family increase. He never advocated any form of contraception for birth control. Although the term 'Neo-Malthusianism' was apparently first used by J. M. Robertson in the 1880s[27], it would seem that it was Francis Place (1771–1854), the Founder of the Birth Control Movement in England and a friend of Thomas Wakley, the Founder and Editor of *The Lancet* (see also p. 354), who expressed the sentiments of neo-Malthusianism. A self-taught jobbing tailor, he became a social reformer. Having fifteen children himself, the refined methods of Malthus were not for him. In his book: *The Principle of Population, including an Examination of the Proposed Remedies of Mr. Malthus*, in which he demonstrated the futility of deferred marriage and complete abstinence, he said plainly in his reply to Malthus:

> He (Malthus) candidly confesses that if people cannot be persuaded to defer marriage till they have a fair prospect of being able to maintain a family, all our former efforts will be thrown away. It is not in the nature of things that any permanent general improvement on the condition of the poor can be effected without an increase in the preventive check[28].

In addition, he suggests that the best method of avoiding promiscuous intercourse is early marriage, in which, however, conception should be prevented until it was medically, socially and economically propitious. As we have seen, he followed his book with the distribution of contraceptive handbills among the working classes, not only in London, but in the industrial North of England. Neo-Malthusianism stresses the importance of birth control not only for medical, but also for social and economic reasons.

In the United States it was, above all, Mrs. Margaret Sanger, who became after 1912, a crusader for family limitation and for a change in the United States legislation concerning birth control. She gained her first hand experience as a nurse in the poor district of the lower East Side of New York. She opened her first contraceptive advice station in the United States in the Brownsville section of Brooklyn, NY in 1916, until the police closed it as a 'public nuisance' and she had to serve a 30-day sentence in jail. In 1917 she became president of the newly-formed 'National Birth Control League'; in that capacity she was still active at the time of the foundation of the New York Birth Control Clinical Research Bureau, set up as a department of the American Birth Control League, which reported on the first 10 000 cases in 1934[29]. She also organized the World Population Conference in Geneva in 1927[30], and the First International Clinical Conference in Zurich in 1931. The proceedings of that conference were published in a volume entitled *The Practice of Contraception*, edited by Margaret Sanger and Hannah M. Stone[31].

The only committee on the subject under medical leadership in the United States was the Committee on Maternal Health, which began its work in 1923. In 1930 it was incorporated as the National Committee on Maternal Health, with offices in the New York Academy of Medicine, and the President of the Academy as Chairman of the Committee for the first five years. The Secretary of the Committee for the first eleven years was a full-time volunteer: Dr. Robert Latou Dickinson, formerly Clinical Professor of Gynaecology and Obstetrics, ex-president of the American Gynaecological Society, the author of many important books, including *Control of Conception* (with Louise Stevens Bryant) in 1931[32]. Dr. Gertrude Sturges, executive secretary of the National Committee, has already been mentioned in her role of observer and medical witness at the British Medical Committee in 1927 (see also pp. 442–443).

We now return to Britain and to the activities of Dr. Marie Stopes. The opening of her first birth control advisory clinic (at 61, Marlborough Road, Holloway) in 1921 was a great success, and so was a public meeting at the Queen's Hall, in London on 31 May 1921. She was next in the public eye on the occasion of the court action against Dr. Halliday Sutherland ('The Birth Control Libel Action' of 1923) who had criticized her (lay) advisory activities at her clinic as potentially harmful. The case was heard before the Lord Chief Justice and went up to the House of Lords, to be won by Dr. Stopes, although not without difficulties. The expert witness for Dr. Sutherland was Professor Anne McIlroy. She had stated that she never had a (woman) patient wearing a check pessary. Marie Stopes disguised herself as a charwoman and attended Professor McIlroy's clinic at the hospital. She walked out with a rubber vagina cap, advised and put in place by Professor McIlroy herself!

In August 1921 the Society for Constructive Birth Control and Racial Progress was formed, with Dr. Stopes as its President. In 1930, a voluntary society founded the National Birth Control Association, to co-ordinate the existing small societies which were running contraceptive advisory clinics, the oldest of which was that of Dr. Stopes. At the beginning of the 1960s, the Association had more than 300 such clinics within its orbit. Dr. Stopes continued her work until her death in 1958, aged 78 years.

The German writers of that period covered more or less the same ground, and Himes compiled a list of many of their names[33]. The Dutch have been in the forefront of population and birth control for a considerable period of time. Dr. J. Ruttgers wrote numerous articles on the subject between 1903 and 1927, and Dr. Aletta Jacobs opened the first systematic advisory office on contraception in Holland in 1881[34]. Dr. S. Van Houten became "one of the most active people in Holland in public instruction, back in the 'eighties and nineties' "[35]. Even more important, Dr. Van Houten became Minister of the Interior and later Prime Minister of the Netherlands! The Dutch League issued a medical pamphlet early on in which contraceptive techniques were well described (by Dr. J. Ruttgers)[36].

In Britain, the Volpar (= *vol*untary *par*enthood) preparations of the British Drug Houses were the result of ten years' research work under the supervision of the Birth Control Investigation Committee. Dr. J. R. Baker, in the Science Department of Oxford University, who had conducted the investigations since 1928, had made a list of requirements for the ideal contraceptive as follows:

(1) It should be inexpensive.
(2) It should require no special appliance for insertion into the vagina.
(3) It should be small.
(4) It should be unaffected by the ordinary range of climate.
(5) It should neither leave any trace on the skin when handled nor stain fabrics.
(6) It should contain no volatile or odorous substance.
(7) It should be non–irritant to the vagina, cervix, and penis.
(8) It should be without pharmacological effect if absorbed into the bloodstream.
(9) It should contain a substance reducing surface tension to ensure the smallest crevices of the folds of the vagina being reached.
(10) It should kill sperms at 5/8 or lower concentration in the alkaline and acid test, and the spermicide should diffuse rapidly out of the vehicle into the semen[37].

Dr. H. M. Carleton, also at Oxford, made a study of the pathology of chemical contraception and suggested work for the group to be planned along four lines:

(1) to devise methods for evaluating the spermicidal powers of pure substances and of contraceptive preparations;
(2) to investigate the principles underlying the killing of sperms by chemical means;
(3) to discover powerful and harmless spermicides;
(4) to produce a scientifically satisfactory contraceptive for general use[37].

On the whole, the number of pregnancies which occurred during the clinical trials with a Volpar product was very small.

Much more exciting, however, and more relevant, was a major research project which took place in Innsbruck, the capital of the Tyrol in Austria, from 1919 to 1932. Professor H. H. Simmer drew attention to it in 1970: 'On the history of hormonal contraception. I. Ludwig Haberlandt (1885–1932) and his concept of "hormonal sterilization"'[38] (see Section II), and 'On the history of hormonal contraception: II. Otfried Otto Fellner (1873–?) and estrogens as antifertility hormones'[39].

Today, Dr. Gregory Pincus, Research Director of Worcester Foundation for Experimental Biology in Massachusetts, is usually referred to as the 'Father of the Pill'. The proper denomination was given, however, to the new effective method of contraception by Alan F. Guttmacher, Professor of Clinical Obstetrics at Columbia Medical School. In the opening speech at a symposium sponsored by G. D. Searle Ltd. (who had devoted much enthusiasm and time to this research), on 18 January 1961, Guttmacher said: It is a technique of birth control which operates by harmlessly altering the physiology of the body, so as to render conception temporarily impossible, at the same time imposing no impediment to the normal physiology of sexual intercourse. The fact that the time of application of such an effective physiologic agent is wholly removed from the time of coitus, bestows an overwhelming advantage, permitting much greater acceptance of contraception the world over[40]. The new drug to which Professor Guttmacher was referring was called Norethynodrel, usually known as 'The Pill' – Physiological Contraception!

One such method had existed for many centuries: women, and, especially, midwives and doctors knew that prolonged breastfeeding of a child gave a high degree of protection from renewed pregnancy. In England, this 'nature's contraceptive' in the form of wet-nursing and prolonged lactation was practised in Chesham, Buckinghamshire, between 1578 and 1601[41], and prolonged lactation was common in China[41a].

Dr. Ludwig Haberlandt (1885–1932), professor extraordinary of physiology (equivalent to the Reader in England) at the University of Innsbruck in Austria, expressed the view that there must be a better contraceptive method than the use of the condom [or of the rubber Dutch cap, or of the gold cervical cap of the Viennese gynaecologist K. Kafka (which he recommended in 1908)]. Haberlandt was familiar with the anatomist Robert Heinrich Johannes Sobotta's (1869–1945) work on 'The formation of the corpus luteum in the mouse' (Ueber die Bildung des Corpus Luteum bei der Maus)[42]. He also knew of the ideas, hypotheses and attempts to elucidate the function of the corpus luteum by Gustav Born in Breslau and his pupils Ludwig Fraenkel and Vilhelm Magnus, which – eventually – led to the discovery of progesterone by Corner and Allen. Haberlandt also knew of the theory of John Beard (1858–1924) in 1897: 'The span of gestation and the cause of birth'[43,44], and of Auguste Prenant (1861–1927) in 1898: 'Sur la valeur morphologique, sur l'action physiologique et thérapeutique possible du corps jaune[45] (see also p. 366). Beard had suggested that the corpus luteum prevented further ovulation. Prenant of Nancy in France added that the prevention of ovulation by the corpus luteum was achieved by means of internal secretion. It was also known that veterinary surgeons successfully treated infertility in cows with persistent corpora lutea by squeezing those and bursting them manually per rectum. Similarly, Joseph Halban described the symdrome of persistent corpora lutea in 1915, which could be treated by effective surgical removal, if it did not regress spontaneously. Leo Loeb (1865–1959) had shown in animals that removal of corpora lutea will speed the next ovulation. Edmund Herman (see also pp. 362, 401) and Marianne Stein in the animal experiment in 1916, demonstrated the prevention of ovulation by giving extracts of corpus luteum[46]. Haberlandt also took due notice of the description and discussion concerning the interstitial cells of the ovarian tissue, which is particularly developed in the pregnant animal. It was assumed that the 'interstitial organ' of the ovary could act like the corpus luteum and occasionally take its place.

This knowledge of the physiology of the corpus luteum and of the theories concerning its function, together with the view that birth control is necessary and that it should be a safe, hormonal, temporary sterilization, fired Haberlandt's imagination. The successful ovarian transplantation experiments by Knauer in Vienna (see also pp. 368–370) and the observation of Eugen Steinach (1861–1944) that the interstitial tissue of the transplanted ovary showed an increase in size, gave Haberlandt the idea of making an animal infertile by implanting the ovary of another, pregnant animal. On 1 March 1919 he performed the first such experiment on a rabbit. The animal, which before had become readily and repeatedly pregnant, did not do so after the experiment, even after repeated copulations. The second experiment failed, but Haberlandt's main problem became lack of funds. Eventually, the Rockefeller Foundation decided to help, and Haberlandt could report in 1921 'On the hormonal sterilization of the female animal' (Ueber hormonal Sterilisierung des weiblichen Tierkoerpers)[47]. He had achieved successful temporary sterilization in five (out of eight) rabbits and in three (out of eight) guinea-pigs. The failures were due to necrosis and resorption of the transplanted ovaries.

A lecture to the Scientific Medical Society of Innsbruck in November 1919 was well received. Even at that time, however, he had in mind to achieve the same result by injections of ovarian extract and, eventually, by giving such extracts by mouth! His first experiments with injections of extract failed mainly because the commercial extract (by Merck) was from non-pregnant ovaries. On

Aus dem physiologischen Institut der Universität Innsbruck.

Ueber hormonale Sterilisierung des weiblichen Tierkörpers*).

(Vorläufige Mitteilung.)

Von Prof. Dr. L. Haberlandt.

Es haben als Erste Beard [1] und Prénant [1a] die Auffassung vertreten, dass das Corpus luteum eine Drüse ohne Ausführungsgang mit innerer Sekretion sei, welche die Aufgabe habe, die Eireifung zwischen den einzelnen Menstrualperioden und besonders während der Gravidität zu verhindern und damit einen ungestörten Verlauf der Schwangerschaft zu gewährleisten. Es ist z. B. eine bei Tierärzten allgemein bekannte Tatsache, auf die auch Tandler [2] besonders aufmerksam gemacht hat, dass beim Rind, bei dem sich nicht selten ein persistierender und hypertrophierender gelber Körper vorfindet, dann die normalerweise alle 3 Wochen wiederkehrende Brunst ausbleibt und erst nach dem Entfernen oder Zerdrücken des Corpus luteum in den nächsten Tagen wieder auftritt. Ferner hat L. Loeb [3] gezeigt, dass beim Meerschweinchen der Eintritt der nächsten Ovulation beschleunigt wird, wenn man die Corpora lutea während der ersten Woche nach einer Ovulation entfernt. Weiters sprechen auch Erfahrungen im selben Sinne, die über die Wirkungsweise von Injektionen von Corpus luteum-Präparaten gemacht wurden. Es haben Pearl und Surface [4] beobachtet, dass bei normalen Hühnern nach genannter Behandlung die Eierproduktion für bestimmte Zeit aufhört. Andererseits konnten Herrmann und Stein [5] in Injektionsversuchen, die sie mit einem aus Corpus luteum hergestellten Reizstoff (Pentaminphosphatid) ausführten, bei noch nicht geschlechtsreifen Kaninchen und Ratten feststellen, dass dadurch die Follikeltätigkeit des Eierstockes zunächst begünstigt, dann aber gehemmt wird, insofern die Follikelreifung und -berstung und damit das Entstehen von Corpora lutea verhindert wird, analog wie es bei trächtigen Tieren der Fall ist. Schliesslich ist mir erst nach Abschluss meiner Transplantationsversuche eine in jüngster Zeit von Naeslund [6] veröffentlichte Arbeit bekannt geworden, der weiblichen Kaninchen ein aus dem gelben Körper gravider Kühe bereitetes Extrakt 2 Wochen lang injizierte und dadurch das Trächtigwerden schon nach 10 Injektionstagen verhindern konnte [1]. Dasselbe Ziel erreichte er auch dadurch, dass er durch Belegen mit vorher vasektomierten, also zeugungsunfähigen Männchen das Entstehen von Corpora lutea hervorrief [2], worauf die so vorbereiteten Weibchen bis zu 6 Tage von zeugungstüchtigen Rammlern nicht trächtig werden konnten.

Andererseits ist es aber auch sichergestellt, dass das interstitielle Gewebe der Ovarien bei Tieren und Menschen in der Zeit der Gravidität mächtig zu wuchern beginnt, wenn das Corpus luteum sich zurückbildet. Es erscheint daher, wie Biedl [7], Aschner [8] u. a. bemerkt haben, die Annahme naheliegend, dass die interstitielle Drüse die Funktion übernimmt, die das Corpus luteum zwar begonnen hat, aber wegen seiner Rückbildung unvollendet lässt. Ist die Eiansiedlung durch den gelben Körper, wie dies von L. Fraenkel [9] festgestellt wurde, gewährleistet und, wie L. Loeb [3] zeigte, die Entstehung der mütterlichen Plazenta veranlasst worden, dann würde von der interstitiellen Drüse für die weitere Ausbildung und Funktion derselben gesorgt werden. Es darf daher wohl auch vermutet werden, dass gleichfalls die ovulationshemmende Wirkung des Corpus luteum verum bei seiner Rückbildung von der inzwischen gewucherten, interstitiellen Drüse allmählich übernommen wird. Da nun Steinach [10 und 11] in transplantierten Ovarien eine hochgradige Wucherung der interstitiellen Zellen gefunden hat, kam ich auf den Gedanken, durch Transplantation von Eierstöcken gravider Tiere in normale Weibchen infolge der Einpflanzung der Corpora lutea einerseits, andererseits durch die Wucherung des interstitiellen Gewebes womöglich eine so weit gehende Ovulationshemmung in den eigenen Eierstöcken des Transplantationstieres auszulösen, dass dadurch eine temporäre Sterilisierung desselben erreicht wird.

Die Versuche führte ich in den Jahren 1919—1921 an gesunden und kräftigen Kaninchen und Meerschweinchen aus, die mindestens schon einmal geworfen hatten und seitdem isoliert gehalten wurden; demnach waren sie sicher nicht trächtig, wenn an ihnen die Ovarientransplantation stattfand. Die Tiere, von denen hiezu die Eierstöcke verwendet wurden, befanden sich durchwegs in der zweiten Hälfte der Gravidität. Selbstverständlich wurden die Ueberpflanzungen streng aseptisch vorgenommen, so dass ausnahmslos primäre Heilungserfolge erzielt wurden. Die Transplantationen erfolgten subkutan und zwar beiderseits unter die Rückenhaut nach Entfernung der Faszien auf den angefrischten Muskelboden, wie dies schon Steinach [10] empfohlen hatte. Das Befinden der Transplantationstiere war gemäss dem reaktionslosen Heilungsverlaufe bei kräftiger Fütterung vollständig

*) Vorgetragen in der Wissenschaftl. Aerztegesellschaft zu Innsbruck. Die ausführliche Abhandlung wird in Pflügers Archiv für die gesamte Physiologie erscheinen.

...andlung verursachte dabei allerdings keine Hemmung ...der Bildung von gelben Körpern, wie sie bei nor... ...nschluss an den Belegakt zustande kommt, sondern ...lung und — Weiterentwicklung. ...uch schon früher P. Ancel und P. Bouin (Compt. ...p. 455 et 506) berichtet.

Figure 67 Front page of Haberlandt's paper [by kind permission of the Royal Society of Medicine, London]

the occasion of the meeting of the German Gynaecological Society in Innsbruck in 1922, he reported on his experiments. At the same meeting there was also a report by the Viennese gynaecologist Otfried Otto Fellner (see Section II) that "After injection of the female sexual lipoid, the active substance of corpus luteum and placenta, animals remain sterile for several months. This confirms similar experiments by Haberlandt"[48–50]. In addition, in his discussion, Fellner was perhaps the first person to suggest that oestrogens may also cause infertility. Haberlandt was obviously grateful for Fellner's acknowledgement of his work. In 1923, Haberlandt could report to the meeting of the German Society of Physiology that he had had success with injections of extracts from ovaries of pregnant cows. Moreover, he could achieve the same (sterilizing) results with placental extracts[51]. He also mentioned that he had attempted to feed ovarian extract to animals, but so far without success. However, in October 1924 he fed two female mice again, and they remained infertile in the presence of effective male animals. He followed this by feeding six mice with ovarian extracts in milk, and five others with placental extracts. They all became temporarily sterile, two of each group permanently so, which latter observation Haberlandt explained by giving a dose which was excessive for the animal. In 1926, Haberlandt had concluded his experiments. Although there was interest in his work, critics did not fail to point out that the results might have been due to non-specific effects of parenterally administered proteins. Fellner came to the rescue and refuted those critics. He recorded that his purified material was free from protein, but caused sterility. Moreover, Haberlandt's feeding experiments which did result in temporary sterility also contradicted the above criticisms. In his experiments Fellner next used mainly oestrogenic material which he called 'Feminin', both by injection and orally, and achieved temporary sterility. Of Fellner's fifteen guinea-pigs treated with Feminin, none became pregnant; of thirty rabbits only three conceived; so did three mice out of 100. One of the animals showed several corpora lutea at autopsy, from which Fellner concluded that his female hormone could not have interfered with the ripening of the follicle and ovulation, but that his 'Feminin' caused damage to the ovum directly[52]. Out of his 30 rabbits, only two became pseudo-pregnant (apart from the three who conceived). No histological proof was offered to demonstrate direct damage to the ovum caused by 'Feminin'.

Fellner, like Iscovesco, had studied the effects of ovarian extracts on the ovaries of experimental animals as early as 1912 and reported on those experiments[53], but the question of hormonal sterilization did not arise at that time. In fact, Ludwig Adler (1876–1958), also a pupil of Schauta of Vienna, reported in 1912 on experiments demonstrating that watery extracts of the ovaries speeded follicular maturation to be followed by degeneration of ovum and follicle[54]. These observations were confirmed by Bernard Aschner in 1913[55], but overlooked in the literature until H. H. Simmer's painstaking studies disinterred them. Unfortunately, these extracts were watery extracts, which are not so soluble as the lipid extracts. Morover, they were, in 1912, not pure extracts but – like those of Edmund Hermann's in Vienna (see p. 362), mixed extracts from the whole ovary. In 1927, however, Fellner summed up his findings as follows[52]:

> Administration of increasing doses of Feminin will give different results in (experimental) animals. (1) Oestrus with enlargement of the womb. (2) Reduced number of offspring, which is mainly female. (3) (?) Destruction of the ova but no inhibition of corpus luteum formation. This leads to hormonal sterility (attempts at nest building without pregnancy = ? pseudopregnancy). (4) Destruction of the ova with inhibition of corpus luteum formation. No pregnancy nor pseudopregnancy. This could, eventually, lead to permanent sterility ('hormonal castration').

Although, at that time, Fellner did not realize that the pharmacological effect of oestrogen did not rule out the existence of a second, different ovarian hormone, he recognized quite correctly that although it seemed paradoxical for the same hormone both to cure and cause sterility, this was only a question of dosage[56]. Alas, as H. H. Simmer points out relevantly, although Fellner demonstrated "the antifertility action of purified oestrogen–containing extracts", he made the same mistake as Robert T. Frank of New York who, in 1922 (see also p. 362 and p. 401) reported his observation on the uterotropic action of follicular fluid in an unsuitable (if not obscure) medical journal. Simmer adds:[39] "It should further be mentioned that Fellner's way of reporting his findings and conclusions was somewhat disorganized and mixed with clinical observations; it failed to conform to the pattern followed in first-rate publications of that time".

We have already mentioned that at that time the question of the existence of two ovarian hormones was not definitely settled. When Haberlandt lectured again on hormone-induced sterility in 1928, he did not distinguish a stimulating hormone from an inhibiting one, although clearly all his early work was based on the concept of an ovulation-inhibiting hormone. He also ignored Fellner's recent publication, but Fellner took pains to bring it to his attention. A certain tension ensued when Haberlandt implied that Fellner's results lacked a solid basis[57]. Subsequently, however, in 1931 he modified his views and admitted that oestrogens might be effective as contraceptive agents[58,59]. Haberlandt was also attacked by the clinicians, who objected to the idea of treating infertility in women by giving ovarian hormone, which – so they argued – cannot at the same time produce infertility! Haberlandt replied that perhaps a lower dosage might act as a stimulus, but the larger dose would have an inhibitory effect. Unfortunately, it seems unlikely that either Fellner or Haberlandt had an opportunity to test their experiments in human patients[60].

Misfortune dogged Haberlandt's footsteps in other respects. Dr. Alfred Greil (1876–1964), anatomist at the same university (Innsbruck), who had been friendly with Haberlandt's father, attacked him personally. He called the idea of sterilization a criminal act and a highly immoral action, which would permit a few 'drones' of society to indulge in love games. There were no such things as hormones of the ovary, he declared. Haberlandt's observations were due to toxic effects. Moreover, if such treatment were to be extended to humans, women treated in such manner would give birth to seriously damaged children. Dr. Greil demanded special legislation for the protection of pregnant women and of propagation. Haberlandt protested that most of the animals made temporarily infertile, regained their capacity for becoming pregnant and produced normal progeny. Finally, he declared that he could not enter into any argument with anyone who still denied the existence of internal secretion of the female gonads. The national newspapers, on the other hand, took up the results of his experiments (in 1927) in their usual exaggerated manner, and made life intolerable for him from a different angle.

In 1924, Haberlandt regarded pulmonary tuberculosis, sugar diabetes, cretinism, Graves' disease, syphilis and chronic heart disease as indications for the use of his physiological method of (temporary) sterilization. In 1930, he extended his ideas towards social and eugenic birth control, and turned his interest towards the application of his method to human beings. After the death of one of the directors of the pharmaceutical firm, Merck, he had to look for support to the Hungarian firm of Richter, who produced for him an extract which he found ten times more potent that those he had received from Merck. It was named 'Infecundin', which he hoped to try out clinically. A year later, one of his gynaecological colleagues mentioned in a discussion that the attempts of hormonal sterilization at the Gynaecological University Clinic at Innsbruck had failed. Whether they had used Merck's or Richter's extract was not clear. Haberlandt died on 22 July 1932, at only 47 years of age. Simmer poses the question why Haberlandt did not succeed. The most likely explanation lies in the poor quality of the extracts he had at his disposal. Fellner argued that until a far greater quantity of hormone could be manufactured synthetically, little success could be expected in the application of the principle of hormonal infertility in women.

Haberlandt died two years before the successful isolation of progesterone. He was less concerned with problems of over-population in the world, but quoted – according to Simmer who restored his memory – a sentence written by Sigmund Freud in 1898: ". . . in theory, it would be one of the greatest triumphs of mankind, . . . if one would succeed to lift the responsible act of procreation to a deliberate and planned activity". I cannot do better than use Simmer's concluding words: "For all those reasons, Haber-landt should be remembered as a pioneer". May I add, however, that the same applies to Fellner.

THE STORY OF INSULIN

Numerous papers and books have been written on the discovery of insulin in 1921, the most spectacular event in the field of endocrino-logy in the first half of this century, apart from the clinical use of cortisone, and perhaps the use of iodized salt for the prevention of goitre, because of the great number of people to benefit from it. This flood of information became an avalanche on the occasion of the 50th anniversary of the discovery. The present writer had the good fortune to listen to Charles Herbert Best (1899–1978) giving an account of the summer 1921, when Sir Frederick Banting (1891–1941) and he had actually succeeded in obtaining insulin. Of the many accounts I have heard or read since then, the one by Dr. John R. Henderson, Reader in Physiology at St. George's Hospital Medical School in London, has appeared to me the most likely one[61], to which should be added Dr. Ian Murray's article on the 'forgotten man', Dr. Nicolas Constantin Paulesco of Bucharest in Roumania (1869–1931)[62].

Before relating the story, we must briefly sketch out the mile-stones since the end of the 18th century, some of which may bear repetition. Matthew Dobson (ca. 1730–1784) reported in 1776 that the sweet taste of diabetic urine was caused by sugar[63]. Dobson (see Section II), a Yorkshireman, had trained in Edinburgh, but practised in Liverpool's Royal Infirmary (see also p. 174). His paper was presented to a London medical society by his colleague and friend Dr. Fothergill at the Mitre Tavern in Fleet Street, London. The description of one of his patients, Peter Dickenson, 33 years old, who was admitted under his care in Liverpool on 22 October 1772, and was found to be suffering from diabetes, is a classic. It was remarkable, however, that Dobson took eight ounces of blood from the arm of his patient. He observed that the serum was sweet to taste, though less so than the urine. In other words, he was the discoverer of hyperglycaemia! From this and various other experiments he deduced that diabetic urine always contains sugar which is not formed in the kidney "but previously existed in the serum of the blood". The final emaciation occurs "from so large a proportion of the alimentary matter being drawn off by the kidney, before it is perfectly assimilated and applied to the purpose of nutrition".

Thomas Cawley observed and reported on diabetes following injury to the pancreas in 1788[64].

We have already discussed the meat diet for diabetics, devised by John Rollo in 1797. He was a Surgeon-General in the Army, who died in 1809; his publication pioneered successful management of diabetes mellitus by restricted diet[65]. Michel Eugène Chevreul (1786–1889) demonstrated in 1815 that the sugar in the urine of diabetics is glucose (Notes sur le sucre de diabètes)[66]. Carl August Trommer (1806–1879) introduced Trommer's test for glucose in the urine in 1841; it was still being taught at German universities in the 1920s, although Fehling's test was the one in common use[67]. Claude Bernard's (1813–1878) experiments with piqûre of the floor of the 4th ventricle have also been mentioned[68] (see p. 376). Bernard's observations on the liver, which stores sugar in the form of glycogen, and that an organ can produce a substance and pass it directly into the blood, the phenomenon of 'internal secretion' (1855) was discussed as the official date of the era of endocrinology. So were Moritz Schiff's (1823–1896) experimental observations on artificial diabetes[69]. Wilhelm Petters, in 1857, demonstrated the presence of acetone in the urine of diabetics[70]. Just a few years before, in 1848, Hermann Christian von Fehling (1812–1885) developed his quantitative test for sugar in the urine[71]. After Fehling and Petters, Carl Adolph Christian Jacob Gerhardt (1833–1902) introduced his iron-chloride reaction for aceto-acetic acid in the urine, when there is acetonaemia[72]. In 1869, Henry Dewey Noyes (1832–1900) in the United States, described eye changes (retinitis) in more advanced forms of diabetes mellitus[73]. Diabetic coma, which has already been mentioned, was first described by William Prout (1785–1850), who is also known for his demonstration of free hydrochloric acid in the gastric juice, and for his claim to have recommended iodine as treatment for goitre before Coindet (see p. 191). Adolf Kussmaul (1822–1902) succeeded in proving that diabetic coma was caused by acetonaemia; he also described the Kussmaul type of respiration in acidaemia with its recurring phase of air-hunger ('Diese grosse Athmung' = this great breathing)[74]. Beta-oxybutyric acid was discovered by Ernst Stadelmann (b. 1853)[75], or rather in 1883 he noticed an acid substance in the urine, when studying the excretion of ammonia in the urine[75]. Stadelmann recognized that the increased production of acids in the blood led to the diabetic coma. It was Oscar Minkowski (1858–1930), however, who identified Stadelmann's acid substance in the diabetic urine as β-oxybutyric acid[76].

Adolf Magnus-Levy (1865–1955) extended the knowledge in this field by his studies of β-oxybutyric acid in diabetic coma[77,78]. Theodor Leber (1840–1917) added to the pathology of the affections of the eye connected with diabetes only a few years after Noyes[79].

Into this period falls an observation which is of great importance but usually overlooked, if not forgotten. In 1884, Charles Louis Xavier Arnozan and Louis Vaillard recorded a 'contribution à l'étude du pancréas du lapin. Lésions provoquées par la ligature du canal de Wirsung'[80] in which they established that after blocking the pancreatic duct, they achieved atrophy of the pancreas in the hare, *without* diabetes. This was in apparent contrast to the most important demonstration by Joseph von Mering (1849–1908) and Oscar Mink-owski (1858–1931), that (experimental) diabetes would be produced by successful pancreatectomy in the dog (see pp. 297–298). Arnozan and Vaillard's paper was also 25 years ahead of MacCallum's paper in 1909 (see p. 298). Joseph von Mering was the first to produce experimental diabetes by means of phloridzin[81], which method proved to be of great importance in the further study of the pathology of the disease.

In 1871, M. Troisier (1844–1919) added the disease entity of diabète bronzé as a sequel of haemochromatosis[82], which was later investigated more extensively by Friedrich Daniel von Reckling-hausen (1833–1910)[83], in 1889; he also gave the disease its name. Carl Harko von Noorden (1858–1944) was, during his long life, a perpetual student of the diabetic patient and – with Naunyn (see p. 297) – was mainly responsible for the most efficient dietetic and general management of the diabetic patient in the pre-insulin era. Some time after the discovery and application of insulin, it was found that many of the general principles laid down by Naunyn and von Noorden still held good[84]. Another physician who deserves special mention was Apollinaire Bouchardat (1806–1886) (see also p. 175) who used a meticulous system of investigations for the assessment of diabetes and devised the most rational dietetic régime for its treatment at the time (1875)[85]. Modifications of Fehling's test were described in 1862 by Frederick William Pavy (1829–1911)[86], who in the course of his researches came to the conclusion that there was a definite causal relation between the degree of sugar in the blood and in the urine, and by A. L. Benedict in the United States, in

1911[87]. The latter should not be confused with Stanley Rossiter Benedict (1884–1936), who, in 1936, published a method for determination of sugar in the blood[88].

Whereas between 1895 and 1914, low carbohydrate and high protein and fat diets were popular, from 1914 until 1921, F. M. Allen's (the well known Boston diabetic expert) prolonged fasting periods became fashionable, although not always of convincing value (cit. after Rolleston)[89]. It was, incidentally, also Allen, who after injection of a pancreatic glycerine extract into normal animals, found sugar in their urine. He concluded, therefore, that pancreatic therapy in diabetes was doomed to failure!

To the important studies of Laguesse, Hedon, Opie, Ssobolew, Frerichs and Lusk we have already referred. Opie, then working in the Department of Pathology of the Johns Hopkins Medical School in Baltimore, also noted that the islands of Langerhans had undergone hyaline degeneration in the case of diabetics who had died of the disease[90]. These observations were confirmed a year later in 1902 by Leonid Ssobolew working independently in St. Petersburg. Based on these two findings, gradually a hypothesis was formulated. This found its final expression by Sharpey-Schafer (among others) in 1916, that diabetes must be caused by the lack of an internal secretion produced by Langerhans's islet cells, the hormone of which Sharpey-Schafer provisionally named 'insulin'.

Meanwhile, a Berlin physician and keen student of diabetes, Georg Ludwig Zuelzer (1870–1949), nearly succeeded, in 1908, in demonstrating that principle. He attempted to obtain extracts of the whole pancreas by various methods. One of them contained what is now known as insulin, with an effect of lowering the blood sugar, but serious hypoglycaemic reactions made him abandon the experiment[91]. Zuelzer also tried his aqueous extracts on human diabetics, but the ensuing pyrexia and hypoglycaemia were as unbearable as the disease itself, although the results were striking. Hoechst Pharmaceuticals gave him a contract for the patent rights of the extract and paid him 6000 marks (= sterling £300) and promised a percentage of the profits; he had, in 1912, taken out U.S. patent No. 1 027 790, although the letters patent said that the extract was too septic to be used for persons[92]. Although Zuelzer got his money, his 'insulin' never reached the market!

Thus, by 1916 the stage was set for the discovery, isolation, synthesis and crystallization of the postulated hormone: insulin. The field was open, the hunt was on, and there were many keen hunters in several countries. In 1907, M. A. Lane, in Chicago, described type α (oxyphil) and type β (basophil) islet cells[93]. 'α' cells were fixed with alcohol; the β cells were fixed with chrome sublimate. Lane's teacher and chief, R. R. Bensley, published a 91-page paper in 1911, on his own studies, using his own gentian violet and orange G stain on the guinea-pig pancreas. He was able to estimate the adult guinea-pig islet organ as containing *ca.* 25 000 (± 5000) islets, corresponding to about 20 per milligram of tissue. This was about 20 times greater than any previous estimate[94,95].

In 1915, J. Homans (b. 1877), one of Cushing's original team members, came to the conclusion that it is the β-cells which secrete the still hypothetical insulin[96]. In his *Pathology of Diabetes*, Dr. Shields Warren (1930), mentioned a third type of cells of the islets, which Bloom called 'D' cells in 1931[97]. The relation of the islet cells to the ordinary cells of the pancreas was discussed as early as 1886, by Lewaschew[98], who believed that exhausted acinous cells become converted into islet tissue. In 1902 A. Mankowski thought that the islands represented the highest stage of activity of the acinous cells[99]. (Sir) Henry H. Dale also believed that starvation, exhaustion and ligature of the duct led to islet formation from the acini[100], but, as Henderson points out, Dale used two techniques: the injection of large doses of secretin into cats and dogs, and fasting toads for several weeks. He claimed to be able to show that in these two situations there was a marked enlargement of islet tissue, the exocrine tissue being converted. Unfortunately, all that really happened was the degranulation of exocrine cells (Henderson[101]) "Dale's scientific career – it was his first publication (1905) – like that of Claude Bernard sixty years earlier, got off to a bad start". Laguesse regarded the alpha-cells as transitional cells and the beta-cells as definitely island cells[102,103]. R. F. Bensley (see above) showed in 1912, that the islands are derived from the epithelium of the pancreatic ducts, which has three developmental potentialities to form ordinary acini, alpha- and beta-cells[94,95].

After the turn of the century, as John R. Henderson elegantly put it:

> In the next twenty years the stage became filled with shadowy figures. The first of them was an extraordinary French physiologist, Eugène Gley (1857–1930).

We came across Gley (see Section II) before as an opponent of Marañon (see also pp. 394 ff.) in Spain; as the outstanding physiologist, who made valuable contributions to the discovery and understanding of the function of the parathyroids independently of, although later than, Sandstroem. But Gley had a great deal of other fundamental research to his credit. To quote Henderson again: "Everything was grist to Gley's mill"; in 1891, he published 12 papers in the French Society of Biology on the thyroid, the adrenals, the pancreas, central nervous system and heart. "At the same time, he was very meticulous concerning definitions, evaluation of facts, and conclusions drawn from the results of carefully designed experiments." He was in accord with the views of Swale Vincent, and the pharmacologist Clark (see also pp. 391 ff.). As regards the present subject, he was impressed by Laguesse's hypothesis that the islets of Langerhans might produce a substance which would normally prevent glucose from being excreted in the urine. To test the theory, he made an aqueous extract of the pancreas and gave it to pancreatectomized dogs. He found that it diminished their glycosuria considerably and improved the diabetic symptoms, but the dogs became otherwise more ill than before (? hypoglycaemia and temperature?). Wondering if that could be caused by the enzymes of the exocrine pancreatic tissue, he then used Bernard's method of injecting gelatine into the duct, and waited for the pancreas to degenerate. He made an extract of the remaining tissue and injected it into diabetic dogs. There followed improvement and the glycosuria decreased. This was the same procedure that Banting and Best carried out 25 years later. Henderson wrote next:

> The only problem is, how should we regard Gley, for it was at this point that he performed one of the more eccentric acts in the history of science. He wrote up his experiments, sealed them in a packet, and in February 1905, deposited them with the French Society of Biology, with instructions that the packet should only be opened at his request. We can only conjecture why a man should do such a thing, but Gley could have no clue as to the significance of his findings, and perhaps was not even quite sure that they were true. But since scientists published at that time a paper on a morning's work, or some odd thoughts they had on the weather, or life force, it would have only been a drop in the ocean if Gley had published his findings. He was clearly a good scientist. . . .

Gley never took up his experiments on the pancreas of the 1890s again. On the occasion of the announcement of Banting and Best's discovery in 1921, he gave instructions to have his packet opened. Although the protocols were not detailed (not more than it was usual at that time), there was no doubt that the experiments would have led to the final results that Gley stipulated. He said that he found the extracts from degenerated pancreas, when administered to completely pancreatectomized dogs, to diminish considerably the urinary sugar content and to alleviate all the other symptoms of diabetes. ". . . because of other researches, the further development of these studies on extracts of degenerated pancreas were laid aside"[104]. Gley, Henderson thinks, "discovered insulin without knowing it"[105].

Starling first used the word 'hormone' in his Croonian Lectures in June 1905; the word 'insuline' (sic) was first used by J. de Meyer in 1907[106], followed by Sharpey-Schafer in 1916[107].

Minkowski, as we have seen, arrived at the result that the dogs in whom the pancreatic duct was tied did not develop diabetes, although the exocrine tissue of the pancreas degenerated, because – during life – the islet cells do not seem affected by the pancreatic enzymes. On the other hand, Minkowski's dogs, which had been completely pancreatectomized, developed severe diabetes; and there Minkowski must have decided to stick, although he lived until 1931, another 41 years after his work with von Mering was published.

In certain fish, the exocrine and the endocrine pancreatic tissue are separated. This is the case in the codfish (*Gadus callurious*). In 1902 in Aberdeen, Rennie and Fraser collected pure islet tissue (the 'Brockman Bodies') from the tip of the gallbladder, where the islet tissue is located[108]; from there it can be removed easily, preserved in acid alcohol and later processed into a potent insulin. Rennie and Fraser, unfortunately, did not realize the real nature of their discovery and their dogs died of what we now regard as hypoglycaemia. E. Clark Noble, a medical student in Toronto and colleague of Charles H. Best, who was originally due to assist Banting together with Best, was sent by Professor Macleod with the late Dr. N. A. McCormick, to spend the summer of 1922 at the Canadian Biological Station at St. Andrew's, New Brunswick, and later with the offshore and deep sea trawlers at Hawkesbury, Nova Scotia. Their work was published in 1922 in two articles under the title 'Insulin from fish'[108]. In 1910, Dr. Erich Leschke, a German physician, whilst denying the existence of an internal secretion, suggested that if an internal secretion did exist, the enzymes of the exocrine secretion might destroy it. As insulin is a protein, it is quite possible that the protein digesting enzymes would destroy it. In 1912, Dr. E. L. Scott in the United States attempted to prove this. He tied the duct and used the extract of the degenerated pancreas tissue. Unfortunately, he missed it by making an alcoholic extract, and insulin is not soluble in alcohol. Although in other experiments he obtained more suggestive results, he concluded: "It does not follow that these effects are due to the internal secretion of the pancreas in the extract"[109]. In 1913, the American physiologists J. R. Murlin and B. Kramer in Rochester postulated that the effective treatment of diabetes must restore to the tissues the power to burn more sugar, as demonstrable in the restoration of the respiratory quotient (carbon dioxide, CO_2, exhaled/oxygen, O_2, absorbed), while the body is burning food. In diabetics with a mixed diet, the respiratory quotient (RQ) is reduced from the normal value of 0.85 to 0.7 (it was, incidentally, Murlin who later coined the word 'glucagon', i.e. 'mobilizer of sugar' for the other hormone of the islet organ, which is produced in the pale cells of the periphery, the alpha-cells, whereas the dark beta-cells contain the insulin). Although Murlin and Kramer obtained some (variable) reduction of the sugar content of the urine by intravenous injection of an acid pancreatic extract (and a more marked one if they used a mixed extract of pancreas and duodenum), the same effect could be achieved by the injection of the same quantity of Ringer's solution. Nor was an increase of the RQ to be observed[109]. Unfortunately, Murlin was sidetracked at the time into making alkaline extracts, because of an observation that diabetic animals, treated with oral or intravenous bicarbonate of soda solution, showed improvement, whereas acid made them worse[110].

Between 1915 and 1919, J. Kleiner and S. Maltzer, using a very dilute emulsion of pancreas, administered it slowly by intravenous injection to completely pancreatectomized dogs; most experiments ended with a fall, sometimes a marked one, of the blood-sugar. Kleiner regarded these results as further evidence for the internal secretion theory of diabetes[111].

A paper by Moses Barron (b. 1883) in 1920, on 'The relation of the islets of Langerhans to diabetes, with special reference to cases of pancreatic lithiasis'[112], gave Frederick Grant Banting (1891–1941) the final inspiration for his successful experiments. Barron confirmed Ssobolew's work. He also suggested that continuation of the experiments on the lines of those of Minkowski and von Mering might lead to the isolation of a substance which could control diabetes.

Banting, after return from war service, had settled down in general practice in London, Ontario, with a slant towards orthopaedics. The practice did not flourish, and he took up a part-time post as Demonstrator in the Department of Physiology in July 1920. On 30 October of that year, while preparing a class on the pancreas for the next day, he came across Moses Barron's paper. On the advice of his friends in London, he went to Toronto, where the Professor of Physiology, Dr. J. J. R. Macleod, was one of the experts on carbohydrate metabolism. He and Ernest Starling had declared as late as 1920:

We do not yet know how the pancreas affects sugar production or utilization in the normal animal. It is generally assumed that it secretes into the bloodstream a hormone, which may, according to the view of the nature of diabetes which we adopt, pass to the tissues and enable them to utilize sugar or to pass to the liver and inhibit the sugar production of this organ. A very small portion of the pancreas is sufficient for this purpose, but we have been unable to imitate the action of the pancreas still in vascular connection with the body, by injection or administration of extracts of this organ[113].

And Starling wrote:

> The most recent work has shown that injection of pancreatic extracts into a depancreatised animal produces no change in the respiratory quotient, although injections of extracts of pancreas and duodenum may cause a temporary fall in the excretion of glucose in the urine on account of the alkalinity of the extract. Neither have experiments with blood transfusions yielded results that are more satisfactory[114].

Thus we arrive at the year 1921, when (Sir) Frederick Grant Banting (1891–1941) (see Section II) and Charles Herbert Best (1899–1978) (see Section II) successfully isolated insulin.

There is, however, one story to be related before we progress to this: the tale of the forgotten man. His name is Nicolas Constantin Paulesco (1869–1931) (see Section II), and he was mentioned in Chapter 16, in the discussion on the first successful attempts of experimental total hypophysectomy. The most complete account of his involvement in the isolation of the anti-diabetic hormone, which he named 'pancréine' (and which seemed identical with the 'isletin' of Banting and Best) was given in 1971 by Ian Murray, on the 50th anniversary of the discovery of insulin: 'Paulesco and the isolation of insulin'[62]. Paulesco was by no means unknown. He received his medical training in Paris, where his outstanding abilities as a student attracted the attention of the celebrated Étienne Lancereaux (1829–1910), whom we have also encountered before (see pp. 311 ff.) concerning his opposition to acromegaly. He was the first to suggest a causal relationship between diabetes and lesions of the pancreas[115], and he gave an account of the 'thin diabetic'[116]. He was then President of the French Academy of Medicine and Chief Physician at the Hôpital Notre-Dame-du Perpétuel-Secours. Paulesco became Lancereaux's intern, and was encouraged by him in his research interests. Paulesco's MD thesis, on the structure and function of the spleen, was classified "extrêmement bien". After qualifying, Paulesco became an assistant in Lancereaux's hospital, where his research work concerned clinical and physiological problems. Apart from his MD, he also obtained diplomas in biochemistry and physiology and became a doctor of science. When - aged 31 – he returned to his native Bucharest in Roumania to take up an appointment as Assistant Professor of Physiology, he had already published a number of papers on endocrine subjects such as the effects of operative and experimental thyroidectomy[117]. He came to the conclusion that the thyroid produced a substance needed for the nutrition of the nervous system. He had also shown that suprarenal gland extracts influenced the nerve endings in muscle[118].

In 1904, he became Professor of Physiology in Bucharest, which he remained until his death in 1931. He also became visiting physician to the Hospital of St. Vincent de Paul, to keep in touch with clinical medicine. He gained his spurs as an outstanding experimental physiologist by designing the first effective method of hypophysectomy in animals by the subtemporal intracranial approach, in collaboration with the surgeon Balacesco in 1907[119]. His technique was adopted – with a slight modification – by Harvey Cushing (see p. 315) who said about Paulesco's work that it was "By far the most important contribution to the subject". His technique of hypophysectomy was surpassed only by Bernhard Aschner (Chapter 16). From his results on 24 dogs and 28 cats, in which he checked the result of removal of pituitary tissue histologically, he was able to show that the pituitary gland was essential to life. As a medical student, he had already become interested in von Mering and Minkowski's work (see pp. 296–298) that the pancreas must manufacture an anti-diabetic hormone. Working with Lancereaux deepened his interest in diabetes. While still in Paris, he began work with Professor Dastre with a view "d'isoler et d'étudier le produit actif de la secretion interne du pancreas"[117]. This research was put aside while he pursued the work on the pituitary; later he was engaged in the study of glycogen formation in the liver, but by 1916 he had resumed his experiments with pancreatic extracts and achieved, by injecting an aqueous solution, an immediate but temporary relief of symptoms in a diabetic dog.

Then Paulesco's work was again interrupted when Roumania became involved in the war, and Bucharest was occupied. Only four years later was he able to resume that particular line of work, but his later experiments confirmed the earlier observations. His results, published in August 1921 (submitted in June)[121], showed that he had succeeded in isolating the anti-diabetic hormone of the pancreas which he named pancréine and which lowered the blood sugar in diabetic and normal dogs. He published his detailed protocols, which allow no doubt that the extract he had obtained from dogs' or beef pancreas contained an active blood-sugar lowering principle. He removed the animal pancreas under as sterile conditions as possible, but did not tie the pancreatic duct because he feared that the side effects seen by previous workers were the result of bacterial infection. After mincing the pancreas and mixing it with distilled water, he stored it in ice for 24 hours. He then filtered it and added 0.7 g of sodium chloride per 100 ml. The extract was then injected into the external jugular vein. His first experiment ended dramatically, when the blood-sugar of the pancreatectomized dog fell from 140 mg% to 26 mg% within an hour: the dog died of hypoglycaemia! In subsequent, more carefully monitored experiments, the lowest blood-sugar level was (less marked and) obtained after two hours; after 12 hours the blood-sugar returned to its level before the experiment. In his 'Conclusions', given in full in Figure 68, with a complete translation, Paulesco stressed that such effects on diabetic hyperglycaemia and glycosuria are not produced either by haemo-dilution with saline, nor by injection with other organ-extracts, nor by fever, experimentally induced. The latter check was carried out because – occasionally – the temperature of the dog was observed to rise after injection of the extract. Although subcutaneous injections also had a marked hypoglycaemic effect, they caused severe local irritation. Attempts to give the extract to human diabetics failed by oral and by rectal administration. Eventually, purification was achieved, enabling a soluble powder of pancréine suitable for sub-cutaneous injections, but only in small quantities. Events had, however, overtaken Paulesco; Banting and Best had made their discovery, and with Macleod's and Collip's energetic efforts, the difficulties of purification had been solved in the United States.

We shall see that Banting and Best's work and conclusions, which were carried out and achieved quite independently, were very similar, except that Banting believed that ligation of the pancreatic duct to cause atrophy was necessary, whereas Paulesco was, by experience, a step ahead. In their report, Banting and Best referred to Paulesco's work, because by then they had his paper in their hands. Unfortunately, as Best admitted in 1971, Banting did not have any knowledge of French and Best's was insufficient; hence they misin-terpreted Paulesco's conclusions and declared that the "injections into the peripheral veins produced no effect and that in his experi-ments second injections do not produce such marked effects as the first"[122].

Paulesco's experiment to which they referred was that in which he observed that injection of extract from one-third of the pancreas resulted in a fall of blood sugar from 140 mg% to 112 mg%, which means a fall of 20%; a subsequent injection of double that amount caused a fall from 210 mg%, which is by 46%. The 'isletin' of Banting and Best produced the same type of severe local reaction so that it could not be used subcutaneously until the extract was purified. In fact, isletin and pancréine must be regarded as having been identical. The contention of Wrenshall, Hetény and Feasby[123] does not hold good, namely:

> While Banting and Best were already at work in July, 1921, Dr. Nicholas Paulesco, in Bucharest, reported very interesting effects of a

(a)

Reçu le 22 juin 1921.

RECHERCHE SUR LE RÔLE
DU PANCRÉAS DANS L'ASSIMILATION NUTRITIVE

PAR LE

Dr N. C. PAULESCO

Professeur de Physiologie à la Faculté de Médecine de Bucarest.

LE rôle physiologique du Pancréas, en tant que glande digestive, a été mis en évidence par CLAUDE BERNARD, et, en tant que glande assimilatrice, par LANCEREAUX. Plus tard, une multitude de chercheurs, de divers pays, ont confirmé et précisé ces géniales découvertes françaises.

A côté des derniers ouvriers qui ont suivi le chemin tracé par LANCEREAUX, je viens apporter une modeste contribution à l'achèvement d'un aussi splendide édifice scientifique.

Je commencerai par exposer mes expériences sur l'*action de l'extrait pancréatique injecté dans le sang*, je continuerai par décrire une *méthode de traitement* du diabète, de l'obésité et de l'acidose, méthode qui est issue de ces recherches expérimentales, et je finirai par donner une *théorie personnelle* sur la pathogénie du diabète et sur le rôle du Pancréas dans l'assimilation.

I. — Action de l'extrait pancréatique injecté dans le sang, chez un animal diabétique

Pour étudier expérimentalement l'action de l'extrait pancréatique injecté dans le sang, il faut avoir :
1o un animal *privé totalement de pancréas*,
2o un extrait pancréatique stérile.

1. Pour pratiquer l'*ablation complète du pancréas*, nous avons eu recours à un procédé personnel qui se trouve décrit dans notre *Traité de physiologie médicale* (1).

(1) PAULESCO. *Traité de physiologie médicale*, II, 313. Paris (VIGOT, éditeur). Ce livre est écrit en français.

(b)

Conclusions.

En résumé :

I. — Si, chez un *animal* **diabétique** par l'ablation du pancréas, on injecte, dans une veine jugulaire, un *extrait pancréatique*, on constate :

a) une *diminution* et même une *suppression* passagère de l'**hyperglycémie**, qui peut être remplacée par de l'**hypoglycémie**, et aussi une *diminution* et même une *suppression* passagère de la **glycosurie** ;

b) une *diminution* considérable de l'**urée sanguine**, ainsi que de l'**urée urinaire** ;

c) une *diminution* notable de l'**acétonémie** ainsi que de l'**acétonurie**.

II. — L'effet de l'extrait pancréatique sur la glycémie et sur la glycosurie, varie avec *le laps de temps* écoulé depuis l'injection. Ainsi, il commence immédiatement après l'injection, atteint le summum au bout de 2 heures, et se prolonge pendant environ 12 heures.

Il varie aussi avec *la quantité de pancréas* employée pour préparer l'extrait.

III. — Si, chez un *animal* **normal**, c'est-à-dire qui n'est pas diabétique, on injecte dans une veine de l'*extrait pancréatique*, on observe une *diminution* sensible de la **glycémie**, ainsi que de l'**urée sanguine** et de l'**urée urinaire**.

IV. — Pareils effets, portant spécialement sur l'hyperglycémie et la glycosurie diabétiques, ne sont produits :

a) ni par une injection intra-veineuse de *sérum physiologique* ;

b) ni par une injection intra-veineuse d'*extrait provenant d'un autre organe que le pancréas* ;

c) ni par une injection intra-rachidienne d'une solution de *nucléinate de soude* qui provoque un accès de fièvre.

Figure 68 Paulesco's paper: (a) front page, (b) conclusions [by kind permission of the Royal Society of Medicine, London]

pancreatic extract on sugar, ketone substances and the urea of the blood and urine of depancreatised dogs. The amounts of these substances were definitely decreased by the extracts. No evidence was presented that the symptoms of diabetes were lessened, the respiratory quotient raised, or that the life of the animal was prolonged.

The respiratory quotient, which was in those days assumed so essential for the assessment of the condition of the diabetic (see also p. 460), is today not regarded to be of such importance. The symptoms of diabetes were not described as being lessened, because Paulesco was desperately anxious to obtain a purified extract. Henderson writes: that "a committee was set up in Bucharest, to investigate ways of purifying the new product, but almost immediately the news came that two Canadians had made such a successful extract". He concludes "So presumably with a few choice Roumanian expletives the committee went home and never met again"[61].

When in 1923 the Nobel Prize was awarded jointly to Banting and Macleod (not to Best and not to Collip), Paulesco's name was not even mentioned. This caused obvious resentment in Roumania. In spite of representations of the French Academy of Medicine, however, nothing was achieved. This was due to the method of selection of Nobel Prize winners, which even today is insufficiently known. Liljestrand, a former Secretary of the Nobel Prize Selection Committee, admitted that although every effort is made to be absolutely fair in selecting the winner of the prize, "no-one could expect that no mistakes would be made"[124]. And Ian Murray quoted: "In a recent private communication, Professor Tiselius, head of the Nobel Institute, has expressed his personal opinion that Paulesco was equally worthy of the award in 1923"[62]. Murray concluded:

> . . . the time has now surely come to abandon controversy and, remembering Pasteur's aphorism, 'To have the fruit, there must have been cultivation of the tree', give grateful recognition to all the many workers in many lands over many years who made the discovery of insulin possible.

To sum up, Paulesco's 'Conclusions' were as follows (see also Fig. 68b) [translation: V.C.M.]:

I. If one injects into a *diabetic* animal (through ablation of the pancreas) a *pancreatic extract* into a jugular vein, one observes:
   (a) a temporary *diminution* and even *suppression* of the *hyperglycaemia*, and also a temporary *diminution* and even *suppression* of the *glycosuria*;
   (b) a considerable *diminution* of the *blood urea*, as well as of the *urinary urea*;

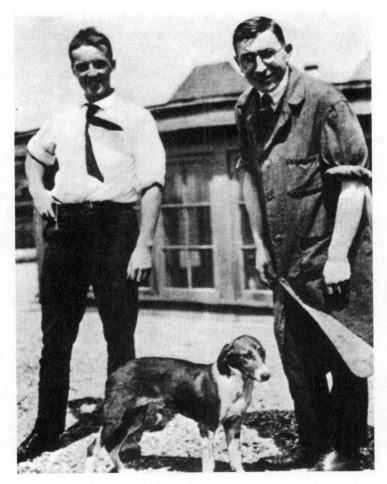

Figure 69   Banting and Best with their dog

(c) a notable *diminution* of the *acetonaemia* and also of the *acetonuria*.

II. The effect of the pancreatic extract on the glycaemia and on the glycosuria varies with *the lapse of time* that has passed since the injection. It commences immediately after the injection, attains its peak at the end of two hours and lasts for about 12 hours.

It varies also with *the amount of pancreas* (tissue) used for preparing the extract.

III. If one injects intravenously *pancreatic extract* into a *normal animal*, which is not diabetic, one observes a fair *diminution* of the *bloodsugar*, also of the *blood* and urinary urea.

IV. Similar effects, especially on the diabetic hyperglycaemia and glycosuria, are not produced: (a) either by an intravenous injection of *normal serum*:

(b) or by an intravenous injection of *an extract obtained from another organ but the pancreas*;

(c) nor by an intra-thecal injection of a solution of *sodium nucleinate*, which produces a rise in temperature.

We can now pick up our thread (from p. 462). As we have seen, Banting – after reading Barron's paper – became obsessed with the thought of doing his own experiment to isolate the hormone of the islet organ. Macleod was discouraging: he told him that the experiment had been tried many times before, by workers much more experienced than Banting, and had always been unsuccessful. Macleod's own account of these events, written in 1922, was eventually published in 1978, having been discovered in 1948, but kept dormant in the Libraries of the Universities of Aberdeen and Toronto since then. It explains his attitude which has been so severely criticized. Perhaps his critics have been too harsh[122a]. Banting was not to be put off; he turned up in Macleod's office the next day, saying that he had not put his case properly: all he was asking for was a work space for two months, some dogs and technical help. Macleod, who was about to go on holiday to his native Scotland, was eventually worn down by Banting; before leaving he lent him a small laboratory, a few dogs, and two final year physiology students, Charles Herbert Best and E. Clark Noble, to assist him. Both had graduated in the Physiology and Biochemistry course at the University of Toronto in June 1921, and had accepted work in the Department of Physiology towards their M.A. degree. As Noble confirmed in his letter to *Guy's Hospital Gazette* of 28 August 1971[125] (see also p. 460):

Best and myself were allocated to work with Banting for two months and to decide between ourselves in what manner we did so; to this end (contrary to most statements, but corroborated by Banting in his Cameron Lecture in Edinburgh, 1928), we did toss a coin to see who would work first, and this happened to be Charles Best. It was also agreed that we should change over at the month's end; however, when this time arrived, Best had become proficient in assisting Dr. Banting in his surgical techniques, so it was mutually agreed, in the best interest of the experiments that Best should continue to work out the full time with him.

Banting and Best first tried duct ligation experiments; like Scott before, they found it difficult to prevent re-canalization of the duct. They were unaware that Lydia de Witt had succeeded in 1906 in ligating the duct in cats. She found that extracts of the surviving islet tissue had glycolytic properties, but she did not pursue the matter further[125a]. Eventually, by putting several ligatures around it, they succeeded in producing almost complete atrophy of the exocrine tissue, made an extract of the remaining material with ice-cold Ringer's solution, which reduced the hyperglycaemia of the pancreatectomized dog. As the limited supply of such an extract soon ran out, Banting remembered a paper by Laguesse stating that foetal pancreas contains a greater amount of islet tissue in relation to the exocrine tissue. He obtained foetal ox pancreas from the local abattoir, the extract of which kept their diabetic dogs alive.

On one occasion, when all the experimental dogs had been used up, Banting sold his Ford car to get some money to buy more animals. On his return from Europe, Macleod realized the importance of Banting and Best's results. After confirming them, Noble relates[125]:

> ... he then outlined the associated major scientific problems that required urgent solution, and to this end turned his whole laboratory staff and facilities over to the problem. To this group shortly afterwards, Macleod added Professor J. B. Collip, who was responsible for the purification of insulin for its safe medicinal use in human beings. It was agreed that all the initial papers should appear under the joint names of 'Banting, Best, Collip, Macleod and Noble', and some ten or twelve of these are to be found in any Medical Library – unlikely activity for 'The Man Who Never Was' – myself.

James Bertram Collip (1892–1965) soon showed that acid–alcohol extracts of whole adult pancreas were more effective than the extracts obtained by the complicated duct ligation[126] (compare also Paulesco's method).

The award of the Nobel Prize in 1923 to Banting and Macleod 'for the discovery of insulin' created something of a stir, heated argument and sadness. Banting refused to allow Macleod's name to be first on the citation (after all, he had been on holiday when the work was being done); Best was not even nominated, so Banting shared his prize with him; Macleod, not to be put to shame, shared his part of the prize with Collip. And Paulesco? He had, of course, not been nominated; it seemed that the University of Bucharest was not among the official bodies who gave information to the Nobel Prize Selection Committee on names of scientists to be put forward for consideration; the French Academy of Medicine, even if they had been willing, would have been too late. No, Paulesco's name was not even mentioned. He was truly 'the Man Who Never Was'. It seems that even in his native country, Roumania, he is today merely regarded as one of the pioneers in the search for insulin. So, who discovered insulin? Henderson answered the question as follows:

> It is probably apparent by now that nobody actually discovered insulin. It existed first as an idea (Laguesse), then as a proven hypothesis (Gley, Zuelzer, Allen, Paulesco – but Henderson had not seen Paulesco's paper at the time of writing), and finally as a practical way of alleviating diabetes [Paulesco and Banting]. J. S. Mill said that a man with a conviction is worth twelve men with ideas. Banting, really, [and before him Paulesco; V.C.M.] was the only man with a conviction, with passion, and all the others (except possibly Paulesco) were just ideas men. When the last insulin syringe has been thrown away, we may find that there were twelve ideas men, for in truth, almost anybody can have an idea. Ideas are the small change of science; it is conviction, – zany, indestructible belief – that is the real pot of gold[61].

GLUCAGON

Banting and Best's team noticed in the early 1920s that injection of pancreatic extracts sometimes resulted in a temporary rise in blood-sugar before hypoglycaemia ensued. This had been observed before them by J. R. Murlin's group in Rochester, Minn.; it will be remembered that in 1913 Murlin had found with Kramer that acid extracts of the pancreas reduced the sugar content of the urine, but he did not follow up his observation (see also pp. 460–461). After the discovery of insulin, Murlin devised a technique which one can only regard as entirely academic: he excluded the exocrine enzymes by perfusing the blood-vessels of the isolated pancreas, and collected insulin from the perfusate. He published details of this method in 1923, with an apparatus designed for the perfusion of a dozen pancreas glands simultaneously. Henderson commented on it:

> There is a magnificent cussedness, a folie de grandeur, about the whole scheme; for Murlin knew at the time with what ease crude insulin preparations could be got from the slaughterhouse pancreases. Yet he claims that the apparatus could produce as much from pig's pancreas as orthodox acid alcohol procedure. Historically, it probably represents the first occasion on which demonstrable insulin was derived from the perfused organ, though as a method it was too cumbersome to be bothered with[94].

During their studies of the solubility of insulin in various solvents, in 1923, Murlin's team found that acetone is not only "not so dependable as ethyl alcohol as an insulin precipitant", but ". . . it throws down a substance, soluble in 95% alcohol, which has hyperglycaemic effect . . . this hyperglycaemic substance has been given the name of *glucagon* and its properties will be described more fully in a later paper"[127]. Henderson continued:

A second pancreatic hormone had tip-toed in from the wings. Even Murlin had no inkling that it was a hormone; after all, there was no deficiency state like diabetes mellitus to give clues, and the substance was possibly a contaminant anyway.

"The results were presented by Gibbs, Root and Murlin to the International Congress of Physiology in Edinburgh in 1923, overshadowed by Macleod, who headed the bill with a lecture on the isolation of insulin"[128]. Development of the recognition and study of glucagon was slow, mainly linked and at the same time confused with the attempts of purification of insulin. Only after John Jacob Abel (1857–1938) had succeeded in obtaining crystalline insulin in 1926[129], proving also that insulin was a protein, could it be established that injection of insulin *never* produced hyperglycaemia. Murlin, continuing his studies of the substance which produced *hyper*glycaemia, could demonstrate that the extract had its maximum effect when injected into the portal vein, rather than in the periphery. We know now that the difference is due to the rapid destruction of glucagon in the body; Murlin, surprisingly, explained it as caused by "the sudden arrival of insulin at the liver". After that broadside, Murlin never published a paper on the subject again, although he carried on his studies on metabolic problems!

THE CONSTITUTIONAL FACTOR

In 1917, there was published in Vienna the first edition of *Die konstitutionelle Disposition zu inneren Krankheiten*[130] (= The constitutional disposition to internal diseases) by Julius Bauer, later Professor of Medicine in Vienna until 1938, and eventually Professor of Clinical Medicine, College of Medical Evangelists, Los Angeles, California. Born in 1887, he died in May 1979 in Los Angeles (see also Section II). With an original training as a neurologist, he became an internist with a special interest in genetics, the constitutional aspects of disease (constitutional pathology) and endocrinology. Like Fuller Albright, he believed that endocrinology was an integral part of internal medicine, which view he later slightly modified to say that it is an integral part of medicine in general (physiology and pathology). The book, which reached several editions, made his reputation. As the name Bauer (meaning farmer) is not uncommon in Germany (there were two Bauers, professors of medicine, in Vienna alone), he was nick-named 'Constitution-Bauer' in German-speaking countries. In 1942, a shorter, up-dated version of the book was published: *Constitution and Disease: Applied Constitutional Pathology* in the United States and in England, which also went into several editions[131]. The following paragraphs, which are self-explanatory, are taken from the 'Preface':

> Tucker and Lessa of Chicago University expressed it as follows: 'In Europe, particularly in Germany, Austria, Italy, and France where the tradition of the endogenous constitutional factors lived in many of the older physicians and scientists, the newer interest in exogenous factors never entirely displaced the constitutional approach to biological problems'.
> . . . The general dislike of speculative approach to biologic problems is justified; but only so far as it is not sufficiently supported by facts. On the other hand the accumulation of facts without an attempt at a synthetic comprehension of all these facts is equally unsatisfactory. Poincaré said that science is composed of facts as a house is built, but a mere piling up of facts is as little a science as a heaping up of stones is a house. (Henry Poincaré 1854–1912)

Bauer's main conception is that the genes act directly on the effector organ, or indirectly through either the endocrine system or the nervous system, which can themselves collaborate. A typical example is the constitutional precipitation of the menopause. Physiological senile involution of the ovaries in the white race in temperate climates occurs between the ages of 46 and 50 years. In some families, however, the menopause sets in at 40 or earlier. The abiotrophic background of such a premature senescence of the ovaries is clearly evident when the constitutional biological inferiority of the gonads can be recognized from other signs, such as late start of the menarche, at the age of 18 or later. 'Abiotrophy' of certain organs was a term coined by Sir William Richard Gowers (1845–1915)[132]. It is the innate degree of perfection, the biological value of the anatomical structure of an organ, which may be constitutionally diminished as compared with other organs in the same individual or with the same organ in other individuals.

> Congenital hypoplasia, structural abnormalities of various kinds, malformations inoffensive in themselves, may be morphological signs of such a biological inferiority. As a matter of fact, abiotrophy corresponds to a certain extent to a precipitated senile involution[133].

A senile cataract, acoustic nerve-deafness, osteoporosis, marked arteriosclerosis in a man of 95, may not be considered abnormal. The same occurring in a person of 45 would be regarded as untimely senile involution. Bauer stressed that too much emphasis had been put upon the endocrine system as an initiator rather than as the mediator between constitution and the effector organ. In agreement with Sir Henry Dale, he pointed out the importance of the receptor capacity of the (effector) organ to hormonal stimulus; this would explain cases where the endocrine lack is expressed in only one organ, which means that the organ has an excessively high threshold for the endocrine stimulus, although the quality and quantity of the hormone production may be normal. The testing time for the biological value of an endocrine system may come later in life; for example, during pregnancy. Some women develop acromegalic features or tetany during pregnancy, both changes disappearing after delivery, though some patients may show some temporary exhaustion afterwards.

Biological inferiority need not mean intellectual or artistic inferiority. Darwin's psychoneurosis is a fair example of intellectual superiority, nay, genius going hand in hand with biological inferiority. But if Bauer demonstrated that a 'normal' man is a mental abstraction because, for example, only 9% of the general (European) population have a greater splanchnic nerve which corresponds to the textbook 'specification', and that only if a variation occurs in less than 4.5% of the population, should it be considered an abnormality, this does not mean that we are unable to do very much for people whose inherited tendencies may be complicated by unfavourable circumstances. Medicine has passed from healing to prevention: if "Heredity determines what one can do, environment determines what one does do". Bauer gave proper consideration to George Draper's careful studies in New York on Human Constitution[134] and to Charles Rupert Stockard's (1879–1939) book: *The Physical Basis of Personality* (1931)[120]. (We came across Stockard's name as a student of neuroendocrinology (p. 417) and joining Papanicolaou's work on oestrus, p. 361). Bauer discussed in detail the "principle of the treble safeguard", meaning that many traits and functions of the organism are

> dependent on and regulated by the proper co-operation of (a) the particular organ ("effector organ", Erfolgsorgan), (b) the endocrine system, and (c) the nervous system. . . . The scheme of figure 2 will clarify the situation. The relationship of the three factors in securing the proper development of a trait or the proper function of an organ may show individual variations. Abnormalities of a trait or function may be produced by abnormalities of one or more of the three factors. Individual differences in the symptomatology of various diseases are frequently accounted for by such differences among the co-operating regulating factors. Cognizance of this fundamental principle of orga-

nization of the vertebrates is not only helpful but sometimes indispensable in order to avoid erroneous conceptions with regard to various pathologic conditions, chiefly of constitutional origin. . . . Many traits and functions ought to be envisaged as complex biological units, and cannot be understood solely by considering single parts of the integrative system[131].

Genes in the chromosomes of the fertilized ovum:

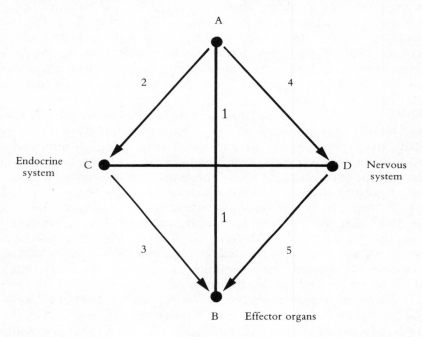

The intricate organization of the human individual requires a broader view by its students than the customary narrow one.[135]

A certain amount of the groundwork had been given by the publication of Rudolf Martin's (1864–1925) *Lehrbuch der Anthropologie* in 1914[135], of which Garrison wrote "the older anthropology ended in a brilliant *fanfare*"[136]. In the same year appeared F. W. A. Martius's important book on *Constitution and Selection*[137]. The First World War came (1914–1918), with its impact on the study of the mental and physical endurance of the fighting men and the development of Mendel's genetics and of endocrinology, the concept of constitution was "in the air". In the view of Keith (1911), (F.G.) Crookshank (1912) and J. Paulsen (1920), race is the outward and visible sign of a definite equilibrium of endocrine secretions, and since the constitutional diseases and insanities are imbalanced states or 'caricatures of the normal' and independent of race, the typology of the constitution is an inter-ethnic phenomenon. Thus Allbutt's (Sir Thomas Clifford, 1836–1925) view of health as a diathesis (like scrofula and syphilis) came into its own and acquired new criteria from a study of the abnormal, even as Freud has illuminated the mechanisms of normal thinking. Salient in this connection was the work of Ernst Kretschmer (1888–1964), on *Koerperbau und Charakter* in 1921, who attempted to correlate body build and constitution with character and mentality (pycnics, extroverts or cycloids versus leptosomics, introverts or schizoids)[138].

THE ADRENAL CORTEX

We discussed in Chapter 15 that Brown-Séquard, Wheeler and Vincent and others established the absolute necessity of the adrenal gland for survival, and especially the existence of the adrenal cortex. We also noted attempts to treat patients suffering from Addison's disease with adrenal extracts, with varying results. We referred to one patient of (Sir) William Osler (when he was still at Johns Hopkins), who died from Addison's disease "during treatment with suprarenal extract" in 1896, but another of Osler's publications of the same year informed the world 'On six cases of Addison's disease

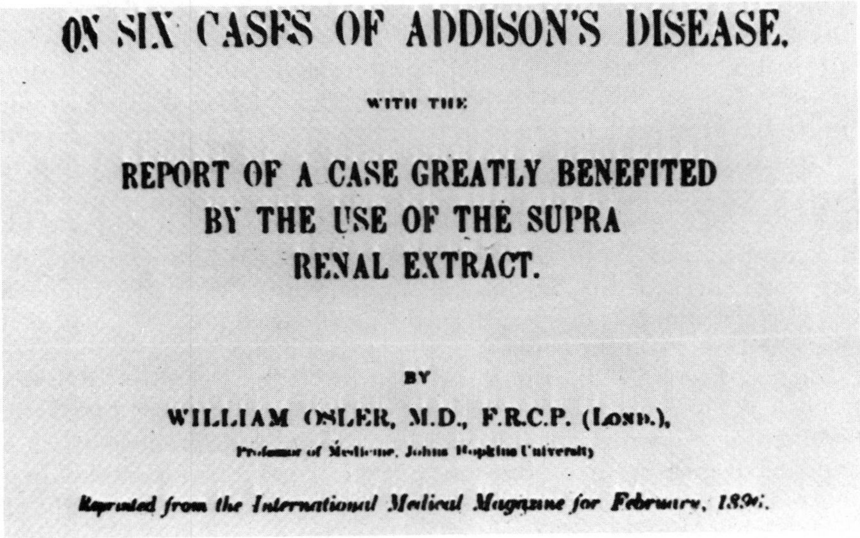

ON SIX CASES OF ADDISON'S DISEASE,

WITH THE

REPORT OF A CASE GREATLY BENEFITED BY THE USE OF THE SUPRA RENAL EXTRACT.

BY

WILLIAM OSLER, M.D., F.R.C.P. (LOND.),

Professor of Medicine, Johns Hopkins University

Reprinted from the International Medical Magazine for February, 1896.

Figure 70   Frontispiece of Osler's paper

with the report of a case greatly benefited by the use of the suprarenal extract'[139,140]. He prepared his extracts from fresh glands only, kept them cold, and he used hog adrenals, which contain a somewhat higher concentration of corticoids. We also mentioned Professor Muirhead's own account of beneficial results of a very dilute solution of mainly epinephrine in saline, administered by rectum on his own Addison's disease. In a survey of those early efforts, F. B. Kinnicutt recorded, in 1897, 36 different reports on the use of adrenal extracts in Addison's disease[141] between 1892 and 1897. It seemed that 28 out of 48 patients showed improvement, if only temporarily (including Osler's). Moreover, Osler recommended extraction of the adrenals with glycerin, which – as Arthur Grollman (b. 1901) later confirmed – was a particularly effective solvent for adrenal steroids. After a comparatively long interval, which was perhaps due to the pre-occupation of many research workers with epinephrine, Julius Moses Rogoff (1883–1966) and George Neil Stewart (1880–1930), working in the Harvey Cushing Laboratory of Experimental Medicine at Western Reserve University, reported in 1927 on results achieved with two different adrenal cortical extracts, one a simple 0.9% sodium chloride and one of glycerol.

These extracts still contained, however, some epinephrine and that fact limited the amount which could be injected without danger[142]. Almost at the same time, Frank Alexander Hartman (b. 1883), Macarthur and W. E. Hartman, at the University of Buffalo, announced a method of extraction of a cortical substance free from epinephrine[143]. It enabled them to keep completely adrenalectomized cats alive for an average of 21 days as compared with the average survival rate of six days for the untreated control. Eventually, in 1929, Joseph John Pfiffner (b. 1903) and Wilbur Willis Swingle (b. 1891) presented the first practical method of preparing a concentrated extract of the adrenal cortex, which made it possible to keep alive indefinitely adrenalectomized cats[144]. It still contained, however, a fair amount of epinephrine and its preparation was slow and cumbersome. In June 1930, Frank A. Hartman and Katharine A. Brownell succeeded in devising a simple process for the preparation of a cortical concentrate, which could also be used intravenously as it contained only a minimal amount of epinephrine[145].

Finally, Frank A. Hartman and George Widmer Thorn (b. 1906) published, in November 1930, a method which was based on maintaining a normal growth curve in adrenalectomized rats with a standard of measurement: one unit of their 'cortin' maintained, when injected daily, the normal growth of animals with an initial weight of 75–150 g[146]. Professor George W. Thorn gave an amusing account in his Thayer Lectures of 1967 on the difficulties he experienced as a young man, when looking after two of those adrenalectomized rats, who were given the extract subcutaneously, when bringing them by rail from Buffalo to New Orleans via New York Central and then the Louisville, Nashville railroads to the A.M.A. Convention in 1932. He added: "Of course, today, with air transportation and automatic syringes the problems would have been greatly simplified!"[147] Only a year later, F. A. Hartman, B. D. Bown, G. W. Thorn and C. Greene could report on the effectiveness of this extract in acute adrenal crisis in man, and the possibility of keeping patients with Addison's disease alive and under control. Difficulties existed at that stage because of the small quantity of extract which could be obtained; moreover, abattoirs, which previously discarded adrenal glands or gave them freely to anyone who wished to come and collect them, suddenly discovered their market value and prices rocketed. In 1936, G. W. Thorn, H. R. Garbut, F. A. Hitchcock and F. A. Hartman showed for the first time that administration of their potent extract would modify the renal excretion of electrolytes in normal subjects[148]. Next followed the classical studies of R. F. Loeb[149], George Harrop[150], and the group of men around them (which included Thorn for a while), which proved the beneficial effect of sodium salts in the treatment of Addison's disease. In 1927, E. J. Baumann and S. Kurland had analysed the inorganic consti-tuents of blood in adrenalectomized cats and rabbits, and found a low level of blood sodium in such cats[151]. In 1932 Loeb observed low serum sodium in patients with Addison's disease, which he then followed by his treatment of such patients with sodium chloride. This was followed by studies in 1933, demonstrating increased excretion of sodium in adrenalectomized dogs[152]. At the same time, R. Truszkowski and R. L. Zwemer pointed to the advantage of a low potassium intake in Addison's disease[153]; this was confirmed by R. N. Wilder, E. C. Kendall, A. M. Snell, E. J. Kepler, E. H. Tynearson and M. Adams[154].

In 1933, both E. C. Kendall[155] and – independently – Arthur Grollman[156] obtained crystals from adrenal cortical extracts, with adrenal cortical hormone-like activity. In 1938, the Swiss Tadeus Reichstein (b. 1897) and J. von Euw reported on the isolation of the substance Q (desoxycorticosterone)[157] having isolated (Reichstein) the compounds F, H and J in 1936[158].

In 1937, M. Steiger and T. Reichstein announced the synthesis from stigmasterol of a steroid compound desoxycorticosterone acetate (DCA)[159].

DCA given for the treatment of Addison's disease produced serious complications if at the same time an increased amount of sodium chloride and a restricted potassium intake was continued, leading to hypertension, oedema and hypokalemia, even to severe hypokalaemic paralysis, involving the extensor muscles of the neck, hands and feet[160]. Thorn, Lewis L. Engel and H. Eisenberg developed pellets of DCA which could be implanted into the skin of the abdomen (125 mg crystalline DCA in a pellet) which were effective for periods as long as eight to ten months, although DCA does not correct the marked abnormality of carbohydrate metabolism (hypoglycaemia) of adrenal cortical insufficiency. Thus it will be seen that a crystalline compound from adrenal cortical extract was produced independently at three research centres, by Reichstein, E. C. Kendall and A. Grollman; this was a phenomenon which was to appear much more often in the years between 1940 and the present, as research has become more and more linked to certain laboratories, 'centres of excellence', and carried on by teams of often a dozen and more research workers. It should also be noted at this point that a great deal of experimental research is carried out by scientists who are not medically qualified; Professor Frank A. Hartman and Katharine A. Brownell, for example, are both physiologists with a Ph.D., Reichstein is a research chemist and the same applies to E. C. Kendall, Sir Charles Harington, Rosalind Pitt-Rivers, Professor Alan S. Parkes and many others. The clinician is today perhaps in a minority in this ever-expanding research activity although, of course, he still has an important role to play in the diagnostic field and in the critical evaluation of modern treatment methods. Last and by no means least, his is and will remain the vital role of co-ordination of so many disciplines in the continually expanding field of what is now called endocrinology.

THE POSTERIOR PITUITARY GLAND

The anatomical situation of the pituitary with its protected position at the base of the brain and within the skull was to a great extent responsible for the delay in its experimental investigation. Added to this is the fact that this small organ, which in man weighs barely more than one gram, is, by development, structure and function divided into three distinct parts. The anterior lobe (pars glandularis or pars distalis) is a higher control centre of metabolic functions, interposited, as we know now, between the individual endocrine glands and the nervous centres of the hypothalamus, and also acting as a regulator within the feedback control system. Extracts of the intermediate lobe (pars intermedia), of greater importance in the animal kingdom, make light frogs become darker by causing dispersion of black pigment in their melanophores, or stimulating –

in mammals – deposition of dark pigment in the skin. The posterior lobe (pars nervosa or processus infundibularis) achieved much later recognition, which is perhaps not surprising, when one reads that (Sir) Henry H. Dale was, as a medical student in 1894, "well pleased at this exclusion of a potential examination subject", when using (Sir) Michael Forster's *Text Book of Physiology* of 1891, in which it was said about the pituitary body: "With regard to the purposes of this organ as a whole we know absolutely nothing"[161]. We have seen that Johann Peter Frank (1745–1821) defined diabetes insipidus in 1794 (see p. 174), but without connecting it with the pituitary. It was his namesake Alfred Erich Frank (1884–1957), who, in 1912, became the first to connect the posterior lobe of the pituitary with diabetes insipidus[162]. He reported on a patient with polyuria, who had been shot. X-rays disclosed that the bullet involved the sella turcica of the man. Similarly, Oliver and Schaefer had demonstrated that the posterior lobe contained a blood-pressure-raising substance (1895)[163], and so did W. H. Howell (1860–1945) in 1898[164].

This observation was further extended by studies of (Sir) Henry Dale in 1906[165] and in 1909[166]. Remarkably, Sir Henry was put on the scent by an accidental observation during experiments on the reversal by ergot of the action of adrenaline.

> I happened in this experiment to be recording also the tone and rhythm of the cat's uterus, an early pregnant one; and thus, by chance, I observed the potent stimulating action on the striated muscle of the uterus, which led to a new and probably the most frequent application of such a pituitary extract – oxytocin.[167]

Thus, Ian Chester Jones says, Dale proved once again Pasteur's celebrated phrase: "Chance only favours the prepared mind"[168]. Dale later recalled (in 1954):

> It is rather remarkable that I seem to have forgotten, in this connexion, the active substances so readily extractable from the posterior lobe of the pituitary – the one chapter of endocrinology to which I had myself made a positive contribution. And my failure is particularly curious, in view of the fact that such an extract had already been in use, for a good many years before insulin, for the successful control of the much rarer and less serious form of diabetes, due to the deficiency of this pituitary lobe, and known as diabetes insipidus.[169]

We have also seen that Paulesco, Cushing and his team, and Aschner had found, experimentally, that removal of the posterior pituitary was not fatal and caused none of the symptoms of 'cachexia hypophysiopriva' (see p. 316) Percy Theodore Herring (1872–1967) first described 'colloid droplets' in the posterior pituitary in 1908[170] (now known as 'neuro-secretory'). He was convinced, as had been

Hubert von Luschka (1820–1875) before him (in 1860)[171] and Peremeschko (in 1867)[172], that this part of the pituitary consisted essentially of neuroglia. In this opinion he was reinforced by Martin Heinrich Rathke's classic description of the origin and development of the pituitary in 1838[173].

Santiago Ramon y Cajal (1852–1934) in 1894, perhaps the greatest modern neuro-histologist, and one of his pupils, F. Tello in 1912, proved the wealth of innervation of the posterior lobe[174,175]. Later studies by I. L. Pines in 1925–1927, and R. Greving in 1926, suggested that most of the nerve fibres of the neurohypophysis were derived from nuclear regions, the supraoptic and paraventricular nuclei in the higher vertebrates[176,177], which observations were subsequently confirmed by numerous workers in the field, from the 1920s to the 1950s. The most up-to-date and painstaking studies on the anatomy and histology of the hypothalamus and the pituitary gland, with special reference to its portal system and the effects of transection of the pituitary stalk are contained in the monumental work by Peter M. Daniel and Marjorie M. L. Pritchard. This covers a period of more than 25 years of research and is being followed up by accounts of further experimental results to the present day[178] (see also pp. 162–163 in Chapter 14). Of particular importance appear the studies of the pituitaries in ferrets and goats after reunion of the severed stalk with regeneration of nerve-fibres of the hypothalamo-neurohypophysial tract and possibly of the tubero–infundibular system, which are now believed to control anterior pituitary activity. They may re-innervate the primary capillary bed of the portal system. If this is correct, the cells in the pars distalis, which these vessels supply, should once again receive the neuro-hormones from the hypothalamus that they require for their proper function. An exciting concept! In fact, as early as 1910, Harvey Cushing and Emil Goetsch (1883–1963) (who later devised an epinephrine skin reaction test for the diagnosis of hyperthyroidism), assumed that Herring's 'colloidal droplets' might, in fact, be hormones of the posterior lobe, which originated in the epithelial cells of the pars intermedia, passed into the neurohypophysis and thence in the ventricle of the brain[179]. R. Collin, however, thought that the colloid moved centripetally along the nerve-fibres of the neuro-hypophysis into the brain itself. Most authors thought up to 1940 that this colloid was formed in the pars intermedia[180].

Meanwhile it had become obvious from the reports of numerous observers, following Oliver and Schaefer, Howell, and Dale that the posterior lobe was the source of pressor, oxytocic and antidiuretic substances and that those substances were polypeptides rich in cystine[181]. More exhaustive studies clarified the picture between

1940 and 1960. It was further established that, firstly, it was unlikely that the pars intermedia was the source of the posterior lobe substances; moreover, E. M. K. Geiling and F. K. Oldham found in 1937, that these principles could be extracted from the posterior lobe of animals who had no pars intermedia, or where the pars intermedia was separated from the neurohypophysis by a thick septum[182]. Once this fact was established, the assumption became likely that the posterior pituitary substances might originate from nervous and not from epithelial tissue. Incidentally, the 'sero-albuminous glands' of the pars intermedia were discovered by W. Thom in 1901[183], and fully described by Jacob Erdheim (1874–1937) in 1904 and have sometimes been named after him[184]. In 1934, Roussy and Mosinger examined over 100 specimens; they are always present at birth and located behind the posterior wall of the hypophysial cleft[185]. The whole issue remained controversial until the very recent investigations by Daniel and Pritchard[178].

Carl Ernst von Baer (1792–1876), of the mammalian ovum fame (see p. 270) believed the posterior lobe to be the anterior extremity of the brain[186]. P. C. Bucy, in 1930, and R. Romeis in 1940[187,188] introduced the idea of a special type of 'adenopituicytes' with a secretory role, which theory, however, could not be verified.

As to the Herring bodies, Geiling found in further investigations in 1935 that they might be, in fact, fixation artefacts. Roussy and Mosinger in 1933[185] (and R. Collin before them in 1928[189]) came to the conclusion that the posterior pituitary hormones may pass by three routes: by the bloodstream (hémocrinie); this may be in general or, in particular, by the portal system, the capillaries of which involve the hypothalamus and its nuclei controlling the sympathetic and parasympathetic system. This was postulated especially by the investigations of G. T. Popa and U. Fielding in 1930[190,191], and confirmed by M. A. Basir in 1932[192]. Daniel and Pritchard state, however:

Popa and Fielding, who first recognized that these vessels form part of a portal circulation, thought that the blood flowed through them from the pituitary to the hypothalamus. However, the true fact that the flow was in the opposite direction, i.e., from the hypothalamus to the pituitary, was soon realized as a result of further morphological studies . . . and visual observations in living animals.[193]

By passing into the cerebrospinal fluid and cerebral ventricles (hydrencéphalocrinie); but further work (Friedman and Friedman 1934[194,195], and Geiling 1935[196]) indicated that the secretion of the posterior lobe is discharged into the blood and not into the cerebro-spinal fluid. Meanwhile, concepts of the physiological role of the neurone and, especially, of the neuronal cell body, had been changing. J. F. Gaskell suggested as early as 1914[197] that certain chromaffin cells in the nerve cords of annelids might have both nervous and endocrine properties. This was followed, as we have seen, by Carl Caskey Speidel's report on 'gland-cells of internal secretion in the spinal cord of the skates'[198] (see also p. 417). It was Ernst Scharrer in 1928, however, who postulated, in a paper on the neurones of the preoptic nucleus of the minnow, the endocrine function of neurones in the hypothalamus[199] (see also p. 419).

Research on all these and related questions became intensified between 1940 and 1977 until it reached the high pitch of the present day. Most importantly, methods have been evolved not only for the identification and isolation of the hormonal peptides involved but also for their measurement by bio-assay and even more objective methods (see Chapter 23). Thus, the recognition and analysis of a number of clinical syndromes was made possible and in some cases their treatment on a scientific basis was established, during what may be regarded as the modern phase of clinical neuro-endocrinology[200].

To return, however, to the earlier phase of these developments: in 1918, F. von Hann demonstrated that the essential pathology in human diabetes insipidus was the destruction of the posterior lobe of the pituitary, which indicated that one of the hormones of the normally functioning gland was probably an antidiuretic principle[201]. A. Konschegg and E. Schuster had already reported in 1915 that posterior pituitary extracts had antidiuretic effect[202]. We have mentioned that Sir Henry H. Dale noted the oxytocic principle in 1906[165]. I. Ott and J. C. Scott, in 1910, recorded a galactokinetic action of posterior pituitary extracts[203]. In 1919, H. W. Dudley[204] and in 1928 O. Kamm and co-workers[205] were able to show the effects of these two major active substances of the posterior lobe. Kamm, who worked for the firm of Parke-Davis in the United States, was the originator of the trade-names of 'oxytocin' and 'vasopressin', which have now been universally accepted. Analysis and synthesis of oxytocin and vasopressin was eventually achieved in 1954–1958, by V. du Vigneaud and his colleagues in the United States[206,207], after Van Dyke et al. had shown in 1942 that there was a high molecular weight peptide[181] in the posterior pituitary which contained both the oxytocic and vasopressin principles. Finally, R. Acher, J. Chauvet and G. Olivry demonstrated, in 1956, that the two hormones are associated in the posterior lobe with a carrier protein called 'neurophysine'[208].

THE PINEAL

In Chapter 13 we discussed the scanty existing knowledge on the pineal. From Galen to Descartes (see p. 129), Wharton (see p. 134), Willis, Gibson, Stensen (pp. 140–141) and Ridley and Cowper's theory of the pineal being a lymphatic gland receiving lympha from the lymph ducts which pass the 3rd ventricle of the brain to the infundibulum and glandula pituitaria (the direction was right!). After that there was no change right up to François Magendie (1783–1855) and beyond, to the beginning of the 20th century. The present situation is still far from satisfactory, in spite of intensive research activity in this field. The gland contains, in mammals, the pinealocytes, which are derived from the neuroepithelial matrix layer, and some modified glia cells. It has a rich blood supply and is surrounded by cerebrospinal fluid. The human pineal usually calcifies after puberty. In cold-blooded vertebrates it is mainly a photoreceptive organ. In mammals, the photo-receptivity is lost and it is a secretory organ. The pineal body is a neuro-endocrine transducer, which means that it secretes a hormone in response to a neural input and not to a circulating substance. It responds to information by light, transmitted by way of the retina to the pineal sympathetic nerves. The direct nervous connection with the brain in the mammalian pineal is lost soon after birth, but the pineal stalk continues to contain commissural fibres which return to the brain without entering the parenchyma of the gland. Instead it is innervated by post-ganglionic fibres from the superior cervical ganglia. The mammalian pineal synthetizes melatonin (5-methoxy *N*-acetyltryptamine). In amphibians, but not in mammals, melatonin has a skin-lightening effect. The role of the pineal in man is still under investigation. A melatonin-free extract of human pineal inhibits gonadotropic secretion. Gliomas which destroyed the pineal have been found in children with precocious puberty, whereas parenchymatous pinealomas may depress gonadal function and delay the onset of puberty. Constant light depressed melatonin production, and the effect of light on the pineal is inhibitory. Melatonin is elevated at the time of menstrual bleeding and it is low at the time of ovulation. C. P. McCord and F. P. Allen showed in 1917 that the pineal of the cow contains a factor that causes the skin of amphibians and reptiles to blanch[209].

THE PARATHYROIDS

Professor Roy O. Greep suggested fairly recently, in 1963, that the parathyroid glands first appeared in evolutionary development in the amphibia, coinciding with the migration from the calcium-rich marine environment to the freshwater or terrestrial one, with its poorer calcium content[210]. Accordingly, the main task of parathyroid hormone in mammals and man is to raise the plasma calcium, and to maintain the plasma and body calcium levels constant.

We have already seen that Sandstrøm and Gley (pp. 277–278) established that the parathyroid glands are essential for the maintenance of life. A description of tetany in children was given by John Clarke (1761–1815), Lecturer in Midwifery at St. Barthomolew's Hospital in London, in 1815[211], with an account of laryngismus stridulus originally mentioned by Nicholas Culpeper (1616–1654). This was soon followed by the account of chronic tetany, with carpo-pedal spasm and spasm of the glottis, by George Kellie (?1770–1866) of Leith in 1816[212]. In Germany, the first description of tetany seems to have been by Salomon Levi Steinheim (1789–1866) of Altona in 1830, which he published under the title of 'Acute rheumatism'[213] (Zwei seltene Formen von hitzigem Rheumatismus). Next appeared Jean Baptiste Hippolyte Dance's (1797–1832), account in his 'Observations sur une espèce de tétanos intermittent', in 1831[214]. More than twenty years after him, François Rémy Lucien Corvisart (1824–1882), nephew of Napoleon's celebrated physician, introduced the word 'tétanie' in his doctor's thesis in 1852[215]. Armand Trousseau (1801–1867) added in 1862 the sign which bears his name, when pressure on the arm is exerted[216]. William Heinrich Erb (1840–1921) discussed the electrical excitability of the motor nerves (leading to the sign named after him) in 1873[217], and František Chvostek (1835–1884) added his sign in 1876[218]. Giulio Vassale (1862–1912) and Francesco Generali showed in 1896 that removal of all four parathyroid glands was followed by severe tetany in the dog[219]. Perhaps the first observation of the effect of parathyroid hormone was that of G. Moussu in 1898, who claimed to have treated successfully the tetany caused by parathyroidectomy in dogs, by injecting an aqueous extract of 12–20 horse parathyroid glands[220]. Later, however, William George MacCallum (1874–1944) and Carl Voegtlin (1879–1960) demonstrated that the main effect of parathyroid hormone was on the calcium level in the plasma, because parathyroidectomy resulted in a greater loss of calcium in the excreta, a fall in blood calcium and the development of tetany. The latter could be alleviated by intravenous injection of calcium chloride[221].

Y. W. N. Berkeley and S. B. Beebe first showed, also in 1909, that an extract of parathyroid gland would relieve hypocalcaemic tetany in man[222]. In 1904 Max Askanazy (1865–1940), in Tuebingen, was the first to realize the causal connection of osteitis fibrosa cystica with tumours of the parathyroid, when he found a parathyroid adenoma at the post-mortem examination of a patient with skeletal disease[223]. This condition was originally described by Gerhard Engel in 1864[224]. A meticulous and full account of the condition was given in 1891 by Friedrich Daniel von Recklinghausen (1833–1910), who also discussed Engel's patient[225]. The condition is often referred to as Engel–Recklinghausen's disease. Jakob Erdheim (1874–1937), the Viennese pathologist and morbid anatomist, observed in 1906 that removal of the parathyroid glands in rats produced tetany and convulsions[226]. In 1907, he described hyperplasia of several or all parathyroid glands in osteomalacia in man. Finally, in 1914, Erdheim described hyperplasia of several or all parathyroids in spontaneous rickets in rats. This is the earliest report of compensatory hyperplasia of the parathyroids, i.e. secondary hyperparathyroidism.

William Stewart Halsted (1852–1922) in Baltimore, was a celebrated surgeon who made important contributions to the improvement of operative technique in thyroid surgery and other major surgical procedures. He attempted 'Auto- and iso-transplantation in dogs of the parathyroid glandules'[257]. He transplanted the parathyroid into thyroid tissue and under the abdominal skin. He found that auto-transplants were effective in 61% of his experiments, but only if sufficient parathyroid tissue had been removed in the first place, to cause hypoparathyroidism; nor should the transplant exceed the amount of parathormone replacement which is needed.

A more important contribution to the treatment of hypoparathyroid conditions in man, we owe to James Bertram Collip (1892–1965) in Toronto, whom we have already come across in 1922/23 as the biochemist responsible for the purification of Banting and Best's insulin (see p. 469 and Ref. 126). His 'parathormone', i.e. "The extraction of a parathyroid hormone which will prevent or control parathyroid tetany and which regulates the level of blood calcium"[229], was followed by his report (together with Douglas Burrows Leitch (b. 1888), on the first patient with tetany successfully treated with 'parathyrin', i.e. the parathyroid hormone[230]. It was published in the same year as his previous paper, but we must note that it was in 1925, sixteen years after MacCallum and Voegtlin had established the connection between tetany, calcium metabolism and the parathyroids! Even so, it took nearly another forty years before a hormone of sufficiently high purity could be prepared for definite chemical characterization and structural analysis.

The four main actions of parathyroid hormone, in chronological order of their discovery, are:

(1) An increase of phosphate excretion in the urine (I. Greenwald)[231].

(2) An increase in the rate of bone resorption mediated by a direct action of parathyroid hormone on bone (N. A. Barnicot)[232].

(3) An increase in the renal tubular reabsorption of calcium, leading to a decreased urinary excretion of calcium (Jahan and Pitts)[233], and similarly of magnesium (at a later date).

(4) An increase in the absorption of calcium from the small intestine (Talmage and Elliott)[234].

Felix Mandl (1892–1957), a Viennese surgeon and pupil of Julius von Hochenegg (see also Section II), was the first person to treat generalized osteitis fibrosa successfully by surgical removal of a parathyroid adenoma in 1925[235]. Two years before Collip's paper in 1925, Adolph Melanchthon Hanson (1888–1959) published 'An elementary chemical study of the parathyroid gland in cattle'[236] (Washington, 1924), in which he described, independently, the isolation of an effective parathyroid extract, and so did L. Berman (New York, 1924)[237]. In 1932, Hans Selye (b. 1907), later of fame for his work on stress, was working in Collip's laboratory. He observed that prolonged injections of small doses of parathormone caused multiplication of osteoblasts and increased bone formation; injection of sublethal doses into rats resulted in multiplication of osteoclasts, absorption of bone and the picture of generalized osteitis fibrosa in man, but once tolerance had developed, there was multiplication of osteoblasts, increased solidity of bone, similar to 'marbled bone' and reduction in the number of osteoclasts[238]. Hanson found that vitamin D, which in many ways has a similar action on calcium metabolism as parathormone, will be effective in parathyroidectomized animals[239]. The evidence available seems to indicate that vitamin D (most likely in the form of 1,2,5-dihydroxycholecalciferol) is needed for parathormone to exert its full effect on bone resorption and intestinal absorption of calcium[240].

Between 1934 and 1938, Fuller Albright (1900–1969) of Boston (see also Section II) and his team published a series of extensive studies on primary hyperparathyroidism, its diagnosis, biochemistry and prognosis[241]. He also described diffuse hyperplasia of all parathyroid glands causing hyperparathyroidism, rather than an adenoma of one gland[242]. His views were summarized in the book with E. C. Reifenstein: *The Parathyroid Glands and Metabolic Bone Disease*[243]. In it, they defined primary hyperparathyroidism simply as "a condition where more parathyroid hormone is manufactured than is needed". Secondary hyperparathyroidism was described as "a condition where more parathyroid hormone is manufactured than is normal, but where the hormone is needed for some compensatory purpose". Later, the term 'tertiary hyperparathyroidism' was introduced for patients who had developed parathyroid tumours because of the existence of prolonged secondary hyperparathyroidism, which – in turn – was caused by glomerular kidney failure or intestinal malabsorption syndrome with osteomalacia. All these groups had originally been regarded as primary hyperparathyroidism. Primary hyperparathyroidism was also equated with a single adenoma of one of the four glands (rarely several adenomas), with parathyroid carcinoma (a rare occurrence), or with primary, water-clear cell hyperplasia, until the description (as above[242]) of primary, diffuse chief cell hyperplasia of all four parathyroid glands.

It was not until 1959 that H. Rasmussen and L. C. Craig succeeded in isolating and purifying parathyroid hormone[244] and elucidating it as a complex polypeptide hormone[245]. The original extraction of the hormone from bovine parathyroid glands by the method of Collip in 1925, by using hot hydrochloric acid, was replaced with other, milder extraction reagents, the most successful of which proved to be phenol[246].

Hypoparathyroidism after thyroidectomy is now rare. Idiopathic hypoparathyroidism, usually occurring in childhood, more often in girls, is also rare, and often associated with other conditions, such as hypothyroidism, hypoadrenalism, hypogonadism, or an auto-immune disorder.

In 1942, Albright and his colleagues[247], described 'Pseudo-hypoparathyroidism' (an example of the 'Seabright–Bantam' syndrome), in which hypocalcaemia is not corrected by the administration of parathyroid hormone and the excretion of urinary phosphates is not increased. The disease is probably transmitted as an X-linked dominant trait and may occur together with thyrotrophin-deficient hypothyroidsm or diabetes mellitus. If the serum calcium and phosphate levels remain normal, the name 'Pseudo-pseudo-hypoparathyroidism' seems appropriate. Pseudo-hypoparathyrodism is thus due to end-organ resistance to parathyroid hormone. Such patients are often short, obese, have a round face and may be mentally retarded; they also often have an impaired sense of smell and taste for bitter or sour. Both disorders are twice as common in the female sex.

To cast a glance into the later stage of new development, it should be mentioned that in 1962, Douglas Harold Copp (b. 1915), E. C. Cameron, B. A. Cheney, A. G. F. Davidson and K. G. Henze reported on 'Evidence for calcitonin – a new hormone from the parathyroid that lowers blood calcium'[248]. In fact, subsequent intensive research disclosed that calcitonin is a polypeptide hormone, produced in the C cells of the thyroid. Its secretion is increased by hypercalcaemia and lowered by hypocalcaemia. It inhibits bone formation and decreases intestinal absorption of calcium and increases urinary calcium and phosphate. It can now be measured and this is important, because medullary carcinomas of the thyroid, both primary and secondary, secrete calcitonin, producing a very high blood level[249].

NEW SYNDROMES

To the 'New Syndromes' (see also Chapter 17), we have now to add one described by Henry Hubert Turner (1892–1970) in 1938, which occurs in girls[250]. In adolescents sexual infantilism is usually present (except for some pubic hair) and also amenorrhoea; webbed neck, short stature and cubitus valgus is also a regular finding. Low posterior hair-line, high arched palate, prominent ears, broad chest, abnormality of the fingernails, micro-gnathia, intestinal telangiectasia and often association with hypertension, co-arctation of the aorta, a pulmonary stenosis and hypoplastic nipples were soon recorded by other observers[251,252]. It has now been established that Turner's syndrome is a form of gonadal dysgenesis, the most common chromosomal anomaly being a 45,XO karyotype[253]. The term 'Turner's syndrome' should really be restricted to those patients with the phenotype described by Turner. Patients with Turner's syndrome with mosaicism are usually taller than the average 142 cm of the former. The buccal smear is chromatin negative in the classic patient with the chromosome karyotype 45,XO. Turner's syndrome must be strongly suspected in any adolescent girl of short stature, without any breast development, but scanty pubic hair growth. Apart from cardiac abnormalities, renal abnormalities are not uncommon (e.g. horse shoe kidney)[254].

In 1942, Harry Fitch Klinefelter (b. 1912), together with E. C. Reifenstein and Fuller Albright, described a "Syndrome characterized by gynaecomastia, aspermatogenesis without A-Leydigism, and increased excretion of follicle-stimulating hormone"[255]. The classic features are, a male phenotype, firm small testicles, gynaecomastia and evidence of decreased androgen production. The XXY form of seminiferous tubule dysgenesis is the most common cause of primary hypogonadism and male infertility. Thus prepubertal boys of tall stature, long legs, small testes, small penis, with (moderate) mental retardation should be suspected of the diagnosis. Bone growth in the lower extremities is greater, but not so in the upper ones; accordingly, the span is less than his height, in contrast to other forms of eunochoidism. Urinary gonadotrophins are usually elevated, plasma testosterone is decreased, which makes the condition a hypergonadotrophic hypogonadism[256].

REFERENCES

1. Borell, Merriley: MS for Workshop on Historical Perspectives on the Scientific Study of Fertility, Am. Acad. Arts and Sciences, Boston, Mass. 9–10 December 1977. Revised for Scientific Workshop: 5–6 May 1978.
2. Himes, N. E.: Medical History of Contraception. p. 256, New York, Gamut Press, 1936.
3. Finch, B. E., Green, Hugh: Contraception through the Ages. London, Peter Owen, 1963.
4. The Practitioner: Special Issue on Contraception. London, July 1923.
5. As 1: pp. 50–51.
6. Fairbairn, J. S.: Birth-control – medical advice. Practitioner **111,** 36–42, 1923.
7. Fairfield, Laetitia D.: The State and birth control. In: Medical Views on Birth Control (ed. Marchant, Sir Jas. introduced by Horder, Sir Thos., pp. 69–88. London, Hopkinson, 1926.
8. Newsholme, Sir Arthur; Hill, L. and Giles, A. E.: Contributions; as 7.
9. Giles, A. E.: The need for medical teaching of birth control. Lancet **1,** 165–167, 1927.
10. Marchant, Sir James (Ed.): Medical Aspects of Birth Control. pp. XVI, 1–183, London, Hopkinson, 1927.
11. As 1: p. 49.
12. As 10: p. xvi.
13. As 1: p. 25.
14. As 10: p. 2–13.
15. Committee on Maternal Health of New York City. Report, pp. 49–50.
16. Ibid.: pp. 57–58.
17. Dickinson, R. L.: Human Sex Anatomy: A Topographical Atlas. Baltimore, Williams & Wilkins, 1933.
18. As 15: p. 37.
19. As 15: p. 65.
20. Stopes, Marie C.: Contraception (Birth Control): Its Theory, History and Practice. A Manual for the Medical and Legal Profession. With an Introduction by Professor Sir William Bayliss. London, Bale Sons & Danielson, 1923.
21. Stopes, Marie C.: The First Five Thousand (being) The First Report of the First Birth Control Clinic in the British Empire. London, John Bale & Sons and Danielson, 1925.
22. Noyes, J. H.: Male Continence. Oneida, New York, pp. 24. Office Oneida Circular, 1872.
23. Stockham, Alice B.: Tokology. A Book for Every Woman. 29th ed. Chicago, Sanitary Pub. Co., 1885.
24. Stockham, Alice B.: Karezza. Ethics of Marriage. Chicago, Alice B. Stockham & Co.
25. As 2: p. 311 ff.
26. Pusey, Wm. A.: Social Problems of Medicine. Presidential Address. Am. Med. Assoc., June, 1924. pp. 1–33, A.M.A. Press, 1924.
27. As 2: p. 257.

28. Place, F.: The Principle of Population, including an Examination of the Proposed Remedies of Mr. Malthus. p. 173. 1822.
29. As 2: p. 315.
30. Sanger, Margaret (Ed.): Proceedings of the World Population Conference in Geneva in 1927.
31. Sanger, Margaret, Stone, Hannah M. (Eds.): The Practice of Contraception. pp. xvii and 3–316. Baltimore, Williams & Wilkins, 1931.
32. Dickinson, R. L., Bryant, Louise Stevens: Control of Contraception: An Illustrated Medical Manual. pp. XII and 1–290. Baltimore, Williams & Wilkins, 1931.
33. As 2: pp. 322–323.
34. As 2: p. 301.
35. As 2: p. 309.
36. Ruttgers, J.: The conscious limitation of offspring in Holland. Med. Pharmacol. Critic (New York). XVII, 174–176, 1914.
37. As 3: p. 45.
38. Simmer, H. H.: On the history of hormonal contraception. I. Ludwig Haberlandt and his concept of 'hormonal sterilization'. Contraception I, 3–27, 1970.
39. Simmer, H. H.: On the history of hormonal contraception. II. Otfried Otto Fellner and estrogens as antifertility hormones. Contraception III (1), 1–20, 1971.
40. As 2: p. 113.
41. MacLaren, Dorothy: Nature's contraception: wet nursing and prolonged lactation. The case of Chesham, Buckinghamshire 1578–1601. Med. Hist. 23, 426–441, 1979.
41a. Short, R. V.: Lactation – the central control of reproduction. CIBA Foundation Symposium, 45 Elsevier/Excerpta Medica/N. Holland, 73–86, 1976.
42. Sobotta, R. H. J.: Ueber die Bildung des Corpus Luteum bei der Maus. Arch. Mikrosk. Anat. 47, 261–308, 1896.
43. Beard, J.: The Span of Gestation and the Cause of Birth. Jena, G. Fischer, 1897.
44. Beard, J.: The rhythm of reproduction in mammals. Anat. Anzeig. 14, 97–103, 1898.
45. Prenant, A.: Sur la valeur morphologique, sur l'action physiologique et thérapeutique possible du corps jaune. Rev. Med. Est. 30, 385–389, 1898.
46. Hermann, E., Stein, Marianne: Ueber die Wirkung eines Hormones d. Corpus luteum auf maennliche u. weibliche Keimdruesen. Wien. Klin. Wochenschr. 29, 778–782, 1916.
47. Haberlandt, L.: Ueber hormonale Sterilisierung des weiblichen Tierkoerpers. Muench. Med. Wochenschr., 68, 1577–1578, 1921.
48. Fellner, O. O.: Discussion. Arch. Gynaekol. 117, 133, 1922.
49. Fellner, O. O.: Ueber die Taetigkeit d. Ovarium in d. Schwangerschaft (interstitielle Zellen). Monatsschr. Geburts. Gynaekol. 54, 88–94, 1921.
50. Fellner, O. O.: Pflueger's Arch. Ges. Physiol. 189, 189–199, 1921.
51. Haberlandt, L.: Ueber die hormonale Sterilisierung weiblicher Tiere. II. Injectionsversuche mit Corpus luteum, Ovarial- und Placenta-Opton. Pflueger's Arch. Ges. Physiol. 202, 1–13, 1924.
52. Fellner, O. O.: Die Wirkung des Feminin auf das Ei. Med. Klin. 23, 1527–1529, 1927.
53. Fellner, O. O.: Experimentell erzeugte Wachstumsveraenderungen am weiblichen Genitale der Kaninchen. Centr. Allg. Pathol. Anat. 23, 673–676, 1912.

54. Adler, Ludwig: Zur Physiologie u. Pathologie der Ovarial-funktion. Arch. Gynaekol. **95,** 349–424, 1912.
55. Aschner, Bernhardt: Ueber brunstartige Erscheinungen (Hyperaemie und Haemorrhagie am weiblichen Genitale) nach subkutaner Injektion von Ovarial-und Plazentarextrakt. Arch. Gynaekol. **99,** 534–540, 1913.
56. As 39: p. 6.
57. Haberlandt, L.: Erwiderung auf obige Bemerkingen O. Fellners. Wien. Klin. Wochenschr. **41,** 741, 1928.
58. Haberlandt, L.: Die hormonale Sterilisierung des weiblichen Organismus. Monatsschr. Geburtsh. Gynaekol. **87,** 326–28, 1931.
59. Haberlandt, L.: Die hormonale Sterilisierung des weiblichen Organismus. pp. 11–12, Jena, Fischer, 1931.
60. As 39: p. 12.
61. Henderson, John R.: Who discovered insulin? Guy's Hosp. Gaz. **85,** 314–318, 1971.
62. Murray, I.: Paulesco and the isolation of insulin. J. Hist. Med. **26** (2), 150–157, 1971.
63. Dobson, M.: Experiments and observations on the urine in diabetes. Med. Obs. Inqu. **5,** 298–316, 1776.
64. Cawley, Thos.: London Med. J. **9,** 286–308, 1788.
65. Rollo, J.: An Account of Two Cases of the Diabetes Mellitus, with Remarks as they Arose During the Progress of the Cure. London, C. Dilly, 1797.
66. Chevreul, M. E.: Ann. Chim. (Paris) **95,** 319–320, 1815.
67. Trommer, C. A.: Unterscheidung von Gummi, Dextrin, Traubenzucker u. Rohrzucker. Ann. Chem. (Heidelberg), **39,** 360–362, 1841.
68. Bernard, C.: Chiens rendus diabétiques. C. R. Soc. Biol. (Paris) **1,** 60, 1849–50.
69. Schiff, M.: Bericht ueber einige Versuche um d. Ursprung d. Harnzuckers bei kuenstlichem Diabetes zu ermitteln. Nachr. Georg-Aug. Univ. K. Ges. Wiss, Goettingen, pp. 243–247, 1856.
70. Petters, W.: Untersuchungen uebr die Honigharnruhr. Vjschr. Prakt. Heilk. **55,** 81–94, 1857.
71. Fehling, Chr. von: Quantitative Bestimmung d. Zuckers im Harn. Arch. Physiol. Heilk. **7,** 64–73, 1848.
72. Gerhardt, J.: Diabetes mellitus und Aceton. Wien. Med. Presse **6,** 672, 1865.
73. Noyes, H. D.: Trans. Am. Ophthalmol. Soc. 71–75, 1869.
74. Kussmaul, A.: Zur Lehre vom Diabetes mellitus. Dtsch. Arch. Klin. Med. **14,** 1–46, 1874.
75. Stadelmann, E.: Ueber die Ursachen der pathologischen Ammoniakausscheidung beim Diabetes mellitus und des Coma diabeticum. Arch. Exp. Pathol. Pharmakol. **17,** 419–444, 1883.
76. Minkowski, O.: Ueber d. Vorkommen von Oxybuttersaeure im Harn bei Diabetes mellitus. Arch. Exp. Pathol. Pharmakol. **18,** 35–48, 1884.
77. Magnus-Levy, A.: Die Oxybuttersaeure u. ihre Bezienhungen zum Coma diabeticum. Arch. Exp. Pathol. Pharmakol. **42,** 149–237, 1899.
78. Magnus-Levy, A.: Untersuchungen ueber die Acidosis im Diabetes mellitus u. die Saeureintoxication im Coma diabeticum. Arch. Exp. Pathol. Pharmakol. **45,** 389–434, 1901.
79. Leber, Th.: Ueber die Erkrankungen d. Auges bei Diabetes mellitus. von Graefe's Arch. Ophthalmol. **21,** Abt. III, 206–337, 1875.
80. Arnozan, Ch. L. X., Vaillard, L.: Arch. Physiol. Norm. Pathol. 3 sér. **3,** 287–316, 1884.

81. Mering, J. von: Ueber experimentallen Diabetes. Verh. Congr. Inn. Med. **5,** 158–189, 1886.
82. Troisier, M.: Bull. Soc. Anat. Paris **46,** 231, 1871.
83. Recklinghausen, F. D. von: Ueber Haemochromatose. Berlin. Klin. Wochenschr. **26,** 925, 1889.
84. Noorden, C. H. von: Der Diabetes mellitus. Wien, A. Hoelder, 1898.
85. Bouchardat, A.: De la glycosurie ou diabète sucré; son tratement hygiénique. Paris, Germer-Baillière, 1875.
86. Pavy, F. W.: Researches on the Treatment of Diabetes. London, J. Churchill, 1862.
87. Benedict, A. L.: J. Am. Med. Assoc. **57,** 1193, 1911.
88. Benedict, S. R.: The analysis of whole blood. II. The determination of sugar and of saccharoids (non-fermentable copper-reducing substances). J. Biol. Chem. **92,** 141–59, 1931.
89. Rolleston, Sir H. D.: The Endocrine Organs in Health and Disease with an Historical Review. p. 433. London, Oxford University Press, 1936.
90. Opie, E. L.: The relation of diabetes mellitus to lesions of the pancreas. Hyaline degeneration of the islands of Langerhans. J. Exp. Med. **5,** 527–540, 1900–01.
91. Zuelzer, G. L.: Ueber Versuche einer specifischen Fermenttherapy des Diabetes. Z. Exp. Pathol. Ther. **5,** 307–318, 1908.
92. ibid.
93. Lane, M. A.: Am. J. Anat., Philadelphia **7,** 409, 1907.
94. Bensley, R. R.: Cit. after J. R. Henderson's unpublished Ms: The Pancreas: Endocrine and Exocrine Functions, Chap. 1: Historical Introduction. p. 17.
95. Bensley, R. R.: Harvey Lectures, NY X, 250, 1915.
96. Homans, J.: Proc. Soc. London B. **86,** 73, 1913.
97. Warren, S.: Pathology of Diabetes, 1930.
98. Lewaschew,: Arch. Mikrosk. Anat. Bonn **26,** 458, 1886.
99. Mankowski, A.: Arch. Mikrosk. Anat. Bonn **59,** 286, 1902.
100. Dale, H. H.: Phil. Trans. R. Soc. London B. **197,** 25, 1905.
101. As 94: p. 16.
102. Laguesse, E. G.: C. R. Soc. Biol. Paris **45,** 819, 1893.
103. Laguesse, E. G.: C. R. Soc. Biol. Paris **65,** 189, 1908.
104. Gley, E.: Letter dated 20 February 1905. C. R. Soc. Biol. Paris **87,** 1922.
105. As 94.
106. Meyer, J. de: Arch. Int. Physiol. **9,** 1, 1910.
107. Sharpey-Schaefer, E. A.: The Endocrine Organs, p. 128. London, 1916.
108. Rennie and Fraser: Cit. after E. Clark Noble, Guy's Hosp. Gaz. **85,** 28 Aug. 1971.
109. Scott, E. L.: Cit. after Wrenshall, G. A., Hetenyi, G. and Feasby, W. R. The Story of Insulin, p. 49. London, Bodley Head, 1962.
110. As 94: p. 22.
111. As 109: p. 52.
112. Barron, M.: Surg. Gynecol. Obstet. **31,** 437–448, 1920.
113. Macleod, J. J. R., Pearce, R. G., Redfield, A. C., Taylor, N. B. *et al.*: Physiology and Biochemistry in Modern Medicine. 3rd ed., St. Louis, C. V. Mosby, 1920.
114. Starling, E. H.: Principles of Human Physiology. 3rd ed. Philadelphia, Lea, 1920.
115. Lancereaux, É.: Notes et réflexions à propos de deux cas de diabète sucré avec altération du pancréas. Bull. Acad. Méd. **6,** 1215–1240, 1877.

116. Lancereaux, É.: Le diabète maigre: ses symptomes, son évolution, son prognostie et son traitement. Méd. Paris **29**, 205–211, 1880.
117. Paulesco, N. C.: Exposé des Titres et Travaux Scientifiques du Dr. Paulesco. Glandes thyroides – physiologie normale et pathologique, pp. 11–14. Paris, 1899.
118. Paulesco, N. C.: Ibid. Recherches experimentales sur la physiologie des capsules surrénales, pp. 17–18.
119. Paulesco, N. C.: L'hypophyse du cerveau. J. Physiol. Pathol. Gen. **9**, 441–456, 1907.
120. Stockard, C. R.: The Physical Basis of Personality. New York, Norton, 1931.
121. Paulesco, N. C.: Recherche sur le role du pancréas dans l'assimilation nutritive. Arch. Int. Physiol. **17**, 85–109, 1921. (Received 22 June 1921.)
122. Banting, F. G., Best, C. H.: The internal secretion of the pancreas. J. Lab. Clin. Med. **7**, 253, 1922.
122a. Macleod, J. J. R.: History of the researches leading to the discovery of insulin. Bull. Hist. Med. **52**, 295–312, 1978.
123. As 109: p. 52.
124. Liljestrand, G.: The prize in physiology and medicine, in 'Nobel, the Man and his Prizes' (ed. Nobel Foundation) p. 153. Amsterdam, 1962.
125. Noble, E. Clark: Guy's Hosp. Gaz. (Letter) **85**, 28 Aug. 1971.
125a. Stevenson, Ll. G.: Sir Frederick Banting. London, Heinemann Medical. p. 68, 1947.
126. Collip, J. B.: The original method as used for the isolation of insulin in semipure form for the treatment of the first clinical cases. J. Biol. Chem. **55**, xl–xli, 1923.
127. As 94: p. 22.
128. As 94: p. 23.
129. Abel, J. J.: Crystalline insulin. Proc. Natl. Acad. Sci. U.S.A. **12**, 132–136, 1926.
130. Bauer, Julius: Die konstitutionelle Disposition zu inneren Krankheiten. Berlin, Springer, 1917.
131. Bauer, Julius: Constitution and Disease. Applied Constitutional Pathology. New York, Grune & Stratton, 1942.
132. Gowers, Sir Wm.: Cited after Bauer: Ref. 131, p. 11.
133. As 131: p. 12.
134. Draper, G.: Human Constitution. Philadelphia, 1926.
135. Martin, R.: Lehrbuch der Anthropologie. pp. 51–52. Jena, G. Fischer, 1914.
136. Garrison, F. H.: An Introduction to the History of Medicine. 4th ed., p. 678, Philadelphia, W. B. Saunders, 1929.
137. Martius, F. W. A.: Constitution and Selection, 1914.
138. Kretschmer, Ernst: Körperbau und Charakter, Berlin. J. Springer, 1921.
139. Osler, Wm.: On six cases of Addison's disease with the report of a case greatly benefited by the use of the suprarenal cortical extract. Reprinted from 'the Int. Med. Magazine' for February 1896.
140. Osler, Wm.: Proc. Johns Hopkins Med. Soc., Hopkins Hosp. Bull., **7**, 208–209, 1896.
141. Kinnicutt, F. P.: The therapeutics of the internal secretions. Am. J. Med. Sci. **114**, 1, 1897.
142. Rogoff, J. M., Stewart, G. N.: The influence of adrenal extracts on the survival period of adrenalectomized dogs. Science **66**, 327–328, 1927.
143. Hartman, F. A., Macarthur, C. G., Hartman, W. E.: A substance which prolongs the life of adrenalectomized cats. Proc. Soc. Exp. Biol. Med. **25**, 69–70, 1927.

144. Pfiffner, J. J., Swingle, W. W.: The preparation of an active extract of the suprarenal cortex. Anat. Rec. **44**, 225, 1929.
145. Hartman, F. A., Brownell, Katharine A.: The hormone of the adrenal cortex. Proc. Soc. Exp. Biol. Med. **27**, 938–939, 1930.
146. Hartman, F. A., Thorn, G. W.: A biological method for the assay of cortin. Proc. Soc. Exp. Biol. Med. **28**, 94–95, 1930.
147. Thorn, G. W.: The adrenal cortex (Thayer Lectures for 1967); Johns Hopkins Med. J. **123**, 49–77, 1968.
148. Thorn, G. W., Garbut, H. R., Hitchcock, F. A., Hartman, F. A.: The effect of cortin upon the renal excretion of sodium, potassium, chloride, inorganic phosphorus and total nitrogen in normal subjects and in patients with Addison's disease. Endocrinology **21**, 202–212, 1937.
149. Loeb, R. F.: The effect of sodium chloride on the treatment of a patient with Addison's disease. Proc. Soc. Exp. Biol. Med. **30**, 808–812, 1933.
150. Harrop, G. A.: The influence of the adrenal cortex upon the distribution of body water. Bull. Johns Hopkins Hosp. **59**, 11–24, 1936.
151. Baumann, E. J., Kurland, S.: Changes in the inorganic constituents of blood in suprarenalectomized cats and rabbits. J. Biol. Chem. **71**, 281–302, 1927.
152. Loeb, R. F., Atchely, D. W., Benedict, E. M., Leland, J.: Electrolyte balance studies in adrenalectomized dogs with particular reference to the excretion of sodium. J. Exp. Med. **57**, 775–792, 1933.
153. Truszkowski, R., Zwemer, R. L.: Cortico-adrenal insufficiency and potassium metabolism. Biochem. J. **30**, 1345–1353, 1936.
154. Wilder, R. N., Kendall, E. C., Snell, A. M., Kepler, E. J., Tynearson, E. H., Adams, M.: Intake of potassium, important considerations in Addison's disease; metabolic study. Arch. Int. Med. **59**, 367–393, 1937.
155. Kendall, E. C.: A chemical and physiological investigation of the suprarenal cortex. Symp. Quant. Biol. **5**, 299, 1937.
156. Grollman, A.: Physiological and chemical studies on the adrenal cortical hormone. Symp. Quant. Biol. **5**, 313, 1937.
157. Reichstein, T., Euw, J. von: Ueber Bestandteile der Nebennierenrinde: Isolierung der Substanzen Q (desoxycorticosterone) und R sowie weitere Stoffe. Helv. Chim. Acta **21**, 1197–1210, 1938.
158. Reichstein, T.: Constituents of the adrenal cortex. Helv. Chim. Acta **19**, 402–412, 1936.
159. Steiger, M., Reichstein, T.: Desoxycorticosterone (21-oxyprogesterone) aus 5-3-oxydatio-Kohlensaeure. Helv. Chim. Acta **20**, 1164–1179, 1937.
160. Thorn, G. W., Firor, W. M.: Desoxycorticosterone acetate therapy in Addison's disease. Clinical consideration. J. Am. Med. Assoc. **231**, 76, 1940.
161. Dale, Sir Henry H.: Evidence concerning the endocrine function of the neurohypophysis and its nervous control. In: The Neurohypophysis, Proc. 8th Symposium, Colston Research Soc., Bristol (Ed. Heller, H.) pp. 1–9. Butterworths Scient. Publ, 1957.
162. Frank, A. E.: Ueber Beziehungen der Hypophyse zum Diabetes insipidus. Berlin. Klin. Wochenschr. **49**, 393–397, 1912.
163. Oliver, G., Schaefer, E. A.: On the physiological action of extracts of pituitary body and certain other glandular organs. J. Physiol., London **18**, 277–279, 1895.
164. Howell, W. H.: The physiological effects of extracts of the hypophysis cerebri and infundibular body. J. Exp. Med. **3**, 245–258, 1898.
165. Dale, Sir Henry H.: On some physiological actions of ergot. J. Physiol. London **34**, 163–206, 1906.

166. Dale, Sir Henry H.: The action of extracts of the pituitary body. Biochem. J. **4,** 427–447, 1909.
167. Dale, Sir Henry H.: Adventures in Physiology with Excursions into Autopharmacology. London, Pergamon Press, 1953.
168. Chester Jones, I.: Evolution Aspects of the Adrenal Cortex and its Homologues. The Sir Henry Dale Lecture for 1976. Proc. Soc. Endocrinol., J. Endocrinol. **71,** 3, 1976.
169. Dale, Sir Henry H.: An Autumn Gleaning. Occasional Lectures and Addresses. London, Pergamon Press, 1954.
170. Herring, P. T.: The histological appearance of the mammalian pituitary body. Q. J. Exp. Physiol. **1,** 121–160, 1908.
171. Luschka, H. von: Der Hirnanhang u. die Steissdruese des Menschen. pp. 1–97. Berlin, G. Reimer, 1860.
172. Peremeschko: Ueber den Bau des Hiranhanges. Virchow's Arch. **38,** 329–342, 1867.
173. Rathke, M. H.: Ueber die Entstehung der Glandula pituitaria. Arch. Anat. Physiol. Wiss. Med. 482–485, 1838.
174. Ramon y Cajal, S.: Algunas contribuciones al concimiento de los ganglios del encefalo. III. Hipofisis. Ann. Soc. Esp. Hist. Rat. **2,** ser. **23,** 195–237, 1894.
175. Tello, F.: Algunas observaciones sobre la histologia de la hipofisis humana. Trab. Lab. Invest. Biol. Univ. Madrid. **10,** 145–184, 1912.
176. Pines, I. L.: Ueber die Innervation der Hypophysis cerebri. Z. Ges. Neurol. Psychiat. **107,** 507–511, 1927.
177. Greving, R.: Beitraege zur Anatomie der Hypophyse und deren Funktion. II. Das nervoese Regulationssystem des Hypophysenhinterlappens (der Nucleus supraopticus und seine Fasersysteme) Z. Ges. Neurol. Psychiat. **104,** 466–479, 1926.
178. Daniel, P. M., Pritchard, Marjorie M.: Studies of the Hypothalamus and the Pituitary Gland. Acta Endocrinol., Suppl 201, **80,** vii–ix, pp. 1–210, 1975.
179. Cushing, H., Goetsch, E.: Concerning the secretion of the infundibular lobe of the pituitary body and its presence in the cerebrospinal fluid. Am. J. Physiol. **27,** 60–86, 1910.
180. Collin, R.: Étude histophysiologique du complexe tuberoinfundibulo-pituitaire. Arch. Morphol. Gen. Exp. **28,** 1–100, 1928.
181. Van Dyke, H. B., Chow, B. F., Greep, R. O., Rothen, A.: Isolation of protein from pars neuralis of ox pituitary with constant oxytocic, pressor and diuresis-inhibiting activities. J. Pharmacol. **74,** 190–209, 1942.
182. Geiling, E. M. K., Oldham, F. K.: Site of formation of posterior lobe hormones. Trans. Assoc. Am. Physicians **52,** 132–136, 1937.
183. Thom, W.: Arch. Mikrosk. Anat., Bonn **57,** 632, 1901.
184. Erdheim, J.: Sitzungsber. Kais. Akad. Wiss., Mathemat. Naturwiss. Kl., Wien, **113,** Abt. iv, p. 537, 1904.
185. Roussy, G. and Mosinger, M.: Ann. Anat. Pathol., Paris **11,** 655, 1934.
186. Baer, C. E. von: 1828, cit. after Rolleston, Ref. 89, p. 53.
187. Bucy, P. C.: The pars nervosa of the bovine hypophysis. J. Comp. Neurol. **50,** 505–519, 1930.
188. Romeis, R.: Hypophyse. In Hdbch. mikroskop. Anatomie der Menschen. (Ed. von Moellendorf, W.), Bd. 6, T1. 3., pp. 389–474, Berlin, Springer, 1940.
189. Collin, R.: La Neurocrinie Hypophysaire. Paris, 1928.
190. Popa, G. T., Fielding, U.: The vascular link between the pituitary and the hypothalamus. Lancet **2,** 238–240, 1930.

191. Popa, G. T., Fielding, U.: A portal circulation from the pituitary to the hypothalamic region. J. Anat. (London) **65,** 88–91, 1930.
192. Basir, M. A.: J. Anat. Cambridge **66,** 387, 1932.
193. As 178: p. 35.
194. Friedman, G. S., Friedman, M. H.: Am. J. Physiol., Boston **103,** p. 244.
195. Friedman, G. S., Friedman, M. H.: Am. J. Physiol., Boston **107,** 220, 1934.
196. Geiling, E. M. K.: J. Am. Med. Assoc. **104,** 738, 1935.
197. Gaskell, J. F.: The chromaffine system of annelids and the relation of this system to the contractile vascular system in the leech. Phil. Trans. B. **205,** 153–211, 1914.
198. Speidel, C. C. Gland cells of internal secretion in the spinal cord of skates. Carnegie Inst. Wash. Publ. No. 13, 1–31, 1919.
199. Scharrer, E.: Die Lichtempfindlichkeit blinder Elritzen (Untersuchungen ueber das Zwischenhirn d. Fische. I.) T./Z. Vergl. Physiol. **7,** 1–38, 1928.
200. Martini, L., Besser, G. M. (eds): Clinical Neuroendocrinology. pp. vi–xvii, 1–610. New York, San Francisco, London, 1977.
201. Hann, F. von: Ueber die Bedeutung der Hypophysenveraenderungen bei Diabetes insipidus. Frankfurt. Z. Pathol. **21,** 337–365, 1918.
202. Konschegg, A., Schuster, E.: Ueber die Beinflussung d. Diurese durch hypophysenextrakte. Dtsch. Med. Wochenschr. **41,** 1091, 1915.
203. Ott, I., Scott, J. C.: The action of infundibulin upon the mammary secretion. Proc. Soc. Exp. Biol. Med. **8,** 48, 1910.
204. Dudley, H. W.: Some observations on the active principle of the pituitary gland. J. Pharmacol. Exp. Ther. **14,** 295, 1919.
205. Kamm, O., Aldrich, T. B., Grote, I. W., Rowe, L. W., Bugbee, E. P.: The active principles of the posterior lobe of the pituitary gland. J. Am. Chem. Soc. **50,** 573–601, 1928.
206. Du Vigneaud, V., Ressler, C., Swan, J. M., Roberts, C. W., Katsoyannis, P. G., Gordon, S.: The synthesis of an octapeptide amide with the hormone activity of oxytocin. J. Am. Chem. Soc. **75,** 4879–4880, 1953.
207. Du Vigneaud, V., Gish, D. T., Katsoyannis, P. G., Hess, G. P.: Synthesis of the pressor-antidiuretic hormone, arginine-vasopressin. J. Am. Chem. Soc. **80,** 3355, 1958.
208. Acher, R., Chauvet, J., Olivry, G.: Sur l'existence eventuelle d'une hormone unique neurohypophysaire. Biochim. Biophys. Acta **22,** 421, 1956.
209. McCord, C. P., Allen, F. P.: Surg. Gynecol Obstet., Chicago **25,** 250, 1917.
210. Greep, R. O.: Parathyroid hormone. In Comparative Endocrinology (Ed. von Euler, U. S. and Heller, H.) Vol. 1, pp. 325–370. New York, Academic Press, 1963.
211. Clarke, J.: Commentaries on some of the most important diseases of children. Part I, pp. 86–97, London, Longman, 1815.
212. Kellie, G.: Notes on the swelling of the tops of the hands and feet, and on a spasmodic affection of the thumbs and toes, which very commonly attends it. Edinb. Med. Surg. J. **12,** 448–452, 1816.
213. Steinheim, Salomon L.: Zwei seltene Formen von hitzigem Rheumatismus. Litt. Ann. Ges. Heilk. **17,** 22–30, 1830.
214. Dance, B. H.: Observations sur une espèce de tétanos intermittent. Arch. Gén. Méd. **26,** 190–205, 1831.
215. Corvisart, F. R. L.: De la contracture des extrémités ou tétanie. Thèse No. 223, Paris, 1852.
216. Trousseau, Armand: Clinique médicale de l'Hôtel-Dieu de Paris. Tom. **2,** pp. 112–114. Paris, J. B. Baillière, 1861.
217. Erb, Wm. H.: Zur Lehre von der Tetanie nebst Bemerkungen ueber die

Pruefung der elektrischen Erregbarkeit motorischer Nerven. Arch. Psychiat. Nervenkr. **4**, 271–316, 1873–4.

218. Chvostek, F.: Beitrag zur Tetanie. Wien. Med. Presse **17**, 1201–1203, 1225–1227, 1253–1258, 1313–1316, 1876.

219. Vassale, G., Generali, F.: Sugli effeti dell'estirpazione delle ghiandole paratiroidee. Riv. Patol. Nerv. Ment. **1**, 95–99, 1896.

220. Moussu, G.: Sur la fonction parathyroidienne. C. R. Soc. Biol. Paris **50**, 867–869, 1898.

221. MacCallum, G., Voegtlin, C.: On the relation of tetany to the parathyroid glands and to calcium metabolism. J. Exp. Med. **11**, 118–151, 1909.

222. Berkeley, Y. W. N., Beebe, S. B.: A contribution to the physiology and chemistry of the parathyroid glands. J. Med. Res. **20**, 149–157, 1909.

223. Askanazy, M.: Ueber Ostitis deformans ohne osteoides Gewebe. Arb. Pathol.-anat. Inst., Tuebingen **4**, 398–422, 1904.

224. Engel, G.: Ueber einen Fall von cystoider Entartung des ganzen Skelettes. Giessen, F. C. Pietsch, 1864.

225. Recklinghausen, F. D. von: Die fibroese oder deformirende Ostitis, die Osteomalacie und die osteoplastische Carcinose in ihren gegenseitigen Beziehungen. In Festschrift R. Virchow, Berlin, G. Reimer, 1891.

226. Erdheim, J.: Tetania parathyreopriva. Mitteilungen Grenzgeb. Med. Chir. **16**, 632–744, 1906.

227. Erdheim, J.: Sitzungsber. d. k. Akad. Wissensch. Math. Naturwiss. Kl. **116**, Abt. iii, 311, 1907.

228. Erdheim, J.: Rachitis and Epithelkoerp. p. 262. Wien, 1914.

229. Collip, J. B.: The extraction of a parathyroid hormone which will prevent or control parathyroid tetany and which regulates the level of blood calcium. J. Biol. Chem. **63**, 395–438, 1925.

230. Collip, J. B., Leitch, D. B.: A case of tetany treated with parathyrin. Can. Med. Assoc. J. **15**, 59–60, 1925.

231. Greenwald, I.: The effect of parathyroidectomy upon metabolism. Am. J. Physiol. **28**, 103–132, 1911.

232. Barnicot, N. A.: The local action of the parathyroid and other tissues on bone in intracerebral grafts. J. Anat. **82**, 233–248, 1948.

233. Jahan, I., Pitts, R. F.: Effect of parathormone on renal tubular re-absorption of phosphate and calcium. Am. J. Physiol. **155**, 42–49, 1948.

234. Talmage, R. V., Elliott, J. R.: Removal of calcium from bone as influenced by the parathyroids. Endocrinology **62**, 717–722, 1958.

235. Mandl, F.: Therapeutischer Versuch bei Ostitis fibrosa generalisata mittels exstirpation eines Epithelkoerperchens. Wien. Klin. Wochenschr. **38**, 1343–1344, 1925.

236. Hanson, A. M.: An elementary chemical study of the parathyroid gland in cattle. Mil. Surg. Wash. **52**, 280–284, 1923.

237. Berman, L.: Proc. Soc. Exp. Biol. Med. **21**, 465, 1924.

238. Selye, H.: Endocrinology **16**, 547, 1932.

239. Hanson, A. M.: J. Am. Med. Assoc., Chicago **105**, 113, 1935.

240. Joffe, B. I., Hackeng, W. H., Seftel, H. C.: Parathyroid hormone concentrations in nutritional rickets. Clin. Sci. **42**, 113–116, 1972.

241. Albright, F., Aub, J. C., Bauer, W.: Hyperparathyroidism – a common and polymorphic condition, as illustrated by seventeen proved cases from one clinic. J. Am. Med. Assoc. **102**, 1276–1287, 1934.

242. Albright, F., Bloomberg, E., Castleman, B., Churchill, E., Churchill, E. D.: Hyperparathyroidism due to diffuse hyperplasia of all parathyroid glands rather than adenoma of one. Arch. Int. Med. **54**, 315–329, 1934.

243. Albright, F., Reifenstein, E. C.: The Parathyroid Glands and Metabolic Bone Disease. Baltimore, Williams & Wilkins, 1948.

244. Rasmussen, H., Craig, L. C.: Purification of parathormone by use of countercurrent distribution. J. Am. Chem. Soc. **81,** 5003, 1959.

245. Rasmussen, H., Craig, L. C.: The parathyroid polypeptides. Recent Progr. Hormone Res. **18,** 269–295, 1962.

246. Aurbach, G. D.: Isolation of parathyroid hormone after extraction with phenol. J. Biol. Chem. **234,** 3179–3181, 1959.

247. Albright, F., Burnett, C. H., Smith, P. H., Parson, W.: Pseudohypoparathyroidism (an example of the 'Seabright–Bantam' syndrome). Report of three cases. Endocrinology **30,** 922–932, 1942.

248. Copp, D. H., Cameron, E. C., Cheney, B. A., Davidson, A. G. F., Henze, K. G.: Evidence for calcitonin – a new hormone from the parathyroid that lowers blood calcium. Endocrinology **70,** 638–649, 1962.

249. Cunliffe, W. J., Black, M. M., Hall, R., Johnston, I. D. A., Hudgson, P., Shuster, S., Sudmundsson, T. V., Joplin, G. F., Williams, E. D., Woodhouse, N. J. Y., Galante, C.: A calcitonin secreting thyroid carcinoma. Lancet II, 63–66, 1968.

250. Turner, H. H.: A syndrome of infantilism, congenital webbed neck, and cubitus valgus. Endocrinology **23,** 566–574, 1938.

251. Brook, C. G. D., Murset, G., Zachman, M., Prader, A.: Growth in children with 45,XO Turner's syndrome. Arch. Dis. Childh. **49,** 789, 1974.

252. Snider, M. E., Solomon, I. L.: Ultimate height in chromosomal gonadal dysgenesis without androgen therapy. Am. J. Dis. Child. **127,** 673, 1974.

253. Lemli, L., Smith, D. W.: The XO syndrome: A study of the differentiated phenotype in 25 patients. J. Pediat. **63,** 577, 1963.

254. Preger, L., Steinbach, H. L., Moskovitz, P. et al.: Roentgenographic abnormalities in phenotypic females with gonadal dysgenesis. Am. J. Roentgen. **104,** 899, 1968.

255. Klinefelter, H. F., Reifenstein, E. C., Albright, F.: Syndrome characterized by gynaecomastia, aspermatogenesis without A-Leydigism, and increased excretion of follicle-stimulating hormone. J. Clin. Endocrinol. **2,** 615–627, 1942.

256. Stewart, J. S. S., Mack, W. S., Govan, A. D. T. et al.: Klinefelter's syndrome: clinical and hormonal aspects. Q. J. Med. **28,** 561, 1959.

257. Halsted, W. S.: Auto- and isotransplantation, in dogs of the parathyroid glandules. J. Exp. Med., **11,** 175–199, 1909.

CHAPTER TWENTY

THE AMERICANS

IT will be obvious from the history of endocrinology so far, that from the 16th century onwards to 1900, most of the dramatis personae lived and worked in Europe – in Italy, France, Germany and in Britain. The majority of the people from whom the modern Americans descended came to the New World from Europe, or were brought from Africa, usually forcibly, mainly after 1600.

We have seen, however, that John B. Davidge, an American medical student in Edinburgh, concluded from Percival Pott's observation that there is a causal connection between the ovaries and menstruation (see Chapter 17). There is no doubt that ideas from Europe were brought back, not only by students from America, but also from medical men from Britain, France and Germany, who worked and settled in North America. We have also seen the great influence Brown-Séquard had in the United States, not only with his organotherapy, but through his lecture tours. In the 1860s, James Marion Sims spent several years in Paris and published his important *Notes on Uterine Surgery* in London, also discussing some problems of infertility and its treatment. So did one of his pupils, Thomas Addis Emmett (1828–1919).

At the time when Oliver and Schaefer began their successful collaboration (in the winter of 1893–1894), and Knauer and Halban in Vienna recorded their ovarian transplant experiments in rabbits (in 1895) and guinea pigs, Robert Tuttle Morris had begun his ovarian graft operations in humans (see p. 369). (Sir) William Osler, encouraged by his chief, Dr. Thayer, attempted to treat Addison's disease with glandular therapy at the Johns Hopkins Medical School in Baltimore in 1896, as did F. B. Kinnicutt (see p. 476); Harvey Williams Cushing and his group, many members of which later achieved international fame, had begun their studies on the pituitary and on experimental hypophysectomy. Other names from the Johns

Hopkins were those of John Jacob Abel (1857–1938) and Albert Cornelius Crawford (1869–1921) (epinephrine, 1897)[1]. We have also mentioned (p. 9) the book on "The internal secretions and the principles of medicine" by Sajous in 1903.

The American line received, however, a real spurt between 1910 and 1920, when there began the involvement of the chemists. We saw the enrolment of Edward Calvin Kendall (1866–1972) into the endocrine field, when he was first assigned the task of isolating the active principle of the thyroid in 1910. David Marine (1880–1976) and William Whitridge Williams (b. 1875) published their study of the relation of iodine to the structure of the thyroid gland in 1908[2]. This was followed by Marine and Kimball's successful Akron experiment in 1917. But this was not the sole difference between the European and American methods of approach. Professor Roy O. Greep, in his Sir Henry Dale Lecture for 1967, said:

> However I may look the part, I am not one of the fathers of endocrine research. The fathers belonged to a generation before me. The names of this small band of pioneering workers spring readily to mind. They were scattered over the face of the globe, but among them I may say that the English, Germans and French had perhaps more than their due. By the time I joined the cast of the gonadotrophin drama, the first act was over and the second had already begun.[3]

Philip E. Smith (1884–1970) bowed himself on to the stage, which he was to grace for so many years, in 1916 and Bennett A. Allen in the same year, as well as several others who have already been mentioned. Walter B. Cannon reported on experimental hyperthyroidism in 1915[4] and on 'Bodily changes in pain, hunger, fear and rage' in the same year[5].

What then was the essential difference between the European – and especially British – flavour of research in this new and vast field, and the American approach? To put it into a single sentence, we should perhaps say that the zest which existed in both camps had added to it the pioneering spirit of the new country of the Americas (if we include people like Houssay and the Canadians).

The natural trend of the élitists, especially in Britain, is towards the centres of excellence, preferably in old established places like University College London, or Cambridge, Oxford and Edinburgh. The élitist in the United States may start at a centre of excellence such as the Johns Hopkins Medical School in Baltimore and remain there, or (like Cushing and Cannon) at Harvard. But he may also go out to a comparatively unknown place, like Berkeley, California, where Herbert MacLean Evans returned to, being born in that State, and build up a new centre of excellence almost from scratch. Hans Lisser (1888–1964) qualified at Johns Hopkins University in 1911 and returned to his native city, San Francisco, in 1914, where he remained for the rest of his life, eventually to become Clinical Professor of Medicine and Endocrinology in the University of California. In 1927, he became President of the Endocrine Society.

In Britain, properly qualified physiologists of the standing of Sharpey-Schafer, Bayliss, Starling, Swale Vincent and Marshall took the lead, with very clearly defined aims and methods. By way of contrast, in the United States, Edward A. Doisy was a biochemist with no previous knowledge of the functions of the ovary. In order to bring about understanding of the differences in outlook and approach, we shall give a few examples of the characteristics of some of the personalities concerned. It should also be noted that in the United States the clinicians were less discouraged to take an open interest in the new field than was the case in Britain. This applied particularly after the work and influence of Fuller Albright, which will be discussed in greater detail. Harvey Cushing was, however, at least at one stage, much more critical.

Even (Sir) Charles Harington was affected by this spirit of adventure on his return from the United States. So was (Sir) Henry Dale, who continually exposed himself intentionally to influences from abroad, by encouraging and inviting young research workers from many countries to work in his laboratory, even late in life (e.g. Feldberg and Bacq).

A further expression of the difference between the British attitude and that in the United States, was the fact that in the United States the 'Association for the Study of Internal Secretions', which after 1952 became the 'Endocrine Society', was founded on 4 June 1917. Hans Lisser told in his paper on 'The First Forty Years (1917–1957)', published in 1967:

> It survived and prospered eventually, but for many years it was hazardous to forecast whether this dashing and intrepid pioneering into a fertile, but suspect field of medicine, would fail or triumph. Hostility towards its earlier meetings was of such nature that it might have been safer to have met in secret – for clinical endocrinology at that time was in disrepute. Meetings were poorly attended, audiences were hard to attract, programs were sparse and speakers were few[6].

In Britain, clinical endocrinology was even more suspect; the present writer well remembers a general medical meeting in London in the 1950s, where clinical cases were presented; one of them was a patient with hyperthyroidism and the merits of medical, radio-iodine and surgical treatment were discussed. A distinguished member got up and warned against attempts of the "Westendocrinologists" (referring to London's Harley Street of medical specialists in the West End of the city), who were suggesting untried diversions when a satisfactory surgical treatment was available! Similarly, Lisser reminds us that Brown-Séquard's testicular extract treatment, Steinach's rejuvenation (and Voronoff's testicular grafts) harmed the reputation of the tender, recently formed Association, so that Herbert M. Evans had felt obliged to remark: "Endocrinology suffered obstetric deformity at its very birth." As late as 1933, a celebrated researcher introduced his paper at a meeting of the Congress of American Physicians and Surgeons in Washington, D.C., with Harvey Cushing presiding, "with the following absurdity: 'To be an endocrinologist among the practising profession today means too often to be primarily concerned with making fat ladies thin.' "[6]

Any young clinician who dared to embark on a career in this field was looked at askance, and considered to be naive and gullible or suspected "of straying into the realm of quackery, and heading for the endocrine gold fields!" Walter B. Cannon put it thus: "He was threatened with ridicule and scorn because of the wild surmise and phantastic claims of brethren whose imagination outran both fact and reason."[6 (p. 6)] The official publication of the Association became *Endocrinology* with Roy Hoskins as Editor for the first twenty-three years.

As for Britain, Peter M. F. Bishop (1904–1979) told, in his Presidential Address to the Section of Endocrinology of the Royal Society of Medicine on 27 October 1954[7], that the *Journal of Endocrinology* came into being in June 1938, after ten founder members had guaranteed a certain sum of money. At Sir Henry Dale's suggestion, Professor (Sir) Alan S. Parkes was appointed Chairman of the Council of Management, Professor F. G. Young its Secretary, and (Sir) Charles Dodds Editor. Owing to the outbreak of war, the overseas subscribers disappeared and the journal nearly foundered. When, in July 1946, the 'Society for Endocrinology' was founded with Professor Parkes as Chairman and Dr. S. J. Folley as Secretary, the journal became its official organ. The Clinicians, on their part, had started the Endocrine Section of the Royal Society of Medicine in January 1946, with Sir Walter Langdon-Brown as President-elect, and – after his death – with Mr. Lennox Ross Broster (1889–1965) as President. One may note that the foundation of the British Society was 29 years behind its North American counterpart! Guy's Hospital Medical School established an Addison Lecture in the same year (1946), the first being given by (Sir) Charles Dodds; among subsequent lecturers, the Americans were well represented. The same applied to the annual Dale Medal and Sir Henry Dale Lecture of the Society for Endocrinology, where the

Americans scored with recipients like George W. Corner, Roy Greep, Charles Best, G. W. Liddle and John D. Everett, to name but a few.

The American Society had to battle hard to justify its existence. Lisser points out that when the Society was founded, there were only two endocrine products available for clinical use: thyroid gland extract and epinephrine. The latter was, however, not effective in true hypoadrenalism; its beneficial effect on asthma did not make asthma an endocrine deficiency disease, or – as Hoskins, the editor of *Endocrinology* remarked, "because adrenalin, used as a drug, raises blood-pressure, and the inference is drawn, that therefore low blood-pressure must be due to 'hypoadrenalism', by the same reasoning constipation might be regarded as 'hypocascarism' "[6] (p. 7). In fact, until the discovery of insulin, which stimulated large scale research into other endocrine organs, clinicians could offer little in the way of effective rational scientific endocrine treatment. Frank Pottenger, a founder and secretary of the (American) society, remarked specifically that

> the existence of the 'Association' depended upon the support of the clinicians. Accordingly, there was more or less disappointment expressed by our members, not only by complaint but too often by resignation. This made the financing of the early years exceedingly difficult. It was necessary to make continual appeals to the friends of our most interested members in order to fill our annually depleted ranks and keep the Association alive.

The 'Association' was founded by a group of men, who were invited by Dr. Henry R. Harrower of Glendale, CA, to a meeting in Detroit in June 1916, at the time of the Meeting of the American Medical Association. This meeting was attended by *ca.* 50 members. Sajous (see Postscript) was elected its first president. It is, however, particularly characteristic for the trend and development of the Association, to pay attention to its fifth annual meeting in Boston, on 6 June 1921. The Presidential Address was given by Harvey W. Cushing, Professor of Surgery at the Harvard Medical School. It was entitled 'Disorders of the Pituitary Gland; Retrospective and Prophetic – an Allegory'. It was published on 18 June (1921) in the *Journal of the American Medical Association*, and not in *Endocrinology*, the official journal of the Association of which Cushing was President, "perhaps with the intent of more widespread dissemination in his scalding ridicule of the endocrinology at that time"[6] (p. 9). It also throws an interesting sidelight on Harvey Cushing, whose zest, enthusiasm and careful planning in endocrine and other research were above board, whose scholarship in general, integrity and literary and historical interests were above reproach, but whose aristocratic (meaning in

503

the sense of 'aristos' = the best) outlook could occasionally be almost intolerant and rigid. He certainly did not suffer fools gladly, although he had a most generous nature. From that address, a few passages are worth quoting:

> We find ourselves embarked on the fogbound and poorly charted sea of endocrinology. It is easy to lose our bearings, for we have, most of us, little knowledge of seafaring and only a vague idea of our destination. Our motives are varied. Some unquestionably follow the lure of discovery; some are earnest colonizers; some have the spirit of missionaries and would spread the gospel; some are attracted merely by the prospect of gain and are running full sail before the trade wind. Traders, adventurers, even pirates, are certain to follow on the heels of exploration. In every profession, even ours, are to be found those who gather up beads of information of little intrinsic value, which are exchanged for the property of credulous people, as gullible as the natives of a new-found land.

Alfred Joseph Clark (1885–1941), Professor of Pharmacology at University College in London, and friend of Swale Vincent, wrote in 1923 in a very similar manner (see p. 390, Chapter 18).

> To our present short sight it would appear that this sudden enthusiasm to put to sea under the pennant of the ductless glands . . . was followed soon after with the establishment a few years ago of this Association whose official organ represents a sort of mariner's almanac of the subject.

In the enthusiasm

> to embark glandward-ho! . . . many of us have lost our bearings in the therapeutic haze eagerly fostered by the many pharmaceutical establishments. . . . Never before has there arisen such an opportunity for polypharmaceutical charlatanism. . . . Surely, nothing will discredit the subject in which we have a common interest so effectively as pseudo-scientific reports, which find their way from the medical press into advertising leaflets where, cleverly intermixed with abstracts or researches of actual value, the administration of pluriglandular compounds is promiscuously advocated for a multitude of symptoms. The Lewis Carroll of today would have Alice nibble from a pituitary mushroom in her left hand, and a lutein one in her right and presto! she is any height desired. . . . No Magellan or Balboa for ductless gland therapeutics in general has yet appeared, though let us hope he may be on the way. Meanwhile there is many an imitator of Cortez or Pizzaro to trade on the superstitious awe of the natives, who will soon come to be fully disillusioned.[6] (p. 10)

Whether Cushing was, at that time, equally critical of his colleague, Walter B. Cannon's 'Emergency Theory' of the action of adrenin as Swale Vincent was (see p. 390), I have not been able to ascertain.

From Hans Lisser's paper it is obvious that the scientific content of the presentations at the early meetings would not be, today, regarded as of a satisfactory standard. His comment on those at the meeting in June 1917, was: "The subject matter almost reminds one of the mystical ancient notion that the pineal gland was the seat of the soul!"[6] [(p. 10)] Progress was made, however. At the 20th Congress, in May 1936, 36 papers were read, spread over 2 days. Lisser remarked in 1967:

> What a striking contrast, when clinicians and investigators 'stand in line' as it were, begging for a chance to appear on the program. Three day sessions, over 60 papers actually presented and almost a hundred more 'read by title'. About 150 contributions where, 30 years ago, one was grateful to obtain ten!

The first issue of *Endocrinology* appeared in January 1917, as a quarterly publication. After 1921, it appeared bi-monthly, and since 1937 it has been a monthly publication. It originally also contained abstracts of the endocrine literature, but this was discontinued after 1940. After 1942, they also discontinued the insertion, inside the title page, of interesting 'mottoes', taken from general or scientific literature. In 1941, a new magazine, *The Journal of Clinical Endocrinology*, was launched to relieve the burden of *Endocrinology* growing to an excessive size and to separate slightly, scientific laboratory research papers from those of clinical research. The *Journal of Clinical Endocrinology* was re-named, in January 1952, *The Journal of Clinical Endocrinology and Metabolism*, and both have flourished. The difficulty in selecting articles submitted to *Endocrinology* will become apparent by the recollection of Bernardo Alberto Houssay (1887–1971) of Buenos Aires. His account of his work (together with Alfredo Biasotti, b. 1903), 'La diabetes pancréatica de los perros hipofisoprivos' in 1930[8], in which he demonstrated the importance of the anterior pituitary in sugar metabolism, namely, that hypophysectomy almost nullified experimental diabetes in pancreatectomized dogs, was turned down by several American scientific journals "because they considered 'surprising' the facts I announced"[6] [(p. 16)]. However, it was accepted and published in *Endocrinology* in 1931[9]. Houssay shared the Nobel Prize for it in 1947. Lisser commented on this in 1967: "Such only-too-human errors are not so likely to occur nowadays, for the advances in endocrinology in the 20 years succeeding the announcement of insulin far outweigh all that was known in the preceding 2000 years, and we are no longer startled by extraordinary achievements." Lisser was wrong on that point. Human nature has not changed fundamentally and "only-too-human errors" continue to occur.

The significance of the success of insulin in the treatment of a disease which was neither uncommon nor easy to control, proved to be a great fillip to the extension of endocrine research. Moreover, many of the great drug companies willingly and meritoriously supported such research in a generous manner, independently of expectation of quick commercial profit.

In 1946, when Dr. Willard O. Thompson was appointed Managing Editor of the *Journal of Clinical Endocrinology*, he was closely associated with the American Goiter Association, of which he became President in 1952. In Britain, the first small group for the study of the thyroid was 'The London Thyroid Club', founded in November 1950, and originally restricted to 18 members. The founders were Sir Thomas Dunhill, the first President, John Wycliffe Linnell (1878–1967), and Dr. (later Lord) Brain (Walter Russell Brain, Baron Russell of Eynsham, 1895–1966). The Club, which began as an informal Dining Club, has now blossomed out into the British equivalent of the American Goiter Association. Dr. Willard O. Thompson successfully coordinated the publications of the American Goiter Association with the *Transactions of the Goiter Association* from 1948 onward, when it was agreed that

> all articles presented at the annual meeting of the American Goiter Association will be published in their *Transactions* regardless of whether or not they appear in *The Journal of Clinical Endocrinology*. At the same time, . . . all articles presented at the annual meeting of the American Goiter Association will be submitted to *The Journal of Clinical Endocrinology*. The decision of the Editorial Board and of the Editorial Office will be final concerning the publication in this Journal.

By these means and agreements a close and important link was forged between the two societies for their mutual benefit.

It is, however, of interest to note that the cost of publishing all those papers became so forbidding that in the Fiftieth Anniversary Issue of *Endocrinology* in January 1967 (Vol. 80, No. 1) a 'Notice to Contributors' appeared on page 229, announcing 'Publication Charges': "To help defray the continually rising costs of publishing this Journal, the Endocrine Society will be obliged to institute page charges". They were US $10.00 for each printed page; $70.00 for a manuscript of average length. Colour illustrations had always been a liability of the author. As a mitigating circumstance, it was added: "Inability to meet the charges will not preclude the publication of acceptable manuscripts".

In 1957, Dr. Lawson Wilkins finished his presidential address as follows:

> Thus, the embryologist, anatomist and cytologist, the physiologist and clever animal experimenter; the enzymologist and geneticist; the chemist skilled in steroidal methodology and synthesis, in protein structure and fractionation or working on the structure of iodinated compounds; the clinical diagnostician or investigator interested in electrolyte or carbohydrate metabolism, in bone disorders and calcium metabolism, or in renal physiology, have all combined to advance endocrinology. I know of no organization other than The Endocrine Society, which combines in common interests so many experts with totally different skills and disciplines as I see before me tonight. Your work has not only elucidated the endocrine disorders and facilitated their diagnosis and treatment, but has contributed greatly to the advancement of all physiology and biochemistry and the understanding and treatment of disease.

"In view of the above, it seems paradoxical to regard so all-inclusive a field of medicine", Lisser concludes, "with wide application, embracing almost every phase of medicine, as a speciality."[6] (p. 28).

Since the publication, in 1967, of Lisser's account of 'The First Forty Years', another fourteen years have passed, during which further great strides have been made in the field of endocrinology. Neuro-endocrinology, the role of the hypothalamus and, indeed, of the brain as the master controller of the endocrine system, to which the kidney and the gut have been added as sources of hormone production, have taken the centre of the field in the last twelve years. But even those recent events are now being eclipsed by the yet more exciting impact of peptide hormone receptor research and the discovery of the enkephalin peptides; the sequence of one of them is a hormone found in the pituitary, called beta-lipotropin. Subsections of it came to be known as β-, α-, and γ-endorphin ("the morphine within", the "poor man's opiate"). These discoveries concern pain, irritability, tranquility and memory; peptides suddenly became all important, and the barriers between research on the function of the brain and on hormones were broken down.

A few brief sketches will illustrate the American scene.

WALTER BRADFORD CANNON

Walter Bradford Cannon (1871–1945) succeeded Henry Pickering Bowditch (1840–1911) – the first full-time Professor of Physiology in the United States – as Professor of Physiology at the Harvard School of Medicine in 1908. He was born at Prairie du Chien,

Wisconsin, and obtained his medical training at Harvard, proceeding to MD in 1900, and subsequently becoming Instructor of Physiology under Bowditch. He was a man who combined a remarkable talent for experimental work with imagination and a span of general knowledge and interest in many fields, now virtually impossible to achieve for one man, and scholarship. He began with studies on digestion, where – among other methods he used bismuth salts which are opaque to X-rays, for the observation of the movements of the stomach of the cat on the fluorescent screen, as early as 1898[10]. Cannon also proved that gastric movements and secretion continue unaffected by the section of the extrinsic fibres of the vagus and splanchnic nerves (1906). He also studied the mechanism of digestion after surgical operations (1905–1909). In pursuing these studies, he wrote later: "In 1905, while observing in myself the rhythmic sounds produced by the activities of the alimentary tract, I had occasion to note that the sensation of hunger was not constant but recurrent, and that the moment of its disappearance was often associated with a rather loud gurgling sound as heard through the stethoscope."[5] (p. 268) These and a great number of other studies over a wide range of subjects led to the publication in 1915 of his book: *Bodily Changes in Pain, Hunger, Fear and Rage*, which gave rise to acclaim and controversy, but has now become a classic of physiology.

Professor Ian Stevenson of the Department of Neurology and Psychiatry of the University of Virginia School of Medicine, had this to say in the Foreword to the 1963 Harper Torchbook edition:

> For me the distinction of the present work lies in the range of material which Cannon's mind contemplated and to which he tried to bring order, always one of the chief tasks of scientists and the accomplishment of the greatest ones. For Cannon was not content with observing smoked drums record gastric movements of his subjects; he seems constantly to have pondered on the meaning of hunger and appetite for man's life. . . . In widening the scope of his thought, Cannon entered considerably into the developing field of anthropology and even more into psychology. . . . Cannon's preoccupation with broad questions he could never solve in his laboratory obviously stimulated the work within it. And that work contributed indirectly to a better understanding of these large problems. . . . This correlating of social stimuli and physical responses made Cannon one of the founders of psychosomatic medicine. And the skill with which he studied and described the correlations he observed has made this book a classic.

In 1926, Cannon outlined for the first time his classic concept of 'homeostasis'. This had a precursor in Claude Bernard's (1813–1878) 'milieu intérieur', "formed by the circulating organic liquid which surrounds and bathes all the tissue elements; . . .[11]. Cannon mentions as first postulate:

> The living being is stable. It must be so in order not to be destroyed, dissolved or disintegrated by the colossal forces, often adverse, which surround it. . . . In a sense it is stable because it is modifiable – the slight instability is the necessary condition for the true stability of the organism.

Thus wrote Richet in 1900[12].

> In an open system, such as our bodies represent, composed of unstable structure and subjected continually to disturbance, constancy is in itself evidence that agencies are acting or are ready to act to maintain this constancy. This has not been proved for all homeostatic conditions. But there are known cases which illustrate the postulate, e.g. homeothermia.[13]

Cannon's whole range of interests resulted, as already stated, in studies in many fields, including the activity of the endocrine organs, the sympathetic nervous system, all that fitting into the concept of homeostasis. In his original postulates[13], he had already stated:

> For example, when the body temperature tends to fall, vasoconstriction checks heat loss, increased adrenal secretion accelerates metabolism, shivering further increases heat production, and a more abundant growth of hair offers further protection. . . .

Subsequently, he and his team carried out further experiments to prove that the adrenal glands were necessary for temperature regulation[14]. All this led to his final summing up in his book *The Wisdom of the Body*[15], where he discussed the role of the adrenosympathetic (neuro-humoral) mechanism in the regulation of hunger, thirst, temperature, body fluids, oxygen supply and water, sugar and protein metabolism. We have already mentioned that Ernest Starling in London gave Cannon's work a special commendation in his Harveian Oration to the Royal College of Physicians in 1923, which was also entitled 'The Wisdom of the Body' (see p. 387). Cannon lived long enough, until 1945, and was still working, so that he could witness the enormous progress of endocrinology and the role his own work had played in this development.

HARVEY WILLIAMS CUSHING

It was of Cushing (1869–1939) that Garrison wrote[16] (p. 731) ". . . he stands *facile princeps* in neurological surgery, particularly in surgery of the head and the pituitary body." He was born in Cleveland, Ohio and educated at Yale and Harvard Medical Schools. After qualifying, he spent 3 years as assistant to William Stewart Halstead (1852–1922), the great surgeon at Johns Hopkins, who introduced so many innovations into major surgery of the breast, the thyroid and also had carried out experimental auto- and iso-transplants of the parathyroids (see Chapter 19). Harvey next spent a year at clinics and research institutions abroad and another 12 years at the Johns Hopkins in Baltimore, before being called to become Moseley professor of surgery at the Harvard School of Medicine in Boston and Surgeon-in-Chief of the Peter Brent Brigham Hospital, from 1912 to 1932.

He was the first in the United States to devote himself to surgery of the brain, which included the experimental study and analysis of its anatomy and physiology. He had done original research before on gallstones, on experimental valvular heart lesions in the dog, on the treatment of facial paralysis in man by anastomosis of the spinal accessory and facial nerves (1903). He had introduced new procedures, such as anaesthetic nerve blocking, leading to the use of local anaesthesia in brain surgery. He had worked in (Sir) Charles Scott Sherrington's (1857–1952) laboratory, when the latter was Professor of Physiology in Liverpool, where he participated in experiments on stimulation of the motor area of the brain in higher apes. Apart from his many contributions to brain surgery, his main work was directed – as already discussed – to the elucidation of the anatomy and functions of the pituitary gland by analysis and experiment, on the success of which his main claim to permanent fame will rest. His monograph, in 1912, *The Pituitary Body and its Disorders*[17], was by no means the end of the road. He continued his research, which led, eventually, to the description of pituitary basophilism[18]. Cushing first described the 'polyglandular syndrome' in 1912[17] (p. 217) and reviewed in detail a number of patients in his paper in 1938[18]. Cushing's syndrome is now defined as the symptoms and signs associated with prolonged exposure to inappropriately elevated plasma corticosteroid levels[19]. The syndrome is divided into two main groups, whether or not the condition is due to exposure to excessive adrenocorticotrophin (ACTH); if it be a pituitary-dependent bilateral adrenocortical hyperplasia (caused by excessive ACTH production in the pituitary), then the condition is conventionally called Cushing's Disease. Apart from iatrogenic and ectopic causes, Cushing's Disease can be regarded as the commonest cause of Cushing's syndrome (in 80% of the cases), but the basophilic adenoma could not be confirmed as the sole cause of the condition. In an independent investigation, the present writer found in a consequential series of 100 apparently-normal human pituitaries histological evidence of basophil micro-adenomas in 6% of the glands investigated in 1937–38 (unpublished)[20]. Among 1000 pituitaries examined in a routine manner, R. T. Costello found in 1935, 72, or 7.2% basophilic adenomas, half as many as the chromophobe adenomas and three and a half times more numerous than eosinophil celled adenomas[21]. W. Susman found 8% of basophil adenomas in 260 pituitaries, rather more frequent than other adenomas[22]; he, therefore, contested the anatomical basis of Cushing's pituitary basophilism.

Cushing was one of the outstanding personalities among the Americans on the endocrine stage at the beginning and during the first 40 years of the century. Aristocratic of appearance, of superb manners, he was a scholar, historian and connoisseur of the fine arts. He wielded a facile and elegant pen; his writings display an unique knowledge of the history of surgery. His *Life of Sir William Osler* is a model of medical biography – or any other for that matter – based on meticulous research and superb presentation[23]. As a book collector, he has also made a name for himself. As we have seen, he did not tolerate fools gladly, and even less did he accept impostors[6]. But, taken all in all, he was a great surgeon, a great teacher, a great medical man, of a generous nature, a great scholar and a great gentleman. For the students, medical and nursing staff of St. Bartholomew's Hospital in London, who were there at the time, he left an indelible impression when as a visiting professor of June 1922, he 'took over' the surgical professorial unit for two weeks from the then professor of surgery, George E. Gask and signed the register as the first 'Honorary Perpetual Student' of the Medical College of that hospital.

DAVID MARINE

David Marine (1880–1976) (see also pp. 254–255), the 'Nestor of Thyroidology', was quite a different type of man. Of French Huguenot descent and of farming stock, he was born at Whitleysburg, Maryland, in September 1880. He and his two younger sisters were orphaned when he was 7 years old. He continued to live on a farm of an aunt until, at 16, he entered Western Maryland College. There the emphasis was on history, literature, English, German and French. On entering Johns Hopkins University, he first studied zoology but soon switched to medicine (in 1901), and qualified in 1905. He had some celebrated teachers in the shape of (Sir) William Osler, William S. Halsted, John Jacob Abel, the pathologist William H. Welch and others. His first appointment was in the Department of Pathology at the Lakeside Hospital in Cleveland. On arrival there, he noticed

> many dogs with swollen necks. I . . . found that the swelling was due to the enlargement of the thyroid gland.[24]

Still under the influence of William Halsted and the latter's interest in thyroid surgery, he decided on the spot to take up that field of research. At that time, however, he had no research experience, experimental or otherwise; nor had he been to Europe, visiting medical centres of excellence, which he succeeded in doing several years later, when he worked with Emil Theodor Kocher, (1841– 1917) (see also pp. 248 and 249) in Bern and his colleague, Karl Wegelin, the expert pathologist in cretinism, during 1913–1914; but by that time, Marine was himself a mainly self-trained thyroid pathologist. The clinical care of thyroid patients he had learned from Dr. William Osler. He also became a voracious reader of scientific and medical literature, in which endeavour his (acquired) knowledge of German and French proved to be of great value. In the thyroid field he found, however, controversy and confusion, reading the works of Coindet, Chatin, von Fellenberg, Felix de Quervain (see also p. 255), and Frederic Rilliet. The latter reported frequent occurrence of hyperthyroidism following iodine treatment[25]. Theodor Kocher coined the sinister term 'Jod-Basedow' for it, in 1910.

Marine, as a scientist, developed four characteristics in his method of work: (a) every problem should be considered from many angles; (b) endemic goitre could not be understood without the study of the anatomy, physiology and pathology of the thyroid; (c) endemic goitre affects animals and man in the same manner; and (d) the effect of treatment in curative medicine is limited. (This was a view fairly generally held by medical representatives of that generation: 'Therapeutic nihilism' was by no means uncommon among the leaders of the profession at that time.) For that reason, prevention of endemic goitre is essential.

Marine next undertook an exhaustive study of the normal thyroid, its structure, anatomy, chemistry and physiology, in a wide range of animals, domestic and wild, and experimental thyroidectomies, partial and total, in dogs and puppies, and the feeding of iodine in varying doses. L. Tait had described a steplike enlargement of the thyroid in multiple pregnancies[26]; this goitre development was preventable by the administration of iodine. Transplants of many endocrine glands were carried out[27]. More than 250 auto- or homografts of thyroid lobes under the skin and in various organs were studied in rabbits from 1913 to 1916. Wherever implanted, thyroid autografts grew, synthesized hormone, and responded to lack of supplement of iodine. Much later (in 1934), thyrotrophin became available and stimulated the auto- and homografts in the guinea pig[28]. Marine came to the conclusion that the identical hyperplastic goitres in euthyroid dogs in Cleveland[28] and in hyperthyroid man[29] are both iodine deficient. After administration of iodine to dogs, the hyperplastic enlarged thyroid becomes a colloid goitre, which grows smaller and functions like a normal thyroid[30]; by inference, iodine should have the same effect on exophthalmic goitre. In 1911 and 1912, Marine recorded the pre-operative use of iodine in 15 patients with exophthalmic goitre[31,32], but it was left to Henry Stanley Plummer (1874–1937) to make this method popular, in 1923[33].

Marine regarded exophthalmic goitre the most common form of hyperthyroidism. This term was coined by George Dock, Professor of Medicine in Tulane, University of Louisiana, New Orleans (and before of Ann Arbor, Michigan) and was preferred by Marine to all other eponyms (see also p. 268). George Dock wrote a paper in 1908 entitled 'The development of our knowledge of exophthalmic goitre'[34]. His introductory remarks were:

> Historical details are not only of interest; they are also instructive. It is, therefore, worth while at times to reconsider them, and even to revise them according to the knowledge of the present. For historical facts, even when authenticated, do not look the same at different epochs, and medical, like political history, has various points of view.

He then discussed in detail the description of the disease described by a number of authors, whether they contributed in any manner to the development of the knowledge of exophthalmic goitre. Contrary to prevailing opinion, he did not find anything in Morgagni's writings suggesting exophthalmic goitre. He discussed Flajani's two patients (see also pp. 259–260), but came to the conclusion that those descriptions did not contribute anything essential towards the knowledge of exophthalmic goitre, but that Flajani's views on surgical treatment of goitre were of importance. Next, Dock discussed C. H. Parry's description (see p. 159) but felt that Parry turned out to be an observer rather than a generalizer, and that his conclusions were not convincing. Nor did Dock think that Graves' description marked a real progress towards the knowledge of exophthalmic goitre; it was only afterwards, when Stokes, and even more when Trousseau, analysed Graves' description that it became meaningful. In Dock's opinion, it was only von Basedow, who not only gave a complete account of the condition, but also drew the correct conclusions, and related the symptoms and signs. Moreover, he added later to the clear description of his patients, a report on the autopsy of such a patient. In his detailed analysis, Dock enumerates 21 eponyms given to the disease between 1835 and 1898.

Thus, the pursuit of Marine's work displays, and continues to display, his step by step exploration of all relevant facts and factors of the problem under analysis. For example, he measured the iodine content of the normal thyroid as well as in the hyperplastic and colloid goitres of dogs, sheep, cattle, hogs and fish. There were numerous investigations and experiments, gradually but inevitably leading up to the Akron experiment. Marine's studies of goitrogens in food became another milestone in the investigation of thyroid disorder. In 1924, in his Harvey Lecture, he said again that "goitre may develop because of relative iodine deficiency caused by the factors which interfere with absorption or utilization of iodine[35]."

Marine lived long enough to see the result of his work develop into an international attempt of goitre prophylaxis. He was a serious man who lived for his work. From 1905 to 1920 he was at the Cushing Laboratory for Experimental Medicine, Western Reserve University in Cleveland, Ohio. From 1920 to 1945 he was Chairman of the Department of Pathology and Director of the Research Laboratory at the Montefiore Hospital in New York, and at the same time Assistant Professor of Pathology at the Columbia University Medical School. He was successful and fortunate in being able to train and assemble a remarkable team of outstanding collaborators from the United States and from abroad. They were: C. H. Lenhart, W. W. Williams, J. M. Rogoff, O. T. Manley, S. H. Rosen, O. P. Kimball, E. J. Baumann, A. Cipra, A. W. Spence (from St. Bartholomew's Hospital, London) and J. Lerman, to name just a few. During the most active phase of his life, right up to the age of 65, he worked 7 days a week. After his retirement he spent his days on his cattle farm or in his garden.

The four main contributions Marine made to thyroid research have already been discussed (p. 255). He was a different personality from Cannon and from Cushing; but he was certainly one of the great American research workers in the endocrine field, whose achievements have had world wide repercussions.

JOHN JACOB ABEL

John Jacob Abel (1857–1938) hailed from Cleveland, Ohio. He was educated at the University of Michigan, but his studies were interrupted because he had to earn a living. This he did by teaching

Latin, mathematics, physics and chemistry at a high school at La Porte, Indiana, for three years. Eventually, he qualified in pharmacy in 1883 and then worked for a year at the Johns Hopkins. This was followed by seven years of 'Wanderjahre' at European universities. He studied anatomy, histology and embryology with Wilhelm His Senior (1831–1904), who was originally from Basel, but at that time Professor of Anatomy at Leipzig. Among His's many contributions to fundamental medicine, he is especially remembered for his classification of tissues based on histogenesis[36]. He also did original work on the ovaries of mammals[37], and became one of the greatest embryologists of his time. (His's 'bundle in the heart' was described by his son, Wilhelm His Junior (1863–1934). Abel learned physiology from Carl Friedrich Ludwig (1816–1895), pharmacology from Johann Ernst Oswald Schmiedeberg (1838–1921), Professor of Pharmacology at Dorpat (1871) and Strasbourg (from 1872), biochemistry from Edmund Drechsel (1834–1897) of the isolation of lysin fame, and from Ernst Felix Immanuel Hoppe-Seyler (1825–1895), who had obtained haemoglobin in crystalline form (in 1864). One of Hoppe-Seyler's pupils and assistants in Strasbourg was Joseph von Mering (1849–1908), whom we encountered, when relating his meeting with Oscar Minkowski (pp. 297–298). These and many other leading scientists became the mentors of young John J. Abel, who qualified as a doctor of medicine at the University of Strasbourg in 1888 and did a tour as a house physician in Vienna before returning to the United States in 1891. There, he became Professor of Pharmacology at the University of Michigan, but accepted a call from Johns Hopkins in Baltimore as Professor of Pharmacology in 1893, to remain there for the rest of his fruitful life.

On his return Abel brought home the new orientation from Europe towards hormone and enzyme research, using the most advanced methods of biochemistry. In the field of endocrinology, his greatest contributions were (1) the isolation of epinephrine, the active principle of the suprarenal medulla, which – together with Albert Cornelius Crawford (1869–1921), he succeeded in isolating as a chemically pure substance in 1897[1]; (2) the crystallization of insulin as a pure substance in 1926, with determination of its chemical composition and properties[38]; at that time, he was 69! He also worked on the elucidation of the function of the posterior pituitary (in 1923–24)[39,40]; he introduced plasmapaeresis, i.e. "Plasma removal with return of corpuscles", with L. G. Rowntree and B. B. Turner in 1914, a method of removing plasma from the living animal, with return of the corpuscles after washing and separation by centrifuging[41]. He investigated the toxins of *Amanita phalloides* together with William Webber Ford (1871–1941) in 1906[42].

Abel was an inspiring teacher and imaginative research worker, who used his thorough experience of European methods in his activities and had a profound influence on the shaping of the emergence of modern American teaching and research. In their paper 'On the blood-pressure-raising principle of the suprarenal capsule[1], Abel and Crawford said:

... There is therefore at present great diversity of opinion as to the chemical character of the blood-pressure-raising constituent of the gland. First, we have found by isolating the blood-pressure-raising constituent in the form of a benzoyl compound and decomposing it, that the active principle is a substance with basic characteristics and that it must in all probability be classed with the pyrrol compounds or with the pyridine bases or alkaloids ...

We have used sheep's glands in large quantity. The medullary substance of the fresh glands was scraped out, dried on the waterbath at 60°C, ground up finely, and extracted with ether for several days until the fats and the substance known as Manase's jecorin were removed. In this way a fine dry powder of a grayish white appearance is obtained, the aqueous extract of which is very active in raising the blood pressure.[1]

EDWARD CALVIN KENDALL

Whereas Cannon, Cushing, Marine and Abel were medical men, Edward Calvin Kendall (1886–1972) was trained as a chemist. He was born at South Norwalk, Connecticut and educated at Columbia University, where he proceeded to MS in 1909 and PhD in 1910. In the autumn of that year, he joined the firm of Parke, Davis & Co., where he was given the task of isolating the active principle of the thyroid. A year later, he joined the staff of St Luke's Hospital in New York, to settle down, eventually, as Professor of Physiological Chemistry at the Mayo Foundation in Rochester, Minnesota, in 1914, where he remained and became Emeritus Professor in 1951. It has already been told how Kendall obtained the crystals of thyroxine (see pp. 422–423) on Christmas Day 1914, and very nearly discovered tri-iodothyronine, as he believed that the thyroid contained a compound more active than thyroxine[43]. The isolation of thyroxine in 1914 was the second time that a pure hormone had been isolated; the first was the isolation of epinephrine (adrenaline) by John Jacob Abel and Albert Cornelius Crawford in 1897. Kendall and his team next turned their attention to the suprarenal cortex (the progress of research on the cortex was discussed on p. 477). Kendall, with H. L.

Mason, B. F. McKenzie, C. S. Myers and G. A. Koelsche, could report on 15 April 1934 at a meeting of the Research Club of the Mayo Clinic, that they had succeeded in isolating in crystalline form 'Cortin', $C_{20}H_{30}O_5$, "the hormone essential to life, from the suprarenal cortex; its chemical nature and its physiologic properties[44]". After reporting it again at a Clinic Staff Meeting on 25 April the essential sentences may be quoted from that paper:

> The isolation of a compound in pure crystalline form is of interest to the chemist, but is not of significance in medicine unless it possesses the essential physiologic activity. In this instance it may be said that administration of the crystalline product will maintain a dog in a normal condition after double suprarenalectomy.[45]

In 1936, E. C. Kendall, H. L. Mason, C. S. Myers, and W. D. Allers followed this with two papers[46,47] in which they recorded the isolation of nine closely related steroid hormones from adrenal cortex extracts, one of them being Compound E ($C_{21}H_{28}O_5$), which in 1939 was renamed 'Cortisone'.

Independently, T. Reichstein and Arthur Grollman (see p. 477), obtained crystals from adrenal cortical extracts, and so did Oscar Paul Wintersteiner (b. 1898) and Joseph John Pfiffner (b. 1903) (see pp. 476–477 and ref. 144 of Chapter 19) (with some limitations).

In 1949, Philip Showalter Hench (1896–1965) together with E. Kendall, C. H. Slocumb and H. F. Polley were able to report on the effect of a hormone of the adrenal cortex and of pituitary adrenocorticotrophic hormone (ACTH) on rheumatoid arthritis[48,49].

James Bertram Collip (1892–1965) of Toronto, with E. M. Anderson and D. L. Thomson, had isolated an impure 'adrenotropin' hormone containing the adrenocorticotrophic principle as early as 1933[50], but it was another ten years before Choh Hao Li (b. 1913), M. E. Simpson and H. M. Evans at Berkeley, California managed to isolate the pure hormone (ACTH) from sheep pituitary[51]. Independently of them, George Sayers (b. 1914) with A. White and C. N. H. Long at Yale, obtained ACTH from swine pituitaries[52].

In 1950, Kendall, Philip Showalter Hench and Tadeus Reichstein (b. 1897) shared the Nobel Prize for their work on adrenal cortical hormones. The three research groups isolated altogether 28 crystalline substances from the adrenal cortex, but only four of them were found to be biologically active.

In 1949, Hench had opportunity to observe the effects of jaundice and pregnancy on rheumatoid arthritis. As a result of these observations, he formed the opinion that rheumatoid arthritis was not primarily caused by infection but was more likely a metabolic disease. For that reason, Hench, Kendall and their collaborators decided, in 1949, to administer Compound E (cortisone) as one of the biologically active substances of the adrenal cortex to a number of patients with rheumatoid arthritis, with dramatic effect. They reported in the *Proceedings of the Mayo Clinics* as follows:

> ... In each of the 14 patients. ... Within a few days there was marked reduction of stiffness of muscles and joints, lessening of articular aching or pain on motion and tenderness, and significant improvement of articular and muscular function.[53]

Kendall thus showed a versatility as a research scientist which is quite remarkable in the much more restricted field of biochemistry than in that of clinical medicine. He was a dedicated and sincere character and well deserved the honours bestowed upon him.

PHILIP EDWARD SMITH

Philip Edward Smith (1884–1970) was born in De Smet in South Dakota and graduated a BS from Pomona College, obtaining a PhD in anatomy at Cornell in 1912. He then joined the Department of Anatomy of Berkeley, California, where he remained until 1926. The next year he spent as an anatomist at Stanford University. He accepted an invitation to become Professor of Anatomy at the College of Physicians and Surgeons at Columbia University in 1927, where he remained until his retirement in 1952. Afterwards he became a research associate at Stanford University, from where he published his last paper in 1963. His career and work represent especially the development of modern endocrinology in the United States.

Smith was a modest, silent, shy but kindly man, who developed an exceptional skill in hypophysectomy in the tadpole and the rat. He developed this difficult operation to a great perfection. As the most important method of investigation in endocrine research from 1925 onwards was the study of responses under varied conditions in hypophysectomized animals, his work became of paramount importance, and one of the most famous of his many papers was 'Hypophysectomy and replacement therapy in the rat'[54], which indicated the probable existence of a pituitary hormone controlling the secretion of the hormones of the adrenal cortex (in 1930). He demonstrated that hypophysectomy, or more correctly, removal of the anterior lobe, not only prevented further development of the adrenal glands but also caused actual regression of the cortex and atrophy of the thyroid and of the gonads. By transplants of active anterior pituitary tissue, Smith could show that these effects were cancelled. Smith's observations formed the basis of the search for the adrenocorticotrophic hormone which – as we have seen – succeeded, eventually, in 1943.

The other important pointer towards a new development in medical education was the fact that Philip E. Smith took a PhD in anatomy and became a Professor of Anatomy without having qualified as a medical man. This trend was particularly noticeable in the United States, but also in Britain, where Sir William Maddock Bayliss became Professor of General Physiology at University College, London, after switching from his original medical studies to a degree in physiology, proceeding to PhD. A similar line was taken by Professor Joseph Needham (b. 1900), whose studies in embryology are outstanding. The present trend of differentiation of salary scales between full-time clinicians in teaching hospitals in Britain and between the pre-clinical teachers, has strongly encouraged this development towards the teaching of anatomy, histology and physiology by non-medical people. This is in contrast to the usual arrangement on the Continent of Europe, although even there, there has been a steady increase in non-medical, but scientifically highly qualified teaching and research staff in the biochemical, nuclear, genetic and social aspects of medicine.

In his paper, in 1927, which was characteristic of his work, 'The disabilities caused by hypophysectomy and their repair'[55], Smith said:

> Hypophysectomy in the rat gives an invariable syndrome, the main features of which are: an almost complete inhibition in growth in the young animal, and a progressive loss of weight (cachexia) in the adult; an atrophy of the genital system with loss of libido sexualis, and in the female an immediate cessation of the sex cycles; an atrophy of the thyroids, parathyroids, and suprarenal cortex; and a general physical impairment characterized by a lowered resistance to operative procedures, loss of appetite, weakness and a flabbiness that readily distinguishes the hypophysectomised from the normal animal. It seems unlikely that they can live a normal life span.
>
> Attempts carried on for the last three years to secure a successful replacement therapy have proved successful as regards all the disabilities arising from hypophysectomy only when the fresh living hypophyseal tissue was administered. The gland material, secured from adult rats, was transplanted intramuscularly. Cushing and his co-workers have reported that pituitary transplantation prolonged the life of their hypophysectomised dogs.

HERBERT McLEAN EVANS

Herbert McLean Evans (1882–1971) was one of the leading figures on the endocrine stage in the first half of this century. In every respect he represented what is best of the American contribution: he was a medical scientist with a number of major achievements to his credit. He was one of the first to bridge the gap between research carried out single handed, or with one or two others, which was common before 1920, and the modern method of large teams in lavishly equipped laboratories.

Evans came from a well-to-do medical family; his father was a surgeon and his uncle Robert was Professor of Surgery and Dean of the University of California Medical School, founded in 1872. Like Herbert, he was a great book collector and a supporter of the opera and theatre. His mother and stepmother both had literary and artistic interests and kept open house. In fact, when Evans, who was born in Modesto, California, where his father practised, first entered the University in San Francisco, he took a regular Bachelor's degree, pursuing literary studies, geology, botany and the fine arts, before entering the California Medical School in 1904. He soon became disillusioned with the mainly clinical teaching and went East in 1905 to enrol at Johns Hopkins, at that period the leading Medical School, especially as far as scientific medicine was concerned.

An excellent and painstaking study of Evans' early years was published by J. D. Raacke of Boston University, in 1976[56], on which this part of the present account is greatly based. Evans soon decided that medical research was his line and not the clinical practice of medicine. This was a great disappointment to his father, who even at the height of Herbert's fame would refer to him as "my son, the rat doctor"[56].

At Johns Hopkins the German view was prevalent, of the importance of basic research and especially of chemical research. At a later age, he modified his views, but on qualifying in 1908, he did not do an internship, but took on a post as an instructor in anatomy. He soon began research in the laboratory of the Professor of Surgery, William Stewart Halsted (1852–1922), whose associate professor was, at that time, Harvey W. Cushing. From there he published, in 1907, three papers which were, however, not the first of his total of 607 papers published.

The first two dealt with the blood supply of the parathyroids and became important for parathyroid surgery; the third concerned the hypertrophy after resection of large intestinal blood-vessels. William Henry Welch (1850–1934), Professor of Pathology until 1916, who then became Professor in History of Medicine, encouraged Evans to participate in medico-historical topics. Evans also briefly met (Sir) William Osler (1849–1919). For the next seven years, Evans worked in the Department of Franklin Paine Mall (1862–1917), who was Professor of Anatomy at Johns Hopkins, and he rose from medical student to Associate Professor of Anatomy. From there he published two papers on the origin of the blood-vessels and lymphatics, which formed a major contribution of his final work. He also got involved in the study of 'vital dyes', first used by Paul Ehrlich in Germany, which stain living tissue without killing it. It seemed particularly important that these 'vital dyes' normally did not cross the blood–brain barrier, except in case of inflammation. By 1911, Evans applied for and received his first Rockefeller Research Grant (6 June 1911) from Simon Flexner, then director of the Rockefeller Institute. Flexner also gave him a grant for a trip to Europe, to visit a number of medical research centres. There, he had a frosty reception from Paul Ehrlich (1854–1915), then Professor of Experimental Therapeutics at the University of Frankfurt, but a better one from Edwin E. Goldmann (1862–1913), a South African, who was Professor of Surgery in Freiburg. Collaborating with a young chemist, Werner Schulemann, he produced a versatile cell dye, named 'Evans Blue', for the definition of macrophages as distinct cell types, to name only one use.

He returned from Germany and wrote a favourable report, especially on German work in basic sciences. He retained this opinion for the rest of his life and he returned there later on several occasions and encouraged his collaborators to visit German medical centres. By 1915, he had 27 important papers to his credit, and was also a research associate at the Department of Embryology at the Carnegie Institution at Washington, which was also located at the Medical School at Baltimore. At that time, he still did most of his work himself, rarely with a collaborator or co-author. He was popular in Baltimore and very happy there, during his 'golden years'.

The Department of Anatomy of the University of California at Berkeley (filled by acting appointments for a number of years) was a poor show compared with the Johns Hopkins. Yet, when Evans received an invitation to return as Chairman and Professor of Anatomy in 1915, he was "profoundly affected", and accepted. However, he did make certain, very carefully thought out, administrative and financial conditions; they were all accepted by the President of the University and by the Board. He could write to Harvey Cushing, now at Harvard:

The die is cast – California has been extremely generous to me. My proposals were met in a hearty spirit. I shall be happy to justify, if possible, their confidence. I feel I ought to go . . .[56].

In planning the shaping of his department, he himself was mainly concerned with research and attempted to organize the teaching, especially of gross anatomy, by securing the services of good associates. Thus, eventually, George Washington Corner (b. 1889) became assistant professor, Katherine J. Scott (1889–1975) instructor, while Dr. Robert O. Moody, who had been associate professor and acting chairman for several years, retained his post as associate. Philip E. Smith was instructor in anatomy, but so overburdened with teaching that his research activities were much curtailed.

With Dr. Katherine Scott, Evans did pioneer work on the relation of nutrition to the oestrous cycle, including the discovery of a dietary factor essential for reproduction[57]. This factor was isolated by Evans and his group 14 years later, in 1936, as Vitamin E[58]. Evans and his team also isolated Vitamin F[59], in 1934, although George Oswald Burr and Mildred M. Burr had already postulated the need of the body for some unsaturated acids in 1930[60].

In their short paper[57], Evans and Dr. Katherine Scott Bishop (as she now was called), had pointed out that rats fed on a diet of 'purified' protein, fat and carbohydrate, to which an appropriate amount of salt and vitamins (fat soluble A and water soluble B) had been added, would thrive, but would be sterile.

> The sterility of dietary origin yields a highly characteristic picture. Animals suffering from it do not differ so profoundly from normal ones in their ovarian function as they do in placental behaviour. Approximately the same number of Graafian follicles mature and rupture per ovulation and the ova are fertilised and implanted. The placentae are abnormal. They may persist almost throughout gestation, but show as early as the second day of their establishment, beginning blood extravasation which increase in extent. Resorption invariably overtakes the products of conception. Natural foodstuffs contain a substance X, which prevents such a sterility or which cures the disorder occasioned by the purified dietary regime. We have thus been able to witness a comparatively sudden restoration of fertility to animals of proven sterility, and whose controls continued sterile, by the administration of fresh green leaves of lettuce. . . .[57] (p. 650)

George Washington Corner was known to Evans as a medical student. He had also worked in Mall's laboratory and he went with Evans to Berkeley. This is not the place to elaborate on the career of this other great American endocrinologist in the field of reproduction; we have already referred to his main contribution in Chapter 18. It may suffice here to say that he was also an adept historian, as could be seen from his Sir Henry Dale Lecture for 1964, (see p. 398 and Chapter 18). He wrote a biography of Herbert McLean Evans[61]. He shared other tastes with Evans, particularly literary interests and book collecting.

Evans' and his group's other great achievement was the discovery and isolation of growth hormone[62], and the isolation of pituitary follicle-stimulating hormone (FSH)[63], in both of which ventures an important share goes to (Professor) Choh Hao Li, one of the important pupils and later collaborators of Evans. Before the isolation of growth hormone in 1945 and of FSH in 1949, Li, Evans and others isolated the interstitial cell stimulating (luteinizing) hormone in 1940[64], which achievement was followed in 1943, by the same group, by the isolation of the adrenocorticotrophic hormone, as already mentioned[51].

Here we must pause, to make a few pertinent remarks. Firstly, it is noteworthy how successful and perhaps fortunate Evans was in the selection of his collaborators, who were of the highest calibre, many of whom achieved great and deserved fame, such as Corner, P. E. Smith and Li, to name but a few. Secondly, that Evans managed to attract women as co-workers, like Mrs. Scott Bishop, and Miriam Simpson. Thirdly, that James B. Collip of Toronto had isolated an impure form of adrenocorticotrophic hormone as early as 1933[50] (see p. 517). Li, Evans and Simpson obtained the pure ACTH from sheep pituitaries; this work was based on Philip E. Smith's fundamental anatomical studies in 1930, to which we have already referred[54] (see p. 519). In their paper, Li, Evans and Simpson declare:

> In order to establish the biological characteristic of a hormone from a complex source such as the pituitary, it must first be isolated in pure form judged both by *chemical* and *biological* data. The present paper presents a method for the isolation of the adrenocorticotrophic hormone which is freed from other active contaminants and behaves chemically as a single substance. . . .
> The importance of a sensitive assay method for the isolation of a hormone hardly needs to be emphasised. . . . The use of hypophysectomised rats in assay of the hormone have allowed the reliable detection of small quantities of the hormone. . . .[51]

To continue, we must note the arrival into endocrine research of a new and most important factor: the demand and ability to measure exactly newly-isolated hormones by bio-assay and – more recently – by radio-immuno-assay methods. Finally, we must take note of the two new facets of modern research in endocrinology: the emergence of team investigations in super-laboratories, which Evans realized and to which he skilfully switched soon after his arrival at Berkeley. In fact, he was one of the prime movers in establishing there, in 1930, the Institute for Experimental Biology, of which he became director. The other point that emerged was the fact that with the creation of several research centres of excellence, but without proper communication or, occasionally, with the existence of a strong competition between such centres, the same or similar results are obtained at two or more centres simultaneously. This occurred, as we have just seen, in the case of the isolation of pure adrenocorticotrophic hormone, when George Sayers (b. 1914), A. White and C. N. H. Long at Yale in New Haven, Connecticut, succeeded in isolating ACTH from hog pituitaries at the same time as Li, Evans and Simpson[52]. Sayers said in the concluding pages of his paper, which was published in the same volume of the *Journal of Biological Chemistry* as Li, Evans and Simpson's paper[51]:

> Although the pure adrenotrophic preparation which has been examined in some detail in the present study has been obtained from hog pituitary glands, highly purified fractions of adrenotrophic hormone have also been obtained from bovine and sheep pituitaries. Preliminary studies of these preparations suggest that they are similar to, if not identical with the product obtained from hog glands. This observation has been supported by personal conversations with Dr. C. H. Li, who has stated that the pure adrenotrophic hormone prepared from sheep glands has many properties identical with those reported here for the hormone obtained from hog pituitaries.[52]

In 1945, Choh Haoh Li and H. M. Evans published their paper on 'Isolation and properties of the anterior pituitary growth hormone'[65], which was followed by the preparation of the crystalline (growth) hormone[66].

Why did Herbert Evans not become a Nobel laureate? This is a question which has been asked by a number of people. It was also discussed by Raacke[56]. Evans' activities as a book collector were recorded by Jacob I. Zietlin, *Herbert M. Evans: pioneer collector of rare books in the history of science*[67]. Regrettably, Evans developed a certain sarcastic trait towards the latter half of his long life, which alienated some of his friends and admirers; but without any doubt, he was one of the greatest American research workers in endocrinology in recent times.

FULLER ALBRIGHT

We discussed some of the important contributions of Fuller Albright (1900–1969) to endocrinology in the previous chapter (see pp. 486–487), and also some of his antics. He graduated MD from Harvard in 1924 and taught there from 1930 to 1956. During his

European travels, he spent a happy year with Jacob Erdheim, the pathologist, in Vienna whom he held in great esteem; he quoted Erdheim's sayings in his celebrated lecture on 'Some of the "Do's" and "Do-nots" in clinical investigation', given in Atlantic City in 1944[68]. His boyish appearance belied his age for a long time. His sense of humour was as famed as were his scientific achievements, but it was a puckish sense of fun without any malice and often directed against himself. His freedom from authority included his own authority. Although many believed that he did not tolerate contradiction, this view was fallacious. His method of work often started from a clinical picture, from which he proceeded to explain each symptom and sign logically, step by step. He would then formulate a theory to explain the unknown elements and each of its possible consequences, leading, eventually, to his famous charting of 'the sequence-of-events'. Progress could be made only (a) by formulating a precise theory, and (b) by challenging that theory. If he could find no one to challenge the theory he had evolved, he would do it himself. His preference was for clinical investigation; but – as he said –

> I think of a clinical investigator as one trying to ride two horses, attempting to be an investigator and a clinician at one and the same time. Whereas such an equestrian manoeuvre is usually considered a bad policy, in this case, probably because of two considerations in particular, experience has shown that it is a very fruitful pastime. In the first place, the ultimate goal of most investigations is to find something of benefit to the human race; where, other than by the bedside of sick patients, could one find so many suggestions of things to be investigated? Secondly, in many instances, nature has arranged an experiment in a sick individual and partly completed; all that is needed are the eyes of the clinician to make certain observations and interpret them. The rider of two horses, however, must remember that there are two horses; he may avoid the danger on one side if he, as a clinician, be swamped with patients and the equal danger on the other side that he, as an investigator, be segregated entirely from the bedside. . . . Let me add one additional point: an intelligent patient, private or otherwise, to whom you have taken the trouble to explain the nature of the investigation, makes the best laboratory animal. . . . Some people can look at a problem and never see that there is a problem; in the words of the late Professor Jakob Erdheim (with whom I spent a very profitable year), 'Die Augen sind gut, aber sie schauen nicht an.' (= "The eyes are good but they do not look at things").[68]

In the 1930s, he developed Parkinsonism, but he carried on his scientific work and tried to ignore his illness. In 1956, he felt that the disease was affecting his thought-processes. He therefore decided to

A HISTORY OF ENDOCRINOLOGY

PROCEEDINGS OF THE THIRTY-SIXTH ANNUAL MEETING OF THE AMERICAN SOCIETY FOR CLINICAL INVESTIGATION HELD IN ATLANTIC CITY, N. J., MAY 8, 1944

READ BEFORE THE SCIENTIFIC SESSION

PRESIDENTIAL ADDRESS

SOME OF THE "DO'S" AND "DO-NOT'S" IN CLINICAL INVESTIGATION

By FULLER ALBRIGHT

When your President and Council decided to hold this meeting, they had to ask themselves the following question put to them by the Office of Defense Transportation in Washington: Is this meeting likely to contribute to the over-all war effort? I, for one, and I think I speak for the majority of the Councillors, had no hesitation in answering the question in the affirmative. All knowledge is interrelated; in times of stress the most scientific nation has a big advantage. Surely a society like ours, where year in and year out some of the most important advances in medicine have first come to the light of day, should carry on through the present unpleasantness. Moreover, with so many of our colleagues scattered over the 7 seas, a big responsibility accrues to us who are left to keep the home fires burning in respect to clinical investigation.

It is perhaps a presumptive symptom of an oncoming intellectual menopause,—indeed, one might say it is evidence of a Young Turk becoming an Old Turk,—when one endeavours to lay down certain precepts for success in a field. It is probably fortunate that no one follows such precepts anyway, that each prefers to learn his own way, though this be the hard way. Be all this as it may, as I look around at those of our colleagues who have attained success in the field of clinical investigation and analyze what methods they have used, I see certain recommendations or "Do's" which may be worth jotting down; furthermore, as I look further, especially into my own past, I see certain "Do-not's" which may be equally worthwhile jotting down as practices to be avoided. I won't attempt to define "success." I do not necessarily mean academic recognition; I do not necessarily mean self-satisfaction; I just mean success.

First let me insert a short digression on what is meant by "clinical investigation." I recently had the pleasure of sitting in on a discussion in which our editor-in-chief, Dr. James L. Gamble, deplored the term "sub-clinical" used in the sense of "pre-symptomatic"; Dr. Chester S. Keefer, who was present, enlarged on this theme and pointed out that "clinical" is derived from the Greek word "klinikos" meaning bed, and that "sub-clinical" (a Latin-Greek hybrid) literally means "under-the-bed." Since animals do not sleep in beds it is quite clear that "clinical investigation" has primarily to do with the investigation of sick people, and is concerned only secondarily, if at all, with sick laboratory animals. But more of that in a minute.

I think of a clinical investigator as one trying to ride two horses,—attempting to be an investigator and a clinician at one and the same time. Whereas such an equestrian manoeuver is usually considered a bad policy, in this case, probably because of two considerations in particular, experience has shown that it is a very fruitful pastime. In the first place, the ultimate goal of most investigation is to find something of benefit to the human race; where, other than by the bedside of sick patients, could one find so many suggestions of things to be investigated? Secondly, in many instances, nature has arranged an experiment in a sick individual and partly completed it; all that is needed are the eyes of the clinician to make certain observations, and the background of the investigator to plan other observations and interpret them.

This rider of two horses, however, must remember that there are two horses; he must avoid the danger on one side that he, as a clinician, be swamped with patients and the equal danger on the other side that he, as an investigator, be segregated entirely from the bedside. In his laboratory, necessarily easily accessible to the wards, his clinical half will be constantly interrupted by such messages as that Mr. Humpty-Dumpty has had a big fall. As a result, his investigative half will find that he cannot compete with the straight non-clinical investigators as regards animal or smoked-drum experiments. To answer a vital question, where such technics are necessary, it is often preferable that he persuade one of his non-clinical colleagues to carry out the observations. You can all look around you and see many examples where a good clinician has gone to the laboratory to get the answer to a question and has gotten it,—more power to him. All I am trying to say is that, if you have acquired the difficult technic of being a fair clinician, you had better use this technic in your clinical investigation.

Let me add one additional point: an intelligent patient, private or otherwise, to whom you have taken the trouble to explain the nature of the investigation, makes the best laboratory animal.

I would not feel quite right addressing this Society without presenting one of what Dr. James H. Means has termed, because of the arrows, my St. Sebastian diagrams. Accordingly, I have arranged one such (Figure 1), depicting the "Do's" and the "Do-not's" which one must pass by in climbing the road which leads to the Castle of Success in Clinical Investigation. You will note that the road is formed by the amalgamation of two paths,

Figure 71   First page of "Do's and Do-not's" by Fuller Albright [by kind permission of the Royal Society of Medicine, London]

undergo chemopallidectomy, which was not successful. He remained an invalid and was for many years, until his death in December 1969, permanently an in-patient at the Massachusetts General Hospital, faithfully looked after by his wife.

He had always stressed (and this was No. 9 of his do-not's), . . .

See to it that you do not wake up some fine morning in an executive capacity. Do not show too much administrative ability. The first time you are asked to serve on a committee, be anything but efficient. Never make the mistake of proposing a new reform; you are apt to be chosen as a committee of one to put said reform through. The desk of the good executive should be clear; that of an investigator should be littered. . . . Whatever else you do, do not become a Professor of Medicine, or the head of a department. Let me make it clear that I do not deprecate the good executive. . . .

And the last of his 'Do's', No. 10:

Do try to reserve some time during the day when you can do some unadulterated thinking. If you salvage a few minutes, you will be doing better than most. . . . Last Lap. . . . Well, you do the 'Do's' and you do not do the 'Do-not's'; you arrive at the door of the Castle of Success. You still need the key to open the door. The key stands for personal equation. 'But personality does not count in pure science', you say. That may be true, but clinical investigation is not a pure science.[68] (pp. 925–926)

In 1961, chronically ill, he accepted the title of Professor of Medicine 'emeritus' at Harvard Medical School. He had been President of the Endocrine Society in 1946–47, and received many honours and medals. In 1965 he was made an Honorary DSc at Harvard University. In 1949, he received the Borden award of the American Association of Medical Colleges for 'monumental contributions'.

In 1928, Albright and his collaborators carried out a number of balance studies concerned with calcium, phosphorus, the bones and the parathyroids. In 1929, he wrote up all these studies, "even the ones he did not, in the end, co-author!" The result was a spate of papers which not only formed the basis for the understanding of parathyroid physiology, but also took the balance technique out of the realm of nutrition and established it as 'solid' scientific methodology. The papers also provided strong support for the new *Journal of Clinical Investigation*, then in its sixth year. The great number of papers that followed had in common the refinement of clinical investigation as an instrument of quantitative analysis. There were studies which showed a 'primary' effect of parathyroid hormone on bone as well[69]. The 'sequence' led, for example, to the first clear

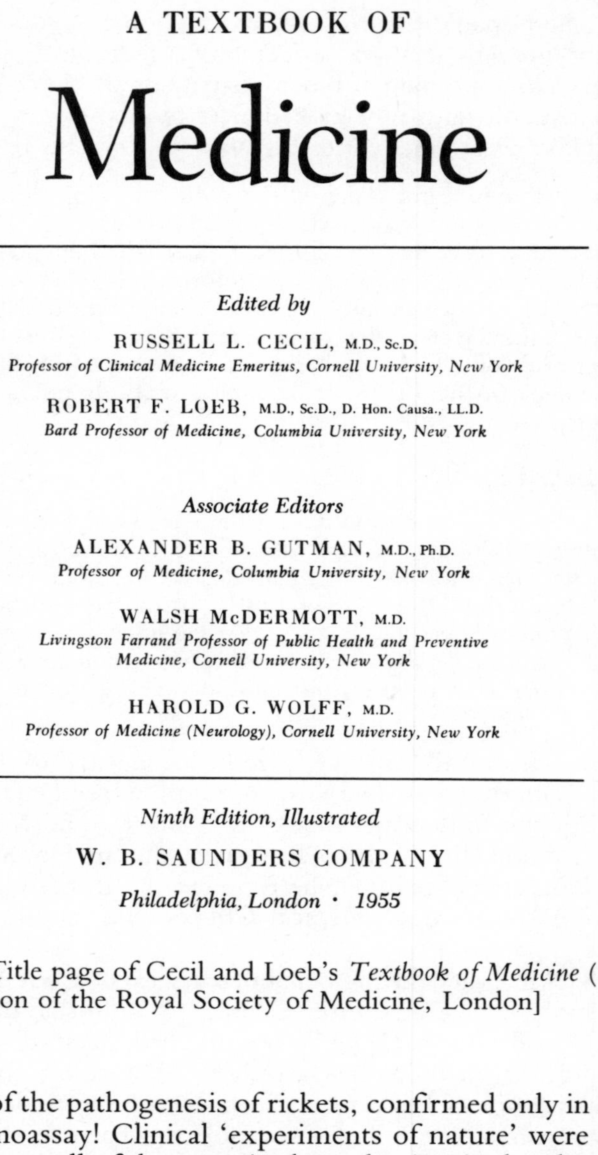

A TEXTBOOK OF

Medicine

Edited by

RUSSELL L. CECIL, M.D., Sc.D.
Professor of Clinical Medicine Emeritus, Cornell University, New York

ROBERT F. LOEB, M.D., Sc.D., D. Hon. Causa., LL.D.
Bard Professor of Medicine, Columbia University, New York

Associate Editors

ALEXANDER B. GUTMAN, M.D., Ph.D.
Professor of Medicine, Columbia University, New York

WALSH McDERMOTT, M.D.
*Livingston Farrand Professor of Public Health and Preventive
Medicine, Cornell University, New York*

HAROLD G. WOLFF, M.D.
Professor of Medicine (Neurology), Cornell University, New York

Ninth Edition, Illustrated

W. B. SAUNDERS COMPANY

Philadelphia, London · 1955

Figure 72 Title page of Cecil and Loeb's *Textbook of Medicine* (1955) [by kind permission of the Royal Society of Medicine, London]

description of the pathogenesis of rickets, confirmed only in 1969, by radio–immunoassay! Clinical 'experiments of nature' were the substrate for almost all of the organized attacks, inspired and systematic (not primarily on disease, but "rather through physiology to disordered physiology of disease"[70]). Practical applications of his discoveries in the fields of metabolism, bone diseases, kidney disorders and ovarian dysfunction, were the use of corticosteroids in asthma, the postmenopausal use of female gonadal hormones, and the treatment of rickets with massive doses of Vitamin D (in the 1930s).

528

In 1937, he described polyostotic fibrous dysplasia, also named Albright's Syndrome[71]. It is a polyostotic type of vascular fibrous tissue replacement of normal bone, scattered throughout the skeletal structure with skin pigmentation and sexual precocity, predominantly occurring in females. Occasionally goitre and hyperthyroidism also occur. Fuller Albright has certainly left his mark on the development of modern endocrinology in general and on American endocrinology in particular. On the humorous side, we have mentioned (see pp. 398–399) his outbursts against the use of history in medicine. The title-page of the 9th edition of Cecil and Loeb's *Textbook of Medicine* of 1955, and Fuller Albright's 'Introduction' to the chapter on the 'Diseases of the Ductless Glands' are included here, just to give the flavour of his humour and his prejudices. It is sad that great men today seem to be less colourful personalities.

OTHER AMERICAN ENDOCRINOLOGISTS

To these few sketches, many more could be added. If Fuller Albright used to stress his opposition to the introduction of history into medicine – perhaps in the hope that his views should be challenged – some of his contemporaries like George Washington Corner were accomplished historians. His lecture on 'The Discovery of the Mammalian Ovum' to the Mayo Foundation in 1933 has become a classic medical historical paper[72]. It covered the works of Aristotle, Herophilus, Galen, Fallopius, Fabricius, William Harvey (who reported his findings to Charles I), Jan Swammerdam, Regner de Graaf and Swammerdam's bitter, though unjustified attack on de Graaf, claiming priority for originating the idea that the female testis is an ovary), van Leeuwenhoek, Albrecht von Haller, Cruikshank (linked with William Hunter), J. L. Prévost and J. B. Dumas (of Geneva) and, eventually, Carl Ernst von Baer. Finally, in 1843, Martin Barry who could observe a spermatozoon inside the ovum, although the union of the two gametes was first demonstrated by Wilhelm August Oscar Hertwig (1849–1922)[73].

There was Oscar Riddle (1877–1968), born and brought up on a farm near Cincinnati, Indiana, the seventh of nine children. His father died when he was five and he had to work hard to get through college, From 1899 to 1901 he taught biological subjects in Spanish at a new school in San Juan, Puerto Rico. He eventually graduated BA of the University of Louisiana at Bloomington. After six months in Chicago, he had to teach in a High School for two and a half years before returning to the Department of Zoology of the University in

Diseases of the Ductless Glands

INTRODUCTION

The author will not write the conventional introduction. He will not give the Greek derivation for the word "hormone," coined by Starling; he will not discuss the experiments of Claude Bernard which led to the concept of an internal secretion; he will not delve into the earliest beginnings of endocrinology which had as their *raisons d'être* such ends as the procurement of a form of manpower safe for the harem, the salvaging of a male soprano voice for the choir, the increased palatability that a rooster attains when he turns into a capon, and so on. He will not trace experimental endocrinology from 1849, when Berthold studied the effect of the gonads on the secondary sex characteristics of fowl, for the next hundred years down to 1949, when attention was focused on cortisone and its pituitary stimulator, adrenocorticotrophic hormone (ACTH). But why mention such prosaic facts in 1955 when we are well into the schizo-atomic era and rapidly approaching, the author fears, the posthistoric era? It would be more in keeping to mention that a pellet of stilbestrol can now replace pregnancy as a promoter of lactation in cows. No, the author will not even list the names of describers of various endocrine syndromes—from Addison with Addison's disease in 1855, down past the almost simultaneous elucidation of hyperparathyroidism in 1926 both by Mandel and by Du Bois to—well—to whom? The author thinks of no recent unmasking of a new syndrome. Are we leaving an era behind?

Instead, he will discuss what endocrinology is, with special emphasis on what endocrinology is not, and then will comment on certain other aspects of the subject.

What Endocrinology Is. Endocrinology is an indivisible division of internal medicine and has to do with certain glands or tissues which secrete highly specific substances into the blood stream for use by other tissues. The only important thought in this definition is contained in the word "indivisible." It is impossible to separate endocrinology from internal medicine; by the same token it is im-

possible to be an endocrinologist without being an internist. The physician who calls himself an endocrinologist and confines his interest to such unfortunate members of society as might appear in the sideshow of a circus, never realizes that pneumonia, a broken leg and a bad burn involve important changes in adrenal cortical function (cf. "Alarm Reaction" of Selye), that the disturbance in homeostasis occasioned by chronic renal insufficiency is ameliorated by a secondary hyperparathyroidism, that the somatotrophic action of testosterone propionate may be made use of in many conditions other than male hypogonadism, and so on.

The author resents the tendency to limit the scope of endocrinology to those disorders of the internal secretions which are not clearly understood. Thus, once some division of endocrinology such as diabetes is put on a firm footing, it is removed from the section on endocrinology to the section on metabolic diseases.

What Endocrinology Is Not. Certain conditions often considered to be endocrinologic are probably not so at all.

First, in order of frequency, comes the fat boy who is slightly late in sexual development and whose genitalia are obscured by excess of fat. This patient, nine times out of ten, is labeled as having Fröhlich's syndrome, whereas in point of fact he is just a fat boy, whatever that is. If left alone, he will develop normally sexually and frequently will cease to be fat after puberty. True Fröhlich's syndrome is exceedingly rare and difficult to diagnose before the normal age of onset of puberty.

Then there comes the child who does not do well in school. There is a feeling among would-be progressive educators that such a situation demands a survey by an endocrinologist. In the author's experience there is only one endocrine abnormality which leads to mental retardation, namely, cretinism. The diagnosis of this condition is a problem for the obstetrician and the pediatrician, not for the endocrinologist. If it is not made in the first few weeks or, at the most, months of life, the damage is already done, and one might just as well not make the diagnosis. Paren-

Figure 73 Diseases of the ductless Glands: Introduction by Fuller Albright (in Cecil and Loeb's *Textbook of Medicine*, 1955) [by kind permission of the Royal Society of Medicine, London]

Chicago. He proceeded to PhD in 1907, his main interest being the study of the anatomy and physiology of birds. He then went to Europe on a travelling fellowship. While he was overseas, his chief in Chicago, Professor Whitman, died. On his return, Riddle joined the laboratories of the Carnegie Institution of Washington, Department of Genetics, at Cold Spring Harbor, where he remained for 35 years, except for a year as Captain in the U.S. Army Sanitary Corps during World War I. His special interest remained the anatomy, genetics and physiology of birds; on the occasion of a somewhat heated discussion at an endocrine meeting, an angry George W. Corner referred to him as "that avian physiologist"! Riddle identified prolactin as the pituitary hormone controlling the secretion of pigeon's milk (see Chapter 14), and helped to establish an assay for its measurement in 1933. His last paper on the subject was published in 1963, when he was 86 years of age (see Chapter 14, p. 197). Evidence of the co-ordination of various specialties in the field of endocrinology, as mentioned in Dr. Lawson Wilkins' Presidential Address in 1957 (see p. 507), was Riddle's active participation in The Endocrine Society, the President of which he was in 1928–29.

Of the Canadians, we have already mentioned Banting, Best and James Bertram Collip (1892–1965). The latter was born at Belleville, Ontario, and studied chemistry at the University of Toronto, where he became a BA in 1912, and PhD in Biochemistry in 1916. He eventually became Professor of Biochemistry at McGill University in 1928 and was Dean of the Medical Faculty of the University of Western Ontario from 1947 to 1961. His important works on the purification of insulin (1922/23), and on the isolation of parathormone in 1925 of the (impure) adrenotrophic hormone in 1933 (see also pp. 485, 517, Chapter 19) have already been mentioned.

Another, somewhat later development has to be fitted into this chapter. We have seen that the beginning of new ideas on hormonal control and prevention of conception originated in Austria in the 1920s (Haberlandt and Fellner; see Chapter 19). These attempts were overlooked, forgotten and not followed up. Haberlandt died young, in 1932, and Fellner disappeared without trace after the fall of Austria to Hitler. It was the Americans who started afresh and brought the idea of hormonal contraception to an effective and practical conclusion. Moreover, in contrast to Haberlandt's and Fellner's experiments, they succeeded in obtaining hormonal contraception by giving hormones by mouth. The search for oral substances to prevent pregnancy has been going on since the publication of the *Book of Changes* in China in 2736 BC. Throughout the ages, it was mainly the taking of dangerous metals, mercury, lead, copper and iron sulphates (?the content of the mysterious 'misy'), which were used; later also arsenic, strychnine and iodine (in the nineteenth century), and even castor oil were used.

We have already seen that in the 1950s new progress was achieved in the United States in the field of physiological contraception, without awareness of the work of Haberlandt and Fellner. In 1951, Dr. Gregory Pincus, the 'Father of the Pill' (see also p. 448), knew that progesterone is increased in the blood at the time of implantation of the fertilized ovum in the womb and prevents the release of further ova from the ovary. He fed, experimentally, a calculated dose of progesterone to female rabbits who were then put together with males of proved fertility. If a dose of more than 5 mg progesterone had been given, not one litter was produced. After further prolonged trials on rabbits and rats, Dr. Pincus selected in 1952, with the co-operation of Dr. John Rock, then Director of the Fertility Clinic of the Free Hospital for Women in Brooklyn, a number of women volunteers. Progesterone was administered orally over a given period of time; the results were sufficiently significant to pursue the line of research, although one in five showed an unsatisfactory response to progesterone itself. Four years later a synthetic substance was eventually manufactured, which was named norethynodrel. It was established that – given orally in a smaller dose – it would produce temporary infertility in quite a high proportion of women. In April 1956, a large scale field trial was organized by Dr. Pincus, using 'Enavid', produced by G. D. Searle Ltd., which contained norethynodrel. First, it was in Rio Piedras in San Juan, Puerto Rico; a second area was set up in Rumaco in 1957; in December 1957, a third testing area was created in Haiti. Social workers took charge of small groups of volunteers, to ascertain that the pills were taken regularly and the course finished. A careful protocol was kept by means of detailed live questionnaires of the progress of the experiments, concerning side-effects, frequency of sexual contacts, the menstrual cycle and other relevant variables.

In 1965, Dr. Gregory Pincus summarized the position (and his own achievement) in his book *The Control of Fertility*[74], still, apparently, unaware of the work of Haberlandt and Fellner on the hormonal control of fertility. In his "over 1400 citations of experimental investigation", which does not cover the whole story, "for in order to assess and select only the publications most pertinent to the subject matter of this book I have examined more than twice this number[74]".

A major German work by Juergen Haller, Professor of Obstetrics and Gynaecology in Goettingen, was first published in the same year: *Ovultationshemmung durch Hormone*[75]. Its third edition of 1971 was translated into English by Herbert Gottfried, PhD, under the title *Hormonal Contraception*[76]. In this work, one early paper of 1921 by Haberlandt is quoted as follows:

> Chapter II. The Inhibition of Ovulation. The Historical Development of a New Method: Inhibition of Ovulation by Hormones. . . . The first observations concerning the temporary inhibition of ovulation by hormones were reported by Haberlandt in 1921; transplantation of ovaries from pregnant animals into sexually mature animals of the same species resulted in temporary sterility of the recipients bearing the transplants. This action was attributed to the large quantities of corpus luteum hormone present in the transplanted ovaries.[76] (p. 17)

Although the book contains 1043 references, the work of Otfried O. Fellner (see Chapter 19) is not mentioned. Much later clinical observations are quoted, by W. Bickenbach and E. Paulikovics in 1944 on 'Hemmung der Follikerlreifung durch Progesteron bei der Frau' (= inhibition of the maturation of the follicle in woman by progesterone)[77], and W. von Massenbach: 'Ueber die unzweckmaessige Anwendung von Corpus-luteum-Hormonen' (= on the inappropriate use of corpus-luteum-hormones) in 1941[78], and by others, which "led to the concept during the 1930s and 1940s that sustained progesterone administration early in the cycle led to a blockade of gonadotrophin secretion and in this way inhibited ovulation"[76] (p. 17).

Gregory Pincus, of the Worcester Foundation for Experimental Biology at Shrewsbury, Massachusetts, published his studies on mammalian fertilization and ovum maintenance, *The Eggs of Mammals*, in 1936[79]. He also managed to obtain rabbit ova in sufficient numbers for experimental work, by stimulating ovaries by administration of gonadotrophic hormones[80]. From a number of such studies by Pincus and his group, and a number of contemporaries, especially in the United States and after 1951, it emerged that there was a possibility of the control of fertility by manipulation of the hormonal environment of the ovum, but the fact (known to Fellner, see p. 451) that oestrogen could prevent ovulation, not only escaped Pincus at that stage (1936), but he and R. E. Kirsch "specifically found (and stated) that estrogen did not prevent ovulation in the rabbit"[74, (p. 4),81].

Although Makepeace, A. W., Weinstein, G. L. and Friedman, M. H. reported in 1937 that progesterone effectively inhibited ovulation in the rabbit – again ignorant of Haberlandt and Fellner – "the logical extension of this observation into a more intensive study of the progesterone action . . . were not reported by us (G. Pincus and M. C. Chang), until 1953"[82]. The reason for this "Latent period of 16 years" was given by Pincus as a shift of interest to studies of adrenocortical function, particularly in relation to physical and mental stress, due to special demands of 'war' research, which was continued for a number of years afterwards. The return to the original line of study with an increasing activity in that field, was attributed by Pincus to two factors: (1) to a visit from Mrs. Margaret Sanger in 1951, and (2) to "the emergence of the appreciation of the importance of the 'population explosion' "[74] (p. 6). Mrs. Sanger was the president of the International Planned Parenthood Federation, and was hoping that a relatively simple and fool-proof method of birth control would be developed through scientific research. The impetus on research by the appreciation of the population explosion was described by Pincus in the August 2nd issue of the *Washington Post* in 1956. Of the many problems following such a request, Pincus said:

> ... the job of the scientist is to undertake experimentation and to publish the results of such experimentation. What happens thereafter is allegedly not his business.

This concept has been dealt demoralizing blows during and since World War II. The rapid transition from the world-wide application of significant discovery has demanded the attention of the scientist to two consequences of his activity ... Willy-nilly, the investigator has had to be also an educator (of fellow scientists, of students, of public health servants, etc.). Secondly ... the research workers' talents have been invoked not only in helping to make sure that the public is properly informed and not grossly misinformed, but also to consider the questions of policy that are inevitably raised with the application of scientific discovery[74] (p. 7).

Although Pincus' book has remained the magnum opus, which covers especially the field of research which he and his numerous collaborators so skilfully and diligently expanded, an explosion of literature on the subject has taken place, parallel to the size of the population explosion in so many parts of the world. This is not only due to the fact that hormonal oral contraception has grown within the short time of only a few years into hundreds of millions of contraceptive pills being manufactured and consumed in all five continents of the globe. The field has not remained limited to the inhibition of ovulation only, but has also been concerned with the role of the semen and with the justifiable hope that a male counterpart of an effective contraceptive pill may also be available soon. In addition, a number of other methods of birth control were studied and assessed, such as ligature of the vas, of the tubes, intrauterine devices and other methods. The side effects of all these attempts at controlling conception created another spate of scientific literature on the side effects. These are not only physical, such as venous thrombosis, but also alleged mental and emotional effects, depression, loss of libido, and those which may cause changing values in the society one lives in, such as promiscuity and the increased danger of sexually transmitted diseases. Proof of this development is also the increasing number of special symposia on the subject. The Nobel Foundation began to organize a series of Nobel Symposia on topics of world importance in the 1960s, and the Fifteenth was held in May 1970, at Sødergarn, Lidingø, Sweden, on 'Control of Human Fertility' with Ulf Borell and Egon Diczfalusy as organizers and editors of the Proceedings. Similar recurrent 'Physicians' Conferences' have been held on the 'Progress in Conception Control' in the United States.

In Britain, the Council for Investigation of Fertility Control began to conduct trials in 1959. To begin with, small scale studies were carried out by Dr. Gerald I. M. Swyer of University College, London, and by Dr. Margaret Jackson of Crediton, Devon. The preparation used was 'Conovid'.

In the trials in the United States it emerged that the results from Puerto Rico were different from those in Los Angeles. In the first year of the trial, 20% of the women had withdrawn from the experiment in Puerto Rico; in California the withdrawal rate was 66%. The side-effects depended on the preparation used. One group concerned menstrual disturbances. There were changes in the menstrual cycle, or the period began before the end of the twenty-day course of tablets ('break-through bleeding'), or even failure of withdrawal bleeding after the course was finished. The subjective side-effects of the early trials were nausea, especially in the first cycle, but later declining; breast discomfort in about 25–30% of the volunteers, and transient fluid retention. The most important complications of oral contraceptive drugs have turned out to be venous thrombosis, leading occasionally to pulmonary thrombo-embolism; rarer, arterial thrombosis in the cerebral or coronary vessels; hypertension and hyperlipidaemia. These depend on the preparation used and on the amount of the hormone content. Today, three main types are in use. 1. Sequential preparations: an oestrogen is taken for two weeks of the cycle, to which is added a progestogen for a further week; they are followed by a withdrawal bleeding, thus closely simulating the phase of a normal menstrual cycle. 2. A combined oestrogen and progesterone preparation is taken for 21 days; the last week there is no therapy, followed by withdrawal bleeding. 3. Progestogen only preparations. It was found that reduction of the oestrogen content below 50 micrograms or even to 30 micrograms reduced the complication of venous thrombosis considerably, without interfering too much with the contraceptive action. In patients where even oestrogen-free pills constitute a risk, other methods have to be used including intrauterine devices (I.U.D.), which have been in use much longer than is often realized. The present writer has seen an English I.U.D., made of 18 carat gold in London in 1807, which was allegedly used by one of the Royal girlfriends. After its (non-sterile) introduction into the cervix, it caused a (painful) low-grade inflammation leading to sterility. There seems evidence that similar dangerous intrauterine devices have been used from time immemorial.

In some patients the use of oral contraceptives may lead to the amenorrhoea–galactorrhoea syndrome, with or without concurrent micro-adenoma of the anterior pituitary, which will be discussed in the next chapter.

DISCUSSION ON THE '*AGE OF THE PILL*', THE PRESENT MAIN METHOD OF CONTRACEPTION

Such a discussion has gained momentum in recent years for a number of reasons. One of them was the increasing frequency of serious side-effects. Another was the fact that the Pill is a contraceptive which is obviously woman-oriented. Attempts at producing an effective 'pill' for the use of the male have not yet been satisfactory. Sterilization of the male has proved quite complicated, difficult to carry out in large populations like India, China or Mexico, and meeting with strong resistance by the male population of developing countries. Apart from thrombotic incidents caused by the female pill, it became apparent that to maintain women during their childbearing period continually in the non-pregnant state with permanent monthly periods may not be an ideal solution. The discovery of prolactin and the study of its actions has added to the re-evaluation of the present situation.

R. V. Short, Director of the Medical Research Council Unit of Reproductive Biology in Edinburgh, and his team have made a number of important contributions to the problem. Short summarized the results in 1976 in a paper on 'The evolution of human reproduction'[83], which deserves special consideration. He had extended his studies to considerations of historical, social and cultural nature among primitive tribes and ancient cultures. His conclusions are so important that they should be quoted in greater detail. If

"psychological development is tied to calendar age, but psychosexual development is determined by nutritional events which control the time of onset of puberty, . . . in developing countries, with a late age at puberty, the acquisition of fertility and intellectual maturity are almost coincident events which complement one another. In developed countries, on the other hand, it seems that we now acquire our sexuality well in advance of the intellectual maturity that enables us to cope with it. Early teenage pregnancies are something quite new in our evolutionary experience, since hitherto they were a biological impossibility."

. . . in primitive communities, sexual intercourse begins at about the time of puberty, but the first pregnancy does not occur for several years thereafter, even though no contraceptive precautions are taken . . . The reason for this . . . seems to be that ovulation does not usually start until a few years after the onset of menstruation.

Historical demographic studies of the time taken for newly weds to conceive, *'fecundability'* (= the probability of conception per menstrual cycle), is another aspect of the study. It seemed rarely to exceed 28% even at the age of 25 in rural populations, although in 1953, 83% of 428 women in New York who were trying to conceive were pregnant within six months at intercourse frequencies of more than four a week.

Lactation in mammals is the other important phase during which reproductive activity has to be restricted because of the considerable increase in energy demands on the mother. The precise mechanism is not yet understood, but

". . . it seems probable that the afferent neural impulses from the teat have an inhibitory effect on the hypothalamus, and this could be the reason for the suckling-induced surges of prolactin secretion. Pituitary prolactin is normally thought to be under inhibitory control from the hypothalamus via prolactin inhibiting factor; . . . it is also possible that prolactin could have a direct inhibitory effect on the ovary itself . . . nutrition itself undoubtedly has a part to play. Even under conditions of frank malnutrition or actual starvation, lactation is scarcely affected . . . In giving preference to the newborn, it is the mother who suffers; . . ."

Man, like other mammals, has relied in the past on lactation as one of the mechanisms for achieving adequate spacing between births (see p. 448). Short quotes examples for this from the Great Apes and the nomadic Kung hunter gatherers of the Kalahari (with average birth intervals of 4 years without abortion or contraception). Since they have become agricultural settlers, the time interval between successive births has dropped by 30%. On the contrary,

"in a typical developed country, menarche begins at 13, cultural infertility breaks down in the late teens, and intercourse before marriage requires the use of contraception or abortion. Lactation is of such short duration that it no longer induces amenorrhoea and birth spacing is dependent on contraception. If the desired family size is 2, contraception, sterilization or abortion is necessary for a further 20 years, after the birth of the second child. The inevitable consequence of this imposed infertility is an enormous increase in the number of menstrual cycles."

This implies a mean blood loss per cycle of *ca.* 43 cc, which may increase with age, and 10% of women may lose 100 cc per month. In a developing country on a marginal protein intake and possible debilitating diseases like malaria, this may amount to danger. Short concluded:

"Since the female is the limiting reproductive resource, it seems sensible that we should emulate nature and concentrate mainly on female-oriented birth control technology. We should also try to recapture what civilization has destroyed, the ability to keep the ovaries and the female reproductive tract in a state of quiescence when reproduction is not desired. Women may be physiologically ill-adapted to spend the greater part of their reproductive lives having an endless succession of menstrual cycles."

As the statistics of breast cancer also indicate that an early menopause decreases the breast cancer risk, Short felt that it would be sensible to develop a non-steroidal contraceptive "that would allow a woman to return to the reproductive state that was the norm for our primitive ancestors – amenorrhoea. The popular belief that such a form of contraception would be unacceptable in developing countries, may be incorrect".

In fact, he and his team have been experimenting in Edinburgh with interesting results with a dosage régime of a conventional contraceptive which reduces the frequency of menstruation to 4 times a year (the '*tricycle pill*'). The experiment also showed "that a number of women were enthusiastic about this approach"[83].

Thus, it appears that research in the field of endocrinology has shifted its gravity to North America, especially since the end of the Second World War. The reasons for this can be readily understood, if one considers the change of the methodology of such research from single researchers or small teams to large groups with many experts in super-laboratories and the cost of such investigations continually increasing. Moreover, there was an interruption of the work in Britain and Europe between 1939 and 1946 with broken lines of communication. However, since the beginning of the 1970s there has been a renaissance of endocrine research in Europe and especially in

Britain – this applies particularly to the clinical field, although experimental research has by no means been neglected. Considerable progress has been made during the last 30 years, partly due to the large scale on which projects can be launched, and partly because exact measurements of hormones have become possible in many instances, revealing the presence of even minute amounts. *Pari passu*, many more pure active hormones have been isolated and prospects of treatment have improved. A brief survey of the progress in the major endocrine fields in those last 30 years will be given in the next chapters, together with a short account of recent promising methods of treatments.

REFERENCES

1. Abel, J. J., Crawford, A. C.: On the blood-pressure-raising constituent of the suprarenal capsule. Johns Hopkins Hosp. Bull. **8**, 151–157, 1897.
2. Marine, D., Williams, W. W.: The relation of iodine to the structure of the thyroid gland. Arch. Int. Med. **1**, 349–384, 1908.
3. Greep, R. O.: The Saga and the Science of the Gonadotrophins. The Sir Henry Dale Lecture for 1967. Proc. Soc. Endocrinol. ii–ix, in J. Endocrinol. **39**, Sept. 1967.
4. Cannon, W. B., Binger, C. A. L., Fitz, R.: Experimental hyperthyroidism. Am. J. Physiol. **36**, 363–364, 1915.
5. Cannon, W. B.: Bodily Changes in Pain, Hunger, Fear and Rage. New York, Appleton, 1915 (First Harper Torchbook edition, New York, 1963.)
6. Lisser, H.: The first forty years (1917–1957). Fiftieth Anniversary Issue, Endocrinology, **80**, 5–28, 1967.
7. Bishop, P. M. F.: The development of British endocrinology. Br. Med. J. **I**, 865–870, 1955.
8. Houssay, B. A. Biasotti, A.: La diabetes pancréatica de los perros hipofisoprivos. Rev. Soc. Argent. Biol. **6**, 251–296, 1930.
9. Houssay, B. A., Biasotti, A.: Endocrinology **15**, 511–523, 1931.
10. Cannon, W. B.: The movements of the stomach studied by means of the Roentgen rays. Am. J. Physiol. **1**, 359–382, 1898.
11. Bernard, C.: Leçons sur les Phénomènes de la Vie Communs aux Animaux et aux Végétaux. Paris. 2 Vols, xxxii, 564 pp. Vol. I, pp. 67: pp. 111–114, pp. 123–124. J. B. Baillière et Fils. 1878/79.
12. Richet, Ch.: Dictionnaire de Physiologie. Vol. iv, p. 721. Paris, Baillière & Cie, 1900.
13. Cannon, W. B.: Physiological regulation of normal states: some tentative postulates concerning biological homeostatics. In À Charles Richet: see Amis, ses Collègues, ses Elèves; 22 Mai 1926. Auguste Pettit, Ed. Paris. Les Éditions Mèdicales, pp. 91–93, 1926.
14. Cannon, W. B., Querido, A., Britton, S. W., Bright, E. M.: Studies on the conditions of activity in endocrine glands. XXI. The role of adrenal secretion in the chemical control of body temperature. Am. J. Physiol. **79**, 466–507, 1926/27.
15. Cannon, W. B.: The Wisdom of the Body. New York, Norton & Co., 1932.
16. Garrison, F. H.: An Introduction to the History of Medicine. 4th ed., p. 731. Philadelphia, W. B. Saunders, 1929.

17. Cushing, H. W.: The Pituitary Body and its Disorders. Philadelphia, J. B. Lippincott, 1912.
18. Cushing, H. W.: The basophil adenomas of the pituitary body and their clinical manifestations (pituitary basophilism). Bull. Johns. Hopkins Hosp. **50,** 137–195, 1932.
19. Besser, G. M., Edwards, C. R. W.: Cushing's Syndrome, in Clinics of Endocrinology and Metabolism, Vol. 1, No. 2, pp. 451–490, 1972.
20. Medvei, V. C.: Histological Investigation of 100 Apparently Normal Human Pituitary Glands. Unpublished study, carried out 1937–38.
21. Costello, R. T.: Proc. Staff Meet. Mayo Clin. **10,** 449, 1935.
22. Susman, W.: Br. J. Surg. **22,** 539, 1935.
23. Cushing, H. W.: Life of Sir William Osler. Oxford University Press, 1925.
24. Matovinovic, Josip: David Marine (1880–1976): Nestor of thyroidology. Perspectives Biol. Med. **21,** 565–589, 1978.
25. Rilliet, F.: Mem. Acad. Med. **24,** 23, 1858/59.
26. Tait, L.: Edinb. Med. J. **20,** 993, 1875.
27. Manley, O. T., Marine, D.: J. Am. Med. Assoc. **67,** 260, 1916.
28. Marine, D., Rosen, S. H.: Am. J. Physiol. **107,** 677, 1934.
29. Marine, D., Lenhart, C. H.: Arch. Int. Med. **8,** 265, 1911.
30. Marine, D., Lenhart, C. H.: Arch. Int. Med. **4,** 253, 1909.
31. Marine, D.: J. Am. Med. Assoc. **59,** 325, 1912.
32. Marine, D., Lenhart, C. H.: Arch. Int. Med. **7,** 506, 1911.
33. Plummer, H. S.: J. Am. Med. Assoc. **80,** 1955, 1923.
34. Dock, G.: J. Am. Med. Assoc. 1119–1122, 1908.
35. Marine, D.: Harvey Lecture, p. 96, 1923/24.
36. His, W. Senior: Die Haeute und Hoehlen des Koerpers. Basel. Schweighauser, 1865.
37. His, W. Senior: Beobachtungen ueber den Bau des Saeugethier-Eierstocks. Arch. Mikrosk. Anat. **1,** 151–202, 1865.
38. Abel, J. J.: Crystalline insulin. Proc. Natl. Acad. Sci., Wash. **12,** 132–136, 1926.
39. Abel, J. J., Rouiller, C. A.: Evaluation of the hormone of the infundibulum of the pituitary gland in terms of histamine, with experiments on the action of repeated injections of the hormone on the blood pressure. J. Pharmacol. **20,** 65–84, 1923.
40. Abel, J. J., Rouiller, C. A., Geiling, E. M. K.: Further investigations on the oxytocic-pressor-diuretic principle of the infundibular portion of the pituitary gland. J. Pharmacol. **20,** 289–316, 1923/24.
41. Abel, J. J., Rowntree, L. G., Turner, B. B.: Plasma removal with return of corpuscles. J. Pharmacol. **5,** 625–641, 1914.
42. Abel, J. J., Ford, W.: The poisons of *Amanita phalloides*. J. Biol. Chem. **2,** 273–288, 1906/07.
43. Pitt-Rivers, Rosalind: The thyroid hormones: historical aspects. p. 412 in Hormonal Proteins and Peptides, Vol. vi, pp. 391–422. New York, Academic Press, 1978.
44. Kendall, E. C., Mason, H. L., McKenzie, B. F., Myers, C. S., Koelsche, G. A.: Proc. Mayo Clin. **9,** 245–250, 1934.
45. Ibid.: Pp. 247–248.
46. Kendall, E. C., Mason, H. L., Myers, C. S., Allers, W. D.: A physiologic and chemical investigation of the suprarenal cortex. J. Biol. Chem. **114,** LVII–LVIII; 613, 1936.
47. Ibid., **116,** 207, 1938.
48. Hench, P. S., Kendall, E. C., Slocumb, C. H., Polley, H. F.: The effect of a

hormone of the adrenal cortex (17-hydroxy-11-dehydro-corticosterone: compound E) and of pituitary adrenocorticotropic hormone on rheumatoid arthritis. Proc. Mayo Clin. **24,** 181–197, 1949.

49. Hench, P. S., Slocumb, C. H., Barnes, A. R., Smith, H. L., Polley, H. F., Kendall, E. C.: The effects of the adrenal cortical hormone 17-hydroxy-11-dehydrocorticosterone (compound E) on the acute phase of rheumatic fever: preliminary report. Proc. Mayo Clin. **24,** 277–297, 1949.

50. Collip, J. B., Anderson, E. M., Thomson, D. L.: The adrenotropic hormone of the anterior pituitary lobe. Lancet **2,** 347–348, 1933.

51. Li, Choh Hao, Simpson, M. E., Evans, H. M.: Adrenocorticotropic hormone. J. Biol. Chem. **149,** 413–424, 1943.

52. Sayers, George, White, A., Long, C. N. H.: Preparation and properties of pituitary adrenocorticotropic hormone. J. Biol. Chem. **149,** 425–436, 1943.

53. Hench, P. S., Kendall, E. C. *et al.*: Proc. Mayo Clin. **24,** 181–197, 1949.

54. Smith, P. E.: Hypophysectomy and replacement therapy in the rat. Am. J Anat. **45,** 205–274, 1930.

55. Smith, P. E.: The disabilities caused by hypophysectomy and their repair. J. Am. Med. Assoc. **88,** 158–161, 1927.

56. Raacke, I. D.: "The die is cast" – "I am going home": The appointment of Herbert McLean Evans as Head of Anatomy at Berkeley. J. Hist. Biol. **9,** No. 2, 301–322, 1976.

57. Evans, H. M., Scott Bishop, Katherine: On the existence of a hitherto unrecognised dietary factor essential for reproduction. Science **56,** 650–651, 1922.

58. Evans, H. M., Emerson, O. H., Emerson, G. A.: The isolation from wheat-germ oil of an alcohol, α-tocopherol, having the properties of vitamin E. J. Biol. Chem. **113,** 319–322, 1936.

59. Evans, H. M., Lepkovsky, S., Murphy, E. A.: Vital needs of the body for certain unsaturated fatty acids. J. Biol. Chem. **106,** 431–460, 1934.

60. Burr, G. O., Burr, Mildred M.: On the nature and role of the fatty acids essential in nutrition. J. Biol. Chem. **86,** 587–621, 1930.

61. Corner, G. W.: Herbert McLean Evans, 1882–1971: a biographical memoir. Biog. Mem. F.R.S. **18,** 83–186, 1972.

62. Li, Choh Hao, Evans, H. M., Simpson, Miriam E.: Isolation and properties of the anterior hypophyseal growth hormone. J. Biol. Chem. **159,** 353–366, 1945.

63. Li, Choh Hao, Simpson, Miriam E., Evans, H. M: Isolation of pituitary follicle-stimulating hormone (FSH). Science **109,** 445–446, 1949.

64. Li, Choh Hao, Simpson, Miriam E., Evans, H. M.: Interstitial cell stimulating hormone. II. Method of preparation and some physico-chemical studies. Endocrinology **27,** 803–808, 1940.

65. As 62.

66. Li, C. H., Evans H. M.: Chemistry of anterior pituitary hormones. In The Hormones (eds, Pincus G, and Thieman, K. V.) New York, Academic Press, 1948.

67. Zietlin, J. I.: Herbert M. Evans: pioneer collector of rare books in the history of science. Isis **62,** 507 ff., 1972.

68. Albright, F.: Some of the 'Do's and Do-Not's' in clinical investigation. J. Clin. Invest. **23,** 921–926, 1944.

69. Albright, F. *et al.*: J. Clin. Invest. **22,** 603, 1943.

70. Bartter, F. C.: Endocrinology **82,** 1109–1112, 1970.

71. Albright, F., Butler, A. M., Hampton, A. O., Smith, P.: N. Eng. J. Med. **216,** 727, 1937.

72. Corner, G. W.: The Discovery of the Mammalian Ovum. Lecture given to the Mayo Foundation in 1933. In Lectures on the History of Medicine, pp. 401–426. Philadelphia, Saunders, 1933.

73. Hertwig, A. O.: Beitraege zur Kenntnis der Bildung, Befruchtung und Theilung des thierischen Eies. Morph. Jahrb. **1**, 347–434, 1876.

74. Pincus, G.: The Control of Fertility, pp. xvii and 360. New York and London, 1965.

75. Haller, J.: Ovulationshemmung durch Hormone. Stuttgart, G. Thieme, 1965.

76. Haller, J.: Hormonal Contraception. Translated from the 3rd German ed. (by Gottfried, H.). Los Altos, California, 1972.

77. Bickenbach, W., Paulikovics, E.: Hemmung der Follikerlreifung durch Progesteron bei der Frau. Zbl. Gynaecol. **68**, 153, 1944.

78. Massenbach, W. von: Ueber die unzweckmaessige Anwendung von Corpus-luteum-Hormonen. Dtsche. Med., Wochenschr. **67**, 513, 1941.

79. Pincus, G.: The Eggs of Mammals. New York, Macmillan, 1936.

80. Pincus, G.: Anat. Rec. **77**, 1, 1940.

81. Pincus, G., Kirsch, R. E.: Am. J. Physiol. **115**, 219, 1936.

82. Pincus, G., Chang, M. C.: Acta Physiol. Latinoam. **3**, 177, 1953.

83. Short, R. V.: Definition of the Problem: The evolution of human reproduction. Proc. R. Soc. London, B. **195**, 3–24, 1976.

CHAPTER TWENTY-ONE

PRESENT TRENDS AND OUTLOOK FOR THE FUTURE – PART I

GENERAL TRENDS AND ACHIEVEMENTS

URING the last fifteen years great progress has been made in many areas of the vast field of endocrinology. This has been due to three major developments. Firstly, to the isolation of a great number of hormones, the existence of which had been suspected and postulated, but not proved. Secondly, to the development of methods which enabled the demonstration of most hormones even in minute amounts. Lastly, to the development of special tests, which have made it possible to measure the amounts of circulating hormones, first by bioassays and lately by the advent of the radio-immunoassay methods, which are replacing many of the indirect tests of endocrine function and give a remarkably accurate measurement of hormones, and some important non-hormonal compounds.

In 1959, S. A. Berson and R. S. Yalow[1] discovered the antigenic properties of proteohormones with relatively low molecular weight. Techniques of labelling organic compounds were then the prerequisite for the development of the radio-immunoassays (RIA). In these, the high specificity of immunological methods and the high sensitivity of the radiochemical techniques are combined. Compared with the bioassay techniques, there are important advantages in sensitivity, precision and specificity in RIA, which is also simple and, therefore, cheaper. RIA is a structure assay, because it quantifies a certain chemical structure. Bioassays, on the other hand, are activity assays (including the sensitive cytochemical assays). In some cases, therefore, RIA and bioassay can be complementary. Fundamentally, however, RIA methods have revolutionized the study of endocrinology.

Thus, early diagnosis and precise localization of abnormal function were made possible, resulting in rational treatment, which can be controlled much more accurately. At the same time, the close interrelationships have been elucidated, not only of the endocrine glands, but of the humoral and nervous regulation of the body, especially of the role of the hypothalamus and, indeed, the whole brain as the 'master-gland', of the feedback mechanism, of releasing and inhabiting factors (hormones) from nervous centres. The 'releasing factors' on first order hormones, elaborated by the hypothalamus, were first named so in 1955, in a paper by Murray Saffran, A. V. Schally and B. G. Benfey[2]. The search for releasing factors corresponding to the other anterior lobe hormones was reviewed ten years later by McCann and Dhariwal in L. Martini's and W. F. Ganong's *Neuroendocrinology*[3], and a tabulated summary revealed the gaps as well as the achievements in the field. In 1966, five releasing factors had already been determined, each being a small polypeptide. Jean-Lambert Pasteels observed in 1962[4] that prolactin was liberated into the surrounding medium, if the rat anterior pituitary lobe was maintained in culture; pituitary stalk extract inhibited this release. This indicated a prolactin inhibiting factor, a new development. The search for the ACTH releasing factor was further complicated by a parallel activity presented by vasopressin, a posterior lobe hormone. It seemed unlikely that the link between the anterior lobe of the pituitary could be entirely nervous because of the scarcity or even complete absence of nerve fibres within the anterior lobe. Professor Peter M. Daniel stressed this in his paper on the 'Anatomy of the hypothalamus and pituitary gland'[5].

The vascular link was discussed in Chapter 14, when we considered the work of Lieutaud (1703–1780) of Aix-en-Provence, of Popa and Fielding in 1930, and the studies of portal systems in the body by Henderson and Daniel in 1978 (see p. 162). The hypothalamus is the main subcortical centre for the control of sympathetic and parasympathetic activities, using the nervous link to the posterior pituitary and the humero-hormonal (portal) one of the anterior lobe. Included in the parasympathetic side are the physiological effects of the activity of the posterior lobe hormones. Stimulation of the posterior region of the hypothalamus may produce sympathetic responses of stress, fight or flight[6]. Destruction of the cortico-hypothalamic connections may lead to sham-rage. Pressure on the hypothalamus, e.g. by craniopharyngiomas (the commonest non-invasive tumours), which grow from the area next to the pituitary stalk and which they may also damage or cut, may result in diabetes insipidus, obesity and hypogonadism, with or without simultaneous pressure on the pituitary[7]. In the efferent direction, the hypothalamus projects through the neighbouring mammillary bodies and through thalamic centres into the frontal lobe.

The anatomical and functional differences of the anterior and posterior lobe of the pituitary were responsible for the different lines along which research proceeded. The secretory products of the posterior lobe can be observed under the light microscope and followed also to the hypothalamus. Releasing hormones from the hypothalamic centres have been demonstrated by other means. Recently, electron-microscopical studies on the hypothalamic arcuate complex revealed synaptic vesicles of the 'dense-cored' variety[8]. Elsewhere in the nervous system such synaptic vesicles can be seen, when the transmitter substances are catecholamines.

In the late 1950s began the study of the chemical composition and structures (i.e. the amino-acid chains) and the assessment of the molecular weight of anterior pituitary hormones, stimulated by the study of the structure of insulin, with a molecular weight of 6000, in 1955, by Sanger and his colleagues[9]. Paul Bell determined the structure of ACTH[10], with a molecular weight of 4500, the smallest of all pituitary hormones. Choh Hao Li and his group gave the structure of growth hormone with a molecular weight of 21 500[11]. These results were complemented by the work of numerous leading research workers on the chemical transmission of nerve impulses (see p. 415 ff). The discovery of the chemical structure of the hormones led to the inquiry as to how such complex chemical molecules could act on other cell complexes and thus to the discovery of receptors and receptor sites. Special interest was focused on manner and location in which hormones act on a single target cell. It was found that the thyroid and lipid-soluble steroid hormones permeate the cell membrane and interact with specific binding proteins in the cytoplasm and the nucleus. Polypeptide hormones, which are water-soluble, and neurotransmitters (and catecholamines) bind to specific receptor sites on the surface of the cell membrane. The hormone–receptor complexes thus formed perform the transmission of the message. This necessitates demonstration of the receptors and receptor sites, which has been achieved by the use of radioactively labelled hormones. The belief that polypeptide hormones do not enter cells has now been challenged in a series of recent studies based on novel techniques. One of these methods uses electron microscopic autoradiography to localize ^{125}I-labelled hormones in target tissues. Thus it was demonstrated that insulin can enter intact liver cells[12] and cultured lymphocytes[13], and that human chorionic gonadotrophin can enter ovarian cells[14]. These observations indicate the possibility that certain actions of polypeptide hormones could be mediated through a direct effect inside the cell of the hormone itself, or of the hormone–receptor complex rather than through conditions on the surface of the cell. It is not yet fully understood how some of these large polypeptide molecules, which may have a molecular weight up to 40 000, permeate the cell, but it seems likely that they do so as hormone–receptor complexes[14]. This mechanism appears to apply especially to insulin, but the purpose of this action is still unknown. Degradation of hormone–receptor and long-term action on the nucleus has been regarded as one of the possibilities[15]. Other polypeptide hormones may have their intracellular effects mediated by the stimulation and increase in concentration of cyclic AMP, localized on the plasma membrane[16].

Morton Grossman of Los Angeles summed up the present position in the following words:

> The concept is rapidly evolving that the body has a single system of chemical messengers comprising an interrelated group of peptides and amines. The same or similar chemical messengers may be utilized for neurocrine, paracrine, and endocrine modes of transmission. The concept is breathtaking in its simplicity and audacity. The major mechanisms for co-ordinating bodily activities can now be viewed as a unified system[17].

Recently, several Symposia have taken place, discussing hormone receptors and their diseases[18].

The use of inhibitors of the synthesis of protein is another method of study, which began in the 1960s as a trickle and has now developed into a flood of research. Labelling has not always been very successful (e.g. in the case of ACTH), but in other instances antagonists could be used, such as in the case of FSH and TSH. In order to identify a hormone receptor, it is essential to show a direct biological response to a receptor occupancy. Peptide hormones are produced in the ribosomes under the control of messenger RNA. They are then packaged at the Golgi apparatus into secretion granules. Some hormones, like insulin, are produced in a larger form, called 'prohormones' (pro-insulin). In the secretion granules these large prohormones are degraded into the active hormone. The granule next migrates to the periphery and fuses with the cell membrane, then discharging its contents into the blood stream. The peptide hormones, which circulate mainly in the free state, fit into specific receptors in the cell wall. They then activate – perhaps through a transducer – cell membrane based adenyl cyclase, which is the catalyst for the conversion of ATP to cyclic AMP. This is turn activates a protein kinase (? through phosphorylation) to an active enzyme, which later passes on the 'message' to the target. The first described example of this, in 1958, was the conversion of inactive phosphorylase to active phosphorylase for the degradation of glycogen in the liver, under the influence of glucagon or epinephrine[19]. Concerning insulin, the most recent studies have just been described. (The same may apply to the action of growth hormone and prolactin.) Steroid hormone action usually differs from the above. Steroid hormones circulate attached to relatively specific proteins and the steroid is then released from its carrier within the blood stream and traverses the cell membrane. Mineral and bone homeostasis seem to involve the action of multiple hormones (parathormone, calcitonin, gluco-corticoids and prostaglandins) at multiple sites (bone, parathyroid glands, gut and kidney)[20]. Receptors may be manufactured within the cell and transported to the membrane surface. Formation of hormone–receptor complexes may be followed by simple dissociation of the hormone from its binding site, or the whole complex may be absorbed into the cell[21].

Research into hormone–receptor interactions has influenced clinical medicine in three ways. First, it has clarified the normal physiology of hormone mechanisms. Secondly, it has allowed the development of important new concepts of aetiology. Lastly, there has been a direct impact on clinical practice, particularly in the fields of diagnostic and prognostic investigations.[22]

This penetration into molecular biology is now a recognized feature of endocrine research. It is recognized that the cellular response to a variety of hormones, both steroids and polypeptides, is conditioned by the presence of protein molecules known as receptors and located on specific cells. They seem to be responsible for the tissue specificity of hormones. Tissues do not respond to a hormone if they do not possess receptors for that hormone. Appropraite receptor proteins have been identified in most target tissues of known steroid hormones (e.g. oestrogen, progesterone, androgens and the corticosteroids). Moreover, in these cases, the receptors have often been found to concentrate them in the nucleus of the cells and bind them to the chromosomes. Such hormone–receptor complexes can stimulate RNA synthesis, leading to synthesis of specific proteins, which implies an influence on the genetic presentation of the cells[23].

Changes in receptor concentration may be a normal mechanism in controlling endocrine function. Occasionally, such changes can be excessive and cause disease[24] (see also pp. 572–575). New developments in the field of genetics give a better understanding of such problems as disorders of sex differentiation. The emergence of the new science of immunopathology made an enormous contribution to the investigation and elucidation of many problems, previously quite inaccessible to systematic research. New chapters were also added by the discovery of new hormones, such as calcitonin. This, together with the intensive study of parathyroid function and calcium metabolism, threw new light on bone disease and related topics. The discovery and study of prostaglandins, of ectopic hormone production by non-endocrine tumours★, added to the enormous expansion of the field. The discovery of circadian variations and specific rhythms in the secretion and circulation of most hormones elucidated – and at the same time, complicated – the physiology and pathology of endocrinology. The more recent work on the role of dopamine and of dopamine agonists, such as bromocriptine, took on special importance, once it was found that the latter can have practical therapeutic effects in a number of pathological conditions, such as acromegaly and gigantism, in the amenorrhoea-galactorrhoea–hyperprolactinaemia syndrome and in Parkinsonism. In the most recent phase, the enkephalins, beta-lipotrophins and beta-endorphins have kept up the excitement of new developments, connected with the brain, the nervous system and a wide range of new hormones.

In all these developments there is, however, one important noticeable difference, which has already been mentioned in the previous chapter. It is the switch from research carried out by one or two people to larger or very large research teams with a manifold coverage by experts, which Herbert M. Evans was one of the first to appreciate and skilfully to apply. Accordingly, the historical development and the anecdotage of the old style disappeared, with a few exceptions. In view of this, we shall adopt in these concluding chapters a different presentation: we shall discuss briefly the main developments under subject headings of the individual endocrine secretions, and some connecting links, although a few personal stories of some of the researchers will be mentioned.

REMARKS ON TESTS AND MEASUREMENTS IN SOME ENDOCRINE CONDITIONS

In the past, only major abnormalities of endocrine function could be recognized, measured, treated, and the results of the treatment were often monitored in a rough and ready manner. Minor degrees of dysfunction were difficult or even impossible to diagnose on clinical evidence alone. Obviously, such minor endocrine dysfunctions which can be demonstrated only by means of several tests and

★ See Postscript.

perhaps with the help of sophisticated dynamic function tests, will need facilities which are available in endocrine centres with specially equipped laboratories. The main groups of common endocrine disorders can often be established by a comparatively small number of special investigations, which are readily available in many hospitals and, therefore, also to general practitioners in Western countries. A good guide for the main types of tests was published in 1974 in the series of *Clinics in Endocrinology and Metabolism* under the title 'Investigations of Endocrine Disorders'[25].

Tests of thyroid function

The table which gives the tests of thyroid function lists fourteen, including four dynamic ones, such as tri-iodothyronine suppression and TSH stimulation tests. There are added tests of peripheral tissue function, e.g. duration of ankle tendon reflex, and electro-cardiograms; moreover, tests of hypothalamic–pituitary function, e.g. serum thyrotrophin (TSH) estimation and thyrotrophin-releasing-hormone (factor) (TSH-RH) test. Tests to establish the cause of thyroid dysfunction are as follows: 1. The detection of thyroid antibodies in the circulation [covering three groups, the third being the long acting thyroid stimulator (LATS), an Ig globulin, for which there was only a bioassay available]. 2. Thyroid scanning and scintigraphy. 3. Radioiodine kinetic studies. 4. Thyroid biopsy. 5. Ultrasonic B scanning, to distinguish between cystic and solid nodules, is only rarely available at present[26]. One of the important, difficult and recently recognized problems is posed by thyrotoxicosis caused by an increased production of tri-iodothyronine (T_3) only, which can occur with diffuse goitre, multinodular goitre and thyroid nodules[27]. The other important, though comparatively rare, condition is ophthalmic Graves' disease, which is clinically euthyroid (T_4 within normal limits, but T_3 often increased). The investigation of the rare dyshormonogenetic goitre is an example of the complexity of modern test methods, which need a specialist centre for such a purpose[28].

Investigation of dysfunction of the parathyroid glands

This[29] is another good example of the problems which research of the last fifteen years has been able to elucidate. As Parfitt put it concisely:

> The essence of precision in endocrine diagnosis is the ability to measure all components of the various feedback loops by which secretion of a

hormone is controlled. For those glands that respond to a pituitary trophic hormone, these feedback loops are entirely hormonal, whereas for glands lacking a pituitary trophic hormone, such as, the pancreatic islets and the parathyroids, the basic feedback loop consists of an effector gland hormone and a non-hormonal plasma (= fluid phase of blood which exists *in vivo*) constituent such as glucose or calcium.[30]

For that reason, the different fractions of calcium in plasma had to be established and analysed, in order to arrive, eventually, at an assessment of ionized calcium. Even so, total protein has to be estimated as well and a protein correction applied to every sample on which calcium is measured.

The parathyroid hormone (PTH) was determined as an 84-amino-acid single-chain polypeptide with a molecular weight of *ca.* 9500, which follows the formation of a prohormone with a molecular weight of about 11 500. (Other workers found a pre-proparathyroid hormone with a molecular weight of *ca.* 13 000, consisting of PTH with six additional amino acids on the NH_2 terminal and an unknown number of additional amino acids on the COOH terminal end[31].) The NH_2 terminal end is most important for biological activity[32]. Its synthesis is mainly controlled by the ionized calcium in the blood which perfuses the gland. The secretion is dependent on the serum concentration of magnesium, which at low concentrations completely inhibits it. Vitamin D also suppresses parathyroid function. After secretion, the hormone has only a short half life of 20 minutes. Chronic hypocalcaemia causes hypertrophy of the para-thyroid glands. Radio-immunoassays have developed slowly and the results are still of a complex nature. They have been interpreted in relation to plasma calcium levels, thus causing problems. Some of those are clarified by the use of dynamic (stimulation and suppression) tests. Additional help in assessing the situation is sometimes given by the changes in bones, which may be recognized by radiological or histological examination. PTH increases the number of osteoclasts, both by increasing their formation and decreasing their transformation. It also increases their bone resorbing activity. To the contrary, PTH decreases the number of osteoblasts and therefore also bone formation. PTH acts on the kidney by increasing the excretion of sodium, potassium, bicarbonate and phosphate, and by decreasing the excretion of calcium and magnesium. These effects are partly mediated by increasing the amount of cyclic AMP in the urine. The formation of 1,25-hydroxy vitamin D in the kidney is also increased.

Disorders of the hypothalamus and of the pituitary

This area of the endocrine field has been "revolutionized once more by the introduction of the synthetic hypothalamic hormones"[33], in 1969, of the tripeptide sequence, causing the release of thyrotrophin and prolactin. This was followed by the decapeptide hormone which releases gonadotrophins (LH and FSH) in 1971[34]. Next came a 14-amino acid peptide in 1973, which inhibits the release of growth hormone (GH)[35] during insulin-induced hypoglycaemia, after exercise, laevo-DOPA and arginine; it also inhibits TSH secretion after TRH and insulin and glucagon secretion in normal subjects, furthermore, it inhibits GH release in acromegalic patients and diabetics[36].

One of the discoveries of the last decade was the fact that many hormones are released into the circulation in pulsatile bursts. This means that hormone measurements of single blood samples are almost useless. In a dynamic test of glucose tolerance load, plasma growth hormone levels in normal people are suppressed; the opposite may be the case in acromegaly and gigantism. There is no space here to discuss all the other tests which are of importance, but it should be remembered that in an attempt to investigate the hypothalamic–pituitary–adrenal axis, three variables have to be taken into account: the circadian rhythm, the response to stress, and the feedback mechanism. Similarly, a number of tests have been introduced to measure the hypothalamic–pituitary–thyroid function[37], the hypothalamic–pituitary–gonadal function[37], the growth hormone release and the prolactin release. Tests of prolactin secretion have become important in the modern treatment of female infertility.

Hyperprolactinaemia needs elucidation, especially when it is caused by prolactinomas. The diagnosis of the latter can be particularly difficult in the case of microadenomas of the anterior pituitary, when even such sophisticated radiological methods as serial linear tomography of the pituitary fossa may fail to give a clear cut interpretation. Complicated tests of anterior pituitary function may have to be added for estimating cortisol, growth hormone, LH and FSH blood levels by means of an indwelling cannula, following an intravenous deposit of soluble insulin, combined with TRH and LH/FSH-RH. This may have to be further combined with dynamic tests of prolactin secretion, such as the assessment of the circadian variation, stimulation tests with intravenous TRH and metoclopramide and suppression tests with laevo-DOPA and bromocriptine[38].

Tests concerning gonadal dysfunction

Gonadotrophins are now measured in the plasma by means of radio-immunoassays, but results may differ with age (FSH and LH increase with age) and with the laboratory in which they are carried out. Plasma oestradiol (oestradiol-17-beta) concentrations can also be measured by RIA, as well as by other methods, and may be helpful in the differentiation of testicular or adrenal tumours producing oestrogens in men from other causes, producing gynaecomastia.

Summing up, present investigations include assays of gonado-trophins in plasma and urine, of oestrogens, progesterone and of androgens. They can be measured at base level and under dynamic conditions. In conjunction with the history of the condition, clinical and X-ray examination, histological (biopsy) investigations and karyotyping, they will lead to the recognition of many gonadal dysfunctions in men and women. The combination of tests for each problem has to be carefully planned. It is by such means that isolated gonadotrophic hormone or even ACTH deficiencies can be detected[39].

The most recent addition is that of cytochemistry. Cytochemical bioassays are the most sensitive as well as the most quantitatively precise methods of assaying polypeptide hormones; the cytochemical bioassay for thyrotrophin, for example, is 10 000 times more sensitive than the radio-immunoassay. These cytochemical micro-bioassay techniques are internationally recommended by the World Health Organisation (WHO) (1975)[40].

Investigating the function of the adrenals

Similar considerations apply to investigating the function of the adrenal glands. Of the hormones of the adrenal cortex, perhaps the most important is cortisol or hydrocortisone. This C-21 steroid is a glucocorticoid, which has properties primarily related to intermediary glucose regulation, although it has some mineral regulating effects as well. Plasma cortisol level curves over 24 hours show circadian periodicity, which means that it is secreted episodically in phase with adrenocorticotrophin (ACTH), which has a dominant circadian rhythm. This applies to normal human subjects as well as to other mammals and sub-mammalian species. The rhythm is not posture dependent, influenced by fasting or over-feeding. The main studies on this question have been carried out during the last twelve years by Professor Dorothy T. Krieger of the Mount Sinai School of

Medicine in New York[41]. In studies based on a sampling frequency of every 24–30 minutes (the half life of cortisol varying between 60 and 90 minutes), Krieger could demonstrate that the circadian rise and fall of plasma corticosteroid concentration and of ACTH did not occur in a linearly smooth manner, but that there were "episodic, relatively synchronous peaks of plasma ACTH and corticosteroid levels . . . evident throughout the day"[42], the majority of such peaks occurring between 3 a.m. and 9 a.m. Krieger and co-workers suggested that this is perhaps a reflection of a circadian, neurally mediated release of a corticotrophin-releasing factor (CRF), because the circadian periodicity of ACTH is also in evidence in adrenalecto-mized animals and in patients with Addison's disease; it cannot be caused, therefore, by the usual feedback process. In spite of the role of light as a synchronizer of adrenal corticosteroid periodicity, in blind persons major alterations do not seem to occur invariably, but "what is actually happening is that periodicity is free-running"[43]. Circadian periodicity of plasma corticosteroid concentrations is not present at birth, but seems to develop with the anatomical develop-ment of the retino-hypothalamic tract[44]. Although – as stated above – periodicity is 'free-running' in animals blinded as adults, it is absent in animals blinded at birth. This indicates that light serves as a synchronizer of periodicity, which, however, is endogenous. How-ever, there are still a number of questions which need to be answered by further research and experiment, before the basic neuroendocrine mechanisms which cause and regulate circadian rhythm can be elucidated. "The CNS location of the 'clock' or 'clocks' that generate(s) such periodicity, is still not resolved"[45].

ACTH is a single chain peptide comprising 39 amino acids. The 24 amino acids at the N-terminal are identical in all species investigated and are required for biological activity[46]. The early morning surge of ACTH primes the adrenal cortex and increases its responsiveness. Apart from the circadian rhythm, ACTH secretion is influenced by stress and by negative feedback. As already stated, ACTH has the smallest molecule of all the pituitary hormones with a molecular weight of about 4500[10]. The adrenocortical steroids are thought to be derived from cholesterol, but the synthesis of cortisol from cholesterol is still under study.

It involves, chemically, a number of hydroxylations and thus the action of multi-enzyme systems. Study of the biosynthesis seems to have slowed down, as since the 1960s there has been a shift of research interest towards the investigation of the receptor sites of the target tissues.

Hypothalamic–pituitary–adrenal function tests were reviewed in 1971 by V.H.T. James and J. Landon[47].

Tests for aldosterone

In 1952, Simpson, Tait and Bush isolated by chromatographic separation a potent sodium-retaining factor from adrenal venous blood[48]. They called it 'electrocortin'. Their group, which at that time included Wettstein, Neher *et al.*[49], determined the chemical structure of 'electrocortin' to be 18-aldehyde of corticosterone, which they renamed 'aldosterone'. It was synthesized a year later by Schmidlin, Anner, Billeter and Wettstein[50], after having been isolated from the urine of patients with nephrosis and heart-failure in 1954[51]. Aldosterone is produced in the zona glomerulosa, in the outermost zone of the adrenal cortex in higher vertebrates. The diagnosis of primary hyperaldosteronism (Conn's syndrome) is notoriously difficult. This is due to the complex mechanism created by excess production of aldosterone. Symptoms of hypertension and hypokalaemia should put one on guard[52, 53]. Moreover, the condition may present itself as nocturia and polyuria, in an attempt to escape from the sodium-retaining effect of aldosterone. The investigations necessary are accordingly complex, although, if suspected, it is now possible to measure the hormone plasma level, although a single measurement is not conclusive. The daily production rate (assessed by intravenous injection of a tracer amount of radioactive aldosterone, followed by collection of urine for 48 hours) is much more important. Even so, a great deal of circumstantial evidence is needed, such as plasma renin assay, to distinguish it from the hypertensive patient on diuretics and with hypokalaemia; sodium balance studies; and response to spironolactone. Plasma electrolyte levels and blood urea assessment are also essential.

Dysfunction of the adrenal medulla

The dysfunction of the adrenal medulla, especially when due to tumours called phaeochromocytomas, can now be detected with greater ease, since, in 1957, Armstrong and McMillan discovered 3-methoxy-4-hydroxymandelic acid (VMA) in human urine. By assaying the urine for the catecholamine metabolites the diagnosis was facilitated[54]. This test is now a justified 'must' in every patient with a definite hypertension, to exclude phaeochromocytomas, which have a poor prognosis unless quickly and successfully treated.

The remarks on tests and measurements in endocrine disorders may be summed up as follows. There is an understandable and growing tendency for more accurate and readily available measurements. Bioassays are being replaced by radio-immunoassays. Urinary assays have become complementary to the assessment of hormone levels in the plasma. Of particular significance is the realization that single blood-hormone measurements are often inconclusive. Once it became evident that many hormones do not function in a smooth linear progress (independently of the method of their production), but in an episodic, pulsatile form, reflecting a circadian, neurally mediated release, test methods had to be adapted to obtain a true picture of their function.

The use of isotopes, first of iodine, in endocrine research stemmed from a lecture by the late President Karl Taylor Compton of the Massachusetts Institute of Technology to the Harvard Medical Faculty in 1937, as J. Howard Means relates[55]. Compton discussed the help physics could offer to biological problems. Among other things, he mentioned the use of artificially radioactive isotopes. The thought arose that if iodine could be made radioactive, it might provide a tool for the study of thyroid physiology and perhaps also a new agent in the diagnosis and treatment of thyroid disease. The question was put to Dr. Compton, who — after making inquiries — replied that Fermi in Italy had made iodine as well as other stable elements radioactive. Accordingly, he invited the thyroid group at the Massachusetts General Hospital to undertake a joint investigation with the Physics Department of the Institute of Technology, of the possible uses of radioactive iodine. A young physicist, Arthur Roberts, was delegated by Robly D. Evans, Professor of Physics, to co-operate in the project with Dr. Saul Hertz, one of Means' young physicians. That was the starting point[56]. As it so often happens in scientific research, at the same time and quite independently, P. C. Leblond, in the Laboratoire de Synthèse Atomique in Paris, under the direction of Professors Lacassagne and Joliot, began making studies with radioactive phosphorus and iodine, which he subsequently carried on "with imagination and distinction" in the United States and in Canada. Early studies on radioactive iodine in relation to the thyroid gland were also carried out by Hamilton and Soley in California[55]. When the studies of the Massachusetts team began in 1937, ^{128}I was used, which was obtained from a radium–beryllium source, before a cyclotron was available. The material had a half-life of only 25 minutes and could be used for experiments not over $1\frac{1}{2}$ hours. In 1940, cyclotron became available and it was possible to make ^{130}I with a half-life of 12.5 hours and with it some diagnostic and therapeutic administrations were made on human beings, in addition to animal experiments. A still more useful isotope, ^{131}I, with a half-life of 8 days, came from the Atomic Energy Laboratory at Oak Bridge, Tennessee, in 1946. C. P. Leblond later (in 1943) applied the method of radioautography, by which location of radiation in tissue could be followed at microscopical level[57].

The advent of chromatography greatly expanded the potentialities of labelled iodine and physiologic studies. It was by means of such a combination, labelled iodine and chromatography, that Gross and Pitt-Rivers, in 1952, discovered tri-iodothyronine (T_3) as the second hormone in the thyroid gland.

This is an excellent example of successful modern endocrine research on a team basis. Conversely, it also illustrates that there is still a place for the single-minded and single-handed investigator like Leblond. Finally, it demonstrates the occurrence of identical vital research projects occurring independently at several places, if the ideas are 'in the air'.

In human recipients, isotopes with a longer half-life were given. Iodine was taken up by the thyroid to saturation point. The top limit was, however, found to be greater in the case of thyroid tissue hyperplasia. Radioiodine was also developed as treatment of the overfunctioning gland and, indeed, for complete ablation of functional thyroid tissue in neoplastic thyroid disease.

As already mentioned, the year 1960 was the watershed in endocrinological research, when the new technique of Rosalyn Yalow and S. A. Berson's 'Immunoassay of endogenous plasma insulin in man'[1] transformed the whole scene. We shall see, when discussing the emergence of kidney and gut hormones, that not only gastrin, insulin and glucagon are measured in this manner, but also ectopic hormones, such as parathormone and adrenocorticotrophic hormone when produced by non-endocrine tumours, and hormones from non-digestive glands, involved in multiple endocrine adenomatosis (see Paul Wermer's syndrome, p. 610). Briefly, all radio-immunoassays are protein-binding methods. The essential principle is the reversible binding of a compound to a specific protein in accordance with the law of mass action. Binding proteins are: serum proteins, hormone receptors and antibodies. For the radio-immunological estimation of a compound, specific antibodies are used against this compound (which is the antigen). The addition of a certain amount of the antibody to an excess of labelled antigen will result in equilibrium, part of the antigen molecules being bound to the antibodies, but the rest being free, because the binding sites are limited. A prerequisite for the analytical application of antibodies is that radioactive and unlabelled molecules of the compound do not differ in their binding properties to the antibody. In a sample with a constant amount of antibodies and radioactive antigen molecules, the portion bound to antibodies is inversely proportional to the amount of unlabelled antigen added. For any given amount of antigens, a certain ratio of 'free/antibody' bound will result which can be calculated as '% free' or in '% bound'[58]. Such radio-immunoassay methods (RIA) could be developed for the exact measurement in urine and/or plasma of peptide hormones, for steroid hormones, for the thyroid hormones and for a great number of non-hormonal compounds, such as drugs (digoxine), plasmaproteins (e.g. IgG), (thyroxine-binding globulin = TBG), and other substances, e.g. cyclic AMP, folic acid, alpha-L-foetoprotein, prostaglandins, morphine and other opiates, vitamin B_{12}, etc.

This implies, however, that the research application of RIA, or its clinical use for diagnosis and control of treatment, necessitates a thorough knowledge of assay theory and practice; it is, therefore, only suitable for use at major centres with specialist laboratories and the results can be interpreted only within the known base values of the laboratories, and only in conjunction with the clinical picture and within the framework of other planned tests.

TECHNIQUES IN ENDOCRINE RESEARCH

All these new developments had changes of technique in endocrine research in their wake. The field of research has been enlarged to incorporate neuro-endocrinology as a major component, as well as comparative ('general') endocrinology, genetic-hormonal relations, the investigation of transport in the blood and at the target cells, and of receptors and receptor sites. This means studies at cellular and subcellular levels and the further extension of techniques from the area of biochemistry to biophysics and such methods as X-ray crystallography. The latter was first used, however, by J. D. Bernal in Cambridge (England) on vitamin D and later on oestrone more than forty years ago! Any substance through which a Roentgen ray is passed will produce diffraction effects. The degree to which these can be used to determine its precise structure will depend upon the regularity of the organization of units within that structure. In the case of biological substances, the best observations can be made in those cases where the substance can be isolated in crystalline form. In the case of hormones, such analytical technique can help to discover the chemical structure of an active substance; this method has become really practicable and rapid since the introduction of automatic data collecting and computing techniques. This applies especially in the case of the complicated structures of steroid hormones, and even more to the extremely complex molecules of peptide and protein hormones. Ule Svante von Euler (b. 1905) of the Karolinska Institut in Stockholm, has been involved particularly in the research of the significance and separation of hormones containing subcellular particles, for nearly thirty years[59, 60]. He isolated and demonstrated these particles from a large number of cells; among others, he showed noradrenaline to be the main transmitter of sympathetic nerve impulses. Von Euler shared the Nobel Prize for 1970.

Another important line of investigation developed in the use of antibodies. Biological macromolecules are found in a high concentration especially in the gamma-globulin fraction of the serum and have a marked reaction with the antigen, i.e. the foreign substance introduced into the animal (or human) body. If an antibody is tagged with a tracer and made to react with an antigen, its specific reaction will make it possible to locate it by detection of the tracer. This technique has been extended to the use of specific antibodies for the localization of antigenic substances in electron microscopy[61].

The reason why neuro-endocrinology has made such an enormous progress in the past twenty years, is mainly the development of new techniques of study with the availability of electron microscopy and the use of radioactive isotopes. These have made it possible to demonstrate neuro-secretion as a special function of the nervous system. As, however, neuro-secretory systems are distributed diffusely, the old established methods of endocrine research, i.e. ablation and replacement therapy, cannot be applied to their study. Moreover, the minute size of many of these systems poses an additional problem to their investigation and biochemical analysis. New techniques, such as micro-analysis and a combination of several lines of investigations, have proved the most promising methods of tackling these problems.

We have already referred to the development of chromatographic methods which have played such an important role in endocrine research during the last 30 years[62, 63]. Although chromatography is, in principle, concerned with molecules in solution, it has been established that subcellular particles, mitochondria and viruses can also be fractionated by this method. Of the various techniques of chromatography, column partition chromatography has proved invaluable for the quantitative separation of steroids, especially vapour-phase chromatography. The most important form from a practical point of view, is paper chromatography[64], which for comparative simplicity and speed can hardly be excelled, again especially in the research on steroids.

It became obvious and essential that the transport and state of hormones in the blood should be investigated. It appears that some of the most important steroids, catecholamines and insulin, circulate in the blood in association with other substances. The transport of insulin, for example, may be responsible for diabetes mellitus if the balance of biologically active and inactive circulating insulin is distorted[65]. Small amounts of corticosteroids are bound to transcortin (a plasma alpha-L-globulin), the excess to albumin. Similarly, small amounts of thyroxin are bound to alpha-L-globulin (= thyroxine-binding globulin, TBG, with a high affinity for thyroxin), larger amounts to albumin.

Since the introduction of relatively pure chemical preparations of hormones, the use of specific antibodies has been developed to sensitive and quantitative immunological methods for the detection of hormones. It has now been demonstrated that hormone molecules can act as an antigen, even when their molecular weight is as low as 3–4000 (as in the case of glucagon). Obviously, purified pig follicle-stimulating or luteinizing hormones with their molecular weight of near 30 000 (and human urinary gonadotrophic hormones) provide excellent antigens. The special role of human thyroglobulin, which can act as an antigen in other human beings or even in the same person, will be discussed together with auto-immune thyroid disease. Immunological methods played an important role in the detection and assay of hormones, using various techniques, e.g. chromato-electrophoresis in the case of insulin and glucagon, or the fluorescent antibody method for ACTH and for growth hormone; but quite a few researchers prefer the radio-precipitin technique with ^{131}I-labelled HGH. For thyrotrophin (TSH) determination the haemagglutination–inhibition method with beef-THS treated cells has been used.

All these sophisticated techniques are now based on the ever increasing use of experimental animals, which poses several problems of its own. It is needless to stress that the maximum humanity is essential when dealing with those animals[66], together with the best possible care and with the utmost economy. This also means the careful selection of questions to which a planned experiment may give a desirable answer. It also means the production of laboratory animals of high quality with adequate scientific control[67].

P. Karlson and his group in Munich was one of the pioneers of the idea that hormones may act at the level of the cell nucleus, thus releasing genetic information, which affects development. Their main experimental work was carried out on insects, and it seems from their studies that a hormone may act as a 'timing device' for the genes which control the development of the insect through several moults. The hormone in this case was ecdysone, produced by the prothoracic gland, which – in its turn – was stimulated by the neurosecretory cells of the brain. Ecdysone is the hormone which induces moulting and metamorphosis[68].

To finalize this excursion into some techniques of endocrine research, two important critical statements must be made. 1. The interpretation of biochemical techniques used in this field can be very difficult, especially in the case of clinical investigations in man. From this it follows that each problem must be carefully defined and the purpose of the study circumscribed in such a manner that a valid answer to a limited objective can be expected. This will dictate the technique(s) chosen for the investigation and also the interpretation of the results. At the same time, a 'straitjacket' plan must be avoided; the interpretation of results must not be so narrow that any unexpected observation is discarded, simply because it does not fit. In a well run laboratory, various techniques must be thoroughly understood by people with a special skill in carrying them out. It is wise, in large laboratories, to have a number of people, experienced in different techniques, to make true team-work possible. This must not imply, however, that all tests are simply carried out on a routine basis. An open mind and free discussion must be kept for unexpected observations, which often lead to new discoveries. Sir Peter Medawar gave, in a B.B.C. serial in the autumn 1963, called 'Experiment: A Series of Scientific Case Histories'[69], a challenging talk, entitled: 'Is the Scientific Paper a Fraud?' By this he did not suggest that the average scientific paper misrepresented facts. He meant that it may be a fraud "because it misrepresents the process of thought that accompanied or gave rise to the work that is described in the paper".

2. This prompts the second critical statement. Each generation of scientific investigators and each phase of such continuing research shows 'trends' of ideas, techniques and of methodology. To assess such trends and to venture to prognosticate future trends is not only difficult, but often impossible. As many of the basic problems remain the same, it is often only the trends which have changed; thus suddenly new light is shed on an old problem which it had not been possible to elucidate before. Marc Klein of Strasbourg presented some valuable and amusing ideas on the subject at a workshop in Stratford-upon-Avon in 1963[70]:

> Everything has its history and to understand a problem fully, one has to know the way it arose and developed, at least through its major landmarks. This would give a solid foundation and show that problems remain fundamentally the same: we grind the same corn and obtain the same flour, but the techniques of grinding have notably changed in the course of time.

> . . .

> It would really not overload the mind or our bibliographies if at least the most basic dates were known. Is it not sad to read in recent

authoritative books that investigations on the corpus luteum began in 1928 with Corner and Allen's paper, reporting the injection of an active glandular extract into ovariectomised pregnant rabbits? . . . further . . . that oestrus is primarily the name of a definite stage of a cycle, introduced by Heape[71] and which applies to the definite period when the female is prepared to accept the male. Thus it is a term defining a behaviour, that is to say, a change of conduct of the whole body under definite natural or experimental conditions. . . . Around the 1890s Lataste, a zoologist of Bordeaux, had discovered by keen observation of laboratory rodents that the female experiences periods of sexual activity, which are connected with a rhythm of the ovary[72, 73].

Lataste and his pupil Morau[74] demonstrated a quite unknown fact: a periodic change of the vaginal epithelium, from a multilayered cornified type, through a cylindrical mucified type, back to the initial stage. Moreover, they were sure that this cylindrical change was correlated with ovarian periodicity. The occurrence of morphological variations seemed incredible to the contemporaries of Lataste and Morau. Their results were disbelieved and scorned. Morau died young, and Lataste, after much discussion with his colleagues from Paris, stopped his investigations and his career in France. "That is why", Marc Klein continues, "the study of behaviour is an essential part of the study of endocrine factors, in this case in reproductive physiology and sex differentiation"[75].

On variations among species, Marc Klein had this to say:

Throughout our sessions, whenever a problem or an answer was questioned, speakers generally sheltered behind the remark: this is true in the species under investigation, and it so happened that nearly every time this species was the rat. This reminds me of seeing, many years ago, in Beach's laboratory at Yale, a cartoon, alluding to the story of the Pied Piper of Hamelin. It showed an enormous rat playing on a flute and behind him a merry crowd of well-known experimental biologists dancing to his tune. I am afraid the moral of the story is true. Species differences impose a heavy load on the whole of endocrinology. . . . We have heard from Professor Dodd, using Rothschild's estimate, that about 4500 species of mammals are known today[76].

The Chinese fable of the meeting of the six blind monkeys and the white elephant is appropriate[77]. "We are six blind monkeys going on a pilgrimage," said the eldest. "I am an elephant." "How is an elephant made?" The monkey who touched the leg, said: "An elephant has the shape of a column like a bamboo tree." "No," said the one who touched the belly. "He is like a huge rough barrel." "An elephant," said another who touched his ear, "has wings like a bat." "No," said one who touched a tusk, "he has a long pointed shell." "Not at all," said the one who was holding the trunk, "an elephant is much like a snake." "Brothers", announced the last who had touched the tail, "let me tell you, an elephant is much like a rope." Thus are false conclusions drawn by those who, absorbed by detail, cannot see the whole.

Thus, the present state of the endocrine field cannot be readily presented like, for example, the Battle of Waterloo is painted, however huge a canvas one may choose. It is still in flux, is still progressing and it is impossible to foresee or foretell the final outcome. All we can do is to take a still photograph, as it were, of the situation, perhaps from various angles, and pick out a few of the contents, pinpoint and briefly discuss them on their present merits. First, let us look at some of the general considerations which have emerged.

Structure of the hormones

Some hormones have already been mentioned (pp. 545–546). The main groups are the peptide, the steroid and the thyroid hormones. We discussed the production of the peptide ones, especially of insulin. The larger molecule of proinsulin, molecular weight 9000–12 000, contains some 30 additional amino acids which connect the A and B chains of insulin. This C-peptide seems to form the proper connection of the disulphide bridges of the insulin molecule, which is, therefore, as an active hormone a double-chain amino acid polypeptide hormone (of a molecular weight of only 6000). Insulin and C-peptide are then secreted together into the blood stream. C-Peptide has no biological activity and proinsulin has only about 10% that of insulin. The assay of C-peptide has been used to assess the integrity of function of the beta-cell in patients on insulin, when insulin antibodies seemed to interfere with the assay of endogenously produced insulin. The islets of Langerhans, estimated to be about one million in the adult human (being *ca.* 1% of the total weight of the pancreas), also contain alpha cells, which secrete glucagon, and delta cells, which secrete gastrin. The secretion granule migrates to the periphery of the cell where it apparently fused with the cell membrane and is then discharged into the bloodstream, as outlined above.

Herbert M. Evans proved convincingly, in 1921, that the interior pituitary contains a growth promoting hormone (growth hormone; somatotrophin, STH, GH); injection of crushed bovine anterior lobe tissue into rats stimulated their somatic growth considerably[78]. Philip E. Smith (1884–1970) found in 1930 that pituitary extracts and implants in hypophysectomized rats restore inhibition of somatic growth and can even cause gigantism (see p. 519). This was followed by Choh Hao Li and H. M. Evans first isolating and then synthesizing the crystalline hormone (see p. 524). Another practical advance was achieved in 1948 by A. Wilhelmi, J. B. Fishman and J. A. Russel, by the introduction of a new procedure of extraction which improved the yield of almost pure crystalline bovine growth hormone[79].

Recent studies have shown that on molecular weight, amino acid composition and partial amino acid sequence, the growth hormone molecules of various species are more similar than had been assumed. The species studied were man, monkey, ox, sheep, horse, pig, dog, rat, rabbit and whale. The average molecular weight was found to be around 22 000. Human GH is a polypeptide of 191 amino acids with two intramolecular bisulphide bonds, in approximately the same position as in most species studied. Reviewing the situation in 1974, Rosalyn S. Yalow could demonstrate by physico-chemical and immunological methods, that peptide hormones do not constitute single molecular species and that, in fact, "many . . . are synthesised in a larger precursor form"[80]. Terminal amino acid residues are remarkably similar among the various species, but immunochemical reactions are highly variable. Physiologically, the release of GH into the circulation is episodic, and highest being 1 or 2 hours after the beginning of sleep. Exercise, relative hypoglycaemia 3–5 hours after meals, and absolute hypoglycaemia after insulin, releases GH into the circulation. The peptidergic neurons of the hypothalamus which release the hypothalamic–hypophysiotrophic peptides are under the control of monoaminergic axons from higher centres of the brain (via the limbic system)[81]. It is probably these connections that cause stress (e.g. hypoglycaemia, exercise, etc.), fright and other emotional stimuli to release growth hormone. One of the most important physiological controls of the endocrine system working through the central nervous system, is the sleep–wake cycle[82]. As the half-life of growth hormone is only 20–25 minutes, it is essential to obtain a time curve for information. Ovine and bovine GHs are fundamentally identical. So are the amino acid sequences of human STH and of human placental lactogen (HPL) or somato-mammo-trophin (HCS). The two hormones each contain 191 residues and 161 of them are identical.

These facts make one appreciate the problems concerning the relations between prolactin and growth hormone. For a long time they could not be separated, until Oscar Riddle managed to achieve it. Recent research has shown, however, that there is a strong similarity between human STH and, for example, ovine prolactin, the latter having 198 amino acids, but also a third bisulphide bridge.

On the other hand, large segments of the molecules of both are homologous. Moreover, prolactin does not merely elicit lactation among the mammals and is essential for stimulation of the rat corpus luteum, but also stimulates growth in many species of vertebrates, from amphibians to mammals. Conversely, GH also has some lactogenic effects. It seems that the prolactins, growth hormone and chorionic somato-mammotrophins (placental lactogens) are phylogenetically ancient hormones in vertebrates, which have evolved from common ancestral molecules.

Growth hormone *in vivo* proved to stimulate sulphate uptake in cartilage cells, except in hypophysectomized rats. The latter observation led to the discovery of 'somato-medin', a GH dependent factor in serum, directly responsible for the stimulation of cartilage cells[83]. A number of such substances have been found and named somatomedins A, B and C. They affect cartilage, adipose tissue, liver and placenta. Somatomedins A and C appear to be the same. They also possess an insulin-like activity, most probably related to their recognition by insulin receptors.

Glucagon (see also pp. 470–471) is a straight-chain amino acid polypeptide (molecular weight 3485). It is secreted by the alpha-cells of Langerhans' islets (and by similar cells in the intestinal mucosa, first reported by Sutherland and De Duve in 1948[84]. There are also the enteric glucagon-like peptide substances of extrapancreatic origin, having a glucagon-like immunoreactivity with or without glucagon-like biological activity[85]. They stimulate glycogenolysis, mediated by the conversion of inactive to active phosphorylase. It is of great interest that cyclic AMP was discovered during the study of the mediation of glycogenolytic effects of glucagon. Continued secretion of glucagon caused stimulation of gluconeogenesis for which, it seems, glucocorticoid interaction is needed.

The steroid hormones are derived from the cortex of the adrenal glands and from the testes and the ovaries. These hormones are embryonically derived from the mesodermal urogenital ridge, which eventually differentiates and forms the tissues which form them. Professor Ian Chester Jones (b. 1916) of the Department of Zoology in Liverpool gave an exciting outline of the 'Evolutionary Aspects of the Adrenal Cortex and its Homologues' in his Sir Henry Dale Lecture for 1976[86]. As Sir Peter Medawar put it in 1953:

For 'endocrine evolution' is not an evolution of hormones, but an evolution of the uses to which they are put; an evolution not, to put it crudely, of chemical formulae, but of reactivities, reaction patterns and tissue competence[87].

This also applies to the evolution of peptide and protein hormones[88]. Historically, Medawar's aphorism has also been claimed to have originated from Fred Hisaw at Harvard, and finally, from Emil Witschi of Switzerland who brought it to his classes in Iowa City[89]. All steroid hormones are derived from cholesterol. Its side-chain is cleaved by an enzyme to form pregnenolone as a precursor. The steroid nucleus is a cyclopentenophenanthrene which is numbered to indicate the carbon atoms to which various keto-, methylaldehyde and other groups are attached, as well as the position of double bonds within the nucleus, all of which give each steroid hormone its specific properties.

The steroid hormones are usually divided into three groups according to the number of carbon atoms they contain. (a) The adrenal cortex produces C-21 steroids: cortisol or hydrocortisone, with the isolation of which Edward Calvin Kendall was concerned (see pp. 517–518). These and related steroids are called gluco- and mineralocorticoids according to their main activities, although cortisol also has an influence on mineral regulation, but as a mineralocorticoid aldosterone is *ca.* 100 times more potent than cortisol. The other important C-21 steroid is progesterone, produced mainly in the corpus luteum in the second part of the menstrual cycle after ovulation has occurred.

(b) The C-19 steroids cover the androgen group, the most active of which is testosterone. These are formed mainly in the testicles, although small amounts are also synthesized in the (male and female) adrenal cortex and in the ovary. Almost all the androgens excreted by the female derive from the adrenal cortex, but the medulla of the ovary may also produce testosterone and andro-stenedione.

(c) The oestrogens are the C-18 steroids oestradiol, oestriol and oestrone, of which oestradiol is the most active prototype. Like phenol they have a 'phenolic' ring with three double bonds (see pp. 396–400)[90]. The oestrogens are manufactured mainly by the ovaries, but small amounts may also be obtained from the testes and adrenals. Thus, it can be seen that the key numbers of the steroid nucleus are positions 3, 11, 17 and 21. Addition or removal of keto- or hydroxyl groups have great influence on their biological action. Hydroxylation at the 11 position in the adrenal cortex will prevent the production of ACTH in the pituitary. Most of the steroids are metabolized to inactive products in the liver. The excretion products in the urine are glucuronide metabolites of cortisol and sulphates of androgens (hydroxy- and 17-keto-steroids). The excretion products are used to a great extent for measurement of the 17-hydroxysteroids. When, towards the end of the 1940s, the active properties of cortisone were discovered, numerous alternatives were attempted in the steroid molecule to achieve or change biological activity. The first one of practical use was prednisone, which was created by a double bond in the 12 position of cortisone. By these means, the glucocorticoid activity was quadrupled in relation to that of cortisone, while the mineralocorticoid activity was reduced to 0.3. The creation of dexamethasone (9-alpha-fluoro-16-alpha-methyl-hydrocortisone) resulted in a glucocorticoid with 30 times the potency of cortisol without any mineralocorticoid activity. In contrast, the addition of a fluorine atom at the 9 position led to the formation of 9-alpha-fluorohydrocortisone, which increased the mineralocorticoid activity of cortisol 250 times, but that of glucocorticoid only 8 times; this has been useful in aldosterone-deficient states for mineral regulation. Similar chemical wizardry was attempted in altering the androgen molecule to reduce the androgenic activity and increase the anabolic one, with somewhat less marked success.

The use of oestrogens for the prevention of ovulation and thus for birth control (see pp. 448, 451, 532–535), led the chemists to the creation of the 19 nor-steroids by removal of the methyl group from the 19 position. These new compounds possess potent progesterone-like activity in addition to the inhibitory effect on ovulation. Other alterations resulted in the formation of compounds with anti-oestrogenic and anti-androgenic properties. The potent anti-oestrogenic compound Clomid-R ('clomiphene') has been used successfully in producing ovulation by stimulating effect on the pituitary or hypothalamus; this will be discussed later, when considering the treatment of infertility.

The structures of the two thyroid hormones, thyroxine (tetra-iodothyronine, T_4) and of tri-iodothyronine (T_3), differ only in the absence of an iodine atom in tri-iodothyronine. Thyroxine is converted into tri-iodothyronine in some peripheral tissues. The thyroid gland is unusual among endocrine glands in that it stores large amounts of hormones within. Thyroxine is usually produced in larger amounts than tri-iodothyronine. When released into the blood stream, the thyroid hormones are bound specifically to serum proteins, named thyroid-binding globulin (TBG) and thyroid-binding pre-albumin (TBPA), and non-specifically to serum albumin. T_4 has a greater avidity for TBG than T_3. Accordingly, a greater amount of T_3 is free in the blood stream than T_4. The synthesis of the two thyroid hormones occurs, as already stated, in four now well-studied and known steps (see pp. 421–428).

The secretion of steroid hormones is more complex; they do not appear in secretion granules.

Mechanism of hormonal action

The main types of hormonal action also seem to depend on the main structural groups. The action of the peptide hormones is as described at the beginning of this chapter.

As we have seen, the steroid hormones, on the other hand, enter the blood, bound to specific proteins, as do the thyroid hormones. They are then released from their carrier proteins, traverse the cell membrane to attach themselves to another receptor protein and travel to the nucleus. There they activate (or repress) genes, thus stimulating production of messenger RNA and protein synthesis. The basic studies on this sequence were done in the oviduct of the chick in response to oestrogen. To complicate matters, the transport of glucose and amino acids into the cell under the action of insulin was found to occur without an increase in cyclic AMP. Moreover, hydrocortisone increases the blood pressure almost immediately, apart from its steroid action, most likely through direct action on the vessel walls. No hormone action can be described unless it is clearly understood that the humoral and nervous actions of the body are not only closely interrelated but indeed, interwoven, inseparable and jointly provide the control of the functions of the body (see pp. 411–421). Oversimplification, however, is not possible. The juxtaglomerular apparatus of the kidneys produces, in its myoepithelial cells around the afferent arterioles of the glomeruli and in the cells of the macula densa of the renal cortex, a proteolytic enzyme called 'renin' (molecular weight *ca.* 40 000), first discovered as a pressor substance by Robert Adolf Armand Tigerstedt (1853–1923) and P. G. Bergman in 1898[91], which enters the circulation by the renal veins. It activates angiotensinogen, a circulating alpha-2-globulin manufactured in the liver as a glycoprotein (molecular weight *ca.* 57 000), to form a decapeptide angiotensin I, which is eventually converted by a blood enzyme into angiotensin II, an octapeptide, which is the most powerful pressor substance manufactured within the body. It acts directly on the smooth muscle of the arteriole and also directly stimulates the production of aldosterone by the zona glomerulosa of the suprarenal cortex. It is destroyed by various peptidases called 'angiotensinases'. Infusion of catecholamines into the renal artery or electrical stimulation of the renal nerves will increase the release of renin, whereas alpha- and, especially, beta-adrenergic blockade will block the renal response to upright posture. Renin release is subject to feedback control by angiotensin II, directly and indirectly, through the effect of the latter on blood volume, blood pressure and sodium balance.

We must now return in greater detail to one part of the action of hormones which is centred on specific receptors. Intensive studies have been carried out in recent years to elucidate their role and influence. At a symposium in London in February 1979[18] the present position concerning receptors and their diseases was summarized. E. Baulieu of Paris claimed:

> Over the past twenty years studies on hormone receptors have materialized the dream of pharmacologists, because for the first time they have provided physico-chemical data on the molecular mechanism by which the target cells receive environmental information[92].

In fact, hormone receptor concentration in a target cell is not of fixed value and its variation depends on many factors. Interaction of a hormone with its receptor, coupling between hormone–receptor and adenylate cyclase and the activity of the latter are all governed by several cellular components. In the case of multiple receptors, various experimental approaches may be necessary. In the brain, for example, there are at least two receptors for opioid peptides according to H. W. Kosterlitz (of Aberdeen University)[93]. The μ-receptors, which represent the preferential binding sites for naloxone, naltrexone or morphine, and the δ-receptors, which represent preferential sites for the enkephalins.

A number of anti-hormones, such as anti-androgens and anti-oestrogens, act by competing for binding to cytoplasmic hormone receptors. Thus, clomiphene and tamoxifen (both non-steroidal triphenylethylenes), the latter being a competitive inhibitor of oestradiol, bind to the cytoplasmic receptor. Moreover, the tamoxifen-receptor complex also transposes to the nucleus, so that antagonism is mediated mainly by nuclear events[94]. The development of abnormal receptors could lead to antibody production (because of abnormal antigen stimulation). On the other hand, a failure of immune tolerance in an autoimmune disease may also cause manufacture of receptor antibodies.

Professor Reginald Hall of Newcastle-upon-Tyne surveyed four receptor-antibody diseases, which have been studied so far[95]. These are as follows.

1. In Graves' disease, thyroid stimulating antibodies are produced (TSAb). These bind to the thyrotrophin receptor, which may sometimes lead to the activation of adenylate cyclase. They may be responsible for the goitre and the signs of hyperthyroidism in Graves' disease.

2. In myasthenia gravis antibodies are produced which react with the acetylcholine (ACh) receptor. The consequence is increased degradation of the receptor and of the occasional binding to the actual receptor site which is involved in the binding of acetylcholine.

This action means a reduction in the number of ACh receptors and alters the structure of the remaining ones. Thus the neuro-muscular transmission is blocked and this leads to the characteristic signs in myasthenia. Interestingly, in animal models of myasthenia, it was demonstrated that alpha-cobratoxin binds to ACh receptors.

3. A rare variety of diabetes mellitus, with insulin resistance and associated with acanthosis nigricans and carbohydrate intolerance was shown to have circulating antibodies to the insulin receptor. This implies that in some instances these antibodies block the action of insulin; in others, an insulin-like action may be accompanied by severe hypoglycaemia. This action of the insulin-receptor antibodies seems to have a similar mechanism as the TSAb action in Graves' disease.

All the above-mentioned conditions of receptor antibody disorders also have immunological disturbances and may be associated with other organ-specific antibodies and auto-immune diseases.

4. A fourth condition, still not clearly defined, is, according to Hall, chronic renal failure with increased amount of immune reactive circulating parathyroid hormone (PTH) antibodies attached to the PTH receptor, thus blocking endogenous PTH action.

G. M. Besser (London), summarized the theoretical, clinical and considerable therapeutic application of recent research on dopamine/growth hormone – dopamine agonists and antagonists[96]. Dopamine and its agonists lower normal and abnormal prolactin secretion in man by direct intervention on dopamine receptors in the pituitary gland. Their other action is on the growth hormone. In normal people, the secretion of GH is stimulated and a (transient) pulse of GH is usually released. In acromegaly and gigantism, however, where GH secretion is pathologically increased, there is a paradoxical fall in GH and inhibition of its secretion as long as dopamine is administered. This seems to be caused by a direct action of the dopamine agonists at the pituitary cell level, whereas in normal individuals the effect is mediated at the median eminence. Dopamine agonists also inhibit TSH and TSH-response to TRH and LH secretion. Above all, dopamine agonists inhibit prolactin secretion by direct action on the pituitary mammotroph cells, and dopamine itself is perhaps the most important physiological hypothalamic prolactin-inhibiting factor (PIF)[97, 98].

Abnormal concentrations of human gonadotrophin receptors may also be directly or indirectly associated with several gonadal disorders. Gonadotrophin receptors may be depleted by pituitary dysfunction or by prolonged treatment with human gonadotrophic hormone[99].

Specific-binding receptor-sites exist for insulin on the surface of many mammalian cells. They are of particular importance for the biological effects; some of those, like lipogenesis and anti-lipolysis, may be activated at the same receptor site. R. H. Jones of London estimated the molecular weight of these receptor sites to be *ca*. 300 000, but he thinks they may well be divisible into sub-units[100]. He does not exclude the possibility of intra-cellular sites as well (see p. 546). The binding affinity seems critically dependent on pH (which may account for insulin resistance in acidosis). Occasionally, insulin resistance may be associated with the existence of anti-receptor antibodies.

David Anderson of Hope Hospital, Salford, Lancs., England, came to the conclusion that osteoporosis is a strong candidate for a receptor disease. There is present a fundamental defect in bone resorption, for which several animal models exist[101].

Thus, the field of receptor studies, and pathological conditions caused by their abnormalities, is steadily expanding[102]. They have to be considered in conjunction with the results of the research on the disorders caused by them and on immunology.

Immunophysiology and pathology in endocrine disorders

In 1900, Paul Ehrlich (1854–1915) anticipated the problems arising from the manufacture of specific antibodies by animals, directed against body constituents similar to their own, such as the antibody response of rabbits to the red blood cells of sheep[103]. He coined the term 'Horror Antitoxicus', to express the seemingly natural revulsion of the animal in reacting against its own self-antigens. With the present knowledge of the immune system and of immune responses, the self-tolerance needs a good deal of explaining.

In the process of distinction between self and non-self, the following facts have to be considered: (1) Animals do sometimes manufacture antibodies with the ability to combine with self-antigens. (2) Tolerance can be artificially induced. (3) Both 'natural' and 'artificial' tolerance can be overcome by appropriate measures.

There might be a case for giving Girolamo Fracastoro (Fracastorius) (1478–1553), some credit in this respect. He was the author in 1530 (publication date; it was written in 1521) of a poetic treatise on syphilis; he also suggested a germ theory of infection. In 1546 his book was published: 'De sympathia et antipathia rerum liber unus. De contagione et contagiosis morbis et curatione.'[104] From studying the text, 'De sympathia and antipathia' could be taken, with imagination, as a suggestion of self and non-self.★ In 1938, John Richardson Marrack (b. 1886) published his study on 'The chem-

★ In 1903, Sajous suggested that the adrenal, pituitary and thyroid glands controlled the immunising mechanisms of the body.

istry of antigens and antibodies'[105]. Soon afterwards, (Sir)
Frank Macfarlane Burnet (b. 1899) and Frank John Fenner (b. 1914)
introduced the 'self-marker' concept[106]. For this and his work on
acquired immunological tolerance, Burnet shared the Nobel Prize
with (Sir) Peter Brian Medawar (b. 1915) in 1960. Burnet and
Fenner's theory of immunity was proved in 1953 by the work
of Rupert Everett Billingham (b. 1921), L. Brent and Peter B.
Medawar[107]. Finally, Ivan Maurice Roitt, Deborah Doniach, P. N.
Campbell and R. V. Hudson demonstrated auto-antibodies in Hashimoto's disease (lymphadenoid goitre) in 1956[108]. They really
pioneered the understanding of auto-immunity as one of the major
causal factors in endocrine disorders; it is by no means restricted to
the thyroid. Deborah Doniach and Gian Franco Bottazzo pointed
out, in a paper on 'Autoimmunity in diabetes mellitus' (which they
kindly allowed me to see before publication), that it was suspected
very soon after the discovery of organ-specific auto-immunity, that
"some cases of diabetes mellitus (DM) might belong to the same
group of disorders, owing to the high prevalence of insulin-
dependent diabetes (Type I) in Addison's Disease, thyrotoxicosis,
myxoedema, pernicious anaemia and hypoparathyroidism".[109] It
should be remembered that the following 'primary' organ-specific
auto-immune diseases have been found, in addition to those mentioned above: Hashimoto's thyroiditis, which was described by
Hakaru Hashimoto (1881–1934) in 1912 as lymphoid infiltration of
the thyroid, 'Struma lymphomatosa'[110]. Before its definition as a
classical auto-immune disease, it puzzled clinicians for several decades, especially as it often begins with signs of hyperthyroidism,
ending in the opposite direction. Equally interesting are the patients
in this group with certain forms of male infertility, premature
menopause, partial hypopituitarism, atrophic fundal gastritis (Type
A) and atrophic antral gastritis (Type B).

Before proceeding with the discussion, especially of auto-immune
forms of male infertility, partial hypopituitarism and auto-immune
diabetes mellitus, the original criteria for 'auto-immune disease'
must be re-stated as originally postulated by Milgrom and Witebsk
in 1962[111]. (a) Antibodies or lymphoid cells reacting specifically
against autologous antigenic target organ tissue must be demonstrated. (b) The auto-antigen must be defined exactly. (c) The
auto-antigen must be able to elicit an immune response in another
organism. (d) Appropriate immunization with this antigen of an
experimental animal must cause lesions which correspond to the
distribution of the antigen in the immunized individual (e.g. development of thyroiditis, but no encephalo-myelitis, after immunization with thyroid material). (e) Passive transfer of the disease

must be possible by serum or lymphoid cells. This postulate should, however, not be regarded as compulsory, as susceptible inbred strains of experimental animals are not always available for use in spontaneous or artificially induced models.

There are several alternative theoretical mechanisms which could explain self-unresponsiveness[112].

Macrophages: Degradation of self-antigen to tolerogenic form.
  B cells: (1) High concentration of antigen may eliminate.
            (2) Low concentration of albumin may block.
            (3) Low concentration may fail to stimulate.
            (4) T cells and/or auto-antibody may suppress.
  T cells: (1) May be eliminated.
            (2) May be blocked by antigen and/or antibody.
            (3) May be supported by other T cells.

None of these mechanisms are mutually exclusive. Professor Deborah Doniach pioneered the study of the humoral and genetic aspects of thyroid auto-immunity. Her conclusions of 1975 still hold good[113]: (1) Thyroid antibody tests provide a reliable indication of lymphoid thyroiditis and should be carried out in all cases of goitre in whom thyroidectomy is contemplated. These tests can also be adapted for antenatal screening of populations, in order to eradicate overt myxoedema, by preventive treatment in predisposed individuals. (2) Thyroid antibodies are a guide in looking for auto-immunity in conditions of unknown aetiology. (3) One of the most interesting aspects is the connection with this group of diseases of the 'immune response' genes, which are still poorly known in the human species. A loss of suppressor T cells has been widely postulated to account for the continued production of autoreactive antibodies. . . . Thyroiditis appears to be the mildest expression of these defects within a group. Niels Jerne concluded in 1973 that the complexity of the immune system could only be compared with that of the brain[114].

The pathogenesis of endocrine exophthalmos was reviewed by Professor Deborah Doniach on the occasion of a discussion on 'thyroid eye disease' in October 1977[115]. Human exophthalmos seems to be caused by a group of auto-immune reactions against the TSH receptors in the thyroid-cell membrane. Some antibodies mimic the actions of (pituitary) TSH. Others fit the receptors incompletely and their activity covers only some of the functions of the thyrotrophic hormone. Formerly grouped as thyroid-stimulating antibodies (TSAb), it is now known that some of them can stimulate only the human thyroid (LATS-P), while others stimulate animal glands (LATS). The exophthalmos-producing immunoglobulin seems able to compete with TSH for the receptor sites which exist on adipocytes[116], harderian gland membranes[117], and human blood polymorphs and monocytes[118]. This means that TSH-receptor antibodies can react on and stimulate certain cells outside the thyroid gland. Indeed, immunoglobulins from people with severe endocrine exophthalmos produced proptosis in animals by stimulating the retro-ocular tissues. The weakness of this theory is that TSH is suppressed in Graves' disease[119], and, especially, that endocrine exophthalmos can occur after hypophysectomy[120].

A separate lesion accounting for the proptosis in exophthalmos, is the myositis of the extraocular muscles. Retro-orbital muscle has no TSH receptors. Inflammatory changes in the extra-ocular ribbon-shaped muscles are commonly observed in thyrotoxicosis when EMI scans of the orbit are carried out. There is oedema, lymphoid infiltration and destruction of the muscle fibres. After the inflammation has subsided, increased fibrosis and loss of contractile tissue remain. Kriss and his co-workers thought that they could prove an anatomical communication between the lymphatic drainage of the thyroid and the orbit, when injecting radioactive colloidal solutions into the former[121]. According to Kriss, it is known that thyroglobulin can be discharged in small quantities in an unhydrolysed form directly into the thyroid. It might find its way into the orbit and set up immunological reactions there. He (and other authors) noted high thyroglobulin antibodies in the serum of patients with malignant exophthalmos. As a result of retrograde flow into the orbit, thyroglobulin may attach itself to extra-ocular muscles. By the same retrograde flow, locally synthesized anti-thyroglobulin antibodies may arrive from the thyroid. Immunological events then occur, such as muscle injury, histamine release, increased vascular permeability, leucocyte migration inhibition. Mullin and his group[122] have confirmed this work, although Takeda and Kriss could not detect thyroglobulin–anti-thyroglobulin complexes in the sera of 21 patients with endocrine exophthalmos, eight of whom had concomitant thyrotoxicosis[123]. Humoral immunity is, therefore, not sufficient to explain the pathogenesis of endocrine exophthalmos. It must result from a combination of both, humoral and cellular immune mechanisms. Lymphocytes become sensitized to extracellular muscle antigen[124]. In 1977 Teng and Yeo found a significant correlation between thyroidal suppression by tri-iodothyronine (T_3) and the TSH-response to TRH[125]; but Solomon and colleagues[126] in the United States found further evidence that ophthalmic Graves' disease is not a single disease entity. One group of patients had TSH stimulating antibodies, with no suppression by (exogenous) T_3, and there were high titres of thyroid antibodies in the serum. These patients were thought to have three auto-immune disorders: Graves' disease, Graves' ophthalmopathy and Hashimoto's thyroiditis! A second group had no TSH antibodies or thyroid antibodies and T_3 did suppress thyroid activity. The diagnosis in these cases was thought to be isolated Graves' exophthalmic disorder without auto-immune thyroid disorder. Professor Deborah Doniach stresses that present evidence suggests that auto-immune lesions are never mediated by just one of the mechanisms of the immune repertoire, but "result from a combination of both humoral and cellular reactions to a variety of related tissue antigens"[115].

The familiar clinical feature that severe diplopia may occur independently of the degree of proptosis, further strengthens the two-prong theory of exophthalmos. There is also evidence for the existence of TSH-receptors (TSH-R) on adipose tissue cells. It is now equally probable that LATS and human-specific thyroid-stimulating antibody are responsible for the hyperactivity of the thyroid in Graves' disease[127]. If endocrine exophthalmos is usually readily diagnosed clinically even if the patient appears euthyroid, the diagnosis can be confirmed by a flat TRH test, by the failure of tri-iodothyronine (T_3) to suppress the uptake of ^{131}I, and/or by the existence of thyroid antibodies.

At this point, we must briefly allude to the long-acting thyroid-stimulator (LATS). It was discovered by D. D. Adams and H. D. Purves in 1956[128], when serum from a thyrotoxic patient, injected into guinea pigs prepared for bioassay of TSH, was found to cause unexpectedly prolonged stimulation of thyroid function. LATS was determined to be an IgG which cannot readily be separated from IgGs. A number of surveys has been published on the incidence of positive LATS' responses in Graves' disease. Some of these demonstrate that LATS is found in unconcentrated serum of approximately half of all patients with the disease. A number of exceptions argue, however, against a sole aetiological role for LATS and imply that additional factors are necessary for the development of hyperthyroidism. Very occasionally patients with LATS are *not* hyperthyroid. Some patients have ophthalmic Graves' disease before hyperthyroidism develops, while others have Hashimoto's disease and post-therapy hypothyroidism. It has also been established that there is *no* increase in positive LATS-responses in patients with exophthalmos. It is highly probable that LATS is synthesized by lymphocytes in the following manner:

$$\text{ATP} \quad \underset{\text{adenyl cyclase}}{\overset{\text{TSH or LATS}}{\cdots\cdots}} \quad \underset{\substack{\text{stimulation of} \\ \text{thyroid cell}}}{\overset{\text{cAMP}}{\downarrow}} \quad \underset{\substack{\text{phosphordiesterase} \\ \text{(After Pat Kendall-Taylor,} \\ \text{1975)}}}{\cdots\cdots\cdots\cdots\rightarrow 5\,\text{AMP}}$$

LATS is a 75 IgG, which conforms to the 4-peptide chain structure for IgG[129]. LATS could not be demonstrated in many grossly hyperthyroid patients, which makes the role of LATS as a cause of Graves' disease questionable. Human thyroid homogenates can neutralize LATS activity, which Adams, Kennedy and Stewart[127] showed to be due to the immunoglobulin G: the LATS-protector (LATS-P), which inhibited the binding of LATS to human thyroid tissue. As LATS-P does *not* inhibit LATS effect in the mouse bioassay, this means that LATS-P binds, by preference, to human, but not to mouse thyroid tissue. LATS-P has been found in up to 90% of patients with Graves' disease, but *not* in the normal population.

We must now return to the discussion of the role of auto-immunity in diabetes mellitus. Diabetes mellitus is, of course, not a single disease, but a heterogeneous group of diseases[130]. The only common factor in the various syndromes is an elevated blood glucose. This multi-factorial disorder has, therefore, many facets of aetiology; some of these facets are themselves multi-factorial. The genetic factor, for example, does not deal with the question of how the disease is inherited, but rather with the nature of the inherited defects which may lead to diabetes. Insulin is the only hormone which can reduce the level of circulatory sugar in the blood. It is able to counteract the action of several hormones which elevate the blood-sugar level by glycogenolysis or gluconeogenesis. The beta-cells of the pancreas, which release insulin, respond to a variety of signals, such as sugars, amino acids and lipid metabolites (substrates), glucagon, ACTH, gastric inhibitory peptides (hormones) and drugs. Somatostatin suppresses the release of insulin. The surface receptors receive the stimulus; this is followed by proinsulin synthesis in the endoplasmic reticulum of the beta-cell.

Ten years ago, cell-mediated immunity became generally accepted, once the development of the leucocyte migration inhibition test (LMT)[131] demonstrated that a proportion of juvenile diabetics were sensitized to pancreas[132]. This juvenile onset diabetes (Type I), which occurs in children and young adults, needs insulin at diagnosis or soon after. Whereas the LMT is positive in recently diagnosed patients, it may become negative after prolonged treatment with insulin. Thirst, polyuria, loss of weight and lassitude are usually marked. The urine contains sugar and acetone. The evidence, however, suggests that these Type I diabetics have normal islet-cell function at birth and normal capacity of insulin production. Nor is there any evidence of the glucostatic mechanism. What is inherited is a susceptibility to exogenous influences which damage the islet cells. In 1972 A. Bloom and his colleagues[133] started a register of newly diagnosed diabetic children, which revealed in the first 1400 questionnaires a history of diabetes in a first degree relation in 11% of the patients, in contrast to 1% in non–diabetic children. This indicates a genetic factor, although not a strong one. Other authors[134], found that possession of certain histocompatibility phenotypes confers a susceptibility to beta-cell destruction by an environmental agent. Next, it seems that diabetes in children will follow viral infection, such as mumps, and that in older children the date of onset of diabetes closely follows the seasonal pattern of infections occurring in normal childhood. Finally, immunological studies have proved the presence of antibodies to islet cells in newly diagnosed juvenile diabetics[135]. Immediately after diagnosis, islet-cell antibodies were found in 85% of Type I patients, but they became less common with the duration of the disease. Thus it seems that inheritance of certain HLA phenotypes confers susceptibility to virus infections pathogenic to the islet cells. When the virus damages the islet cells, it releases antigenic products which, in turn, leads to the production of antibodies. The antigen–antibody reaction then destroys the beta cells, producing diabetes. Huang and McLaren[136] studied the effect of peripheral lymphocytes from juvenile diabetics on cultured insulinoma cells. They demonstrated cytotoxic effects after 4 days' contact with sensitized lymphocytes, whereas no such results could be produced with normal lymphocytes or with the sera of the diabetic patients. Direct T-cell cytotoxicity also seemed to be involved in some instances of diabetes. Direct T-cell effects may occur when virally altered cell-membrane antigens are involved. With native tissue antigens, antibody-dependent killer (K)-cell cytotoxicity is usually observed.

Another group of insulin-dependent diabetes is associated with diseases which are now regarded as caused by auto-immunity. These may be alopecia, Addison's anaemia, Addison's disease, hypogonadism and thyroid disorders, in which case antibodies to the appropriate organs are often found. The only common-link factor in these diseases is organ specific humoral and cellular auto-immunity. The additional presence of permanent antibodies to islet cells proves that in these patients diabetes is merely one aspect of a primary immunity disorder. Experiments with passive transfer of diabetes from man to mouse are not quite completed as yet, but are promising enough to expect that it will eventually be possible to find out how activated lymphocytes injure beta cells.

Intensive and promising research in this field is going on at present. This permits the hope that the multi-factorial disorders which are covered by the generic term 'diabetes mellitus' will be analysed in a more satisfactory manner in the not too distant future.

Distinct antibodies to glucagon (A) – somatostatin (D) – cells and pancreatic polypeptides (H-PP) cells seem now to be nearer to definition. Somatostatin is secreted in various parts of the central nervous system, in the spinal cord and beta cells along the entire length of the gastro-intestinal tract, where it acts as a paracrine hormone and inhibits the secretion of other intestinal polypeptides[137]. It is clear from histocompatibility antigen (HLA) studies, that two diabetic genes can be inherited, which increase the likelihood of disease expression. Types HLA B8 and D3 and DWR3 are found more frequently in subjects with auto-immune disorders, including thyrotoxicosis, Addison's disease, myasthenia gravis and pernicious anaemia, when associated with endocrinopathies.

Auto-immunity against steroid producing organs was discussed by W. J. Irvine, Edinburgh[138]. There is a very low prevalence of adrenocortical antibodies in the general population. People with adrenocortical antibodies in the serum but without Addison's disease may have an impaired reserve of adrenocortical function. In idiopathic Addison's disease, the presence of IgG antibodies in the serum of 67–70% of patients, reactive with the cytoplasm of adrenocortical cells and evidence for cell-mediated immunity by the migration inhibition test, together with the histological appearance of the adrenal cortex, all indicate the possibility of an auto-immune pathology in this disorder.

In women of reproductive age, idiopathic Addison's disease is usually associated clinically with hypergonadotrophic amenorrhoea or marked oligomenorrhoea. Atrophy of the ovaries may be present with high prevalence in the serum of a group of IgG antibodies which react with the steroid-producing cells within the ovary, which also react with adrenocortical antigens. These steroid-cell antibodies occur only rarely in patients with primary hypergonadotrophic amenorrhoea without associated idiopathic Addison's disease. Interestingly, men with idiopathic Addison's disease rarely develop antibodies to steroid-producing cells in the Leydig cells and have rarely evidence of hypogonadism. It seems that most patients with auto-immune Addison's disease develop an immune reaction against antigens in the adrenal cortex, but a fair number develop such reactions against antigens, shared between the adrenal cortex and the steroid-producing cells in the gonads and placenta.

Male infertility has, for a long time, been assumed to be a group of disorders rather than one; recently, it has become clear that even impotence in the elderly male is not a homogeneous condition from the physiological, endocrine and psychological point of view. To present the situation in a nutshell, auto- and iso-antigens of spermatozoa have been found in the sera of infertile men and women, and auto-immunity to sperm in men can cause aspermatogenesis. Anti-sperm antibodies may be detected in the serum as IgG, but they only interfere with fertility if they are present in the genital secretions as IgA[139]. They have an immobilizing effect on normal donor sperm, causing them to clump together head-to-head (H–H), tail-to-tail (T–T), or tail–tip-to-tail–tip (TT–TT); it seems that these various positions are due to different antibodies. Women's sera almost always contain H–H agglutinins, those from men usually have tail agglutinins. Technical details of the tests were defined by a WHO workshop in 1976[140] and the results of an extensive international study were reported by the WHO Reference Bank for Reproductive Immunology in 1977[141]. W. F. Hendry (London) stressed that the additional test of sperm–cervical mucus contact (SCMC) has helped to define the 10% subfertile men in whom there is an auto-immune barrier to sperm penetration, although the treatment of anti-sperm antibodies is still not very successful[142]. It should be noted that the presence of antibodies reacting with antigens of sperm of the female ovum was observed as early as 1961[143]! In some patients the antibody response disappeared and fertility was restored[144]. In animals, immunological interference with pregnancy was achieved by passive administration of antibodies. Whether such an immunologically produced prevention of pregnancy is safe, reversible and generally applicable, has to be further investigated. In the case of the average human, it is assumed that there are about 10^{12} lymphocytes and 10^{20} (a hundred million times more) antibody molecules. These antibodies inactivate the target molecules by binding with it.

Most antigens possess several receptors with which antibodies can bind. Such an antigen–antibody complex can be of an aggregate type and lead to precipitation of the molecule which is, eventually, disposed of by the phagocytes. In some cases, however, antibodies can be directed to irrelevant portions of the molecule, in which case they do not neutralize the activity of the antigen and may even enhance it. This had been observed in the case of antibodies against some steroid hormones and of TSH[145]. When there are membrane-associated antigens, antibodies can bind with them; if complement is available and the antibody is suitable, cell lysis will occur; however, secretory antibodies of the IgA class do not have attachment sites of the complement and their combination with the membrane-bound antigens cannot cause cell lysis.

There are also genetic controls for the ability of an animal to respond to an antigen[146]. The human being is *not* an inbred animal, there is heterogeneity of the antibodies formed to a polymer, and the antigen and the set of antibodies formed to the same antigen differ from one individual to another. Antigens with a limited number of immuno-determinants do not always produce effective antibodies in order to block the biological activity of the target hormone. Tolerance (non-responsiveness) to antigens can also occur at very low doses or very high concentrations of the antigen. It is thought to be caused by an elimination of the clone of the immuno-competent cells recognizing the antigen (or by suppressor cells blocking the immune response).

Immunization against the pituitary gonadotrophins and sexual steroid hormones or against LH-RH, the decapeptide produced in the hypothalamus which controls the release of LH and FSH, may lead to disruption of the reproductive processes.

Factors which prevent or promote the access of spermatozoa to the upper female genital tract also play a part in the sperm being made available for fertilization.

Spermatozoa possess auto- and iso-antigens. Sperm agglutinins in the serum, causing male infertility, were described 25 years ago by P. Rümke[147], and also by L. Wilson[148]. These were the first definite reports of natural infertility caused by immunological factors. Moreover, up to 75% of vasectomized men develop anti-sperm antibodies within a few months after the operation, perhaps as a result of the escape of sperm into the blood circulation at the time of the vasectomy. In normal healthy men, it seems that the blood–testis barrier and the inability of the lymphoid cells to get to the tubular compartments containing the sperm-borne antigens prevents the manufacture of auto-antibodies. J. Freund and his colleagues induced aspermatogenesis, anaphylaxis and cutaneous sensitization in the guinea pig by homologous testicular extract, in 1955[149]. Antibodies could be produced with sperm antigens only, but to achieve aspermatogenesis, Freund and his colleagues used a potent adjuvant (Freund's complete adjuvant = FCA), to produce auto-immune allergic orchitis. It is not permissible to use such adjuvants on human subjects. On the other hand, Professor G. P. Talwar and his team have been able to block the sperm development beyond the stage of primary spermatocytes, with the germinal epithelium remaining apparently undamaged, and Leydig cells remaining functional and responding normally to gonadotrophins; they have been able to prove this in rats, guinea pigs, rabbits, dogs, rams and rhesus monkeys with almost 100% effectiveness[146].

Although the sperm carries several antigens foreign to the female, normally, a rejection-type of immune response does not seem to occur. There have been, however, occasionally clinical observations in which the female genital tract contains sperm-agglutinating, cytotoxic, complement-fixing and immobilizing antibodies[150]. This was found by several groups of researchers, independently. In many such patients this abnormal immune behaviour causes infertility. It is enhanced by continuing repeated deposits of sperm. A certain number of prostitutes have been reported to carry anti-sperm antibodies[151]. Active immunization, i.e. injection into the recipient of the antigens and elicitation in her of the antibodies (and CMI) against the antigens, will be, according to Talwar, the obvious choice for prevention of pregnancy in large-scale family planning programmes. Passive use of injected preformed antibodies is effective for only as long as the life span of the antibodies and may be of use, occasionally, in a singular intervention for the termination of pregnancy.

This whole field of research is in an exciting phase of progress and holds important possibilities for the future as regards its clinical application. It includes the study and investigation of the placental products and, especially, human chorionic gonadotrophin (hCG), manufactured as early as the 9th day after fertilization[152]! It sustains early pregnancy corpus luteum function and steroidogenesis and thus prevents menstruation. If antibodies intercept the hCG function, this may result in the loss of the impregnated ovum.

hCG is also synthesized at ectopic sites in very small amounts in normal tissues (testes, sperm, non-endocrine tissues), and in a greater quantity in tumours, such as testicular embryonic carcinomas, breast cancer, GI tract tumours[153]. The use of anti-hCG immunization as treatment for hCG-producing tumours is by no means clear, and needs to be evaluated.

G. Franco Bottazzo and Professor Deborah Doniach reviewed pituitary autoimmunity[154]. Although clinical polyendocrinopathies are not common (see also p. 556), patients with two endocrine diseases together or following one another are not particularly rare. In such patients circulating antibodies or cell-mediated reactions can occasionally be found for all endocrine organs, the pancreas and pituitary included. In four previous publications, lymphocytic hypophysitis was described histologically, and an auto-immune pathogenesis was postulated in two of the four patients, owing to the association with thyroiditis, gastritis and adrenalitis.

Systematic examination by immunofluorescence on all endocrine glands of sera from Addisonian and hypoparathyroid patients gave the lead to the first description of the islet-cell antibodies in 1974[155, 156]. They have proved to be of clinical importance for the distinction and prediction of various types of diabetes mellitus[157]. The same series of (stored) polyendocrine sera were applied to normal human pituitary glands, obtained by hypophysectomy, for relief in patients with carcinoma of the breast. In 19 out of 287 cases, antibodies were found, reacting specifically with the prolactin-secreting cells (PRL) of the anterior pituitary[158]. No antibodies were found in patients with panhypopituitarism, but PRL-cell antibodies were described in two patients with mild or partial pituitary deficiencies. The second specific pituitary antibody to be identified was against the human growth-hormone secretory cells, in a young girl with retarded growth since the age of 6, whose mother had Addison's disease and thyroiditis. Finally, Gleason and colleagues reported on another patient with a possible auto-immune hypophysitis in a 59-year-old woman[159], with attacks of hypoglycaemia and unexplained arthralgias, who – at post-mortem – had an enlarged pituitary gland with the features of an auto-immune lesion, i.e. lymphoid follicles, interstitial round cell collections, fibrosis and focal collections of pituitary cells. The condition had not been diagnosed during life.

REFERENCES

1. Berson, S. A., Yalow, Rosalyn S.: General radioimmunoassy, in methods in investigative and diagnostic endocrinology, pp. 84–120. Peptide Hormones (eds. Berson, S. A. and Yalow, R. S.). Vol. 2A. New York, American Elsevier, 1973.
2. Saffran, Murray, Schally, A. V., Benfey, B. G.: Stimulation of the release of corticotropin from the adenohypophysis by a neurohypophysial factor. Endocrinology. **57,** 439–444, 1955.
3. McCann, G. M., Dhariwal, A. P. S.: Hypothalamic releasing factors and the neurovascular link between the brain and the anterior pituitary. In Neuroendocrinology (eds. Martini, L., Ganong, W. F.), pp. 261–296. New York, 1966.
4. Pasteels, Jean-Lambert: Administration d'extraits hypothalamiques à l'hypophyse de rat *in vitro*. C. R. Hebd. Séanc. Acad. Sci. Paris **254,** 2664–2666, 1962.
5. Daniel, P. M.: Anatomy of the hypothalamus and pituitary gland. In Hypothalamic and Pituitary Hormones, pp. 1–7. Assoc. Clin. Pathologists, supplement, **30,** 1977.
6. Hughes, A. F. W.: A history of endocrinology. J. Hist. Med. Allied Sci., **32,** 292–313, 1977.
7. Daniel, P. M., Treip, C. S.: Pathology of the hypothalamus. Clin. Endocrinol. Metabol. **6,** 1–19, 1977.
8. Zambrano, David: The arcuate complex of the female rat during the sexual cycle. Z. Zellforsch. **93,** 560–570, 1969.
9. Ryle, A. P., Sanger, F., Smith, L. F., Kitai, R.: The disulphide bonds of insulin. Biochem. J. **60,** 541–556, 1955.
10. Bell, P. H.: Purification and structure of B-corticotropin. J. Am. Chem. Soc. **76,** 5565–5567, 1954.
11. Li, Choh Hao, Dixon, J. S., Chung, David: Adrenocorticotropins. XXI. The amino acid sequence of bovine adrenocorticotropin. Biochim. Biophys. Acta **46,** 324–334, 1961.

12. Gorden, P. *et al.*: Science **200,** 782, 1978.
13. Science **202,** 260, 1978.
14. Conn, P. M.: Nature **274,** 598, 1978.
15. Br. Med. J., **I,** 773, 1979.
16. Pastan, I. H., Johnson, G. S., Anderson, W. B.: Annu. Rev. Biochem. **44,** 491, 1975.
17. Grossman, M. I.: In the 'Foreword' to Gut Hormones (ed. Bloom, S. R.), p. v. Edinburgh, London and New York, Churchill Livingstone, 1978.
18. Hormone Receptors and their Diseases. Section of Endocrinol. R. Soc. Med., Soc. for Endocrinol., Br. Diabet. Ass. 27th and 28th February 1979, at the Roy. Soc. Med. in London.
19. Robison, G. A., Butcher, R. W., Sutherland, E. W.: Cyclic AMP. New York, Academic Press, 1971.
20. Anderson, D. C.: Hormone Receptors and Bone Disease. In Ref. 18, Presentation No. 25.
21. Davies, T. F.: The impact of peptide hormone receptor research on clinical medicine. J. R. Coll. Physicians **12,** 379–397, 1978.
22. Ibid. p. 383.
23. Hill, S. R., Jr.: Endocrinology revisited. Alabama J. Med. Scis. **14(1),** pp. 1–9, 1977.
24. As 21: p. 385.
25. Bayliss, R. I. S. (ed.): Investigations of endocrine disorders. In Clinics in Endocrinology and Metabolism. Vol. 3, No. 3. London, Philadelphia, Toronto, W. B. Saunders, 1974.
26. Ibid.: Section on Diseases of the Thyroid Gland by Evered, D., pp. 425–450.
27. Hollander, C. S., Shenkman, L.: T$_3$ toxicosis. Br. J. Hosp. Med. **8,** 393–395, 1972.
28. As 26: p. 447.
29. As 25: Section on Investigation of Disorders of the Parathyroid Glands by Parfitt, A. M., pp. 451–474.
30. Ibid.: p. 451.
31. Cohn, D. V., Macgregor, R. R., Chu, L. L. H. *et al.*: Biosynthesis of proparathyroid hormone and parathyroid hormone chemistry, physiology and role of calcium in regulation. Am. J. Med. **56,** 767, 1974.
32. Brewer, B. H., Jr., Fairwell, T., Rittell, W. *et al.*: Recent studies on the chemistry of human, bovine and porcine parathyroid hormones. Am. J. Med. **56,** 759, 1974.
33. As 25: Section on Diseases of the Hypothalamus and Pituitary Gland, by Edwards, C. R. W., Besser, G. M., pp. 475–505.
34. Schally, A. V., Arimura, A., Baba, Y., Nair, R. M. G., Matsuo, A., Redding, T. W., Debeljuk, L., White, W. P.: Isolation and properties of the FSH and LH releasing hormone. Biochem. Biophys. Res. Commun. **43,** 393–399, 1971.
35. Brazeau, P., Vale, W., Burgus, R., Ling, N., Butcher, M., Rivier, J., Guillemin, R.: Hypothalamic polypeptide that inhibits the secretion of immunoreactive pituitary growth hormone. Science **179,** 77–79, 1973.
36. Hall, R., Besser, G. M., Schally, A. V., Coy, D. H., Evered, D., Goldie, D. J., Kastin, A. J., McNeilly, A. S., Mortimer, C. H., Phenekos, C., Tunbridge, W. M. G., Weightman, D.: Action of growth hormone release inhibiting hormone in healthy men and in acromegaly. Lancet **II,** 581–584, 1973.
37. As 33: p. 486.
38. Cowden, E. A., Thomson, J. A., Doyle, D., Ratcliffe, J. G., Macpherson, P.,

Teasdale, G. M: Tests of prolactin secretion in the diagnosis of prolactinomas. Lancet **I,** 1155–1161, 1979.

39. Burke, C. W., Moore, R. A., Rees, L. H., Bottazzo, G. F., Mashiter, K. and Bitensky, L.: Isolated ACTH deficiency and TSH deficiency in the adult. J. R. Soc. Med. **72,** 328–335, 1979.
40. World Health Organisation: WHO Tech. Rep. Ser. **565,** 5–72, 1975.
41. Krieger, Dorothy T.: Factors influencing the circadian periodicity of ACTH and corticosteroids. Med. Clin. N. Am. **62,** 251–259, 1978.
42. Ibid.: pp. 251–252.
43. Ibid.: p. 257.
44. Krieger, D. T.: Circadian rhythms. Abstracts, pp. 13–14. Int. Symposium on Endocrine Function of the Human Adrenal Cortex. Florence, 4–7 October 1977.
45. Ibid.: p. 14.
46. Rees, Lesley H.: ACTH and related peptides. Abstracts, p. 9. Int. Symposium on Endocrine Function of the Human Adrenal Cortex. Florence, 4–7 October 1977.
47. James, V. H. T., Landon, J.: Hypothalamic-pituitary-adrenal Function Tests. Horsham (Sussex). Ciba Laboratories. 1971.
48. Simpson, S. A., Tait, J. F., Bush, P. G. G. were quoted by George Widmer Thorn (b. 1906) as the group who isolated 'electrocortin' (=aldosterone): Johns Hopkins Med. J. **123,** 49–77, 1968. In fact a publication by Grundy, Hilary M., Simpson, S. A. and Tait, J. F.: Isolation of a highly active mineralocorticoid from beef adrenal extract. Nature, London **169,** 795–796, 1952, is regarded as the first publication.
49. Simpson, S. A., Tait, J. F.: Recent progress in methods of isolation, chemistry, and physiology of aldosterone. Recent. Progr. Hormone Res. **11,** 183–210, 1955.
50. Cited after Thorn, G. W.: The adrenal cortex. I. Historical aspects. Johns Hopkins Med. J. **123,** 49–77, 1968.
51. Conn, J. W.: Primary aldosteronism, a new syndrome. J. Lab. Clin. Med. **45,** 6–17, 1955.
52. Conn, J. W., Conn, E. S.: Primary aldosteronism versus hypertensive disease with secondary aldosteronism. In Recent Progress in Hormone Research (ed. Pincus, G.), Vol. XVII, Section III, pp. 389–414. London, Academic Press, 1961.
53. Mills, I. H.: Clinical Aspects of Adrenal Function. Oxford, Blackwell, 1964.
54. Armstrong, M. D., McMillan, A.: Identification of a major urinary metabolite of norepinephrine. Fed. Proc. **16,** 146, 1957.
55. Means, J. H.: Historical background of the use of radioactive iodine in medicine. N. Eng. J. Med. **252,** 936–940, 1955.
56. Hertz, S., Roberts, A., Evans, R. D.: Radioactive iodine as an indicator in the study of thyroid physiology. Proc. Soc. Exp. Biol. Med. **38,** 510–513, 1938.
57. Leblond, C. P.: Localization of newly administered iodine in the thyroid gland as indicated by radioiodine. J. Anat. **77,** 149, 1943.
58. Raith, L.: Introduction to Radioimmunoassay Methods. Dietzenbach-Steinberg, Byk-Mallinckrodt, 1975.
59. Euler, U. S. von: Conference on structure and function of biologically active peptides. Ann. N.Y. Acad. Sci. **104,** 449, 1963.
60. Euler, U. S. von: A specific sympathomimetic ergone in adrenergic nerve fibres (sympathin) and its relations to adrenaline and nor-adrenaline. Acta Physiol. Scand. **12,** 73–97, 1946.
61. Pepe, F. A., Finck, H.: J. Biophys. Biochem. Cytol. **11,** 521, 1961.

62. Heftmann, E.: Chromatography. New York, Reinhold, 1962.
63. Lederer, E., Lederer, M.: Chromatography. In Comprehensive Biochemistry, vol. **4**, p. 32. Amsterdam, Elsevier, 1962.
64. Arx, E. von., Neher, R.: J. Chromat. **8**, 145, 1962.
65. Antoniades, H. N., Bougas, J. A., Pyle, H. H.: N. Eng. J. Med. **267**, 218, 1962.
66. Harington, C. R.: J. Anim. Tech. Assoc. **13**, 3, 1962.
67. Lane-Petter, W.: Revision of Laboratory Animals for Research: A Practical Guide. Amsterdam, Elsevier, 1961.
68. Karlson, P., Sekeris, C. E.: Nature, London **195**, 183, 1962.
69. Medawar, P. B.: Is the Scientific Paper a Fraud? pp. 7–12. In Experiment. A Series of Scientific Case Histories. London, BBC Publication, 1964.
70. Klein, M. In Techniques in endocrine research. Proceedings of a NATO Advanced Study Institute at Stratford-on-Avon, pp. 289–302. Eds Eckstein, P., Knowles, F. London, New York, Academic Press, 1963.
71. Heape, W.: Q. J. Micros. Sci. **44**, 1, 1901.
72. Lataste, F.: C. R. Soc. Biol. Paris. **44**, 765, 1892.
73. Lataste, F.: Recherches de Zooéthique. Bordeaux, Durand, 1887.
74. Lataste, F., Morau, H.: J. Anat., Paris. **25**, 277, 1889.
75. As 70: p. 295.
76. As 70: p. 161.
77. As 70: pp. 301–302.
78. Evans, H. M., Long, J. A.: The effect of the anterior lobe administered intraperitoneally upon growth, maturity and oestrus cycles of the rat. Anat. Rec. **21**, 62–63, 1921.
79. Wilhelmi, A. E., Fishman, J. B., Russel, J. A.: A new preparation of crystalline anterior pituitary growth hormone. J. Biol. Chem. **176**, 735–745, 1948.
80. Yalow, Rosalyn S.: Heterogeneity of peptide hormones. Rec. Prog. Hormone Res. **30**, 597–633, 1974.
81. Daughaday, W. H.: The adenohypophysis. In Textbook of Endocrinology (ed. Williams, R. H.). Philadelphia, W. B. Saunders, 1974.
82. Weitzman, E. D., Boyer, R. M., Kapen, S., Hellman, L.: The relationship of sleep and sleep states to neuroendocrine secretion and biological rhythms in man. Rec. Prog. Hormone Res. **31**, 399, 1975.
83. Van Wyk, J. J., Underwood, L. E., Hintz, R. L. *et al.*: The somatomedins. A family of insulin-like hormones under growth hormone control. Rec. Prog. Hormone Res. **30**, 259, 1974.
84. Sutherland, E. W., Duve, C. de: Origin and distribution of the hyperglycaemic–glycogenolytic factor of the pancreas. J. Biol. Chem. **175**, 665–670, 1948.
85. Holst, J. J.: Extraction, gel filtration pattern and receptor binding of porcine, gastro-intestinal, glucagon-like immuno-reactivity. Diabetologia **13**, 159–169, 1977.
86. Jones, I. C.: Evolutionary Aspects of the Adrenal Cortex and its Homologues. Sir Henry Dale Lecture for 1976. Proc. Soc. Endocrinol. in J. Endocrinol. **71**, 3P–32P, 1976.
87. Ibid.: p. 26P.
88. Geschwind, I. I.: Molecular variation and possible lines of evolution of peptide and protein hormones. Am. Zool. **7**, 89–108, 1967.
89. Witschi, Emil: Cit. in 86: p. 26P.
90. Browne, J. S. L.: Chemical and physiological properties of crystalline oestrogenic hormones. Canad. J. Res. **8**, 180–197, 1933.

91. Tigerstedt, R. A. A., Bergman P. G.: Niere und Kreislauf. Scand. Arch. Physiol. **8,** 223–271, 1898.
92. Baulieu, E.: Hormone Receptors and Historical Perspective. As 18: Presentation No. 1.
93. Kosterlitz, H. W.: Opioid Peptides and their Receptors. As 18: Presentation No. 7.
94. Wakeling, A. E.: Anti-oestrogens. As 18: Presentation No. 12.
95. Hall, R.: The Receptor Antibody Disease. As 18: Presentation No. 14.
96. Besser, G. M.: Dopamine/Growth Hormone – Dopamine Agonists and Antagonists in Clinical Practice. As 18: Presentation No. 16.
97. McLeod, R. M.: In Frontiers of Neuroendocrinology **4,** 169–194, 1976.
98. Takahara, J., Arimura, A., Schally, A. V.: Endocrinology **95,** 462, 1974.
99. Davies, T. F.: Human Testicular Gonadotrophin Receptors. As 18: Presentation No. 17.
100. Jones, R. H.: Insulin. As 18: Presentation No. 26.
101. As 20.
102. Schulster, D.: Post-Receptor Events in the Cell Membrane. As 18: Presentation No. 3.
103. Ehrlich, P.: Gesammelte Arbeiten ueber Immunitaetsforschung (Collected works on research on immunity). Berlin, A. Hirschwald, 1904.
104. Fracastoro, Girolamo: De sympathia et antipathia rerum liber unus. De contagione et contagiosis morbis et curatione. Venetiis, apud heredes L. Iuntae, 1546.
105. Marrack, J. R.: The chemistry of antigens and antibodies. Spec. Rep. Ser. Med. Res. Council, London, **230,** 1–194, 1938.
106. Burnet, Sir Frank M., Fenner, F. J.: The Production of Antibodies. 2nd ed. Melbourne, Macmillan, 1949.
107. Billingham, R. E., Brent, L., Medawar, P. B.: Actively acquired tolerance of foreign cells. Nature, London **172,** 603–606, 1953.
108. Roitt, I. M., Doniach, Deborah, Campbell, P. N., Hudson, R. V.: Autoantibodies in Hashimoto's disease (lymphadenoid goitre). Lancet **II,** 820–821, 1956.
109. Bottazzo, G. F., Doniach, Deborah: Autoimmunity in diabetes mellitus. In Secondary Diabetes (ed. Podolsky). New York, Raven Press, 1979.
110. Hashimoto, H.: Zur Kenntnis der lymphomatosen Veraenderung der Schilddruese (Struma lymphomatosa). Arch. Klin. Chir. **97,** 219–248, 1912.
111. Milgrom, F., Witebsk, E.: Autoantibodies and autoimmune diseases. J. Am. Med. Assoc. **181,** 706–716, 1962.
112. Playfair, J. H. L.: The distinction between self and non-self. In Clinics in Endocrinology and Metabolism, Vol. 4, No. 2, Autoimmunity in Endocrine Disease (ed. Irvine, W. J.). London, Philadelphia, W. B. Saunders, 1975.
113. Doniach, Deborah: Humoral and genetic aspects of thyroid autoimmunity, pp. 267–285. In Clinics in Endocrinology and Metabolism, Vol. 4, No. 2: As 112.
114. Jerne, Niels: Scientific American, July 1973, cit. from 113.
115. Doniach, Deborah: Thyroid eye disease. Proc. R. Soc. Med. Lond. **70,** 695–698, 1977.
116. Hart, I. R., Mackenzie, J. M.: Endocrinology **88,** 26, 1971.
117. Winand, R., Kohn, L. D.: J. Biol. Chem. **250,** 6522, 1975.
118. Chabaud, O., Lissitzky, S.: Molec. Cell. Endocrinol. **7,** 79, 1977.
119. Kourides, I. A. *et al.*: J. Clin. Endocrinol. Metab. **40,** 872, 1975.
120. Furth, E. D. *et al.*: J. Clin. Endocrinol. Metab. **22,** 518, 1962.

121. Kriss, J. P., Konishi, J., Herman, M.: Rec. Prog. Hormone Res. **31,** 533, 1975.
122. Mullin, B. R., Levinson, R. E., Friedman, A., Henson, D. E., Winand, R. J., Kohn, L. D.: Endocrinology **100,** 351, 1977.
123. Takeda, Y., Kriss, J. P.: J. Clin. Endocrinol. Metab. **44,** 46, 1977.
124. Munro, R. L. *et al.*: J. Clin. Endocrinol. Metab. **37,** 286, 1973.
125. Teng, C. S., Yeo, P. P. B.: Ophthalmic Graves's disease: natural history and detailed thyroid function studies. Br. Med. J. **I,** 273–275, 1977.
126. Solomon, D. H. *et al.*: N. Eng. Med. **296,** 181, 1977.
127. Adams, D. D., Kennedy, T. H., Stewart, R. D. H.: Aust. N.Z. J. Med. **6,** 300, 1976.
128. Adams, D. D., Purves, H. D.: Abnormal responses in the assay of thyrotrophin. Proc. Univ. Otago Med. School **34,** 11–12, 1956.
129. Cohen, S., Porter, R. R.: Structure and biological activity of immunoglobulins. Adv. Immunol. **4,** 287–349, 1964.
130. Bloom, A.: The nature of diabetes, J. R. Soc. Med. London **71,** 170–179, 1978.
131. Bendixen, G., Soberg, M.: A leucocyte migration technique for *in vitro* detection of cellular hypersensitivity in man. Dan. Med. Bull. **16,** 1, 1969.
132. Nerup, J., Andersen, O. O., Bendixen, G., Egeberg, J., Gunnarson, R., Kromann, G., Poulsen, J. E.: Cell-mediated immunity in diabetes mellitus. Proc. R. Soc. Med. **67,** 506, 1974.
133. Bloom, A., Hayes, R. M., Gamble, D. R.: Register of newly diagnosed diabetic children. Br. Med. J. **II,** 580, 1975.
134. Cudworth, A. G., Woodrow, J. C.: Evidence for HL-A linked genes in 'Juvenile' diabetes mellitus. Br. Med. J. **II,** 133, 1975.
135. Irvine, W. J., McCallum, C. J., Gray, R. S., Campbell, C. J., Duncan, L. J. P., Farquhar, J. W., Vaughan, H., Morris, P. J.: Pancreatic islet-cell antibodies in diabetes mellitus correlated with the duration and type of diabetes, coexistent autoimmune disease and HLA type. Diabetes **26,** 138, 1977.
136. Huang, S. W., MacLaren, N. K.: Insulin-dependent diabetes: a disease of auto-aggression. Science **192,** 64, 1976.
137. Orci, L., Baetens, D., Ravazzola, M., Malaisse-Lagae, F., Amherdt, M., Rufener, C.: Somatostatin in the pancreas and the gastrointestinal tract. In Endocrine Gut and Pancreas (ed. Fujita, T.). New York, Elsevier, 1976.
138. Irvine, W. J.: Autoimmunity against steroid producing organs. Abstracts, pp. 39–40. Int. Symposium on Endocrine Function of the Human Adrenal Cortex. Florence, 4–7 Oct. 1977.
139. Hendry, W. F.: Male infertility. Br. J. Hosp. Med. **22,** 47–60, 1979.
140. Rose, N. R., Hjort, J., Rümke, P., Harper, M. J. K., Vyazov, O.: Clin. Exp. Immunol. **23,** 175, 1976.
141. WHO Reference Bank for Reproductive Immunology: Clin. Exp. Immunol. **30,** 173, 1977.
142. Hendry, W. F.: Br. J. Urol. **49,** 752–762, 1977.
143. Nakabayashi, N., Tyler, A., Tyler, E. T.: Immunological aspects of human infertility. Fertil. Steril. **12,** 544, 1961.
144. Franklin, R. R., Dukes, C. D.: Anti-spermatozoal antibody and non-explained infertility. Am. J. Obstet. Gynecol. **89,** 6, 1944.
145. Nieschlag, E., Usadel, K. H., Wickings, E. J. *et al.* Effects of active immunisation with steroids on endocrine and reproductive functions in male animals. In Immunization with Hormones in Reproduction Research (ed. Nieschlag, E.). Amsterdam, N. Holland, 155, 1975.

146. Talwar, G. P.: Immunology in reproduction. J. Reprod. Med., **22,** No. 2, 61–76, 1979.
147. Rümke, P.: The presence of sperm antibodies in the serum of two patients with oligozoospermia. Vox Sang **4,** 135, 1954.
148. Wilson, L.: Sperm agglutinins in human semen and blood, Proc. Exp. Biol. Med. **85,** 652, 1954.
149. Freund, J., Thompson, G. E., Lipton, M. M.: J. Exp. Med., **101,** 591, 1955.
150. D'Almeida, M., Eyquem, M. A.: Antisperm activity in cervical mucus of infertile women. In Abstract of Papers of 3rd International Symposium on Immunology of Reproduction, Varna, Bulgaria, 1975: p. 83. Copenhagen, Scriptor, 1976.
151. Schwimmer, W. B., Ustay, K. A., Behrman, S. J.: An evaluation of immunologic factors of infertility. Fertil., Steril. **18,** 167, 1967.
152. Catt, K. J., Dufau, M. L., Vaitukaitis, J. L.: Appearance of hCG in pregnancy plasma following the initiation of implantation of the blastocyst. J. Clin. Endocrinol. Metab. **40,** 537, 1975.
153. Vaitukaitis, J. L.: Human chorionic gonadotrophin as a tumour marker. Am. Clin. Lab. Sci. **4,** 276, 1974.
154. Bottazzo, G. F., Doniach, D.: (Review of pituitary autoimmunity) J. R. Soc. Med. **71,** 433–436, 1978.
155. Bottazzo, G. F., Florin-Christensen, A., Doniach, D.: Lancet **II,** 1279, 1974.
156. Maccuish, A. C., Barnes, E. W., Irvine, W. J., Duncan, L. J. P.: Lancet **II,** 1529, 1974.
157. Irvine, W. J., McCallum, Gray, R. S., Duncan, L. J. P.: Lancet **I,** 1529, 1977.
158. Bottazzo, G. F., Pouplard, A., Florin-Christensen, A., Doniach, D., Lancet **II,** 97, 1975.
159. Gleason, T. H., Stebbins, P. C, Shanahan, M. F.: Arch. Pathol. Lab. Med. **102,** 46, 1978.

CHAPTER TWENTY-TWO

PRESENT TRENDS AND OUTLOOK FOR THE FUTURE – PART II

RHYTHM IN THE PHYSIOLOGY AND PATHOLOGY OF ENDOCRINE SECRETION

BIOLOGICAL rhythms have been known of for a long time. The alternation of light and darkness, the sleep–wake pattern in moderate climates, the pattern of feeding and digestion (excretion), are generally accepted. Less obvious are the rhythmic variations in blood pressure, pulse rate, temperature and almost all bodily and mental functions. It has now also been established that hormonal secretion is subject, to a great extent, to rhythmic control. This maybe of various types. It is advisable to define a few terms which are in common use in this subject.

A regularly recurring event is 'rhythmic' or 'periodic'. If presented in the form of a curve, it can be 'sinusoid'. It may be a symmetrical or asymmetrical curve and display a peak. A 'cycle' is the shortest part of such a curve which repeats itself indefinitely, in a time which is called the 'period' of the cycle. Amplitude is usually defined as the distance from the peak to the trough. If the rhythm depends wholly on an external event like daylight and darkness after sunset, it is 'exogenous'; if it is not influenced by such external events, it is 'endogenous'. When the exogenous rhythm is suspended, the endogenous rhythm may continue independently as 'free-running'. If one special factor influences a rhythm, J. Aschoff, in 1958, coined the term 'Zeitgeber' (= time determinant) for it[1]. 'Phase' refers to any particular point on the curve, and 'phase-shift' indicates that the periodicity, without change in form, is delayed or advanced. The term 'diurnal', now only rarely used, defines a daily rhythm. In 1959 Franz Halberg, of the University of Minnesota, introduced the term 'circadian' (from the Latin = 'circa diem', covering periods from 20 to 28 hours)[2]. From the ancient Greek was taken the term 'nykthemeral' ($\nu\acute{\upsilon}\xi$ = night; $\acute{\epsilon}\mu\acute{\epsilon}\varrho\alpha$ = day); meaning the alternation of night and day. Endogenous and exogenous control often interact. The mechanism is perhaps located in the brain, which seems to act as time recorder and controller of the biological rhythms of the body, and it is called the 'clock'. Clocks need adjustment, as they cannot usually keep exact time for long periods; this is done by the 'Zeitgeber'.

Apart from circadian rhythms, there are, of course, weekly, monthly, seasonal and even annual cycles. Biological rhythms are thus exogenous, endogenous and genetically determined and also influenced environmentally by social conditions, feeding habits, etc. Franz Halberg and his colleagues (Chronobiology Laboratory of the University of Minnesota Medical School) are of the opinion that psychiatric and physical disorders will occur if some cycles move out of phase and out of synchrony with the normal sleep–activity schedule of the usual 24-hour unit of activity. Dr. Halberg's team developed fundamental methods for detecting and defining rhythms and for analysing their characteristics. In the last ten years, a considerable number of circadian rhythms has been detected in body chemistry, organic function and related aspects. Rex B. Hersley of the University of Pennsylvania found in 1929, in a course of study of factory workers, that emotional variations take place daily. Moreover, psychological changes occur in cycles ranging from four to six weeks.

There is a circadian rhythm in the activity of desoxyribonucleic acid (DNA) and ribonucleic acid (RNA) as Dr. Halberg and colleagues could demonstrate. Dr. Curt P. Richter of Johns Hopkins has studied the connection between drug action, potentially harmful exposures (PHE) and activity rhythms, for over 40 years. He found that some commonly-used drugs leave, after prolonged (ab-)use, disrupted physiological rhythms, which are often observed in behavioural changes after medication has stopped. In fact, just as phase-shifts may alter drug response, drugs can alter physiological circadian rhythms.

Dorothy and Howard Krieger have led this field of study for a number of years. Dorothy T. Krieger is Professor of Medicine and Director, Division of Endocrinology and Metabolism at the Mount Sinai School of Medicine in New York. As one of the first observers she pointed out that the circadian rise and fall of plasma ACTH and corticosteroid concentrations did not occur in a linear, smooth manner, but that there is episodic secretion superimposed upon the circadian pattern. Such episodic, relatively synchronous peaks were evident throughout the day, the majority occurring between 3.00

a.m. and 9.00 a.m., with a gradual upward trend[3]. The fact is that secretion of most hormones and production of other biologically active substances does not occur in a continuous smooth line, but in a pulsating manner, similar to many forms of radiation, and only partly influenced by the circadian rhythm. The demonstration of a circadian periodicity in plasma ACTH levels in patients with Addison's disease and in the adrenalectomized animal, strongly suggests that such circadian periodicity cannot be due merely to feedback processes. Development of circadian periodicity is age related and endogenous (genetic), but is influenced by the sleep–wake, light–dark cycle; it can be abolished by drugs which affect serotonin action. Periodicity is present in blind persons, with some evidence that it is free-running[4]. Circadian periodicity remains normal in depressed patients, yet the magnitude and frequency of the episodic secretion is increased. It is also normal in obese patients. In patients with Cushing's disease (or syndrome), circadian periodicity disappears. In Cushing's disease this periodicity remains abnormal after remission achieved by pituitary irradiation; in Cushing's syndrome periodicity returns to normal after surgical removal of the adrenal tumour. At present, it is assumed that the circadian variation of the pituitary–adrenal function reflects the circadian variation of the central nervous mechanism involved in the control of the corticotrophin-releasing factor (CRF). As already stated, the periodicity of ACTH concentrations persists in adrenalectomized animals, and a periodicity of brain CRF concentrations is present in hypophysectomized animals. Light is generally accepted as the most important synchronizer of the phase (the clocktime of peaks) of circadian rhythm, but the mechanism of this procedure has not yet been elucidated. Lesions of the supra-chiasmatic nucleus (and posterior to it) abolish adrenal circadian periodicity. It seems that they disrupt the excitatory pathway "which is responsible for the firing of cells which secrete CRF"[5]. Circadian periodicity of corticosteroids in the plasma does not exist at birth and appears only with anatomical (and physiological) development of the retino-hypothalamic tract, arising from the ganglion cells of the retina and ending in the supra-chiasmatic nuclei. Administration of dexamethasone in the newborn can delay, but not prevent, the development of such periodicity, the 'Zeitgeber' (or synchronizer) of which is light; the periodicity is, however, exogenous. If adult animals are blinded, the periodicity will become 'free-running'; in animals blinded at birth, periodicity is absent. In humans, the circadian increase of plasma corticosteroid levels is blocked by the administration of cyproheptadine (an antiserotonergic agent), when given near to the time of the expected circadian rise.

Limitation of food and water intake to a 2-hour period during the morning in nocturnal animals produces a phase-shift in the time of the peak of plasma concentration of corticosteroid levels. Whether the change in the sleep–wake habits or the altered time of food–intake is responsible, has not been established yet. Eating and drinking patterns in animals do make use of neuro-transmitter mechanisms; they could, therefore, be the cause for the change in corticosteroid periodicity. Once this periodicity is established, however, it is remarkably resistant to change. In humans, it will persist under varied feeding or fasting conditions, bed rest, and 48–72 hours sleep-deprivations; but in conscious patients with (radiologically and clinically) localized hypothalamic disease, over 50% showed abnormal corticosteroid patterns. In one of two, clinically endocrine-normal, non-obese patients with radiological evidence of a hypothalamic tumour and normal sella turcica, Dorothy Krieger found irregular oscillatory patterns of ACTH and plasma corticoid levels, similar to those in Cushing's disease[3].

It is also obvious that the species differences in the neuro-transmitters will need explanation. Krieger poses, accordingly, a number of critical questions:

> Is the circadian rhythm preparatory, as has been suggested, for awakening, with the consequent increased steroid levels available for stresses that ensue? Is the circadian rise in corticosteroid level a by-product of other neural mechanisms, which are coupled to neuro-endocrine function, but whose prime role is with regard to other neural processes? Does its presence make for increased susceptibility to various stimuli at different times of the day? Is the differential desynchronization of circadian periodicity of various bodily constituents responsible for the symptoms of 'jet-lag'?

The answers to these questions should bring us several steps nearer to the understanding and critical analysis of neuro-endocrine mechanisms. They may be achieved sooner than expected at present.

Meanwhile, circadian variations have also been investigated in the case of circulating thyrotrophin, thyroid hormones and prolactin by Professors John Landon and G. M. Besser and their colleagues in London (England)[6]. Significant circadian changes in serum TSH, thyroid hormone uptake test, serum and urine total thyroxine and serum prolactin were shown in all six clinically euthyroid male volunteers between 25 and 35 years of age. TSH displayed a reciprocal pattern to serum thyroxine, and THUT: the evening and night-time levels were higher than those during the day. The TSH and PRL patterns did not correlate. No consistent circadian changes were observed in serum or urinary T_3. This seems to imply that free T_3 (tri-iodothyronine) levels are maintained by a fairly constant peripheral conversion from T_4 (thyroxine), whereas TSH has a centrally determined circadian rhythm. As we have seen, the circadian pattern of the hormones of the hypothalamic–pituitary–adrenal axis are well established. It was found that the increase in TSH occurred *ca*. 4 hours before sleep, with the highest level between 23.00 and 02.00 hours. When the patient's sleep–wake cycle was reversed, De Costre and his colleagues found[7] that a reversed circadian pattern of serum total thyroxine (T_4) resulted. Chan and her colleagues found, however, that the abolition of circadian rhythms of endogenous plasma corticosteroids with 2 mg daily dexamethasone for 24 hours, did not alter the circadian pattern of TSH, which was, therefore, *not* dependent on the corticosteroid circadian rhythm. The practical lesson from this follows that blood collection for TSH and other thyroid hormone estimations and for PRL should be performed between 09.00 a.m. and noon, at mean basal level; one should also bear in mind circadian rhythm variations when conducting prolonged tests.

The hypothalamic–pituitary–gonadal axis is also subject to rhythmic variations. Seasonal and maturational variations in the field of reproductive function have been observed and described for many centuries and were, in fact, the first such observations. It is, therefore, not surprising that the integrated systems influencing all aspects of reproduction show a periodic pattern and are bound to demonstrate variations in the levels and effects of the circulating hormones. The particularly important result of recent investigations is, however, that the gonadotrophic hormones have shown not only the seasonal variations for such a length of time, but also that these larger, but relatively sluggish changes are "the result of variation in the briefer, minute-to-minute episodic releases of gonadotrophins and steroids, which occur throughout the day and night in all animal species"[8]. The present view is that the pattern of blood gonadotrophins and of many other hormone levels is pulsatile, in addition to being circadian. Episodic increases may vary in size, duration and frequency and are superimposed on the gonadotrophins (or other hormones) already present in the circulation. This means that the 'level' of the gonadotrophin (or other hormone) found in any individual measurement at a given time, is the result of the interaction of secretion, distribution and clearance at that moment. 'Pulses' of gonadotrophin may occur at 30–240 minute intervals, the rate and magnitude of the pulses being dependent upon sex, hormonal milieu, and many other pharmacological and environmental conditions. In addition, there is always a constant 'leakage' or 'obligatory' secretion, and an absolute cessation of gonadotrophin secretion has not been found. However, whereas before puberty, LH-pulses are small (no doubt due to a weak response to the LH-RH (releasing factor), after puberty the pulses of LH released during sleep increase in magnitude and are answered by gonadal function. There is certainly a late-sleep-rise of testosterone after late-sleep-rise of LH in men. The fact that young castrates and children with gonadal dysgenesis also show slow increases in gonadotrophin levels at puberty, indicates the role of a central mechanism in the pubertal increase of gonadotrophins.

During the menstrual cycle, the pattern of pulsatile release varies and reaches a peak, both in magnitude and in frequency, during the mid-cycle pre-ovulatory surge, and a nadir during the luteal phase. The secretion of gonadotrophins in men also occurs in a series of pulses. Reports of episodic releases of LRF make it seem likely that the pulsatile release of gonadotrophins is in response to a central trigger in the brain. This does not mean, however, that the pituitary is merely a repository for gonadotrophins, or any other hormones for that matter, as the response to administration of LRF can be modified ('pituitary sensitization'). This 'quantum theory', as it were, of pulsatile hormone release appears to apply to most known hormones. Its connection with the central trigger mechanism in the brain puts the whole question of neuro-hormonal relations or neuro-endocrinology on an entirely new level. To this must be added the fact that some of the most basic biological processes, such as mitochondrial function, and some of the most ungoverned ones, such as ectopic hormone secretion by some tumours, have displayed inherent periodicity and pulsatile, episodic release. The indication of intensive research in these directions is, therefore, not surprising.

The matter may appear even more complicated when one has to take into account the results of the research of Martha McClintock, a Harvard psychologist. She showed in 1971 that women living in close contact, such as nuns, hospital nurses in residence, women university students living in colleges, may develop a menstrual synchrony phenomenon. In social animals, a similar oestrous synchrony can occasionally be observed. Martha McClintock, in her study of 135 woman college residents in Boston, and later, Cynthia Graham in Canada in 1979, found that it takes about 4 months to come into synchrony. Common environmental factors do not seem to have influence, but only interpersonal factors. It appeared that a dominant personality in a female group would also dominate the timing of her room-mates' cycles, which became synchronous to hers as long as they lived together[9]. Michael Russell at Stanford could demonstrate that this 'Leader effect' was caused by the influence of axillary secretions on the olfactory system of the recipient. Ms. F. Roegel concluded from this that, as in primates, these 'pheromones' caused the menstrual synchrony. According to Cynthia Graham, the substance responsible could be isovaleric acid, which was also one of the 'copulins' isolated from vaginal secretions by Richard Michael. If the odour is suppressed by strong deodorants (perfumes), resistance to synchrony may be observed. In contrast, menstrual synchrony can be disrupted by male smells, especially by the male pheromones in the 16-andestrone group. Martha McClintock noticed that women in regular contact with men had shortened cycles. When nuns were persuaded to sleep on pillows impregnated with sweat from a nearby men's prison, they lost the synchrony, and their cycles were speeded up. Although in higher mammals females show disruption of their oestrous synchrony in the presence of a new male ('Strange male effect'), that disruption is connected with fertility, whereas menstrual synchrony may be the opposite. Are there neuro-transmitters at work from the olfactory receptors to the hypothalamus ? We shall have to await the results of further research.

Four normal young adults (three nulliparous women and one man), aged between 20 and 30 years, voluntarily underwent partial or complete inversion of their sleep–waking cycles, to investigate the connection between nocturnal release of prolactin with sleep. The result of the experiment was that in each of the four subjects on each baseline night, plasma prolactin concentration began to rise shortly after sleep onset and continued to rise in an episodic manner throughout sleep. With shifts of sleep onset of 3, 6 and 12 hours respectively, prolactin release shifted immediately and completely in all persons participating in the experiment, and prolactin levels did not begin to rise until sleep had begun. Nor did increase of prolactin secretion occur at the same time of night as it had done on baseline nights. This means that the 24-hour pattern of prolactin secretion cannot be regarded as circadian. At the same time it was proved that the nocturnal release of prolactin is similar to that of growth hormone from the point of view of sleep dependency, except in two respects.

(1) Prolactin release continues in a pulsatile manner in significant quantities as sleep goes on, showing the highest concentrations towards the end of the period of sleep, while the bulk of growth hormone is released in the early sleep period.

(2) Episodic release of prolactin continues during waking hours (at about 1 p.m. and 6 p.m.) unrelated to sleep. This obviously means that several central nervous system mechanisms may be involved in producing the 24 hour patterns shown in the case of these two hormones[10]. At the same time, a study published from the Johns Hopkins Hospital related that no significant

circadian rhythm could be demonstrated of plasma LH and no significant correlation between testosterone and LH levels, in the case of six normal young adult men, aged 21 to 26, in hourly determinations by RIA during 24 hours of normal activity and sleep[11].

Circadian variation in blood glucose levels, in glucose tolerance and in plasma immunoreactive insulin levels was reported by Richard J. Jarrett (London)[12], both in the fasting state and after meals and during glucose tolerance tests, which is important for investigative procedures. These variations were found to be associated with changes in plasma insulin levels and assumed to be secondary to a diurnal rhythm in the beta-cell response of the pancreas. Variations in sensitivity and involvement of other hormones could not be excluded.

A fairly comprehensive account of human circadian rhythms was compiled by R. T. W. L. Conroy, Professor of Physiology at the Royal College of Surgeons in Ireland and J. N. Mills, Professor of Physiology of the University of Manchester[13], with applied aspects, such as shift-working, time-zone transitions and astronautics, and important clinical implications, which included temperature, endocrinology, psychiatry, malignancy, pharmacology, therapeutics, mortality and susceptibility. Of particular interest appeared the chapter on 'experiments with abnormal time schedules', especially on 'non-24-hour days' and 'phase-shifts'; the latter we have just mentioned when discussing the experimental phase-shift in the study of prolactin secretion.

'The synchronization and maintenance of human circadian rhythms' with the discussion of an 'endogenous circadian clock', is another subject of controversy and importance. The fact that there are dissociations between various circadian rhythms in the same person raises the possibility of the existence of more than one 'biological clock' in the same individual. As we have seen, circadian rhythms exist in many cells and organs of the body; the function of transmitter mechanisms, such as the hormones and their nervous connections seems more likely to be the task of synchronizing various rhythms rather than to impose a specific rhythm on a non-rhythmic tissue. As an example may be quoted the eosinophil rhythm, controlled by the circadian variation in the corticosteroid rhythm which in turn is controlled by the ACTH rhythm. This itself is moderated by CRF, presumably governed by a higher centre in the brain, which in its turn is influenced by sensory input from the external environment, such as awareness of the alteration of day and night.

The study of insect hormones has shown rapid progress and has become of great interest, not merely in terms of comparative anatomy and physiology, but because insects have a neuro-secretory system, which may shed light on our own. In fact, a great deal of the work of the Scharrer's was carried out on the prothoracic glands and especially on the corpora allata of *Leucophaea maderae* (Orthoptera); the corpora allata could be controlled by neuro-secretory factors. Berta and Ernst Scharrer presented an interesting comparison between the intercerebralis–cardiacum–allatum system of insects and the hypothalamo-hypophyseal system of the vertebrates[14]. But is nervous control the only possibility? And in what ways does it operate? Scharrer favours a neuro-hormonal relationship between the CNS and the corpora allata in *Leucophaea*, partly based on his electron microscope study of the corpora allata and also because elementary neurosecretory granules are abundant in the glands. In addition, it could be shown that some of the hormones are steroids or mixtures of them, some of which (ecdysone) have now been synthesized. As insects cannot synthesize steroids from simple precursors, such as acetate, they must be manufactured from cholesterol (in the case of ecdysone, for example), which must be obtained from the diet. Cholesterol is, therefore, an important growth factor for many insects. Ecdysone, the hormone of the prothoracic glands, is the "moulting hormone" and also a "growth and differentiation hormone"[14]. In insects, the same hormones can have developmental, physiological and behavioural effects in the same animal, but may be at variance in a different species. Thus insect hormones may be useful for pest control, as insects cannot readily develop immunity to such compounds as they do against some chemical pesticides.

To sum up, the control of the secretion of adrenal corticoids is mainly affected by the variability in the release of ACTH. The latter depends on three variables:

(a) The nykt–hemeral rhythm, influenced by the person's exposure to light and by sleeping habits, the highest blood levels occurring at waking time and the lowest during early sleep.

(b) The feedback mechanism. This will reduce ACTH secretion when corticosteroids in the circulation are high, and vice versa.

(c) Physical or psychological stress will increase corticosteroid and ACTH secretion considerably, and may obliterate the effects of the feedback mechanism and of the nykt–hemeral rhythm. All these three variables are mainly controlled through the hypothalamus, which controls especially the production of ACTH by secretion of CRF (corticotrophin-releasing factor). Cortisol has often been called the 'stress hormone'.

'Stress' is a concept which was first introduced into medicine by Hans Selye (b. 1907) of Montreal in 1936 (see Section II). The terms stress and strain were taken from the dynamics of physics, although in an inverse meaning:

> The term stress is applied to the mutual actions which take place across any section of a body to which a system of forces is applied.[15] The term strain is applied to any change occurring in the dimensions, or shape of a body when forces are applied.[15]

Selye described the "stress syndrome"[16] in connection with the "general adaptation syndrome", which is a stereotyped non-specific response of the body to all noxious influences. Selye was, in his conclusions, mainly influenced by Artur Biedl, whose pupil he had been in Prague, and by Claude Bernard, and also by Walter B. Cannon, with whom he had spent a year as a Rockefeller scholar in Baltimore. In 1950, he summarized his views and the results of his research in his major work: *The Physiology and Pathology of Exposure to Stress*[17]. He told how, during his studies on the causation of collagen disorders, he stumbled on the idea that animals (and man) respond to stress or injury with a certain sequence of physiological reactions and adapt themselves (with the "general adaptation syndrome"). Selye is a great believer in carefully thought out and planned methods of experimentation, using the simplest possible technique. Above the door of his Institute in Montreal is written in French:

> Neither the prestige of your theme
> Nor the power of your tools
> The breadth of your knowledge
> The care of your planning
> Will ever be able to take the place of the originality of your thought.
> And the acuity of your power of observation.

The most valuable clinical dynamic test for answering the question: "Can the patient respond adequately to stress?", is the insulin test[18]. It is safe, sensitive and reliable and causes less disturbance to the patient than, for example, the lysine–vasopressine test. An impaired response to hypoglycaemia means that the patient may need corticosteroid replacement in order to stand up to stress. Moreover, the test will also help to determine whether cortisol cover may be needed for carrying out a surgical procedure. The hypogly-caemia test seems, at present, the most convenient diagnostic tool for estimating the adequate function of the hypothalamic–pituitary–adrenal axis, except in case of epilepsy and ischaemic heart disease, when it is contra-indicated.

As already stated, there is a circadian rhythm of the secretion of ACTH, prompted by the hypothalamus. It controls the variation of the cortisol output from the adrenals. The plasma cortisol is normally at its peak at about the time of waking, at its lowest at about the time of going to bed. It usually begins to rise at about 3 a.m. Depressive illness, heart failure, Cushing's syndrome and other forms of stress cause disturbance of this rhythm; it does not occur in Addison's disease.

The present understanding of disordered function being a multifactorial phenomenon seems also to apply to the corticotrophin release (CR) mechanism. Stimulating, inhibiting and stressful factors can exert their influence acting independently or together and in different ways. This results in a situation which appears confusing and is difficult to analyse.

Selye defined the General Adaptation Syndrome (GAS) as the "Physiological mechanism which raises resistance to damage as such"[19]. The endocrine system has to play an important role in these reactions which occur independently of the nature of the damaging agent. The sum of all those non-specific systemic reactions to long-continued exposure to stress is the GAS, with enlargement of the adrenal cortex, increased manufacture of cortisol, involution of the thymus and peptic ulceration. Selye distinguished three stages of GAS:

(1) Alarm Reaction: Some of it passive = shock = signs of damage;
(2) Stage of Resistance = protracted counter-shock; adaptation to one agent may be gained "at the expense of resistance" to other agents;
(3) Stage of Exhaustion: In cases of very prolonged exposure to stimuli to which adaptation had been developed, but could no longer be maintained. 'Hypertension', nephrosclerosis and 'rheumatic diseases' may represent by-products of endocrine reactions which are at play at the GAS. Its primary biological purpose is to raise resistance to non-specific stress.

The history of the concept can be traced back to Walter Cannon's "Homeostasis", the "milieu interieur" of Claude Bernard and to the development of the knowledge of shock during the last 50 years.

Hibernation is also influenced by the anterior pituitary, the thyroid gland, the gonads and the adrenals. The development of the islets of Langerhans seems, however, to be stimulated. Winter-sleep-like conditions can be induced in some animals by insulin, when blood-magnesium rises as in hibernation.

NEW HORMONES

The heading to this section is misleading. It is true that some hormones, such as calcitonin, were not discovered until 1962. On the other hand, the existence of a pressor substance in the kidneys, which enters the circulation by the renal veins, was postulated by Tigerstedt as early as 1898[20]. The title of this section means, therefore, merely that the substances to be mentioned briefly, are today accepted as being on the ever expanding list of hormones, because their functions fit within that definition.

The kidney hormones

Let us continue with the kidney hormones. According to J. W. Fisher[21], it was Goormaghtigh, who suggested in 1939, that renin, "the first kidney hormone" (but see also pp. 567–568 on the role of renin, a proteolytic enzyme) might be secreted by the cells of the juxtaglomerular apparatus[22]. Although it was shown to be connected with the intracellular granules of the juxtaglomerular cells, it seems that it might also be produced in other cells in the vascular pole region of the glomeruli. This is an important observation of general application. We shall see that a similar arrangement applies in the case of the gut hormones; this principle has, in fact, a general value concerning the majority of hormones.

The actual discovery of 'haemopoietin' was made by P. Carnot and G. Déflandre in 1906[23]. They achieved a significant increase in peripheral red cell counts in normal rabbits injected with plasma, which had been made anaemic by bleeding. It was given the new name, 'erythropoietin' by the Finnish researchers E. Bonsdorff and E. Jalavista in 1948[24], who felt that this name is more indicative of its effects on erythroid cells. Professor P. Carnot was a professor of the Faculty of Medicine in the University of Paris in 1903, and Head of the Medical Clinic at the Hôpital Hôtel de Dieu in Paris in 1927. More intensive research was carried out by Kurt Reissmann, who in 1950 could definitely confirm the existence of an erythropoietic factor by an ingenious experiment[25]. One of a pair of parabiotic rats was exposed to lowered oxygen-tension, while the other inhaled normal air. Erythropoietic stimulation was observed in both rats, implying to Reissmann that a humoral erythropoietic factor had been transmitted from the hypoxic animal to stimulate the erythro-poiesis in the non-hypoxic rat. Fred Stohlman, Jr. (died in 1974 in a plane accident) and his colleagues showed convincingly[26] the erythropoietic effect in plasma from a patient with regional hypoxia and polycythaemia secondary to a patent ductus arteriosus. Albert S. Gordon and colleagues[27], made further early contributions to this field with work on humoral influences on erythropoiesis and on the biogenesis and assay of erythropoietin. But it is only 22 years since Jacobson and his colleagues, in 1957[28], demonstrated the existence of the second renal hormone, 'erythropoietin'. The kidney is regarded as the primary organ in the production of the hormone and concerned with the daily regulation of erythropoiesis. The actual cytological site of production in the kidney has not yet been established. After removal of the kidneys in humans and related species, extra-renal erythro-poietin can be manufactured. Almost simultaneously, the same discovery was made by the Polish team of Mme. Z. Kuratowska, B. Lewartowski and E. Michalak[29], and by a third group of J. W. Fisher and B. J. Birdwell[30,31] – that the "isolated perfused kidney is capable of producing erythropoietin when triggered by hypoxia and/or cobalt". This almost coincided with the CIBA Foundation Sympo-sium on Haemopoiesis[32], the first of many meetings on the subject to follow, to obtain a synopsis of the extensive research in this field during the last 20 years. The last International Conference on Erythropoiesis in Tokyo, was reported on in 1975[33], showing the importance this subject has achieved. Albert Gordon and his col-leagues have recently investigated the renal erythropoietic factor, 'erythrogenin', in an attempt to clarify the mechanism of the role of the kidney in manufacturing erythropoietin, such as, for example, the production of erythropoietin in kidney tissue cultures. A great number of questions have emerged, showing the close links with the rest of the humoral regulation; for example, the role of the adrenergic nervous system in regulating kidney production of erythropoietin and as messenger substances in the response of the erythroid cells to erythropoietin; in fact, demonstrating the influence of the anterior pituitary and of the adrenal cortex (the pituitary-adrenal axis) on erythropoietin formation, and of erythropoiesis and mechanisms of anaemia in renal disease.

Apart from renin, erythropoietin and erythrogenin, the other humoral agents produced by and isolated from the kidneys are the renomedullary prostaglandins (PGE_2 and $PGF_2-\alpha$) and the angioten-sins. Angiotensin I is a deka-peptide, formed by the action of renin on a plasma globulin, which belongs to the α-2 fraction. Angiotensin II is an octa-peptide with aldosterone releasing effects on the adrenal cortex, and with even more marked pharmacological effect on the smooth muscle of the blood-vessels. It is produced by the action of a plasma-converting enzyme on angiotensin I. Thus, the complex renin–angiotensin and aldosterone relationships have a profound influence on normal and abnormal renal function, sodium and potassium metabolism, neuro-muscular dysfunction and the aetiology of hypertensive vascular disease.

Growth hormone

Growth hormone was discussed on pp. 562–564 and p. 569. It will be discussed again on pp. 654–655.

Prolactin

The release mechanism and the secretion of prolactin was discussed in the previous section (see pp. 595–596). John Hunter and Oscar Riddle's role in the discovery of prolactin have also been mentioned (pp. 530–531). Prolactin, growth hormone, and chorionic somatomammotrophin are related to one another. Human prolactin is very similar to ovine prolactin, structurally and immunologically. As many as six areas of the prolactin molecule are identical with growth hormone and chorionic somatomammotrophin. The primary function of prolactin in the human is the initiation and maintenance of lactation. Up to the age of and during puberty, a significant male–female difference does not seem to occur in the prolactin level in the blood. Normal adult women, however, do have a significantly higher level than adult men. In women, it is also higher during the luteal phase of the menstrual cycle than during the follicular phase. There is a progressive increase in the plasma concentration throughout pregnancy. Stimulation of the breast causes prolactin release in women only, but not in men[34]. Although in the eight years since human prolactin was isolated and defined[35], the causal relations between increased secretion and certain disorders of reproduction have been established, we still do not understand the function of prolactin in males. Absence or marked reduction in the plasma level of prolactin, e.g. after hypophysectomy or after prolonged treatment with bromocriptine, a dopamine agonist, does not show any biochemical or pathological changes in the male. Excess of prolactin in the blood may cause impotence. The mechanism seems to be direct gonadal suppression[36], but in normal non-lactating subjects, no gonad-inhibiting action was observed. Hyperprolactinaemia is associated with an increase in the secretion of adrenal androgens, particularly of dehydroepiandrosterone (DHA). A connection has been shown between serum-prolactin and nocturnal DHA in boys before puberty[37]; perhaps it is part of the mechanism of the pituitary control of adrenarche. As well as drugs and lactation, stress, rhythm (see pp. 595–596) and diet also influence prolactin secretion. Physical stress increases blood-prolactin concentration, e.g. running, admission to hospital, venepuncture and surgical operations[38]. Dr. Halberg found, in addition to the circadian rhythm of secretion, the existence of a circannual rhythm[39]. A change to a vegetarian diet abolished the nocturnal peak of prolactin in the blood[40] and peak is delayed in massive obesity[41].

In the best up-to-date review on prolactin in 1974, Nicoll[42] enumerated 85 different actions, to which more have been added since. In a number of species, including some mammals, four important control functions could be demonstrated, namely growth, electrolyte balance, gonadal function and parental care, but this is not so in man. The chronobiologists (Halberg and colleagues) would like to rename prolactin and call it 'versatilin' for its wide diversity of roles in many species, except in the non-lactating human female and in the male. In the white-throated sparrow, A. H. Meier found that prolactin seems to be one of the controlling factors of migration and fat deposition[43,44].

Gut hormones

Today, gastro-enterological endocrinology has acquired a large corner of the field, with well defined physio-pathological concepts, specific biological, biochemical and immunological assay methods, and well defined diseases. It is, however, a fairly recent development, which may be said to have begun with the description of a new syndrome, associating gastric hypersecretion, primary peptic ulcerations of the jejunum with islet cell tumours of the pancreas, by Robert Milton Zollinger (b. 1903) and Edwin Homer Ellison (b. 1918)[45]. John Sidney Edkins (1863–1940) had first described gastric secretion (gastrin) in 1906[46]. He showed that extracts of the pyloric mucous membrane caused increased production of an acid gastric juice. Baron E. Maydell confirmed, in 1913, that subcutaneous injection of extracts of pyloric mucous membrane increased secretion in a dog with chronic gastric fistula[47]. R. W. Keeton and F. C. Koch further confirmed the specific nature of this gastric secretin or 'gastrin' in 1915[48]. They obtained equally active extracts from the fundus of the stomach.

The isolation of gastrin and definition of its structure was achieved by R. Gregory in 1966; but it was Friedrich Feyrter (1895–1973), Professor of Pathology in Danzig, who made a special study of and described the peripheric (parakrine) endocrine glands of man[49, 50]. He was the first to postulate the presence of distinctive endocrine cells in the gastro-intestinal tract, but in the early (1938) and intermediate (1953) stages of his work, he did not attempt to identify the argentaffin, argyrophil and clear cells, which composed this system, with any of the known polypeptide hormones. Later (in 1969), he added a number of speculations, but always considered that the cells were 'parakrine' in nature, that is to say, acting on their immediate neighbours. He considered, furthermore, that they arose by a process called 'andophytic' or budding from the enterocytes of the gastro-intestinal tract or from similar cells, lining the ducts of foregut origin. A single alternative theory is that the endocrine cells are all derivatives of the neural crest and thus neuro-ectodermal and, strictly speaking, neuro-endocrine[51]. This was put forward by A. G. E. Pearse in 1966, within the framework of a unifying hypothesis.

All this time, we have to bear in mind that Starling introduced the newly coined word 'hormone' in 1905 when he was reporting on his discovery, with Bayliss, of 'secretin', first reported by them in 1902[52] (see pp. 340–341). When the two turned their attention to the pancreas, they were still under the influence of the views of Ivan Petrovich Pavlov (1849–1936), the great man from St. Petersburg, who assumed a nervous control of the secretion of the glands within the gastro-intestinal tract. After their brilliant experimental work, Bayliss and Starling came to the conclusion that the regulation of secretin production must be humoral. It was another 40 years before it was established that both control mechanisms are in action and form a neuro-humoral regulation in the body. Today, the view is almost universally held, that the endocrine cells of the gut and pancreas arise from enterocyte stem cells or from duct cells (of embryologically entodermal or foregut origin).

The mammalian gastro-intestinal tract and pancreas contain at least 13 ultra-structurally and cyto-chemically distinguishable endocrine cells, all of which possess the 'amino-handling' and other characteristics of the polypeptide hormone-secreting cells of the APUD series. The term APUD stands for the initial letters of the three most constant characteristics: Amine content, amine-Precursor Uptake and amino-acid Decarboxylase content. The series include the medullary carcinomas of the thyroid, bronchial and intestinal carcinoids and phaeochromocytomas. G. U. Foster, Ian MacIntyre and A. G. E. Pearse first suggested in 1964 that the parafollicular (or

C) cells of the thyroid were the site of origin of calcitonin. These C-cells are derived from the neural crest. That is why phaeochromocytomas and medullary carcinomas of the thyroid, which are both of neuro-ectodermal origin, contain a variety of amines and are sometimes associated with the familial medullary carcinoma syndrome. The C-cells are members of the APUD cell series, six of which have now been shown to be derived from the neuroectoderm. It has been postulated that all the endocrine cells of the pancreas and of the gut have the same origin; there seems to be a great deal of evidence in favour of this assumption (pp. 487, 675).

Radio-immunoassay and immuno-histo-chemical methods have succeeded in identifying at least seven distinct gastro-intestinal polypeptides in various regions of the gut. A comprehensive review of gut hormones (of xiv + 664 pages!) was published in 1978[53], the idea arising from a meeting held in Lausanne in the Summer of 1977, to celebrate the 75th Anniversary of the discovery of secretin. Since that date, progress seems to have been so fast, "that even conventional journal articles were lagging far behind"[53]. The present information does not go beyond that date. Correlation of a given cell type in the gut with a specific peptide was then possible only for the gastrin (G) cell and the entero-glucagon-producing EG and AL cells. As regards the islets of the pancreas, the correlation of the beta-cells with insulin and of the alpha-cells with glucagon, are absolutely certain. The difficulty of obtaining biopsy material from the pancreas, explains the problem of elucidating some of the endocrine abnormalities of that gland.

In the Zollinger–Ellison syndrome, the gastric hypersecretion and the severe peptic ulceration are caused by the liberation of a large amount of gastrin by the tumour. For this reason, the name of 'gastrinoma' has been suggested, but Z–E syndrome is still commonly used. The tumour is located mainly in the pancreas, but is found sometimes in the wall of the duodenum. All the endocrine gut cells can develop tumours. After the discovery of hypoglycaemic symptoms caused by excessive doses of insulin administration, the diagnosis of spontaneous hypoglycaemia was soon reported. Seale Harris recorded four patients with spontaneous hyperinsulinism in 1924[54], but did not connect it with adenomas of the islets of Langerhans. Russel Morse Wilder (1885–1959), F. N. Allan, M. H. Power and H. E. Robertson reported in 1927 on a surgeon who had acute attacks of severe spontaneous hypoglycaemia; operation disclosed a primary carcinoma of the islets of Langerhans with metastases in the liver, which contained large amounts of insulin[55]. In fact, adenoma of the beta-cells of Langerhans's islets is the common cause of spontaneous hypoglycaemic attacks, although some much more complex forms may occur without tumour formation. In 1928 W. V. McClenahan and G. W. Morris described a patient with adenoma of the islets of Langerhans, which was diagnosed during life, with a persistent low blood-sugar-curve and attacks of spontaneous hypoglycaemia[56]. By 1933, it was clear that spontaneous hypoglycaemia could be the result of multi-factorial conditions. It could be caused by an excess of insulin-production due to tumours or to hyperplasia of the islet-tissue, or simply by functional overproduction. It could be caused by the lack of opposing secretions, such as in Addison's disease, Simmonds's disease, pituitary tumours, or in myxoedema (glucagon deficiency was not recognized at that time); lack of glycogen; in hepatic disease (cirrhosis), muscular atrophy; abnormal excretion of sugar in renal glycosuria and during lactation; depletion of stores, such as in excessive muscular exercise and in starvation; interference with the regulating centre, which may occur in cerebro-pontine disorder, or overaction of the vagus nerve[57]. In 1934 Charles Herbert Best (1899–1978) himself was of the opinion[58], that the causes of hypoglycaemia were (a) damage to the liver cells; (b) inhibition of gluconeogenesis by insulin; and/or (c) diminished gluconeogenesis due to underfunction of the pituitary, the thyroid or the adrenals. He thought that formation of sugar in the liver was mainly under control of the anterior pituitary, as he found that hypophysectomy in the animal experiment may cause hypoglycaemia (see also Houssay and Biasotty's experiments, p. 505). Allen Oldfather Whipple (b. 1881) and V. E. Franz, who had collected 62 patients with adenoma of the islet cells, found in 1935, somewhat to their surprise, that in 30 of them there was no hypoglycaemia present[59]. They also felt that the diagnosis of adenoma is not made easily and the new growth might well be in reality a slowly growing carcinoma. Of patients showing clinical hypoglycaemia caused by hypersecretion of the gland as a whole and without tumour formation, Best collected four, which were regarded as functional, moderate and different from organic hyperinsulinism. Foetal hyperinsulinism was reported in the case of diabetic mothers and regarded as a compensatory hypertrophy[60].

The fact that many of the symptoms of hypoglycaemia may mimic neurological and psychiatric conditions, makes it understandable that some leading authors, for example, J. Wilder, classified hypoglycaemias as follows: hypoglycaemia caused by (1) disorder of the vegetative nervous system; (2) organic disease of the nervous system; and (3) frank psychiatric disorder[61,62]. Insulinomas may, therefore, produce severe hypoglycaemic symptoms, due to their inability to suppress insulin secretion in response to the hypoglycaemia. There must be high plasma-insulin levels present, when there is spontaneous fasting hypoglycaemia. A high plasma pro-insulin-like component/insulin ratio will provide additional support.

We have seen that glucagon was found to be the second pancreatic hormone (see pp. 470–471). It was discovered in 1923, two years after insulin. In contrast to the discoverers of insulin, Murlin and his colleagues received little recognition for naming it (glucagon = mobilizer of glucose), and for suggesting that it was a glucoregulatory hormone. Although it was purified and found to be produced in the A_2 cells of the pancreatic islets (the A_1 or D cells manufacture gastrin) and also in the A_2-like cells of the gastro–intestinal mucosa (gut-glucagon), the exact physiological role of glucagon was little understood. It was B. Peterson and B. Hellman who showed that it was the alpha-2 cells (and not the silver-positive cells) which were the glucagon-secreting cells in the islet tissue, and this occurred as late as 1963[63]. Yet even so, histological proof of alpha-2 cell hyperplasia has never been reported in the islets of human diabetics. It was only the introduction of RIAs by S. A. Berenson and Rosalyn S. Yalow in 1958[64], which made R. M. Unger and colleagues apply its principles to the measurement of blood glucagon and find[65] that the plasma glucagon levels of diabetic patients are increased at all times throughout life in relation to the prevailing glucose concentration. E. W. Sutherland, G. A. Robison and R. W. Butcher pointed out[66] that the study of the origin of glucagon hyperglycaemia has provided several interesting general biological considerations. This was also found by E. G. Krebs and his group[67]. These research teams demonstrated the interconversion of the enzyme phosphorylase between an active and inactive form. When glucagon is secreted in response to lowered blood-sugar levels, it increases the conversion of inactive liver phosphorylase B into active phosphorylase A, which, in turn, increases the breakdown of liver glycogen. This is brought about by the actions of a kinase and a phosphatase which catalyse phosphorylation and dephosphorylation of the catalytic enzyme. This was the first observation, in 1968, of a regulatory mechanism, probably not uncommon in metabolic systems. The most important result proved to be the discovery that glucagon enhances the production and/or release of cyclic adenylate (3′,5′-cAMP), which mediates the effects of many of the known mammalian hormones, as it is an essential co-enzyme for the phosphokinase. The glycogenolytic effect increases the blood-glucose level, but glucagon itself has no obvious effect on the extra-hepatic utilization of glucose. Its function was developed by Sutherland in his 'second messenger' concept. According to this idea, glucagon binds a specific receptor on the cell surface and this activates the enzyme adenylcyclase. As a result, the cAMP within the cell, the 'second messenger', increases and causes changes in the main enzymes of many metabolic systems, which include those concerned with glycogen synthesis. These rate changes may occur within seconds or within hours. However, glucagon does not produce breakdown of muscle glycogen because it cannot activate muscle phosphorylase.

The isolation and crystallization of porcine pancreatic glucagon was achieved by A. Staub and colleagues in 1953[68,69]. It is a small, single-chain polypeptide, comprising 29 amino-acid residues, and has a molecular weight of 3485. Its structure is quite different from that of insulin. It was synthesized in 1956 by the team of the Lilly Research Laboratories in Indianopolis, based on the structure analysis by Bromer and his colleagues[70]. The actual synthesis was successfully carried out after several attempts and hard work over seven years (1961–1968) by E. Wünsch of the Max Planck Institute in Munich and his group[71,72]. Whereas insulin is essential for life, glucagon is not. The actual role of glucagon was re-defined by Ellis Samols of Augusta, Georgia and his colleagues, between 1965 and 1971[73] and V. Marks[74]. According to their theory, "a major role of glucagon in man, is to regulate insulin secretion in response to the ingestion of food without the necessity for comparatively large changes in substrate concentration in the blood". This would possibly be wasteful and harmful as a result of major changes in the 'milieu interieur'. To sum up, according to their hypothesis, glucagon "acts as a signal sensor and amplifier of certain stimuli to insulin secretion, thereby enormously increasing the sensitivity of the insulin-secreting system to insulin requirements"[75]. At this point, we must remember the classical efforts of Piero P. Foà and his team in the 1950s and 1960s[76,77]. He was one of the pioneers of the study of endogenous glucagon. Moreover, glucagon's present use in the identification of cell receptor sites, promises that it might continue to be used as a model hormone-tool for the further study of cell biology. An important observation has connected glucagon release with stress and anxiety, although a rise in blood-sugar has been known to occur under stress as long ago as 1877! (Claude Bernard, 1813–1878)[78]. Stress was brought about by a variety of external stimuli, including sudden noise, which acted on the nervous system. This was carried out in a variety of animals, including baboons and rhesus monkeys[79].

Glucagonomas have rarely been diagnosed clinically, as there are usually no striking abnormalities associated with hyperglucagon-aemia. When a pancreatic tumour is suspected, the possibility should be borne in mind. The true incidence of glucagonomas is thus not really known. In a number of instances, post-mortem examination revealed a pancreatic islet cell adenoma, without any clinical symptoms, except that about half of the patients had been diabetics. Histo-chemical and immuno-fluorescent staining disclosed the presence of glucagon in some of those post-mortem studies (about eight were described between 1946 and 1960), although L. Grimelius, G. T. Hutquist and B. Stenkvist reported in 1975 that they had found eleven A_2-cell adenomas in autopsy material from 1366 adults[80]. In 1974, C. N. Mallinson, S. R. Bloom, A. P. Warin, P. R. Salmon and B. Cox reported on nine patients with a peculiar skin rash, necrolytic migratory erythema, who all had pancreatic tumours. In four patients, examination of the tumour tissue revealed A_2-cells containing glucagon and there were very high glucagon levels in the plasma[81]. The fact that the main presenting sign of severe hyperglucagonaemia in man was a peculiar skin rash, was perhaps the reason why the syndrome was neglected after its first description in 1966 by McGavran and colleagues[82]. As the condition is potentially curable if detected early, the diagnosis is of importance. Glucagonomas are now included into the group of apudomas of the pancreas, because this ugly term of abbreviation includes all the hyperplastic and neoplastic lesions of APUD cells and these lesions often demonstrate the APUD features more definitely than their parent cells. Hyperplasia, adenoma, carcinoid and carcinoma all occur in the pancreas and involve the endocrine (APUD) cells in the islets and those between the acinar cells. S. R. Bloom, A. G. E. Pearse and colleagues classified the apudomas on a functional basis as (a) orthoendocrine (secreting the normal pancreatic peptides); (b) paraendocrine (secreting peptides, amines or other substances which are normally produced by other glands or tissues); and (c) multiple hormone-secreting lesions, when the pancreatic apudoma is associated with multiple endocrine adenopathy (MEA)[83]. Glucagonomas have also been found as part of MEA.

S. Oberndorfer in 1907 first introduced the word 'Karzinoide' (carcinoid)[84]. He described a group of intestinal tumours which grew slowly and seemed to run a more benign course than the more common intestinal adenocarcinomas. In 1928 P. Masson published a survey of the carcinoid syndrome[85]. The remarkable clinical signs of severe flushing, wheezing diarrhoea and valvular lesions are tell-tale signs of such patients. They were described again by G. Biörck, O. Axén and A. Thörson in 1952[86]. They arise from the argentaffin cells of the intestinal mucosa near the bases of the crypts of Lieberkühn. These cells were described by Nikolai Kultschitzky (1856–1925) in 1897[87]. They often contain granules which show a staining affinity for silver or chromium compounds, hence the name argentaffinoma. Embryologically, they belong to the mid-gut structures. The majority are found in the ileo-caecal region (in the appendix or in the terminal ileum), but occasionally they may occur elsewhere in the gut, or in the biliary system. Some adenomas and oatcell carcinomas of the bronchus may show a certain similarity, but without the argentaffin reaction. Metastases are more frequent in the bronchial carcinoids, although local involvement of neighbouring lymphnodes and organs (liver) may occur. The original view that the symptoms, especially the flushing, is caused by the liberation into the circulation of 5-hydroxytryptamine and other vaso-reactive peptides, is no longer popular. It is thought that kallikrein (bradykinin), histamine and perhaps prostaglandins are involved as humoral agents in the production of the symptoms and signs of the syndrome. The propensity of atypical carcinoid tumours (e.g. at bronchial sites) to secrete ectopic hormones, such as ACTH and/or insulin, is now also recognized as a possible feature of the disease.

The symptoms of the carcinoid syndrome, especially diarrhoea and episodic facial flushing (provoked by ethyl alcohol), have also been reported in thyroid carcinoma. The latter stems from the parafollicular (C) cells of the thyroid, between the follicular epithelium and the basement membrane, in a similar position as the Kultschitzky cells in the intestine. The medullary carcinoma cells may manufacture prostaglandins, serotonin and kinin-forming enzymes. This implies that this tumour may be part of the carcinoid group of tumours, producing a related range of vaso-reactive substances[88]. Additional evidence supporting such a view is the fact that both may produce ectopic ACTH, and calcitonin secretion in carcinoid has also been observed[89]. Incidentally, the term 'apudoma' was coined by Szijj and her colleagues in 1969 "to describe a medullary carcinoma of the thyroid, secreting ACTH"[83].

The rare pancreatic cholera syndrome with its watery diarrhoea (WDHA syndrome) may bear a brief note, in which vaso-reactive intestinal peptides (VIP) play an important role.

Finally, the multiple hormone producing tumours, multiple endocrine adenomatosis, a familial syndrome, must be mentioned. It was studied by Paul Wermer (1898–1978) of the College of Physicians and Surgeons, Columbia University, New York, during the past two decades[90] (see also p. 556). The two hereditary syndromes are both caused by tumours and hyperplasia of endocrine glands. They are: multiple endocrine neoplasia, type 1 (MEN type 1), also called Wermer's syndrome, and MEN, type 2, also called S. Pale's syndrome. The former name for type 1, multiple endocrine adenomatosis (MEA) should not be used, because, as we know, carcinomas and carcinoids occur frequently in patients with Wermer's syndrome; this syndrome represents, therefore, a pleiotropic autosomal gene, activated in the diseased tissues.

The seven gastro-intestinal polypeptides in various regions of the gut which have, at present, been defined as gut hormones (see also p. 605) are gastrin, secretin, cholecystokinin-pancreozymin (CCK), pancreatic polypeptide (PP), gastric inhibitory peptide (GIP), motilin and enteroglucagon (GLI). Pancreatic polypeptide (PP) was first detected accidentally, as an impurity of insulin. It is found almost entirely in the pancreas of man, in whom it may circulate in high concentration especially after a meal, when its level increases rapidly. This is caused by neuro-humoral signals from the gut (entero PP axis). Its physiology is now the subject of intensive research.

Gastric inhibitory peptide (GIP) is a hormone secreted and released in the jejunum stimulated particularly by fat and carbohydrate. Its structural amino acid sequence is related to those of secretin, glucagon and VIP. Apart from inhibiting gastric acid, it stimulates insulin release, an action which is, however, glucose dependent. It has a major role in the regulation of carbohydrate metabolism by the gut. It has been suspected that GIP release is much increased in diabetes mellitus and in obesity, perhaps due to a failure in normal feedback control.

Motilin is also a jejunal hormone, with potent pharmacological effect on the motor activity of the upper alimentary tract. Its existence was postulated by J. C. Brown and colleagues in 1966, based on studies of alkalinization of the duodenum of dogs[91]. It is found in the enterochromaffin cells of the duodenum and jejunum, and has been isolated and synthesized. It has a potent effect on gastric emptying and lower oesophageal-sphincter pressure, but there seem to be major species differences.

Cholecystokinin (CCK) is the gallbladder-emptying factor, discovered as early as 1928 by A. C. Ivy and E. Oldberg[92]. It has been isolated and it emerged that there are several molecular forms of this polypeptide. The COOH-terminal sequence resembles those of the gastrins. Apart from gastrin, it is the gut hormone with a clear cut and well known physiological action. The pathology is, as yet, less well understood, which is perhaps not entirely surprising.

In 1948, E. W. Sutherland and C. de Duve detected a hyper-glycaemic glucagon-like substance in the gastric mucosa of dogs[93]. In 1961, Unger and his colleagues discovered glucagon-like im-munoreactivity in various parts of the intestine[94]. This substance is chemically and biologically different from pancreatic glucagon and was named 'enteroglucagon', 'gut glucagon' or 'intestinal glucagon-like immuno-reactivity' (GLI). The cells containing it were found mainly in the ileum and colon, where they were located with the immuno-fluorescence technique[95]. In all these areas, intensive research is going on.

Prostaglandins

Prostaglandins are a ubiquitous group of substances, produced in nearly all tissues. These essentially fatty acid derivatives show close interaction with the endocrine system by their control over the concentration of cyclic AMP. The original discovery of these lipid-soluble, smooth muscle stimulating compounds, occurred in the seminal fluid in 1933, by M. W. Goldblatt[96,97], and by U. S. von Euler in 1934[98-100]. At that time, some sensitive but non-specific bioassays were available, so that there followed a long interval of inactivity in the study of prostaglandins. Eventually, in 1960, prostaglandins were isolated in crystalline form by S. Bergström and his colleagues in the 1960s[101,102]. The chemical structures were determined in 1962 and 1963, again by Bergström and his group[103,104]. This renewed study became possible when ultraviolet spectro-photometry, gas–liquid chromatography, mass spectrometry and especially, RIA became available.

Prostaglandins are not normally stored in tissues. They are biosynthesized from essential fatty acids when required. The biosynthesis is a complex process of many steps which involve a variety of enzymes and co-factors. As prostaglandins participate in so many physiological and pathological processes, inhibition of prostaglandin biosynthesis has become an important study. One of the most important results of these studies has been the demonstration that non-steroidal anti-inflammatory drugs inhibit prostaglandin synthesis in a number of tissues. Moreover, the antipyretic, analgesic and anti-inflammatory effects of salicylates and indomethacin, seem to be the result of inhibition of prostaglandin synthesis. These inhibitors, indomethacin, aspirin and fenamates, have also been proved effective in the treatment of some varieties of dysmenorrhoea, premature labour, and diarrhoea occurring after irradiation of the large bowel. The relation of prostaglandins and cyclic AMP is, however, complex. Prostaglandins are regarded in the role of modulators of noradrenergic transmission. Prostaglandins in their relation to cerebral circulation seem, in animal experiments, to be constrictor agents. Prostaglandins have a depressant action on behaviour, ranging from mild sedation to catatonia; this depends on the compound used and on the method of administration. This vast field is expanding so rapidly that the subject, a review of which was covered in 1972 in a single volume, was presented four years later (in 1976) by the editor, S. M. M. Karim, Research Professor of Obstetrics and Gynaecology, University of Singapore, in three volumes of several hundred pages each![105–107] The role of prostaglandins in relation to reproduction is concerned with induction of labour by prostaglandins, and interruption of pregnancy with them, but also with the application of prostaglandins in animal husbandry. Another important practical application may result from recent observations of two research teams, one in Charleston, SC, and the other in Seattle. *In vitro* experiments suggest that aspirin interrupts the conversion of arachidonic acid to prostaglandins, thus curbing the abnormally accelerated platelet aggregation in diabetes and in some other vascular conditions[108].

Hypothalamic factors and other neurosecretory substances

We now have to consider the discovery of the releasing- and inhibiting-factors produced in the hypothalamus. Before discussing them briefly, a few critical remarks must be made.

1. In the same manner as the discovery of gut hormones, of immune-body reactions, of the receptors and receptor-sites, the factors (or hormones) of the hypothalamus have extended the field of endocrinology. At the same time, they have also blurred it. It reminds one of a parlour game on television, which seems popular at present: a classic 'group' painting is shown, by the Elder Breughel, for example; one has to look at it for 30 seconds, after which time a number of questions have to be answered, such as: How many men, women and children were in the picture? How many dogs and cats? And so on. Erwin Schroedinger, the Viennese physicist of Nobel Prize fame, remarked somewhere (I believe it was in his lectures in Dublin on 'What is Life?' in 1945[109]) that one may analyse the colours of a master-painting according to the laws of optics and of chemistry; this does not, however, reflect the impression of the painting, nor can it help to explain why it is a masterpiece. At the present juncture, we have to ask ourselves whether the meaning of hypothalamic 'factors' is the same as that which Ernest Starling had in mind, when he introduced the term of 'hormones' at the beginning of the century? Similarly, when Pflueger and later Sharpey–Schafer originally thought that menstruation was under nervous control, their theories were modified in favour of the glands with internal secretion. At present, the idea of combined nervous *and* humoral control has gained ground and has become the 'new' (?) theory of neuro-endocrine control. Are we still taking in the field (painting) or are we

merely looking at and counting the number of people who are sitting down or standing?

2. It must be clearly understood that the hypothalamus is now regarded as a single, interrelated entity. In the 1930s it was customary to talk about the 'endocrine orchestra' and (Sir) Walter Langdon-Brown was the first to state that "the pituitary is the leader of the endocrine orchestra"[110]. When (Sir) Douglas Hubble delivered the Fourth Langdon-Brown Lecture on 'The Endocrine Orchestra' at the Royal College of Physicians in London in 1960, the picture had already changed considerably[111]. He himself said:

> When I was asked to deliver this Langdon-Brown Lecture, I was therefore naturally attracted by the subject of the influence of emotional factors on the control and function of the endocrine system. Experimentalists have, however, in this generation been mainly concerned with the hypothalamus, the pituitary and the hormones themselves, and a relatively small amount of time has been given [in 1960] to the exploration of the extensive neural connections of the hypothalamus with the cerebral cortex, basal ganglia, and the thalamus. New analytical techniques are now being developed, which will eventually map out this enormous field, and, although the early results undoubtedly indicate that these higher centres have a profound effect in modifying hormonal output, I decided that it would be premature to try to review the relations of the nervous system with the endocrine system. I must hope that some successor of mine in the Langdon-Brown Lectureship will embrace the opportunity which no one would have seized more eagerly than Langdon-Brown himself.

Hubble readily admitted that the organization and control mechanisms of the endocrine system were more complex than those of any other system, with the exception of the cerebral one; but he looked in vain for a more approximate biological analogy than that of an orchestra.

> An orchestra is a group of individuals harmoniously loyal to their higher control and playing with a common purpose towards a common end – the best possible interpretation of the piece of music in front of them. In the endocrine system is a group of individual organs, with much more complicated relationships and with controls which although complex, are yet unified, working with a common purpose towards a common end – the maintenance of homoeostasis in the body.

The hypothalamus is integrated into the control mechanism of the hypothalamic–pituitary–adrenal axis, of the hypothalamic–pituitary–gonadal axis and of the hypothalamic–pituitary–thyroid axis. ACTH release from the pituitary is under control of the (hypothalamic) corticotrophin-releasing factor (CRF), but the level of plasma corti-sol plays a major part in the release, by means of the feedback mechanism. Increased cortisol levels inhibit, and decreased plasma-cortisol levels stimulate, the release of ACTH. The cortisol concen-tration probably acts at both sites, at the hypothalamus and at the pituitary.

We have discussed growth hormone and its release under normal conditions and in acromegalics (see pp. 562–563, p. 569 and p. 602). There is also a growth-hormone-release inhibiting factor (GH.RIH., G.I.F., SRIF, also called 'somatostatin'), in the hypothalamus. Somatostatin plays perhaps a greater role in the regulation of the endocrine system, because it inhibits also the release of insulin and glucagon[112]. It is, furthermore, active in its cyclisized disulphide bridged form as well as in its non-cyclisized form. As GH-release is so related to the onset of sleep, delay of sleep means also delay of release of GH. Prolactin secretion, as we have seen, also coincides with the onset of sleep, but in contrast to GH, the first release is followed by even greater bouts of episodic discharges during sub-sequent stages of sleep. We must be, however, quite clear in our definitions: these substances are of neural origin, but are real hormones[113]. They are secreted into the pituitary portal vessels and in that manner transported to their target organ. Their correct definition has to be, therefore, 'releasing hormone', although the word 'factor' is often used to avoid confusion with the pituitary hormones which they release, or the release of which they inhibit. Moreover, experimental evidence is now available in the case of a number of releasing and inhibiting hypothalamic neurohormones, concerning their mode of secretion, transport and chemical struc-ture. Thus, the structure of porcine thyrotrophin-releasing hormone has been established to be Glu-His-Pro(NH$_2$)[114]. Apart from the corticotrophin-releasing hormone (CRF), thyrotrophin-releasing hormone (TRH), growth hormone-releasing hormone (GH.RH), GH-release-inhibiting hormone (GH.RIH), prolactin-release-inhibiting hormone (PRIH) and prolactin-releasing hormone (PRH), the following have been established: follicle-stimulating-hormone-releasing hormone (FSH.RH), luteinizing-hormone-releasing hor-mone (LH.RH), a melanocyte-stimulating hormone-release-inhibiting hormone (MR.IH) and a melanocyte-stimulating hor-mone-releasing hormone (MRH). The luteinizing-hormone-releasing hormone (LRF, LH.RH) is a dekapeptide and antibodies made against it block ovulation and inhibit the release of gonadotrophins[115]. Some of these hormones also have unexpected effects, unrelated to their releasing or inhibiting activities on pituit-ary hormones. TRF can achieve prolactin release in women. Somatostatin, as we have seen, also inhibits the release of insulin and glucagon at the level of the endocrine pancreas.

There is direct evidence that the episodic, pulsatile pituitary release of luteinizing hormone is caused by a similar pulsatile release of LH.RH from the hypothalamus[116]. In the prepubertal period, girls and boys present a sleep-augmented pattern to LH-release, whereby the secretion is finished near the beginning of the REM phases of the sleep period. In adult man, the enhanced night secretion pattern of plasma testosterone-release carries on into the periods of daylight, so that the strong circadian pattern to the episodic release of LH disappears[117]. In the adult woman the course of the menstrual pattern of LH and FSH blurs the study of the circadian pattern; this implied the need for careful assessment and planning when comparing women during like periods of the menstrual cycle. The episodic nature of LH and FSH secretion from the pituitary is an intrinsic characteristic of the medial basal hypothalamus and due to the pulsatile release of LH.RH[118].

Prolactin secretion is normally inhibited by dopamine. Hyperprolactinaemia, often accompanied by amenorrhoea, can be corrected by dopamine-agonists, such as bromocriptine (see section on treatment, pp. 658–659).

It is not surprising that the hypothalamic regulatory mechanisms have become one of the most important areas of endocrine research.

Anorexia nervosa

Richard Morton (1637–1698) (see also p. 298 concerning Morton's view on heredity in diabetes mellitus) gave, in his classical treatise on tuberculosis in 1689, the first account of anorexia nervosa, including in his list of patients a boy of 16[119].

The condition was described and named by (Sir) William Withey Gull (1816–1890), the great physician at Guy's Hospital, London, who also gave the classic description of myxoedema in 1873 (see pp. 244–245) and a year before (1872) of the arteriolosclerotic atrophy of the kidney. He mentioned amenorrhoea, bradycardia and hypothermia first in 1868[120]. He called it 'anorexia nervosa' (also known as apepsia hysterica, anorexia hysterica) in 1874[121]. On the Continent, Joseph Jules Déjerine (1849–1917), the great French neurologist, called it 'anorexie mentale'[122], but in the German-speaking countries the terminology did not become popular. Ernst von Bergmann (1836–1907)[123], and E. Kylin[124] claimed successful treatment of this 'functional' condition with transplants of animal anterior pituitary tissue. Julius Bauer (1887–1979), Max Schur and V. C. Medvei[125] suggested a classification of anterior pituitary insufficiency in 1936, as follows: caused (1) by anatomical destruction of the gland; (a) due to tumours, infection, vascular damage, (?) primary atrophy; (b) due to encroachment from neighbouring structures (tumours, infection, trauma). (2) Pituitary insufficiency caused by disturbances of 'correlation'. By this term, Schur and Medvei implied that prolonged mental (nervous, neurotic) stress could influence the function and secretion of endocrine organs (i.e. of the ovary, the anterior pituitary) in persons who are constitutionally conditioned (J. Bauer), thereby thinking along the lines of H. Selye's general adaptation syndrome (pp. 598–599), without having any knowledge of it at the time. The present view is that the syndrome, which occurs mainly in adolescent girls, consists of amenorrhoea and self-induced extreme loss of weight. Classical examples are teenage girls who were overweight or who believed they were, and started off on a downward path of obsessional dieting, often combined with excitable overactivity. Such patients often have a distorted perception of their own body size.

The apparent similarities to hypopituitarism are, however, usually restricted to amenorrhoea, low LH and FSH levels, low–normal thyroid function, delayed TSH-response to TRH, and, of course, depressed ovarian function. In severely-ill patients the blood pressure may be low, and so is the fasting blood-sugar. The pubic and axillary hair are usually normal. If successful re-feeding takes place, the above-mentioned symptoms all seem reversible. The psychological features have been extensively studied by the psychiatrists and need no repetition here. In the light of modern trends of neuro-endocrinology, and especially of the two-way influence of hormones and behaviour, the present writer feels that Schur's and his own observations in 1937 may still have some validity.

This view is supported by the following observations by other workers. Col. Eugene C. Jacobs of the Medical Corps, USA, reported on the the effects of starvation on sex hormones in the male[126]. Of nine thousand American Prisoners of War, captured on Bataan and Corregidor in April–May, 1942 and kept at Cabanatuan, Nueva Ecija Prison Camp, more than 2400 died after eight months, of diseases (malaria, dysentery, vitamin deficiency and diphtheria) aggravated by starvation. A total of 40 months of food deprivation was interrupted only by four months (after December 1943) when Red Cross parcels of food and vitamins were received. The effects of starvation on the sex hormones appeared identical to those on animals, and produced a 'castration syndrome'. Subsequent adequate diet (December to April 1943, and after Liberation) caused recovery from the syndrome, with transient gynaecomastia in 6% of the prisoners. This had been noted by other observers and attributed to the effect of vitamin B complex deficiency on the inactivation of oestrone in the liver[127, 128]. After 40 months of severe starvation, the survivors recovered normal sexual function after adequate feeding.

More recently, Srebnik and Nelson[129] recorded that pituitary LH concentrations were reduced after malnutrition. These observations confirmed the concept of functional hypopituitarism, induced by starvation, by Perloff et al. in 1954[130]. They were also in agreement with the findings in 1976 of Beumont et al.[131], that circulating LH levels were reduced in anorexia nervosa and so was the response to gonadotrophin-releasing hormone. Moreover, Davies and Lewis could show[132] in male rats and guinea-pigs, that these animals lost half of their LH receptors after dietary deprivation, and their response to hCG stimulation was also reduced. They felt that the weight reduction probably caused reduced pituitary LH output, causing the loss of ovarian and testicular LH receptors, which may be the explanation of the amenorrhoea and infertility in some of these patients. They think that this concept of functional hypopituitarism may be explained by changes in oestrogen metabolism associated with the loss of body fat, which alter the gonadotrophin dynamics[133], and result in excessive LH suppression. Such a concept would also explain the close association between menarche and body weight[134] and food intake and infertility[135].

Peter J. Dally, a London (England) psychiatrist, who wrote a comprehensive monograph on anorexia nervosa in 1969, has just published what he seems to wish to be regarded not a second edition, but a new monograph under the same title, *Anorexia Nervosa*, together with two colleagues at Westminster Hospital, London, Joan Gomez and A. J. Isaacs[136]. In their 'Conclusions' (pp. 197–202) of their book, they not only say "There is thus clear evidence of hypothalamic dysfunction in anorexia nervosa, . . ." but also mention:

Four decades have elapsed since Sheldon's (1939) characterisation of anorexia nervosa as 'functional Simmond's disease', and although he suspected hypothalamic involvement, it is only within the last few years that neuroendocrine studies have permitted confirmation of this concept. Certainly, there is evidence of deficient secretion of pituitary hormones in anorexia nervosa, particularly in respect of LH and, to a lesser extent, FSH, and more subtle defects may exist in relation to TSH and prolactin, but ACTH secretion is relatively unimpaired and growth hormone may indeed be produced excessively.

Their reference to J. H. Sheldon is to a remark made by him in a discussion on anorexia nervosa, in 1939 at the Royal Society of Medicine of London[137]. It is obvious that the above-mentioned paper by Max Schur and V. C. Medvei of 1937[125] escaped their attention and, equally, that of Sheldon.

G. M. Besser found in twelve women patients with anorexia nervosa that the LH/FSH-RH test will cause secretion of LH and FSH in the majority of the patients,

> even though these patients show hypogonadism under basal conditions. It will not differentiate between primary pituitary and hypothalamic disease since in the latter condition absent gonadotrophin secretion may be seen. Gonadotrophin releasing hormone appears to be required for synthesis of gonadotrophins as well as their release.[138]

According to this view, the endocrine dysfunction of anorexia nervosa originates in the hypothalamus and not in the anterior pituitary. The amenorrhoea in women often precedes the loss of weight. Moreover, the administration of LH-RH can restore the cyclical secretion of gonadotrophin by the pituitary and induce normal ovulatory cycles, but the weight-loss must also be restored and the mental state improved, for the treatment to be successful.

Interlude — The psychology of teams[139]

Before continuing the discussion on the discovery of other hormones of the hypothalamus, an observation of principle must be recorded. It will have become obvious in the course of our journey through the centuries, and especially through the last 50 years, how often discoveries are 'in the air', as it were (see also Brown–Séquard, pp. 292 and 329). How very often they are the result of a number of individual scientists, or – in more recent years – a number of laboratories or of teams working on the same problem, proceeding in the same direction, although often unknown to one another. Ideally, once it is known that two or more teams are working on the same projects, they should get together, co-ordinate and co-operate and by sharing their experience, arrive at the goal more readily and more quickly. The question then arises, however, of sharing the credit in the eventual discovery. These discoveries are really often the result and the sum total of the previous contributions of a host of research workers. In endocrinology, as elsewhere in the field of science or the arts, the person(s) who first pass the winning post are the recognized winners in a specific race and receive perhaps greater credit than is their due. Moreover, it happens quite often that two persons or two or more teams pass the winning post together, neck and neck; we have noted several examples of this in the course of our history. Sadly, it can even happen that the real winner does not receive any credit, if, for example, his findings are published in a difficult language (Polish, such as was the case of Oliver and Schaefer's discovery of the pressure substance of the adrenal medulla and concurrently Cybulski and Szymonowicz discovery of the same principle in Cracow (pp. 329–330), or even when published in French as in the case of Paulesco, or in a scientific journal with limited publication and readership (Gregor Mendel, or Robert T. Frank in New York, p. 275).

Hostility between scientists is not unusual. It has been encountered in the previous chapters of our narrative. We have also outlined (in Chapter 20) the difficulties that may arise in the relations of two otherwise amiable persons, such as Herbert M. Evans and Oscar Riddle, although I did not reproduce literally the crucial dialogue which was remarkably heated, even in the expurgated form of the official record of the meeting[140].

Intense competition between two modern research teams, of 21 years duration and "particularly highly charged by a combination of scientific frustration and barely restrained personality conflict" has rarely been described. It was eventually done by Nicholas Wade, a staff-writer for *Science* magazine in Washington, DC[141–143]. He gave his articles the titles: 'Rough journey to a Nobel prize'; 'Three-lap race to Stockholm', and 'A race spurred by rivalry'. They are of particular interest, because they give an insight into the stresses of present-day group research (apart from the problems of funding such research). The articles appear to be of special importance, because contemporarily, three well known neuro-endocrine physiologists, Joseph Meites of Michigan, Bernard T. Donovan of London (England) and Samuel M. McCann of Dallas, Texas, edited a book: *Pioneers in Neuroendocrinology*[144]. The editors selected a number of research workers in the field, to give an account in the first person, of their personal involvement and history of their main line research. Each such chapter is headed by a photograph and a mini-biography. Two of these accounts are: 14. 'Pioneering in Neuroendocrinology 1952–1969', by Roger Guillemin, MD, PhD, born in 1924 in Dijon, France[145], who is at present Head of the Laboratories for Neuroendocrinology, The Salk Institute, La Jolla, California; and: 21. 'In the Pursuit of Hypothalamic Hormones', by Andrew Victor Schally, PhD, born in 1926 in Wilno, Poland[146], who is in charge of the Endocrine and Polypeptide Laboratory, Veterans Administration Hospital and the Department of Medicine, Tulane University School of Medicine, New Orleans. These two very different men, as regards background, outlook and temperament are the two main protagonists in Nicholas Wade's narrative; they eventually shared the Nobel Prize in physiology in 1977 with one another and with Rosalyn

Yalow, of radioimmunoassay fame, for their work on peptide hormones of the brain. This is not the place, nor does space permit, to relate the whole history of 21 years of sometimes bitter competition in detail, but to answer a few questions which seem of importance for the critical evaluation of modern methods of team research and their justification.

First, let us look briefly at the two personalities who were leading the teams, after first working together for five years. Here are a few remarks by people, some of them their team mates, who observed them at close range. "They are unusual types of individuals, to say the least", remarked Schally's colleague Abba Kastin:

> At first impression, you think they are just two entirely different people. You see Guillemin as sophisticated, urbane and charming, Andrew [Schally] as very candid, caring little for social amenities. Neither impression is inaccurate, yet underneath they are in many ways identical.[147]

This view was also expressed by Cyril Bowers, another member of Schally's team: "Guillemin and Schally have very similar personalities"[148]. Although Guillemin maintains that the relationship with Schally was, in fact, no different from the ordinary forms of scientific competition and cannot even be called a race; this may seem correct to people who know conditions of scientific competition in France, where fierce rivalry often begins at the stage of first year medical students. Joseph Meites, for example, says:

> They were bitter rivals, to put it mildly. It was well known among endocrinologists and could be observed right out in the open at public meetings. Essentially it was a fight as to who was going to get there first.

Schally described the relationship as a "Race" consisting of "many years of vicious attacks and bitter retaliation".

It all began in 1955, when each discovered that the interaction between brain (hypothalamus) and pituitary gland could be demonstrated in tissue culture. After five years of co-operation, Schally achieved his own team. The isolation of TRH in 1969 marked the first lap of the race and it was, substantially, a draw. Identification of LH-RH two years later was the second lap, in which Schally had gone ahead. The third was the isolation of somatostatin (GH-RIH), which was achieved by Guillemin's team in 1973 and by Schally's in 1976. In 1977, "they arrived neck and neck at the finishing post, which Alfred Nobel set up for aspiring scientists, in Stockholm" (Wade). Wade poses three important questions:[149] 1. Why did Guillemin and Schally succeed when others failed? 2. How did their rivalry differ from the usual forms of scientific competition? 3. Did it hasten or impede their progress? *Answers*: 1. It was Geoffrey Harris of Cambridge who had established the theory of hypothalamic releasing factors. He was a most elegant physiological experimentator. He and Samuel M. McCann (born 1925), (now of Dallas, Texas), postulated the existence of LRF. McCann also pointed the way to somatostatin; but neither he nor Geoffrey Harris was willing to give up the investigations of other problems in the field and concentrate all his resources and energy on the isolation programme. Cyril Bowers, the Tulane University endocrinologist, who assisted Schally to solve the structure of TRF, remarked: "Most intelligent people won't do isolation work – I think my IQ went down about 20 points, while I was doing it." These isolation programmes not only demand strict intellectual discipline, but also that no portion of the critically small amount of isolated material must be diverted to other experimental use. Guillemin admitted that "for years I refused to do elegant physiological work on TRF because I knew that whatever I took for physiological studies, would be subtracted from the world supply available for determining the structure". Moreover, Harris and McCann were academic scientists, whereas neither Guillemin nor Schally was at an academic institution. They had to build up strong teams, the physiologist working "humbly with the chemist" (Guillemin), especially, to provide quick answers whether a (new) fraction is biologically active, so that the chemist can go on with the next step. This means the use of speedy, if not elegant, assays.

> I knew Harris could never isolate LRF because he had chosen the wrong assay. With his method . . . it took four months to get an answer.

McCann said that to operate on the Guillemin–Schally scale, he would have to put all his money into buying hypothalami; which would have meant jettisoning everything. An interesting corollary of the Guillemin–Schally method was that they developed very few of the methods they used, as Murray Saffran, Schally's former teacher, noted. Schally's comment was:

> I spent many years devising better systems before I realized that fiddling with methods had very few rewards. I decided, our aim was isolating the structure[149].

Roger Burgus, Guillemin's chemist, said: "We have not developed any revolutionary new techniques, although we were the first to apply certain techniques to our field." Guillemin and Schally each realized that strong teams with specialist expertise were essential and also that the hypothalamic material had to be obtained and processed on an industrial scale. "Neither operation is within the customary experience of an academic biologist", says Wade. The cost was considerable: In Guillemin's laboratory between 1964 and 1967, more than 50 tons of fresh frozen tissues were handled, processed, lyophilized and extracted (at 40 US cents per sheep hypothalamus). Schally was lucky, because the meatpackers Oscar Mayer & Co. donated him one million pig hypothalami. Between them, they spent easily one million dollars (Guillemin ca. 650 000, Schally ca. 350 000, for reasons given above[150]), which, after the negative results of many years (until the mid-1960s) led their financial backers to the conclusion that no more money could be wasted. Fortunately, at that moment, TRH was isolated and defined and nobody could laugh at them again.

2. Thus, dedication, determination, concentration, single-mindedness and high cost were all important factors in their progress and eventual success.

3. Was the intense competition beneficial for their final achievements? The bad features of this competition were: "Sniping at each other's errors or wrong proposals, citing as little as possible of each other's work". Because Guillemin worked on material from sheep, Schally decided to use pigs. Exchange of material was not practised; Schally commented:

> It is like giving someone a gun so he can shoot you . . . He was an opponent and an enemy at that time. Also, I simply didn't have enough material for my own use.

Such a policy was more that of the leaders of the two teams than that of other members. Meites's opinion is, however, that the rivalry was beneficial, because it stimulated both men to do their best and to check each other's work; but Saffran said: "Perhaps a little more interchange might have helped a great deal"[151]. Concerning the incentive or disincentive of the Nobel Prize, the view of one of the team-mates also coincides with the personal opinion of the present writer:

> Despite what either may say about not caring about the Prize, they've been after it for years. . . .
> . . . both of them would be happier people if the Prize didn't exist. It has its negative features and the world might be better without it.

As to the far reaching results of their achievements, Wade concludes his study with the following words:

> Guillemin and Schally became the first to decipher the language in which the brain says to the body 'keep warm', 'reproduce', 'grow no more'. For their single-mindedness and persistence, a fitting reward.[151]

Elsewhere Meites says:

> The 'chemotransmitter hypothesis' of Geoffrey Harris had indeed been
> vindicated. Andrew Schally and Roger Guillemin had made the
> isolation of the elusive hypothalamic hormones their major goal, and
> rightfully were rewarded with many honours for their success. I know
> that even right up to the time of the announcements of the structure
> of TRH, there still was considerable scepticism as to whether hypo-
> thalamic hormones really existed and whether they would ever be
> isolated by any of the individuals working on them[144].

Joseph Meites (born 1913), BS, MA, PhD, is himself a distinguished contributor to the study on neuro-endocrine control of
prolactin and other anterior pituitary hormones. Since 1953, he has
been professor and head of the Department of Physiology, Neuro-
endocrine Research Laboratory of the Michigan State University. He
served on the Endocrinology Study Section of the National Institutes
of Health (NIH) from 1965 to 1970. He was greatly influenced by
Geoffrey Harris whom he knew well and admired very much. He
was the first President of the International Society of Neuroendocrinology from 1972 to 1976.

The hormones of the hypothalamus (continued)

The neurons of the hypothalamus which release the hypophysiotrophic peptides are themselves controlled by the higher centres of the
brain via the monaminergic axons. It seems that it is in this manner
that emotional factors like fright and stress operate to regulate the
endocrine system. Samuel McDonald McCann (born 1925) of Dallas, Texas, successfully induced hypertension in Norway rats, by
subjecting them to the sound of an air jet[152]; what is more, adopting
Selye's stress concept, they then adrenalectomized the animals, to
show that the hypertension disappeared! It was at that time that his
interest in the hypothalamic regulation of the anterior pituitary was
aroused. He was even more stimulated by reading Geoffrey W.
Harris's paper on 'Neural control of the pituitary gland'[153]. No
wonder he became one of the leading protagonists of the hypothalamic neuro-endocrine research; after his involvement in the search
for the structure of CRF, he and his colleagues described the
LH-releasing activity in medium eminence-extracts of the
hypothalamus[154]. They later found that dopamine, norepinephrine
and epinephrine (all three catecholamines) can release LH-RH under
the influence of oestrogen[155]. More recently, McCann and his group
have also shown interest in the control of adenohypophyseal sec-

retions by prostaglandins. Come to think of it, what a progress since 1914, when the Danish investigator Knud Sand spoke of "X-substances" as indispensable for gonadal development and function, thus anticipating gonadotrophic stimuli, and since 1925, when A. Lipschuetz found that ovarian grafts grow better in spayed than in intact animals and concluded that extra-gonadal trophic influences must be important regulators of ovarian growth![156]

To these influences of emotional factors and stress must be added the important circadian pattern of the sleep–wake cycle[157]. The stages of normal sleep in adult, healthy people are determined by the changes in the electro-encephalogram recurring in different degrees during the four cycles of normal sleep in the night.

The central regulation of the hypothalamus is affected by chemical neuro-transmitters. These include the three monamines, dopamine, norepinephrine and serotonin[158].

Stresses such as exercise, emotions, illness, trauma, surgery and hypoglycaemia will overcome the circadian rhythm and produce great increase in ACTH and plasma cortisol levels. These results are modulated through the central nervous system (CNS) and can be suppressed by exogenous glucocorticoids[159]. There now seems to exist evidence that an excess of counter-regulatory ('stress') hormones is a necessary condition for severe hyperglycaemia or keto-acidosis, while absolute insulin–deficiency is not. According to David S. Schade of the University of the New Mexico School of Medicine, the stress hormones like glucagon, the catecholamines, cortisol and growth hormone, are secreted in different patterns during stress, e.g. anxiety, exercise, fasting, infection, fever or trauma. In man, sufficient insulin is normally produced to neutralize most of the diabetogenic activity of these hormones. In the case of diabetics, who secrete only limited amounts of insulin, their effects are marked; but insulin deficiency is not absolute in all cases of diabetic keto-acidosis, although the stress hormones may show a four-fold elevation. Norepinephrine circulates in comparatively high concentration in every type of stress, except in hypoglycaemia. It is also the only stress hormone which suppresses endogenous insulin production in man, but stimulates that of glucagon. In diabetics, it produces marked metabolic decompensation, which is obviously not due to its suppression of insulin, as there is little endogenous insulin to suppress. Glucagon and catecholamines increase cyclic AMP levels rapidly, steroids are transported in the cells to the nuclei, inducing the formation of a new RNA. This in turn causes the formation of new protein and the diabetogenic effect, hours after the introduction of the original hormone[160].

It has been established that highly purified ACTH from beef, sheep, pig and human pituitaries, is a straight-chain polypeptide of 39 amino-acid residues with phenylalanine at the C-terminal and serine at the N-terminal. Their molecular weight is *ca*. 4500. In spite of some structural species differences, they are all able to stimulate the adrenal cortex; the species variations, which are confined to the amino acids in positions 25 to 33, are not essential for biological activity, as can be shown by their removal. During the research into the structure of ACTH, the compositions of three types of MSH (= melanocyte-stimulating hormone) were demonstrated. Recent theory assumes that similar cell types in the pars distalis and pars intermedia of the pituitary are capable of synthesizing both β-lipotrophin and ACTH, which then are secreted intact from the pars distalis. There are, however, certain enzymes in the pars intermedia which cleave ACTH and β-LPH and modify them to the smaller peptides, typical of the secretion from the pars intermedia.

Studies on various types of vertebrates seem to indicate that the hypothalamus receives information from the general environment and other parts of the brain; it then translates this neural information into the language of the chemical messenger-interpreters (neuro-hormones), which act as release factors. They are passing via the pituitary portal system to the anterior pituitary, where they accelerate or inhibit the output of specific hormones. Thus was laid the foundation to the present neuro-humoral theory, which conceptual formulation is now in the process of being transformed to a factual formulation. What a development in 25 years! Joseph Meites summarized it in a useful table[161]: (opposite).

There were, of course, many other research workers involved in making important contributions to neuro-endocrinology, unfortunately too numerous to give a full list of them in the present book. A good account of them and their work is given in the two volumes already mentioned, *Pioneers in Neuroendocrinology*[144], the first volume of which was published in 1975, the second in 1978. They contain autobiographical sketches (and the photographs), of about fifty such pioneers, who were still alive at the time of writing, and they cover many nations. There is Claude Aron (b. 1917) in Strasbourg, talking on 'Neuroendocrine Feedbacks' with an important valedictory quotation from the Cahiers de Valéry: "Do not tend to deny what one cannot affirm". Another French scientist, J. Benoit (b. 1896), writes on 'My Research in Neuro-endocrinology: Study of the Photo-Sexual Reflex in the Domestic Duck'. John W. Everett (b. 1906), Professor of Anatomy at Duke University School of Medicine, Durham, North Carolina, discusses the concept of a diurnally rhythmic physiological clock in the rostral hypothalamus, governing the ovulatory discharge of gonadotrophin. Hans

Investigators First Reporting Evidence for Presence of Hypothalamic Releasing Factors

Factor (Hormone)	Year	Investigator
1. Corticotrophin-releasing factor (CRF)	1955	Saffran and Schally; Guillemin and Rosenberg
2. Luteinizing hormone-releasing factor (LRF)	1960	McCann et al; Harris et al.
3. Prolactin-releasing factor in mammals (PRF)	1960	Meites et al.
PRF in avian species	1965–66	Kragt and Meites; Nicoll
4. Prolactin-release inhibiting factor (PIF)	1961–63	Talwalker, Ratner and Meites; Pasteels
5. Thyrotrophin-releasing factor (TRF)	1961–62	Schreiber and Kmentova
6. Growth hormone-releasing factor (GRF)	1963–64	Deuben and Meites
7. Follicle-stimulating hormone-releasing factor (FRF)	1964	Igarashi and McCann; Mittler and Meites
8. MSH-release-inhibiting factor (MIF)	1965	Kastin et al.
9. MSH-releasing factor (MRF)	1965	Talesnik and Orias; Kastin et al.
10. GH-release inhibiting factor (GIF)	1968	Krulich and McCann

Heller (1905–1974), who came via Prague and Vienna to become Professor of Pharmacology in Bristol (England), was editor of the *Journal of Endocrinology* from 1963 to 1974, and well known for his work on comparative endocrinology and the neuro-hypophysis. Hudson Hoagland (b. 1900), a physiologist, was co-founder and one time president of the Worcester Foundation for Experimental Biology. The other co-founder and co-director was Dr. Gregory Pincus, of contraceptive pill fame. Hoagland's studies on human stress and on the influence of hormones on behaviour are well known. Another Austrian scientist, Walter J. M. Hohlweg (b. 1902), who also worked in Berlin for many years, finally became director of the Hormone Laboratory at the Women's Hospital of the University of Graz (Austria). His work was mainly concerned with the regulatory centres of the endocrine glands in the hypothalamus. He attempted to elucidate the neuro-endocrine basis of the adreno-genital syndrome, and postulated the Hohlweg Effect, which is sex specific for females: the injection of oestrogen into men does not cause secretion of LH (ICSH), as was proved by experiments by G. Doerner and F. Doecke[162]. Walter R. Ingram (b. 1905), English by birth, but American by upbringing and training, was Professor of Anatomy in Iowa from 1940 to 1966. He is best known for his studies of the neuro-hypophysis and its actions. Dora Elizabeth Jacobsohn (b. 1908) was born in Berlin, proceeding to MD in 1933. After emigrating in 1934, she settled in Lund (Sweden), where she received a personal professorship in 1964. She became a post-graduate student of Geoffrey W. Harris at Cambridge in 1949, and remained his close collaborator and friend until his death in 1971. He often went to Lund to discuss the problems of their joint experiments, and, indeed, argue hotly about them! The role of the hypophyseal portal vessels and the demonstration of their capacity of regeneration was the most important result of that co-operation[163]. Dorothy Price, born in November 1899 in Aurora, Illinois, Professor of Zoology in Chicago, was mainly working in the field of the endocrinology of reproduction; her particular interest was the feedback control of gonadal and hypophysial hormones. On the husband and wife team, Ernst Scharrer (1905–1965) and Berta Scharrer (b. 1906), both originally from Munich (Bavaria), we have already reported. They both became Professors of Anatomy at the Albert Einstein College of Medicine in New York. Their work on neuro-secretion was early and fundamental. Another woman scientist in the field was Marthe Vogt (b. 1903), originally from Berlin, who retired in 1968 as Head of the Pharmacology Unit, Agricultural Research Council Institute of Animal Physiology, Babraham, Cambridge. She studied the interaction between cortex and medulla of the adrenal gland, and the action of noradrenaline in the brain, which had first been shown by von Euler in 1946.

Beta-lipotrophin (β-LPH) was first isolated in 1965, by C. H. Li and his group[164]. Although it has remained a peptide of somewhat uncertain function, it is known to be manufactured in the pituitary gland in the same cells as ACTH and, in fact, the two peptides are always released together[165]. β-Endorphin comprises the CO_2.H-terminal of β-LPH (β^{61-91}-LPH). β-Endorphin, the most potent of the three (α-, β- and γ-endorphin) was first isolated by A. F. Bradbury and his colleagues in 1975[166]. Endorphins are long-chain polypeptides derived from lipotrophin, but are not so quickly destroyed in the body. β-Endorphin binds powerfully to opiate receptors (see also Kosterlitz, p. 568); and displays morphine-like activity *in vivo* and *in vitro*. F. Bloom, D. Segal, N. Ling and R. Guillemin[167] declared it to be a central neurotransmitter.

The NH$_2$-terminal fragment, γ-LPH, has proved to be more elusive. W. J. Jeffcoate and colleagues[168] reported that their observations with three separate RIAs in human plasma and cerebrospinal fluid, obtained between 9 and 10 a.m. from 14 normal persons and from 11 with disease of the pituitary–adrenal system and increased plasma ACTH, were as follows. In normal people the NH$_2$- and CO$_2$H-terminal β-LPH were about equal, but in patients with increased plasma ACTH and β-LPH levels, there was also an excess of NH$_2$-terminal (γ-LPH) immuno-reactivity, representing γ-LPH in the circulation. In the cerebrospinal fluid (CSF) of 32 patients, three were suffering from pituitary-dependent Cushing's disease, the other 29 from non–ACTH-related pituitary or non-endocrine neurological disease. The levels of the CSF were raised in both γ-LPH and of β^{61-91}-LPH, not simply as a result of diffusion from the plasma. This was regarded as evidence that these small peptides are important neuro-transmitters in man.

Recent studies imply that β-LPH may be the precursor of the endorphins. W. J. Jeffcoate *et al.*[169] developed a RIA for human β-endorphin in plasma and CSF, and a second antiserum one, which measured β-LPH alone. By these means they could establish the presence of β-endorphin in a higher concentration in CSF than in plasma, also in patients with hypopituitarism and undetectable plasma-β-endorphin, indicating that β-endorphin was manufactured in the brain rather than in the pituitary.

These findings were supported by the results of D. T. Krieger and her group, who reported dissociation in the distribution of ACTH, β-endorphin, and β-LPH immuno-reactivities in the bovine brain[170]. It has been shown that the human brain contains receptors which will bind opium specifically. It appears that under normal conditions these receptors deal with pain perception by reacting with a natural substance produced in the brain. In 1975, J. Hughes and his colleagues in Aberdeen reported the identification of two small peptides, obtained from pig-brain, which possess pain-killing and pain-receptor-binding activity[171]. These substances are the enkephalins, each of which contains five amino-acids, and differing from one another by only one amino-acid. The structure of one of these enkephalins was identical with one fragment of β-LPH, a large pituitary peptide hormone, which may be, as stated, the precursor of the endorphins. One of the three latter, β-endorphin, has at least 30 times more affinity for the opiate receptors in the brain than the enkephalins. An important factor concerning the pharmacological potency of the enkephalins is their rapid enzymatic destruction in the body. These pentapeptides are, indeed, destroyed so quickly that even when they are injected into the cerebral ventricles, they exert at most short-lasting weak analgesic activity. But if protected against degradation by protein-cleaving enzymes, they acquire a long-lasting analgesic activity[172].

Prolonged opium addiction would mean chronic suppression of β-endorphin production. Attempts to wean an opium-addict will cause the pain-receptors to be unoccupied, causing the well known exquisitely painful stage as part of the withdrawal symptoms. It is known, especially in China and Hong Kong, that acupuncture alleviates the very painful sensations during withdrawal. A joint project of studying 'Acupuncture in heroin addicts: changes in met-enkephalin and β-endorphin in blood and CSF'[173], was undertaken in London and Hong Kong. The first report is exciting: basal β-endorphin was found to be elevated in both blood and CSF, but did not change during electro-acupuncture, although the therapy suppressed the clinical features of withdrawal. Met-enkephalin levels were not elevated in blood or CSF before treatment, but successful electro-acupuncture was accompanied by an unequivocal rise in all patients in the CSF, although blood-levels did not change. "This is the first specific evidence for a physiological basis for the efficiency of electro-acupuncture treatment of the heroin withdrawal symptoms".

The same team followed this up by treating 10 patients with recurrent pain with low-frequency electro-acupuncture. The pain was effectively alleviated. Basal levels of β-endorphin and met-enkephalin in the lumbar CSF of these patients were not different from those in pain-free controls. After electro-acupuncture in the patients with pain, CSF β-endorphin levels rose significantly in all subjects, but met-enkephalin levels were unchanged[178].

Although enkephalins have been isolated from the brain and are, as their name testifies, associated with the brain, they have also been detected throughout the gastro-intestinal tract[174]. The studies were stimulated by the discovery of the enkephalins in the gastro-intestinal tract and by the fact that this tract is "a very important target for the powerful actions of opiates".

Of other brain/gut hormones, serotonin should be mentioned briefly. It was identified as 5-hydroxytryptamine (5-HT) in 1954. As a gut hormone, it activates mucous secretion from goblet cells and from pyloric mucous cells and suppresses gastric acid output. The fact that instillation of acid into the duodenum produces marked inhibition of gastric acid secretion was first demonstrated in 1901[175]. The fact that serotonin is released from the duodenum either by acidification or, independently, by instillation of hypertonic glucose into the duodenum, suggested that the ensuing inhibition of gastric acidity is due to the physiologic action of serotonin. This could be proved experimentally, once RIA was available. In 1968, A. Feldstein and O. Williamson found serotonin metabolism in the rat brain, which established it as a brain/gut hormone[176]. Its exact physiological activity, apart from the control of gastric acid secretion, is at present not clear.

Recent observations in a slightly different direction have revealed that excessive and prolonged (chronic) alcohol intake may stimulate excessive corticosteroid secretion, followed by hypercortisolaemia, simulating Cushing's syndrome (*alcohol-induced-pseudo-Cushing's syndrome*)[177]. The underlying mechanism of alcohol-induced severe hypercortisolaemia is unknown. When the alcohol abuse is stopped, the symptoms disappear.

The modern research worker in the endocrine field faces an exciting vista. Yet the target area is not really narrowed down because neuro-endocrinology has taken up such an important position. The search for the understanding of achievement of homoeostasis in the living being covers every aspect of the biological sciences. No wonder that ever larger teams of experts in many disciplines are needed, and ever larger funds, in attempting to answer the increasing number of questions which emerge daily. Honesty, dedication and optimism will have to remain the guidelines for the future as they have been in the past.

REFERENCES

1. Aschoff, J.: Tierische Periodik unter dem Einfluss von Zeitgebern. Z. Tierpsychol. **15**, 1–30, 1958.
2. Halberg, F.: Physiologic 24-hour periodicity: General and procedural considerations with reference to the adrenal cycle. Z. Vitamin-, Hormon-. Fermentforsch. **10**, 225–296, 1959.
3. Krieger, Dorothy: Factors influencing the circadian periodicity of ACTH and corticosteroids. Med. Clin. N. Am. **62**, 251–259, 1978.
4. Orth, D. N., Besser, S. M., King, P. H., Nicholson, W. E.: Free running circadian plasma cortisol rhythm in a blind human subject. Clin. Endocrinol. **10**, 603–617, 1979.
5. Krieger, Dorothy: Circadian Rhythms. Abstracts, pp. 13–14. Int. Symposium on Endocrine Function of the Human Adrenal Cortex. Florence, 4–7 October 1977.
6. Chan, V., Jones, Ann, Liendo-Ch., P., McNeilly, A., Landon, J., Besser, G. M.: The relationship between circadian variations in circulating thyrotrophin, thyroid hormones and prolactin. Clin. Endocrinol. **9**, 337–349, 1978.
7. Decostre, P., Buhler, V., Degroot, L. J., Refetoff, S.: Diurnal rhythm in total serum thyroxine levels. Metabolism **20**, 782–791, 1971.
8. Naftolin, F.: Gonadotrophin Rhythms. Abstracts, pp. 10–11. In The Hypothalamic–Pituitary–Gonadal Axis. Meeting at the R. Soc. Med. London, 25–26 February 1975.

9. Clark, T.: Vaginal power or menstrual synchrony phenomenon. World Med. **15,** No. 9, 39–44, 1980.

10. Sassin, J. F., Frantz, A. G., Kapen, S., Weitzman, E. D.: The nocturnal rise of human prolactin is dependent on sleep. J. Clin. Endocrinol. Metab. **37,** 436–440, 1973.

11. Lazerda, Luiz de, Kowarski, A., Johanson, Ann J., Athanasiou, R., Migeon, C. J.: Integrated concentration and circadian variation of plasma testosterone in normal men. J. Clin. Endocrinol. Metab. **37,** 366–371, 1973.

12. Jarrett, R. J.: Circadian variation in blood glucose levels, in glucose tolerance and in plasma immunoreactive insulin levels. Acta Diabet. Lat. **9,** 263–275, 1972.

13. Conroy, R. T. W. L., Mills, J. N.: Human Circadian Rhythms. pp. I–IX, 1–236. London, Churchill, 1970.

14. Scharrer, B., Scharrer, E.: Neurosecretion. VI. A comparison between the intercerebralis–cardiacum-allatum system of the insects and the hypothalamohypophyseal system of the vertebrates. Biol. Bull. **87,** 242–251, 1944.

15. Duncan, J., Starling, S. G.: A Textbook of Physics. p. 153. London, Macmillan, 1959.

16. Selye, H.: Stress syndrome. A syndrome produced by diverse noxious agents. Nature, London **138,** 32, 1936.

17. Selye, H.: The Physiology and Pathology of Exposure to Stress. Montreal, Acta Inc., 1950.

18. Jacobs, H. S., Nabarro, J. D. N.: Tests of hypothalamic–pituitary–adrenal function in man. Q. J. Med. **38,** 475–491, 1969.

19. Selye, H.: General adaptation syndrome, pp. 837–839. In Textbook of Endocrinology, 2nd ed. Montreal. Acta Endocrinol., 1949.

20. Tigerstedt, R. A. A., Bergman, P. G.: Niere und Kreislauf. Scand. Arch. Physiol. **8,** 223–271, 1898.

21. Fisher, J. W.: Kidney Hormones (ed. Fisher, J. W.) London, Academic Press, 1970.

22. Goormaghtigh, A.: Proc. Soc. Exp. Biol. Med. **42,** 688, 1939.

23. Carnot, P., Déflandre, G.: C. R. Acad. Sci. Paris **143,** 384–386, 432–435, 1906.

24. Bonsdorff, E., Jalavista, E.: Acta Physiol. Scand. **16,** 150–155, 1948.

25. Reissmann, K. R.: Blood **5,** 372–380, 1950.

26. Stohlman, F. Jr., Rath, C. E., Rose, J. C.: Blood **9,** 721–733, 1954.

27. Gordon, A. S., Piliero, S. J., Kleinberg, W., Freedman, H. H.: Proc. Soc. Exp. Biol. Med. **86,** 255–258, 1954.

28. Jacobson, L. O., Goldwasser, E., Fried, W., Plzak, L.: Trans. Assoc. Amer. Phys., Philadelphia **70,** 305–310, 1957.

29. Kuratowska, Z., Lewartowski, B., Michalak, E.: Bull. Acad. Pol. Sci. **8,** 77–80, 1960.

30. Fisher, J. W., Birdwell, B. J.: Acta Haematol. **26,** 224–232, 1961.

31. Fisher, J. W. (ed.): Kidney Hormones. Vol. II. Erythropoietin. London and New York, Academic Press, 1977.

32. CIBA Foundation Symposium on Haemopoiesis (eds. Wolstenholme, G. E. W., O'Connor, M.). Boston, Little, Brown & Co, 1960.

33. Nakao, K., Fisher, J. W., Takaku, T. (eds.): Erythropoiesis. University of Tokyo Press, pp. 1–516, 1975.

34. Kolodney, R. C., Jacobs, L. S., Daughaday, W. H.: Mammary stimulation causes prolactin secretion in non-lactating women. Nature (London) **238,** 284, 1972.

35. Hwang, P., Guyda, H., Friesen, H.: A radioimmunoassay for human prolactin. Proc. Natl. Acad, Sci. U.S.A. **68**, 1902, 1971.
36. Thorner, M. O.: Prolactin: clinical physiology and the significance and management of hyperprolactinaemia. In Clinical Neuroendocrinology (eds. Martini, L., Besser, G. M.) pp. 319–361. New York, Academic Press, 1977.
37. Popp, J., Klein, A., Grueters, A., Korth-Schutz, S.: Nocturnal serum androgen concentrations and prolactin in boys with delayed puberty. Acta Endocrinol., Suppl. 225, 123, 1979.
38. Noel, G. L., Suh, H. K., Stone, J. G., Frantz, A. G.: Human prolactin and growth hormone release during surgery and other conditions of stress. J. Clin. Endocrinol. Metab. **35**, 840–851, 1972.
39. Tarquini, B., Gheri, R., Romano, S. Costa, A., Cagnoni, M., Lee, J. K., Halberg, F.: Circadian mesor-hyperprolactinaemia in fibrocystic mastopathy. Am. J. Med. **66**, 229–237, 1979.
40. Hill, P., Wynder, E.: Diet and prolactin release. Lancet **2**, 806–807, 1876.
41. Kopelman, P. G., Pilkington, T. R. E., White, N., Jeffcoate, S. L.: Impaired hypothalamic control of prolactin secretion in massive obesity. Lancet **1**, 747–749, 1979.
42. Nicoll, C. S.: Physiological actions of prolactin. In (eds. Knobil, E., Sawyer, W. H.). Handbook of Physiology, Sect. 7, Vol. IV, Part 2, Chap. 32, pp. 253–292, 1974.
43. Meier, A. H.: Temporal synergism of corticosterone and prolactin controlling seasonal conditions in the white throated sparrow, Zonotrichia albicollis. In Scheving, L. E., Halberg, F., Panly, J. E. (eds.) Chronobiology, pp. 647–651. Tokyo, Igaku Shoin, 1974.
44. Lancet: Leading Article – What does Prolactin do in Man? Lancet **2**, 234–235, 1979
45. Zollinger, R. M., Ellison, E. H.: Primary peptic ulcerations of the jejunum associated with islet-cell tumours of the pancreas. Ann. Surg. **142**, 709–728, 1955.
46. Edkins, J. S.: On the chemical mechanism of gastric secretion. J. Physiol. (London) **34**, 133–144, 1906.
47. Maydell, E.: Zur Frage des Magensekretins (= on secretin of the stomach). Pflueger's Arch. **150**, 390–404, 1913.
48. Keeton, R. W., Koch, F. C.: The distribution of gastrin in the body. Am. J. Physiol. **37**, 481–504, 1915.
49. Feyrter, F.: Ueber die peripheren endokrinen (parakrinen) Druesen des Menschen, Wien-Duesseldorf, Maudrich. 1953.
50. Feyrter, F.: Ueber diffuse endokrine epitheliale Organe. Leipzig, Barth, 1938.
51. Pearse, A. G. E., Welsch, I.: Z. Zellforsch. **92**, 596–609, 1968.
52. Bayliss, W. M., Starling, E. H.: On the causation of the so-called 'peripheral reflex secretion' of the pancreas. Proc. R. Soc. London **69**, pp. 352–353, 1901–1902.
53. Bloom, S. R. (ed.): Gut Hormones. Edinburgh, London, New York, Churchill Livingstone, 1978.
54. Harris, S.: J. Am. Med. Assoc. **83**, 729, 1924.
55. Wilder, R. M., Allan, F. N., Power, M. H., Robertson, H. E.: Carcinoma of the islands of the pancreas; hyperinsulinism and hypoglycaemia. J. Am. Med. Assoc. **89**, 348–355, 1927.
56. McClenahan, V., Morris, G. W.: Trans. Assoc. Am. Phys. Philadelphia **43**, 168, 1928.
57. Wauchope, G. M.: Q. J. Med. Oxford, n.s. **2**, 117, 1933.
58. Best, C. H.: Lancet I, 1157, 1934.

59. Whipple, A. O., Franz, V. E.: Ann. Surg. Philadelphia 101, 1299, 1935.
60. Dubreuil, G., Anderodias, A.: C. R. Soc. Biol. Paris 83, 1490, 1920.
61. Wilder, J.: Dtsch Z. Nervenheilkunde, Leipzig. 112, 192, 1930.
62. Wilder, J.: Med. Klin. 26, 192, 1930.
63. Peterson, B., Hellman, B.: Acta Endocrinol. 44, 139–149, 1963.
64. Berenson, S. A., Yalow, R. S.: General radioimmunoassay, in methods of investigative and diagnostic endocrinology, pp. 84–120. Peptide Hormones (eds. Berenson, S. A., Yalow, R. S.). Vol. 2A. New York, American Elsevier, 1973.
65. Unger, R. H., Eisentraut, A. M., Keller, S., Lanz, H. C., Madison, L. L.: Proc. Soc. Exp. Biol. Med. 102, 621–623, 1959.
66. Sutherland, E. W., Robison, G. A., Butcher, R. W.: Circulation 37, 279–306, 1968.
67. Walsh, D. A., Perkins, J. P., Krebs, E. G.: J. Biol. Chem. 243, 3763–3765, 1968.
68. Staub, A., Sinn, L. G., Behrens, O. K.: Science 117, 628–629, 1953.
69. Staub, A., Sinn, L. G., Behrens, O. K.: J. Biol. Chem. 214, 619–632, 1955.
70. Bromer, W., Sinn, L. G., Staub, A., Behrens, O. K.: J. Am. Chem. Soc. 78, 3858–3860, 1956.
71. Wünsch, E., Zwick, A., Fontana, A.: Chem. Ber. 101, 326–335, 1968.
72. Wünsch, E., Zwick, A., Jaeger, E.: Chem. Ber. 101, 336–340, 1968.
73. Samols, E., Marri, G., Marks, V.: Lancet II, 415–417, 1965.
74. Marks, V.: Proc. of European Day on Glucagon, pp. 63–71, Padua, 1971.
75. Samols, E., Tyler, J. M., Marks, V.: p. 152, in chap. 9: Glucagon–Insulin Relationships in: Glucagon (eds. Lefebvre, P. J., Unger, R. H.). Oxford, Pergamon Press, 1972.
76. Foà, P. P., Galansino, G., Pozza, G.: Recent Progress in Hormone Research (ed. Pincus, G.), Vol. 13, pp. 473–510. New York, Academic Press, 1957.
77. Foà, P. P.: In The Endocrine Pancreas. Handbook of Physiology (eds. Freinkel, N. Steiner, D.). Am. Physiol. Soc., 1971.
78. Bernard, Claude: Leçons sur le diabète et la Glycogenèse Animale. Paris, Baillière, 1877.
79. Bloom, S. R., Daniel, P. M., Johnston, D. I., Ogawa, Olivia, Pratt, O. E.: Release of glucagon, induced by stress. Q. J. Exp. Physiol. 58, 99–108, 1973.
80. Grimelius, L., Hutquist, G. T., Stenkvist, B.: Cytological differentiation of asymptomatic pancreatic islet-cell tumours in autopsy material. Virchow's Arch., Pathol. Anat. Histol. 365, 275–288, 1975.
81. Mallinson, C. N., Bloom, S. R., Warin, A. P., Salmon, P. R., Cox, B.: A glucagonoma syndrome. Lancet II, 1–5, 1974.
82. McGavran, M. H., Unger, R. H., Recant, L., Polk, H., Kilo, C., Levin, M. E.: A glucagon-secreting alpha-cell carcinoma of the pancreas. N. Eng. J. Med. 274, 1408–1413, 1966.
83. Welbourn, A. B., Polak, J. M., Bloom, S. R., Pearse, A. G. E., Galland, R. B.: Apudomas of the Pancreas. In: Gut Hormones (ed. Bloom, R. S.), p. 561. Edinburgh, Churchill Livingstone, 1978.
84. Oberndorfer, S.: Karzinoide: Tumoren des Duenndarmes. Frankf. Z. Pathol. 1, 426, 1907.
85. Masson, P.: Carcinoid (argentaffin-cell) tumours and nerve hyperplasia of appendicular mucosa. Am. J. Pathol. 4, 181–211, 1928.
86. Bioerck, G., Axén, O., Thörson, A.: Am. Heart J. 44, 143, 1952.
87. Kultschitzky, N.: Zur Frage ueber den Bau des Darmkanals. Arch. Mikrosk. Anat. 49, 7–35, 1897.
88. Williams, E. D.: Proc. R. Soc. Med. 59, 602, 1966.

89. Milhaud, G.: In Proc. Fourth Parathyroid Conference (eds. Talmage, R. V., Munson, P. L.). Amsterdam, Excerpta Medica, 1972.
90. Wermer, P.: In Clinics in Gastroenterology. Vol. 3, No. 3, London, W. B. Saunders, 1974.
91. Brown, J. C., Johnson, L. P., Magee, D. F.: Effect of duodenal alkalinization on gastric motility. Gastroenterology, 50, 333–339, 1966.
92. Ivy, A. C., Oldberg, E.: Hormone mechanism for gallbladder contraction. Am. J. Physiol. 85, 381–383, 1928.
93. Sutherland, E. W., Duve, C. de: Origin and distribution of the hyperglycaemic–glycogenolytic factor of the pancreas. J. Biol. Chem. 175, 665–670, 1948.
94. Unger, R. H., Eisentraut, A. M., Sims, K., McCall, M. S., Madison, L. L.: Site of origin of glucagon in dogs and humans. Southern Soc. Clin. Res. 9, 53, 1961.
95. Polak, J. M., Bloom, S. R., Coulling, I., Pearse, A. G. E.: Immunofluorescence localization of secretin and enteroglucagon in human intestinal mucosa. Scand. J. Gastroenterol. 6, 739–744, 1971.
96. Goldblatt, M. W.: A depressor substance in seminal fluid. J. Soc. Chem. Ind. (London) 52, 1056–1057, 1933.
97. Goldblatt, M. W.: Properties of human seminal plasma. J. Physiol. (London) 84, 208–218, 1933.
98. Euler, U. S. von: An adrenaline-like action in extracts from prostatic and related glands. J. Physiol. (London) 81, 102–112, 1934.
99. Euler, U. S. von: A depressor substance in the vesicular gland. J. Physiol. (London) 84, 21P, 1935.
100. Euler, U. S. von: On the specific vaso-dilating and plain muscle stimulating substances from accessory genital glands in man and certain animals (prostaglandin and vesiglandin). J. Physiol. (London) 88, 213–234, 1936.
101. Bergström, S., Sjövall, J.: The isolation of prostaglandin F from sheep prostate glands. Acta Chem. Scand. 14, 1693–1700, 1960.
102. Bergström, S., Sjövall, J.: The isolation of prostaglandin E from sheep prostate glands. Acta Chem. Scand. 14, 1701–1705, 1960.
103. Bergström, S., Ryhage, R., Samuelson, B., Sjövall, J.: The structure of prostaglandin E, F_1 and F_2. Acta Chem. Scand. 16, 501–502, 1962.
104. Bergström, S., Ryhage, R., Samuelson, B., Sjövall, J.: Prostaglandins and related factors 15. The structures of prostaglandin E_1, $F_{1\alpha}$ and $F_{1\beta}$. J. Biol. Chem. 238, 3555–3564, 1963.
105. Karim, S. M. (ed.): Prostaglandins, Physiological, Pharmacological and Pathological Aspects. Lancaster, MTP Press, 1976.
106. Karim, S. M. (ed.): Prostaglandins and Reproduction. Lancaster, MTP Press, 1976.
107. Karim, S. M. (ed.): Prostaglandins: Chemical and Biochemical Aspects. Lancaster, MTP Press, 1976.
108. Colwell, J. A.: Diabetes Outlook 14, (4) 7, (April–May) 1979.
109. Schroedinger, E.: What is Life? Cambridge University Press, 1945.
110. Langdon–Brown, Sir Walter: Practitioner 127, 614, 1931.
111. Hubble, Sir Douglas: The endocrine orchestra. Br. Med. J. i, 523–528, 1961.
112. Boss, B., Vale, W., Grant, G.: Hypothalamic hormones. In Biochemical Actions of Hormones, Vol. III, p. 87 (ed. Litwack, G.), New York, Academic Press, 1925.
113. Schally, A. V., Arimura, A., Kastin, A. J.: Hypothalamic regulatory hormones. Science 179, 341, 1973.

114. Bowers, C. Y., Schally, A. V., Enzmann, F., Bøler, J., Folkers, K.: Endocrinology **86,** 1143, 1970.
115. Saffran, M.: Chemistry of hypothalamic hypophysiotropic factors. Handbook of Physiology and Endocrinology, Vol. IV, Part 2, p. 563, 1974.
116. Carmel, P. W., Araki, S., Ferin, M.: Endocrinology **99,** 243, 1976.
117. Weitzman, E. D.: Biologic rhythms and hormone secretion patterns. Hosp. Pract. p. 79, 1976.
118. Krey, L. C., Butler, W. R., Knobil, E.: Surgical disconnection of the medial basal hypothalamus and pituitary function in the rhesus monkey. I. Gonadotropin secretion. Endocrinology **96,** 1073, 1975.
119. Morton, Richard: Phthisiologia, seu exercitationes de phthisi. Cap. I. Londini, imp. S. Smith, 1689.
120. Gull, Sir Wm. W.: The address in medicine. Lancet ii, 171, 1868.
121. Gull, Sir William, W.: Anorexia nervosa (apepsia hysterica; anorexia hysterica). Trans. Clin. Soc. London **7,** 22–28, 1874.
122. Déjérine, J. J.: Anorexie mentale. In: Les manifestations fonctionelles des Psychonevroses, cit. after Schur, M., Medvei, V. C., Wien. Arch. Inn. Med. **31,** 67–98, 1937.
123. Bergmann, E. von: Dtsch Med. Wochenschr. I, 123, 157, 159, 1934.
124. Kylin, E.: Ergebn. Inn. Med. Khk. **49,** 1, 1935.
125. Schur, M., Medvei, V. C.: Ueber Hypophysenvorderlappeninsuffizienz (= on insufficiency of the anterior pituitary); Wien. Arch. Inn. Med. **31,** 67–98, 1937.
126. Jacobs, E. C.: Effects of starvation on sex hormones in the male. J. Clin. Endocrinol. **8,** 227–232, 1948.
127. Biskind, M. S., Biskind, G. R.: Effect of vitamin B complex deficiency on inactivation of estrone in the liver. Endocrinology **31,** 109–114, 1942.
128. Trentin, J. J., Turner, C. W.: Inanition and mammary gland response. Endocrinology **29,** 984–989, 1941.
129. Srebnik, H. H., Nelson, M. M.: Endocrinology **70,** 723, 1962.
130. Perloff, W. H., Lasche, E. M., Nodine, J. H., Schneeberg, N. G., Vieillard, C. B.: J. Am. Med. Assoc. **155,** 1307, 1954.
131. Beumont, P. J. V., George, G. C. W., Pimstone, B. L., Vinik, A. I.: J. Clin. Endocrinol. Metab. **43,** 487, 1976.
132. Davies, T. F., Lewis, M.: Cit. after T. F. Davies, J. R. Coll. Phycns. (London), **12,** 379–397, 1978.
133. Howland, B. E., Ibrahim, E. A.: J. Reprod. Fertil. **35,** 545, 1973.
134. Frisch, R. E., McArthur, J. W.: Science **185,** 949, 1974.
135. Frisch, R. E.: Science **199,** 22, 1978.
136. Dally, P., Gomez, Joan and Isaacs, A. J.: Anorexia Nervosa, London. Wm. Heinemann, 1979.
137. Sheldon, J. H.: Proc. R. Soc. Med. **32,** 738–741, 1939.
138. Besser, G. M.: LH-RH tests in patients with pituitary and hypothalamic tumours and anorexia nervosa. In 4. Pituitary Tumours. Symposium on Some Aspects of Hypothalamic Regulation of Endocrine Functions. Vienna, pp. 241–243. June 1973.
139. Medvei, V. C.: Teams and their leaders. Some implications for scientific work. Lancet i, 1213–1214, 1964.
140. Greep, R. O.: History of research on anterior hypophysial hormones. In Handbook of Physiology, Sect. 7, Endocrinology, Vol. IV, Part 1, Chap. 21, pp. 1–27; Am. Physiol. Soc. 1974.
141. Wade, N.: Rough journey to a Nobel Prize. New Scient. 219–221, 1978.
142. Wade, N.: Three-lap race to Stockholm. New Scient. 301–303, 1978.

143. Wade, N.: A race spurred by rivalry. New Scient. 358–360, 1978.
144. Meites, J., Donovan, B. T., McCann, S. M. (eds.): Pioneers in Neuroendocrinology, 2 Vols. New York, London, Plenum Press, 1978.
145. Ibid.: Vol. II, pp. 221–239.
146. Ibid.: Vol. II, pp. 347–366.
147. As 143: p. 359.
148. As 141: p. 219.
149. As 143: p. 358.
150. As 141: p. 221.
151. As 143: p. 360.
152. McCann, S. M., Rothballer, A. B., Yeakel, Eleanor H., Shenkin, H. A.: Adrenalectomy and blood-pressure of rats subjected to auditory stimulation. Am. J. Physiol. **155**, 128, 1948.
153. Harris, G. W.: Neural control of the pituitary gland. Physiol. Rev. **28**, 139, 1948.
154. McCann, S. M., Tadeisnik, S., Friedman, H. M.: Proc. Soc. Exp. Biol. **104**, 432, 1960.
155. McCann, S. M., Ojeda, S. R., Martinovic, J., Vijayan, E.: Rôle of catecholamines, in particular dopamine, in the control of gonadotrophine secretion. Adv. Biochem. Psychopharmacol. **16**, 109, 1977.
156. Sand, Knud: Cit. after H. Selye, p. 323, In Textbook of Endocrinology. 2nd ed. Montreal. Acta Endocrinol. 1949.
157. Weitzman, E. D., Boyer, R. M., Kapen, S., Hellman, L.: The relationship of sleep and sleepstates to neuroendocrine secretion and biological rhythms in man. Rec. Prog. Hormone Res. **31**, 399, 1975.
158. Frohman, L. A.: Neurotransmitters as regulators of endocrine function. Hosp. Pract, p. 54, April, 1975.
159. Nelson, D. H.: Regulation of glucocorticoid release. Am. J. Med. **53**, 590, 1972.
160. Schade, S. D.: Diabetes Outlook **14**, (4), 1, 8, 1979.
161. As 144: Vol. II; pp. 289–310, 18. Studies on Neuroendocrine Control of Prolactin and other Anterior Pituitary Hormones, p. 298.
162. Doerner, G., Doecke, F., Geschlechtsspecifische Reaktion des Hypothalamus–Hypophysenvorderlappensystems der Ratte nach einmaliger oestrogen applikation. Z. Gynaekol. **86**, 1321, 1964.
163. Jacobsohn, D.: Regeneration of hypophysial portal vessels and grafts of anterior pituitary glands in rabbits. Acta Endocrinol. (Kbh) **17**, 187, 1954.
164. Li, C. H., Barnafi, L., Chretien, M., Chungi, D.: Nature **208**, 1093. 1965.
165. Jeffcoate, W. J., Rees, L. H., Lowry, P. J., Besser, G. M.: A specific radioimmunoassay for human β-lipotrophin. J. Clin. Endocrinol. Metab. **47**, 160–167, 1978.
166. Bradbury, A. F., Smyth, D. G., Snell, C. R.: Biosynthesis of β-MSH and ACTH. In: Chemistry, Structure and Biology (eds. Water, R., Meienhofer, J.), pp. 609–615. Ann Arbor, Science Inc., 1975.
167. Bloom, F., Segal, D., Ling, N., Guillemin, R.: Science **194**, 630, 1976.
168. Jeffcoate, W. J., Rees, L. H., Lowry, P. J., Hope, J., Besser, G. M.: β-lipotrophin in human plasma and cerebrospinal fluid, radioimmunoassay evidence for γ-lipotrophin and β-endorphin. J. Endocrinol. **77**, 27P–28P, 1978.
169. Jeffcoate, W. J., McLoughlin, Lorraine, Hope, J., Rees, Lesley H., Ratter, Sally J., Lowry, P. J., Besser, G. M.: β-Endorphin in human cerebrospinal fluid. Lancet II, 119–121, 1978.

170. Krieger, D. T., Liotta, A., Suda, T., Palkovits, M., Rownstein, M. J. B.: Biochem. Biophys. Res. Commun. **76,** 930, 1977.
171. Hughes, J., Smith, T. W., Kosterlitz, H. W., Fothergill, L. A., Morgan, B. A., Morris, H. R.: Identification of two related pentapeptides from the brain with potent opiate agonist activity. Nature **258,** 577–579, 1975.
172. Feldberg, W.: 79. Pharmacology of the central actions of endorphins, pp. 495–500. In: Gut Hormones (ed. Bloom, S. R.). Edinburgh, Churchill Livingstone, 1978.
173. Clement-Jones, Vicky, Wen, H. L., McLoughlin, Lorraine, Lowry, P. J., Besser, G. M., Rees, Lesley H.: Acupuncture in heroin addicts: changes in met-enkephalin and β-endorphin in blood and CSF. Lancet **2,** 380, 1979.
174. Konturek, S. J., Pawlik, W., Tasler, J., Thor, P., Waluś, K., Król, R., Jaworek, J., Schally, A. V.: 81. Effects of enkephalin on the gastrointestinal tract. pp. 507–512. In Gut Hormones (ed. Bloom, S. R.). Edinburgh, Churchill Livingstone, 1975.
175. Shemaikin, A. I.: Thesis, St. Petersburg, 1904. Cited in Babkin, B. P.: Secretory Mechanisms of the Digestive Glands. 2nd. ed. New York, Paul B. Hoeber Inc., 1950.
176. Feldstein, A., Williamson, O.: 5-Hydroxytryptamine metabolism in rat brain and liver homogenates. Br. J. Pharmacol. **34,** 38–46, 1968.
177. Rees, Lesley H., Besser, G. M., Jeffcoate, W. J. Goldie, D. J., Marks, V.: Alcohol-induced pseudo-Cushing's syndrome. Lancet I, 726–728, 1977.
178. Clement-Jones, V., Tomlin, Susan, Rees, L. H., McLoughlin, Lorraine, Besser, G. M., Wen, H. L.: Increased β-endorphin, but not met-enkephalin levels in human cerebrospinal fluid after acupuncture for recurrent pain. Lancet **2,** 946–949, 1980.

CHAPTER TWENTY-THREE

PRESENT TRENDS AND OUTLOOK FOR THE FUTURE – PART III

OCCUPATIONAL ENDOCRINOLOGY: DEVELOPMENT OF A NEW SUBSPECIALTY

D R. Malcolm Harrington, senior lecturer in occupational medicine at the London School of Hygiene and Tropical Medicine, estimates that there might be ten to twenty thousand people in the British pharmaceutical industry directly involved in the manufacture of biologically active materials[1]. Not all of these materials pose endocrine hazards. On the other hand, some non-endocrine chemical compounds may do: heavy metals, e.g. mercury and lead, may cause infertility in the male; the Occidental Chemical Company's plant in California manufactured the pesticide dibromochloropropane: at that plant male infertility was recorded in 1977. The present writer observed temporary male infertility in a tester of a refrigerator factory, who had to work in deliberately overheated testrooms[2] and the same principle applies to all men who have to work in a small enclosed space with high temperature and no air movement. Similar effects on testicular function were found to be caused by diathermy[3]. Some plants and mycotoxins can be oes-trogenic and so can certain chlorinated hydrocarbons, e.g. DDT and polychlorinated biphenyls. Moreover, biologically active prepara-tions may be hazardous in infinitesimal amounts, in contrast to heavy metals, for example. Oestrogen in dust levels can, according to Harrington's calculations, be dangerous in excess of $0.1\ \mu g$ per cubic metre, at short term exposure. The main hazards occur, of course, in pharmaceutical establishments which manufacture oral contraceptives. In one case of personal observation, while working for the United States Public Health Service, Harrington noted in one such plant synthesizing pure diethylstilboestrol (DES), where particular care had been taken over oestrogen dust control, that 20% of the male workers had gynaecomastia, impotence and loss of libido, and one man was lactating. Women production workers had a fourfold greater risk of intermenstrual bleeding. Another factory under investigation had a better record, apparently because all the production line staff were post-menopausal women, but gynaecomastia in men did occur. Occupationally-caused gynaecomastia in men is not a new discovery, but has been recognized for 30 years. From our previous considerations, it should be obvious that the occurrence of these hazardous defects is dependent on end-organ response and not simply a measure of the biologically active dose of the noxious substance. Reduced sperm counts due to suppression of testosterone levels do not necessarily equate with sterility, and oestrogenic suppression of testosterone over a short period is usually reversible. In addition, it must be borne in mind that under clinical conditions, post-menopausal oestrogen therapy is strongly associated with corpus carcinoma of the womb, and DES with cancer of the breast.

There is a great deal of investigation and research to be carried out in this largely uncharted field, and really effective preventative measures will have to be designed and carried out.

ADVANCES IN TREATMENT (SINCE 1940)

General considerations

When the long-lived Michel Eugène Chevreul (1786–1889) first described cholesterol in Paris in 1815[4], he could not possibly foresee what developments would eventually result from his observation. (Incidentally he proved, in 1815, that the sugar in diabetic urine is glucose[5], and he also isolated creatine from muscle in 1832.) When its correct structural formula was finally established, it became the basis for the evolution of the many steroid hormones which came into therapeutic use: oestrone (1929)[6], oestriol (1930)[7], androsterone (1931)[8,9], oestradiol (1933)[10], progesterone (1934)[11], testosterone (1935)[12], cortisone (1935)[13], deoxycortone (1937)[14], methyltestosterone (1938)[15], ethisterone (1938)[16], ethinyloestradiol (1938)[17]. A non-steroid chemical compound with oestrogenic activity was synthesized in 1938 by (Sir) Edward Charles Dodds (Bart.) (1899–1973) and his team in London[18].

The thyroid

Hyperthyroidism. Edwin Bennett Astwood (b. 1909) introduced in 1943 the antithyroid compounds thiourea and thiouracil[19], which originated in David Marine's discovery that cabbage contained a goitrogen (see p. 255) in 1928–1929. In fact, it was A. M. Chesney and B. P. Webster of Johns Hopkins Medical School, who made the first observation of endocrine goitre in rabbits[20] and were put on the right scent after consulting Marine[21]. Webster and Chesney next showed that the goitrogenic effect was preventable, if cabbage and iodine were given at the same time[22]. Marine, Baumann and Cipra[23] described seasonal variations of the goitrogenic effect of cabbage and other Brassica plants (cauliflowers and turnips). After Webster had joined Marine's team, they found that the thiocyanates, which were characteristic constituents of Brassicaceae, caused goitre when injected into rabbits, and that methylcyanide was goitro-genic[24].

Radioactive iodine treatment for hyperthyroidism followed the pioneering studies of Hertz (see also pp. 555–556) in Boston (1938–1939) and in Berkeley in 1940[25]. Further development occurred particularly after 1946, with the availability of the atomic pile, when ^{131}I was used in diagnosis and treatment, although mainly in the older age groups (over the age of 60) until proved that it was not excessively carcinogenic.

The advent of effective medical and radioactive iodine treatment caused a major change in the structure of the therapy of hyperthyroidism. From the 1920s onward, surgical technique had developed to cope with this difficult medical condition. This development was helped considerably when the physicians had learned how to prepare such patients for the operative treatment, especially after Henry Stanley Plummer (1874–1937) and William Meredith Boothby (1880–1953) had introduced the pre-operative administration of iodine[26] in exophthalmic goitre, and the supervision of the aftercare was improved. The surgical technique also became much more sophisticated and the so-called 'subtotal' removal of the gland achieved better results. This was only possible, however, as special surgical centres became established, where the famous leading surgeons acquired great skill in performing the operation in the great number of patients they dealt with. Another vital factor was the development of anaesthesia, which had to be particularly skilled during subtotal thyroidectomy in patients with toxic goitre. The names of famous thyroid surgeons became household words in many countries. We have already mentioned that Emil Theodor Kocher (1841–1917) in Switzerland was reputed to have carried out 2000 thyroidectomies; he was one of the pioneers of thyroid surgery and received the Nobel Prize in 1909. Several names of celebrated performers of the art emerged in the United States. In Britain, the Australian-born (Sir) Thomas Dunhill was supposed to have performed 15 000 thyroidectomies[27] and Thomas Albert Hindmarsh in Newcastle 6000[28]. It has also been mentioned that in Vienna, Austria, von Eiselberg and von Hochenegg were interested in the operation. Professor F. Kaspar, a pupil of von Hochenegg (1880–1945) was credited with 12 000 thyroidectomies and Professor Paul Huber (1901–1975) of Innsbruck, was credited with 12 000 of these operations[29]. Cecil Augustus Joll (1885–1945) of London, who pioneered the subtotal thyroidectomy and was a contemporary of Dunhill, is also said to have carried out more than 10 000 such operations. Each of these surgeons built up a highly effective team of anaesthetists, assistants, physicians, pathologists and nursing staff. No wonder that when the present writer attempted to give an assessment of the result of treatment of toxic goitre in 1959[30], the results were heavily weighted in favour of expert surgery at special centres.

With the establishment of medical and radioiodine treatment, surgery went into decline and the virtuosos and their teams disappeared. As radioiodine treatment came of age and no special danger of carcinogenic effects was observed, it has become a popular alternative to medical treatment. It must be stressed, however, that the incidence of hypothyroidism following such treatment is very high, and that long-term follow-ups by a number of observers, including the present writer[31], showed that hypothyroidism may occur as late as 10 and 15 years after the last treatment, and that 20 years after treatment the number of patients who become hypothyroid may reach 65–70%. This result does not depend solely on the dosage administered, but obviously also on the target organ response. There seems to be no definite correlation between the thyroid–antibody titre before therapy and the occurrence (frequency) of hypothyroidism following radioiodine treatment[31]. Smith and Wilson reported in 1967 that by using small doses of ^{131}I coupled with antithyroid drugs, they found that 85% of their patients were euthyroid at 5-year follow-up and did not require any drug therapy[32]. This state of affairs means that patients treated with radioiodine need a life-long medical follow-up of their thyroid condition.

Methimazole (=Mercazole) was synthesized by R. G. Jones, E. C. Kornfeld, K. C. McLaughlin and R. C. Anderson in 1949[33]; it is not only less toxic than methyl-thiouracil, but possesses ten times its antithyroid potency. Two years later, in 1951, A.

Lawson, C. Rimington and C. E. Searle synthesized carbimazole (='Neo-mercazole'), a modified methimazole[34], which was first used by A. Lawson and C. Barry[35]. It proved to be as potent as methimazole, but less toxic[36]. Moreover these drugs, when used pre-operatively, have considerably reduced surgical mortality rate and lessened the danger of thyroid crisis.

In order to control nervousness and tachycardia, especially before surgical treatment of toxic goitre, recently β-adrenergic blockers have been used successfully, such as propranolol (except when asthma or complete heart block are present)[37]. Propranolol on its own or combined with iodides has been used for a restricted time in the case of pregnant women. The question of thyroid surgery is still to be considered, especially in the young. Thyroidectomy is still the most common cause of parathyroid deficiency. Fourman stressed the insidious onset of symptoms of partial hypoparathyroidism, which are not necessarily related to the absolute value of the calcium in the plasma[38]. Today, patients over 50 are often prepared with neo-mercazole for radioiodine treatment. The dosage of the latter is still not definite; there does not seem to exist a preference for any hard and fast rule for calculations. After an estimate of the gland size by a scan, some prefer a single dose around 7000 rads, others two smaller doses with an interval and followed with carbimazole until euthyroid. Carbimazole does not make the gland radio-resistant.

Progressive exophthalmos may be unilateral, especially in patients who are euthyroid. The association with lid retraction indicates endocrine causes. The same applies to the clinically obviously thyrotoxic patient. Asymmetry in endocrine exophthalmos is usually not very marked and rarely exceeds 6 mm. Since the real cause is unknown, the primary aim of treatment must be the prevention of ulceration of the cornea and of panophthalmitis. The occurrence of retro-orbital infiltration and papilloedema also need immediate treatment to avoid optic atrophy. In addition to these strictly medical indications for immediate intervention, the human aspect must not be forgotten or underrated; that is, the extreme apprehension in the patient created by the disfiguring nature of the condition, much aggravated by the nervous symptoms of toxic goitre.

The most effective treatment of malignant exophthalmos is orbital decompression, by the technique of Naffziger, introduced in 1931. In less extreme situations, high-dosage systemic corticosteroid treatment and even a heroic retrobulbar injection of depot-corticosteroid has been reported successful[39]. The rationale for the use of systemic steroids is that they may act as an immunosuppressive agent in a condition which is assumed to have an autoimmune basis. On the other hand, the high doses of steroid needed (up to

140 mg of prednisone daily), may produce side-effects (hypercortical symptoms). The use of intravenous ACTH did not give a convincingly good result in the average patient[40,41]. Arthur Jones (London) observed improvement in many cases following orbital irradiation[42]. Thyroid ablation was also considered, on the (not very convincing) hypothesis that the thyroid causes the condition by manufacturing LATS. This is, however, not an easy measure to achieve, either by operation followed by radioiodine treatment, or by repeated doses of radioiodine to a total of 300 millicuries! Its success could not be generally confirmed. I. T. Boyle and colleagues put forward a renewed suggestion in 1969 that "steroids with or without orbital decompression" are the most effective available treatment at present[43].

Hypothyroidism: (a) Screening for neonatal (congenital) hypothyroidsim (CHT) by hormone determinations is already in existence on a large scale in the USA and in Canada; also in various parts of Europe and in Japan. In England, there is an East Anglian Regional Neonatal Metabolic Screening Unit at the Peterborough District Hospital, where an International Discussion on the subject was held on 5th October 1978. Hormone determinations are performed in cord blood or in dried blood spotted on filter paper.

Once it had been realized that cretins were suffering from similar hormone deprivation as patients with myxoedema (before the turn of the century), attempts were made to detect and to treat them. Although success was achieved occasionally in individual cases, little real progress was made until the mid-1970s, the advent of the CHT screening programme. S. Raiti and G. S. Newns reported in a retrospective study in 1971, that in children clinically diagnosed and treated before the first month of life, 74% achieved an IQ in excess of 90, whereas in those diagnosed between the fourth and sixth months, only 33% came into this category[44]. The first result of cord-blood screening appeared in 1976[45]. It showed low thyroxine, normal triiodothyronin values and high TSH in the blood of neonates in whom congenital hypothyroidism (CHT) was diagnosed. The advantage of cord-blood is the relatively large amount of plasma obtained, which permits the whole spectrum of hormones to be assayed by the radioimmunoassay (RIA) methods, and this during the first few days of life. The improved RIA techniques make it possible to measure hormones in very small amounts of blood spotted and dried on filter paper.

In 1845 Beaupré stated: "Cretinism usually remains unrecognized until the child is eighteen months or two years of age"[46]. The same author gave, in the same dissertation, one of the best classic clinical descriptions of a cretin.

I see a head of unusual form and size, a squat bloated figure, stupid look, bleared, hollow empty eyes, thick projecting eyelids and a flabby nose. His face is of a leaden hue, his skin dirty, flabby, covered in tetters, and his thick tongue hangs over his moist livid lips. His mouth is always open and full of saliva, shows teeth going to decay. His chest is narrow, his back is curved, his breath asthmatic, his legs short and misshapen, without power. The knees are thick and inclined inward, the feet flat. The large head droops listlessly over the breast; the abdomen is like a bag.

In the Quebec Screening Network for Metabolic Diseases, new-born screening for CHT began in 1974, with the spotted and dried blood on filter paper. It was based on thyroxine screening, followed by TSH, if necessary. In 2½ years, 212 000 neonates were screened and 46 diagnosed as having CHT and 16 as having deficiency in thyroid binding globulin (TBG)[47].

In Switzerland, it was decided to use TSH screening (by an adaptation of the routine RIA for TSH to dried blood spotted on filter paper)[48]. Since 1977, this test has been added to the mass neonatal screening programme for metabolic disorders (begun in 1965), which includes practically all newborn infants in Switzerland. This method proved most suitable for a large scale screening programme, but it detects only primary hypothyroidism and not hypothalamic pituitary forms, nor TBG deficiency and some other (rare) disorders with low thyroxine values. If possible, a combined thyroxine and TSH assay should be attempted. Although it is important to make hypothyroid neonates euthyroid as soon as possible, caution is needed in the presence of severe CHT, because of the possible existence of a myxoedematous myocardium; if such is the case, very energetic treatment may cause heart failure and/or serious arrhythmias. The initial single dose of thyroxine in the CGT is 0.05–0.1 mg.

(b) Thyroxine: The most important progress, especially in the treatment of hypothyroidism, proved to be the commercial synthesis of laevo-thyroxine sodium[49], which was highly active when given orally (0.1 mg being equal to *ca.* 60 mg of thyroid tablets BP). The two main advantages were that it could be produced cheaply in large quantities and that it had a constant biological potency.

After 1952, when Gross and Pitt-Rivers identified and synthesized the second thyroid hormone, triiodothyronine (T_3) (or liothyronine, BNF) (see pp. 427–428), it was found to be four or five times more effective by mouth than L-thyroxine-sodium (in terms of weight), with a more rapid but much less prolonged action[50], 30 μg of liothyronine being equal to 60 mg of crude thyroid extract. Yet, thyroxine has remained the main effective treatment of hypo-

645

thyroidism. Whether a combination of both thyroxine and triiodo-thyronine is more effective than thyroxine, has not been proved[51]. On the other hand, according to Smith, Taylor and Massey[51], the rapid action of liothyronine (T_3) has proved to be of great value in myxoedoematous coma, when injected intravenously every 12 hours until consciousness is regained; after that point, it is given orally together with thyroxine for about four days, after which time thyroxine is continued in the usual manner. Because of the frequent concomitant adrenocortical insufficiency in myxoedematous coma ('Schmidt's syndrome'), it is advisable to give intravenous hydro-cortisone at the same time[52].

The adrenals

Cortical insufficiency (Addison's Disease). It took a long time after (Sir) William Osler's early attempts and Professor Muirhead's de-scription (see pp. 235–236 and p. 475), before a treatment could be devised which was at least partially satisfactory. It consisted of sodium chloride, given by mouth, and cortical extract (or deoxycor-tone acetate in oil) injected daily, intramuscularly. After stabiliza-tion 'depot therapy' could be used, i.e. pellets of deoxycortone acetate could be implanted subcutaneously, or an aqueous solution of its crystals injected intramuscularly. The problems and dangers of this treatment were discussed in Chapter 19. Although Oscar Paul Wintersteiner (b. 1898) and Joseph John Pfiffner (b. 1903) had isolated cortisone in 1935[53,54] – i.e. 'compound F', which was identical with E. C. Kendall's 'compound E' – it was another ten years before L. M. Sarett achieved the partial synthesis of cortisone acetate from desoxycolic acid[55], and even then supplies were very limited. A major improvement occurred in 1949 when the joint efforts of the Mayo Clinic and Messrs. Merck & Co. Inc. succeeded in producing 'compound E' (cortisone) on a large enough scale to be used in the treatment of rheumatic fever[56].

There is an interesting corollary to the last-mentioned paper[56], published in 1949 by Philip Showalter Hench (1898–1965), his colleagues and E. C. Kendall. We discussed George Redmayne Murray's (1865–1939) important contribution to the treatment of myxoedema in 1891 (see pp. 292–296). At that time, Murray was pathologist to the Hospital of Sick Children in Newcastle-upon-Tyne, England. Newcastle has also put a claim to Addison, because his family hailed from the region and because, after his tragic end in Brighton, he was eventually buried there. We have also mentioned Hindmarsh, who specialized in thyroid surgery in Newcastle

(p. 642). In spite of this, the spirit of Swale Vincent and the pharmacologist A. J. Clark (see pp. 389–392) must have reached Newcastle, because Dr. Charles Nathaniel Armstrong, (born 1897), himself a Newcastle man, found on his appointment to the staff of the Royal Victoria Infirmary in 1931, that his interest and enthusiasm in endocrine disorders was looked upon with indifference if not suspicion[28]. He remarked that the students taught by him at that time knew more about Cushing's syndrome than his senior colleagues wished to know. That attitude changed dramatically, however, with Hench and Kendall's publication on the effects of adrenocortical hormone on rheumatoid arthritis! Be it as it may, Newcastle today has become one of the major centres of thyroid research in England, and Dr. Armstrong not only contributed to this development, but has lived to witness it.

The first to use cortisone acetate in Addison's disease were George Widmer Thorn and P. H. Forsham in 1949[57]. The treatment had to be supplemented with sodium chloride or deoxycortone acetate to achieve a satisfactory electrolyte balance, as cortisone has a poor sodium retaining capacity.

In the 1950s, preliminary stabilization with deoxycortone acetate was followed by monthly intramuscular injections of the long–acting deoxycortone trimethylacetate[58,59].

The natural secreted cortical hormone is cortisol (hydrocortisone), which was synthesized in 1950 by Wendler and colleagues[60]. Intravenous hydrocortisone sodium succinate is life saving in an Addisonian crisis. The estimated half-life of endogenous cortisol (at normal concentrations) is about 66 minutes. Its secretion is episodic[61]. The patient must be maintained with hormone replacement therapy for life. The usual adult dose is 30 mg per day (20 mg at 9 a.m. and 10 mg at 5 p.m.) of hydrocortisone or 37.5 mg/day of cortisone acetate. Additional mineral-corticoid therapy is needed in more severe deficiency in form of 0.1–0.2 mg daily of 9α-fluorohydrocortisone, which has minimal glucocorticoid effect in that dose.

In 1952, *aldosterone* was isolated from the adrenal cortex (see p. 554) by Grundy, Simpson and Tait and provisionally named 'electrocortin'[62]. Simpson *et al.*[63] determined its chemical structure. The name 'aldosterone' was selected because it is a steroid containing an aldehyde group. Its sodium-retaining power was 25 times more potent than that of deoxycortone, its effect on the excretion of potassium five times more. Curiously enough, it occasionally had enough glucocorticoid activity to make an attempt of treating (two) patients with Addison's disease successful with daily intramuscular injections in 1954[64], but this cannot be recommended as a safe or satisfactory treatment in general. The development of fludrocortisone, however, in 1961, which was much more effective taken orally, displaced aldosterone from its role in the treatment of Addison's disease.

Fried and Sabo observed, in 1954, that the introduction into the steroid ring of cortisone acetate of one of the halogens (e.g. bromine or fluorine) at the 9α position resulted in a compound more active than the parent hormone[65]. G. W. Liddle, M. M. Pechet and F. C. Bartter demonstrated in the same year, that 9α-fludrocortisol acetate (fludrocortisone) was the most active of these compounds, especially as regards the sodium-retaining effect, and was almost equal to that of aldosterone[66,67]. In England in 1955, O. Garrod, J. D. N. Nabarro, G. L. S. Pawan and G. Walker pioneered the combined treatment of Addison's disease with cortisone acetate and fludrocortisone with a normal sodium intake[68]. This was paralleled in the United States by Goldfien et al.[67] in the same year.

Congenital adrenocortical hyperplasia (CAH): presenting as pseudohermaphroditism in young girls and as macrogenitosomia praecox ('Infant Hercules') in young boys, it is now regarded as an inborn error of metabolism caused by deficiency of one or more enzymes which are necessary for normal steroid biosynthesis. There may be deficiency of 21-hydroxylase (the commonest form), 11-hydroxylase, 3-β-HSD, which may all cause virilization in newborn females. All types are transmitted by autosomal recessive genes[69]. Until 1950, there was no effective medical nor surgical treatment for these conditions. L. Wilkins and colleagues found early in 1950[70] a much increased excretion of 17-ketosteroids in the urine, whereas cortisol synthesis is impaired. Treatment of the milder forms (with virilism) with cortisol often considerably reversed the symptoms of virilism[71]. In women, the breasts begin to develop, a menstrual cycle is established and fertility may even occur; alas, the hirsuties, although stopped from progression, often remains noticeable. A. S. Mason and C. J. O. R. Morris also suggested in 1953[72] (and, independently, J. W. Jailer[73]), that the condition (CAH) was, indeed, due to a defect in the enzyme system; Jailer could demonstrate that the defect was in the conversion of 17-hydroxyprogesterone into cortisol. This is caused, according to Dorfman, by deficiency in the above-mentioned enzyme 21-hydroxylase[74], which causes the postnatal virilization and salt loss (but no hypertension) in small girls. The circle of events was given by L. Wilkins and colleagues in 1955, as follows[75]: 21-hydroxylase deficiency may be mild or severe. There is no deficiency of aldosterone production. Cortisol synthesis is deficient. This causes, via feedback, increased ACTH secretion. ACTH, in turn, stimulates the adrenal cortex to hyperplastic function with production of androgen and oestrogen in excess. The latter inhibit, via feedback, the secretion of pituitary gonadotrophins, causing gonadal hypoplasia and sterility. Administration of cortisone reduces the secretion of ACTH to normal amounts, thus preventing the other sequelae. Similar considerations apply to the other enzyme deficiencies causing CAH, e.g. 3-β-hydroxydehydrogenase (3-β-HSD)[76].

Cushing's Syndrome: A. W. Spence pointed out[77] that, as recently as 1946, L. J. Soffer wrote authoritatively that adrenal cortical tumours could be removed surgically only at great risk[78]. Death usually occurred within 48 hours after the operation, due to shock. This was caused by acute adrenal insufficiency as the contralateral adrenal gland was often small and atrophic. For the same reason, Frank A. Hartman and Katherine A. Brownell wrote in 1949 that, usually,

> removal of the tumour includes removal of the adrenal on that side. Therefore, the condition of the other gland must be determined first. If there is doubt to the healthy condition of the second adrenal, the operation is questionable since adrenal insufficiency may ensue.

The excessive amount of cortisol manufactured by the adenoma diminishes, by feedback mechanism, the production of ACTH, which, in turn, depresses the function of the adrenocortical tissue. Injection of cortisone acetate before the operation and intravenous infusion of cortisol with dextrose and saline during the operation, followed by intramuscular cortisone acetate for a day or two afterwards and, eventually, cortisol by injection or by mouth, transformed that gloomy situation, especially when, later, fludrocortisone also became available. Cortisone was gradually reduced in order to promote secretion of ACTH. In the event, the arrival of cortisol (hydrocortisone) on the scene in 1953[79], achieved the present, much happier, state of affairs. The prevailing surgical treatment of Cushing's syndrome today is total bilateral adrenalectomy, the patient being permanently dependent afterwards on complete glucocorticoid and mineralocorticoid replacement. In children, normal growth usually occurs[80]. The danger after surgically successful bilateral adrenalectomy is the development of a pituitary chromophobe adenoma with hyperpigmentation, visual field defect, enlargement of the sella turcica and a marked rise in plasma ACTH, as first described by D. H. Nelson, J. W. Meakin and G. W. Thorn[81] (Nelson's syndrome), in 1960. It is more likely to occur in children than in adults (27% as compared with 10% in adults)[82]. G. W. Liddle reported, together with D. N. Orth in 1971, on the successful prevention of Nelson's syndrome by conventional external pituitary irradiation, to suppress the source of ACTH production[83].

In his Sir Henry Dale Lecture for 1973[84], Professor Grant W. Liddle, at present Chairman of the Department of Medicine, Vanderbilt University Medical School at Nashville, Tennessee, discussed 'Blueprints for the Solution of Three Endocrinological Enigmas'. The second was entitled: 'Does the hypothalamus play a role in the aetiology of Cushing's disease? In it, he posed the question: "Why in Cushing's disease, does the pituitary secrete so much ACTH?" Beginning with the distinguished work of the late Geoffrey Harris, there have been numerous studies ... indicating that the secretion of ACTH is controlled by a releasing factor, originating in the hypothalamus. Hypothetically, excessive stimulation of the pituitary by CRF could lead to Cushing's syndrome.

In comparing two groups of patients, those with Cushing's disease after bilateral adrenalectomy and substitution therapy with 10 mg cortisol every eight hours, and a control group of Addison's disease patients, also with 'normalized' plasma cortisol of 10 mg eight hourly: Liddle and his colleagues found that the second group had low ACTH levels like healthy subjects, while the patients with normal cortisol levels after surgical treatment for Cushing's disease, had markedly raised ACTH levels.

It was suggested that medical treatment in pituitary-dependent Cushing's disease was not feasible. The obvious use of adrenal blocking drugs appeared ineffective because they caused rise in the plasma ACTH, and it was assumed that they would break through the blockade. In fact, W. J. Jeffcoate, Lesley Rees, Susan Tomlin, A. E. Jones, C. R. W. Edwards and G. M. Besser could demonstrate that in 13 patients with pituitary-dependent bilateral adrenal hyperplasia (Cushing's disease), the long-term use of metyrapone (2–66 months) achieved long-term clinical control with improvement, in spite of increased serum-ACTH levels. Eight of the patients had additional external pituitary irradiation. Slight hirsuties was the only definite side effect[85].

In simple adrenal hyperplasia, bilateral adrenalectomy was recommended, in the absence of an adrenal tumour, in 1957 by J. D. N. Nabarro[86] and by A. W. Spence[87], in preference to external pituitary irradiation[88].

The use of adrenal inhibitors of cortisol biosynthesis has been attempted as treatment of inoperable adrenocortical carcinomas[89].

In *ectopic ACTH syndrome*, the ideal therapy is the removal of the ACTH secreting tumour. The majority of these are, however, malignant and inoperable.

Conn's Syndrome (primary aldosteronism): In 1955 Professor Jerome

W. Conn (born 1907) of Ann Arbor, Michigan, published the description of 'Primary aldosteronism, a new clinical syndrome'[90], which was named after him. It is caused by excessive secretion of aldosterone, usually as a result of a benign adrenocortical adenoma. There was hypernatraemia, excessive loss of potassium with hypokalaemic alkalosis, renal dysfunction (polyuria, nykturia and albuminuria), hypertension, headaches, intermittent tetany and periodic muscular weakness. He presented the case of a 34-year-old woman with tetany and periodic paralysis with excessive amounts of aldosterone in the urine. His diagnosis of an aldosterone containing tumour was confirmed by surgery. Coincidentally, I. J. Mader and L. T. Isery reported on a similar patient, where a large aldosterone producing tumour was also found[91]. B. M. Evans and M. D. Milne, in Britain, described in 1954 a patient with 'Potassium-losing nephritis presenting' as a case of periodic paralysis'[92]. Conn, who read the paper in the *British Medical Journal*, suggested the diagnosis in a letter to the Journal. It was confirmed subsequently by operation, as C. L. Cope related[93].

According to Conn's review of 150 patients by 1960[94], a single benign adenoma was found in 70% of them, and in 15% more than one adenoma was present. In about 9%, primary aldosteronism was caused by bilateral adrenocortical hyperplasia. In these cases, subtotal adrenalectomy and cortisol substitution therapy may be necessary[95]. In aldosteronism, short stature and poor weight gain may also exist; Chvostek's and Trousseau's signs may be present (due to hypokalaemia), but not oedema. In *primary* hyperaldosteronism there is a decreased level of circulating renin. In *secondary* aldosteronism, circulating renin is increased. There is also a syndrome of *pseudoaldosteronism, or Liddle's syndrome*, due to a defect in the sodium/potassium exchange at the tissue membrane, which seems familial[96]. Potassium loss, sodium retention, renin suppression and aldosterone synthesis will result.

Recently, it was reported that an aldosterone-suppression test based on a simple method of extracellular-fluid volume expansion over three days reliably discriminated between patients with aldosterone-producing adenomas, idiopathic adrenal hypoplasia, and essential benign hypertension. In patients with primary hyperaldosteronism adrenal-vein plasma aldosterone/cortisol concentration ratios successfully lateralized all 21 adenomas. In such patients (with an adenoma) "the contralateral gland was always suppressed, as indicated by a ratio, which was less than that seen in the lower inferior vena cava, whereas in patients with hyperplasia the adrenal-vein aldosterone/cortisol concentration ratio from each adrenal was always greater than that seen in the lower inferior vena cava"[260].

In 1962 F. C. Bartter and colleagues described 'Bartter's syndrome', which consists of hyperplasia of the juxtaglomerular complex with hyperaldosteronism and hypokalaemic alkalosis, and which is, in fact, one of the groups of secondary hyperaldosteronism. There may be short stature, but the blood-pressure is usually normal. The juxtaglomerular kidney cells show hypertrophy and hyperplasia. It is sometimes a familial condition[97,98].

Steroid chemists have, in the last 30 years, produced a number of *synthetic corticosteroid analogues*, with the aim that they should possess the main beneficial actions of cortisone without sodium retention, osteoporosis and other undesirable side effects. Some of them, like prednisone (from cortisone) and prednisolone (from cortisol)[99] have a therapeutic effect five times greater than that of cortisone, but their side effects are the same, except for their much diminished sodium-retaining action. Dexamethasone (=16α-methyl-9α-fluoro-prednisolone) is seven times more active than prednisolone[100]; it has a minimal sodium-retaining effect, and has become particularly well known by its use in the evaluation of adrenocortical function, mainly to study cortisol suppression. G. W. Liddle showed that administration of 0.5 mg of dexamethasone every six hours caused a decrease in urinary 17-OHCS to less than half of the initial value within two days in the case of healthy adults[101]. Synthetic ACTH analogues are also available, both for evaluation and screening tests and for treatment of status asthmaticus, anaphylactic shock, allergic disorders, ulcerative colitis, but also to wean patients from corticosteroid therapy.

Phaeochromocytomas. These are functioning hyperplasias or tumours of the chromaffin tissue. They are found most commonly in the adrenal medulla, but they also exist in aberrant tissue, especially along the sympathetic chain, the para-aortic area, the aortic bifurcation, and the bladder. The clinical signs and symptoms are caused by the production of excessive amounts of catecholamines and are due to their pharmacological effects.

After Felix Fraenkel's description in 1886 (see Chapter 16), the condition was next mentioned, without recognition of its cause, by Jacob Pal (1863–1936) of Vienna, in his book *Gefaesskrisen* (=vascular crises) in 1905[102], and – nearly 30 years later – by Pierre Bernal of Paris, in 1934, in his book *Crises Hypertensives*[103]. Bernal described (in the first chapter) a 'Hypertension paroxystique pure', which he identified with the syndrome of the 'surrenalome' or 'medullo-surrenalome hypertensif'. Such patients with essential paroxysmal hypertension, where operation or post-mortem examination revealed tumours of the adrenal glands, were also described by Berdez of Lausanne in 1892[261], by Johannes Orth (1847–

1923) (in Prussia) in 1914[104], but especially by Ernest Marcel Labbé (1870–1939), J. Tinel and E. Doumer in Paris in 1922[105], by Manasse (1866–1927) in 1893[262], by Louis Henry Vaquez (1860–1936), E. Donzelot and E. Géraudel in 1929[106], by Charles Mayo in 1927[107], and in the same year by Ch. Oberling and G. Jung, the latter a pupil of Lériche[108]. There was a report from A. M. Shipley in 1929[109] and other authors at about the same time.

The present writer observed, diagnosed and studied such a patient in 1933, who was later reported on by Julius Bauer (1887–1979) of Vienna and René Lériche (1879–1955) of Lyon[110]. A second operation carried out by Professor Lériche confirmed the diagnosis of phaeochromocytoma of the right adrenal medulla in a man of 40. These operations were of great risk until 1949, when it was demonstrated that phaeochromocytomas contain not only adrenaline, but large amounts of noradrenaline[111,112]. The latter seems to be responsible for the main symptoms. During operation, the release of noradrenaline into the bloodstream causes the sudden rise of hypertension, followed by the dramatic drop of blood-pressure on clamping the adrenal vein. Ulf Swante von Euler (Nobel Prize: 1970) had shown noradrenaline to be the main transmitter of sympathetic nerve impulses in 1946[113]. It should be remembered that dihydroxyphenylalanine (DOPA) is, in turn, decarboxylated to dopamine, which is one of the important neurotransmitters within the central nervous system (CNS). The adrenal medulla is of ectodermal origin (the cortex is mesodermal); it responds, therefore, mainly to nervous stimuli and is not under feedback control. The medullary hormones are called catecholamines, because of their catechol nucleus and amine side chain. The mortality rate during surgery of phaeochromocytomas in the early days was very high. Today, definitive diagnosis is made (1) by detection of elevated catecholamines in the urine and in the blood. 30–50% are excreted as 3-methoxy-4-hydroxy-mandelic acid)= vanillyl-mandelic acid or VMA) and some 25% are excreted as metanephrine and normetanephrine. Catecholamines act through receptors; those of the alpha-type respond to norepinephrine and mediate the contraction of vascular smooth muscle and diminish cyclic AMP synthesis. Beta-type receptors respond to epinephrine and, by contrast, relax vascular smooth muscle and increase the synthesis of cyclic AMP. Recently developed substances are capable of blocking the alpha and beta effects of the catecholamines (phenoxybenzamine being an alpha-blocker and propranolol a widely used beta-blocker). These have proved to be useful not only for the study and function of the catecholamines, but essential for the pre-operative preparation of patients. The type of blockade depends on the type of catecholamines produced by the tumour and the response to the alpha and beta blockers. R. Meier introduced phentolamine as alpha-adrenergic blocker in 1948[114], but phenoxy-benzamine (= dibenzyline) has longer action and fewer side-effects.

Small phaeochromocytomas have been found often to have normal urine VMA, metanephrines, free catecholamines and plasma noradrenaline, but the plasma-adrenaline was persistently at least three times higher than normal. Increase of plasma-adrenaline was measured by sensitive radioenzymatic or high performance liquid chromatographic methods. Increase of plasma-adrenaline caused by fear or anxiety was excluded by taking a blood sample before and after intravenous 2.5 mg pentolinium. After pentolinium both plasma-noradrenaline and adrenaline fell by more than 50%, but in phaeochromocytoma patients there was no change[114a].

Drugs have also been used to inhibit the synthesis of catecholamines, by blocking the conversion of tyrosine into DOPA; thus, catecholamine synthesis is reduced and hypertension diminished[115]. Careful management of the anaesthetic has become essential in all phases, before, during and after the operation. In case of a diagnosis of bilateral phaeochromocytomas, glucocorticoid therapy must be begun three days before bilateral adrenalectomy. As phaeochromocytomas have occurred in families[116], it is essential that all members of the family of a patient should be examined.

The combination with medullary thyroid carcinoma was described by J. H. Sipple[117]. This makes it necessary to have a calcitonin estimation carried out, to exclude such a possibility. Phaeochromocytomas may also participate in multiple endocrine neoplasia, type 2 (MEA II), as described by Steiner and his colleagues[118].

The Pituitary Gland

Growth hormone disorders: the fact that growth hormone (GH) is species-specific has made treatment with porcine and bovine preparations disappointing. In 1959 M. S. Raben reviewed metabolic balance studies with human growth hormone (HGH) in over twenty people, in which he was also able to note its marked anabolic effect[119]. Since then multiple effects on many cell types have been demonstrated[120], but many of these effects can be demonstrated only *in vivo*. The effects are, apart from being anabolic, on carbohydrate and on lipid metabolism. Raben, incidentally, was the first to treat successfully a 17-year-old boy with pituitary infantilism and short stature, with HGH; he grew $3\frac{1}{4}$ inches in 16 months, compared with

½ inch during the previous 18 months; but the infantilism remained unchanged[121]. Other authors confirmed these findings, especially J. M. Tanner and R. H. Whitehouse, who found a satisfactory result in 26 dwarfed children and adolescents, with or without hypopituitarism[122]. Similarly good results were obtained in three patients with hypopituitarism following surgical treatment of craniopharyngiomas, and in ten out of sixteen patients, who were hyposomatotrophic dwarfs (dwarfism due to lack of growth hormone without evidence of an organic lesion). In four of the unsuccessful treatments, antibodies had developed to the HGH.

Although adult height is mainly determined by genetic factors, differences in the timing of the growth process (which includes the timing of the amount of growth hormone release), are of importance, and this should be assessed as early as possible, as delay may be accompanied by a discrepancy between growth in height and advancing bone age[123].

In 1957, W. D. Salmon, Jr. and W. H. Daughaday discovered a hormonally controlled serum factor which stimulates sulphate incorporation by cartilage (in hypophysectomized rats) in vitro[124], which they called 'the sulfation factor', but which has now been renamed 'somatomedin' (A, B and C), which affect cartilage, muscle, adipose tissue, liver and human placenta; the somatomedins are controlled in their activity by growth hormone[125].

Disorders of growth hormone may occur, of course, in the opposite direction, when an excess of HGH may produce gigantism and acromegaly. Medical treatment of the latter condition has now also been attempted successfully, instead of, or in addition to, attempts at surgical or radiological treatment (many of the anterior pituitary tumours being relatively radio-resistant). Pituitary surgery is usually carried out transfrontally or transphenoidally (see also Chapter 16, pp. 321–327). Radiotherapy entails irradiation (from cobalt or proton sources), a linear accelerator, or intrasellar implants of yttrium seeds. Transphenoidal surgery renders 25% of the patients deficient of one or more pituitary hormones. Recently, the development of transphenoidal microsurgery has meant great progress, by making it possible to remove very small tumours, such as microadenomas, without any of the side-effects encountered before. External irradiation rarely causes hypopituitarism, but any fall in HGH may often be delayed up to 4 years! Implantation of ^{90}yttrium produces a good clinical response in 50% of patients, but after one year the serum GH is under 5 μg/l in only 20%, and 25% will become hypopituitary.

G. M. Besser, J. A. H. Wass and M. O. Thorner of London (England), reported on the long-term treatment of 73 patients with active acromegaly with bromocriptine (= 2-bromo-α-ergo-kryptine), which stimulates dopamine receptors. The observation covered periods from three to twenty-five months (see also p. 569)[126]. By January 1978, Besser and Wass had extended the series to 87 patients, observed up to 42 months[127]. Whereas dopamine and dopamine agonists cause a rise in HGH in normal subjects, Liuzzi and colleagues found in acromegalics a paradoxical fall in plasma GH levels following bromocriptine[128]. In 71 (82 by January 1978) of the above-mentioned patients, carefully observed by Besser and colleagues, there was not only biochemical evidence of considerable improvement, but clinical improvement, especially in the first four months of treatment when it often appeared to be dramatic. Recurrent headaches and excessive sweating disappeared (the latter in 60 out of 63 patients); the facial appearance improved in 26 patients within a few weeks, size of hands and feet diminished in 17 patients, potency improved in 17 male patients, 15 of whom had excessive serum prolactin before treatment, which became undetectable afterwards. Two patients had had no surgery, in spite of upper quadratic field defects for red vision; these disappeared within three months on bromocriptine. The discrepancy between clinical response (97%) and the biochemical one (79%) is perhaps explained by the fact that bromocriptine seems to suppress the monomer form of circulating growth hormones, which is the most biologically active, and less the biologically inactive oligomers, which produce clinically inactive disease in the presence of abnormally raised immunoreactive growth hormone. There were few side effects apart from nausea and postural hypotension, and occasional peptic ulcers.

Infertility due to isolated gonadotrophic hormone deficiency is now amenable to treatment. In women, in certain cases of failure of ovulation an advance was achieved in the treatment of the condition with the synthesis of clomiphene citrate ('Clomid'), in Cincinatti in 1960[129], when D. E. Holtkamp et al. showed that this orally active, non-steroidal compound, which is chemically related to the oestrogen chlorotrienese (TACE), inhibited the secretion of pituitary gonadotrophins and suppressed ovulation[130]. It was, therefore, expected to become an oral contraceptive, but R. B. Greenblatt and his group in the United States[131], and D. Charles in England[132], demonstrated that in some anovulatory women it induced ovulation. C. A. Paulsen and W. I. Herrmann suggested in 1962, that clomiphene may act by stimulating secretion of the pituitary gonadotrophins[133]; this does not apply in the case of women with secondary amenorrhoea without hypothalamic or pituitary lesions. Peter M. F. Bishop (1905–1979) of London, reported in 1965 on a clinical trial in 102 anovulatory women between 1962 and 1965[134], that there was 50% chance in inducing ovulation in women with longstanding secondary amenorrhoea, in amenorrhoea following pregnancy (although he did not distinguish between patients with or without hyperprolactinaemia) and in oligomenorrhoea and metropathia; 12 pregnancies occurred among 68 women so treated, who wished to conceive.

In hypopituitary infertility, treatment with human FSH and human chorionic gonadotrophin may induce ovulation and excretion of oestrogens and progesterone in the urine (FSH being obtained from human pituitaries or from human menopausal gonadotrophin in the urine (HMG) or Pergonal); but careful regulation of the dosage is necessary to avoid over-stimulation, resulting in multiple ovulation. FSH preparations also contained a certain amount of LH. The pioneers in the use of human pituitary gonadotrophins in this respect were C. A. Gemzell, Professor Egon Diczfalusy (b. 1920) (a Hungarian, who is Head of the Reproductive Endocrinology Research Unit of the Swedish Medical Research Council and was Dale Medallist and Lecturer in 1978) and G. Tillinger in 1958[135]. Two years later they recorded the first pregnancy following treatment with human FSH followed by human chorionic gonadotrophin (HCG)[136]. In Britain, the techniques of the dosage and timing of the treatment have been studied and developed by A. C. Crooke and his team in Birmingham since 1963[137].

A promising line as a diagnostic aid and a treatment for the future was the development of the synthetic luteinizing hormone-releasing hormone of the hypothalamus (LH-RH), the combination of LH-RH/FSH-RH, the serum levels of which can be measured by radio-immunoassay (RIA). In women with infertility or amenorrhoea and normal or low gonadotrophin levels, it is a useful test to define the underlying endocrine condition, although the distinction between hypothalamic and pituitary hypogonadotrophic hypogonadism may not be established. In men, the test may be helpful in diagnosing hypogonadotrophic hypogonadism. It has shown special promise to be used as a therapeutic possibility in certain selected cases of infertility, such as Kallman's syndrome (the association of eunuchoidism and anosmia) with low gonadotrophin excretion, or with pituitary tumours, where spermatogenesis was achieved in some patients[138].

Of particular interest has proved, however, the study of *the hyperprolactinaemia-hypogonadism syndrome* which occurs in men and women. The reasons for the importance of these studies, especially intensive since 1972[139], are:

1. Women with inappropriate galactorrhoea consisted of about 30% of those having been discovered to have hyperprolactinaema[140],

although G. M. Besser and his colleagues found it in 80% of such women[141]. In women, secondary amenorrhoea is the most common menstrual disorder (although menorrhagia and/or regular periods may occur with anovular cycles). Characteristically, Hippocrates says in his *Aphorisms*, Section V, no. 39: "If a woman who is neither pregnant nor has given birth, produce milk, her menstruation has stopped", thus describing the clinical signs of the galactorrhoea-hyperprolactaemia syndrome in women 24 centuries before our time![142].

Anton de Haen (1704–1776), Professor of Medicine at the University of Vienna, was one of the founders of the annual reports on clinical observations together with post-mortem findings and progress in medicine: 'Ratio medendi in noscomio practico Vindoboniensi'. In volume 6, pp. 264–272; 1759, amenorrhoea is mentioned in connection with the finding of a pituitary tumour, although the causality of the syndrome was not established.

Remarkably, Galen's idea that waste products from the brain flow down to the base of the brain, down the pituitary stalk and to the pituitary gland and are passed by ducts through the sphenoid and ethmoid bones to the nasopharynx, to emerge as pituita or nasal mucus, was disproved, as we have seen (pp. 65, 138 and 150), at least under normal conditions. Yet, it has now emerged, under abnormal conditions cerebrospinal fluid rhinorrhoea does, rarely, occur. These conditions may be spontaneous, traumatic, following nasal surgery, but especially in the case of some intracranial tumours, particularly of pituitary tumours, and, among them, prolactinomas, often quite small. In fact, Willis (in 1664)[251] and Morgagni (in 1761)[252] were among the first to mention the abnormal passage of cerebrospinal fluid from the nose. This was confirmed at post-mortem by Miller in 1826, in a patient with hydrocephalus[253] and by Tillaux in 1877, proven by chemical analysis[254]. St. Clair Thompson discussed it in 1899 in his monograph[255], and the present position is carefully assessed in a recent paper, adding three more patients with CSF rhinorrhoea due to pituitary tumours, by I. E. Cole and Malcolm Keene[256].

In men, relative or absolute impotence is usually the presenting symptom, together with reduction of the seminal volume in some cases. Male galactorrhoea is, however, less frequent. Gonadotrophin deficiency in such men and women occurs mainly in patients who have had surgical or radiotherapeutic ablation of pituitary tumours.

2. Male and female patients usually resume normal gonadal function, if the circulating prolactin levels can be reduced to normal.

3. It seems that in certain target tissues, prolactin can induce its own receptors[143]. In other target tissues, steroid hormones may alter

the number of receptors and thus the presentation of prolactin action.

4. It is of importance that hyperprolactinaemia has been found in a large number of women who have been on the contraceptive pill for some length of time and developed secondary amenorrhoea. It is, however, known that oestrogens and thyrotrophin-releasing hormone will raise prolactin levels.

5. Prolactin-secreting pituitary tumours (prolactinomas) will raise the serum prolactin level. Many of these tumours are micro-adenomas which, certainly at first, cannot be defined radiologically.

6. Prolactin secretion is normally controlled by dopamine. Accordingly, dopamine agonists will also inhibit prolactin secretion. Such an inhibitor is 2-bromo-α-ergocryptine, which is a synthetic, long acting, orally effective, ergot alkaloid.

7. In nearly all patients, lowering serum prolactin levels with bromocriptine will result in speedy return of menstruation and ovulation. The highest success-rate occurs in women with post-pill amenorrhoea and anovulation, even if they are apparently normo-prolactinaemic.

8. It is of importance to avoid pregnancy after such treatment, unless a pituitary micro-adenoma (prolactinoma) has been excluded or successfully treated, because such tumours can rapidly enlarge during pregnancy with danger to neighbouring structures, and especially to the optic chiasma and to vision.

Treatment of infertility due to irreversible blockage of the Fallopian tubes by extracorporeal fertilization

A new and exciting line of experimental research reached fruition after twelve years of painstaking and laborious work, carried out in spite of many false trails and setbacks by the English gynaecologist Patrick Steptoe at Oldham and District Hospital, Lancashire, and the physiologist Robert C. Edwards, with the support of his wife, Dr. R. E. Fowler. It was begun to overcome the problem of infertility in women suffering from irreversible blockage of the Fallopian tubes. Every single step of the complicated process had to be evaluated by trial and error and by most meticulous judgement. Eventually, Mr. Steptoe succeeded in obtaining a human oocyte by means of laparoscopy from the side rather than from the top of a ripe Graafian follicle, in a natural cycle, just about four hours before ovulation would have occurred spontaneously. The monitoring of the natural surge of LH (= luteinizing hormone) in the 24-hour urine was used to indicate the time when the oocyte was due to be released in ovulation. A period of 24–27 hours after the surge was determined as the correct time for the recovery of the oocyte. Mr. Steptoe's technique developed to a stage where he could obtain an oocyte within 80 seconds after introduction of the laparoscope. Dr. Edwards then achieved the transfer of the oocyte into the culture medium with the sperm in the incubator in less than 60 seconds. Five years after completing this part of the study, which included the maturation of the fertilized oocytes, the first attempts were made of re-implanting the fertilized ovum into the mother's womb and monitoring the ensuing pregnancies. It was found that the 8–16 cell stage was best suited for re-implants. It was also found that the re-implants were only successful when carried out in the late evening, perhaps because of a diurnal rhythm variation or perhaps because the stimulation of the mother's adrenal may be less in the quiet of the night. The re-implantation had to be carried out in a very gentle manner. After exposing the cervix, a 1.4 mm plastic cannula was introduced through it under strictly sterile conditions; then using a very small syringe, the embryo was re-introduced into the mother.

Eventually, of the 68 who had been laparoscoped, four women became pregnant. By the end of January 1979, when Steptoe and Edwards reported to the Royal College of Obstetricians and Gynaecologists in London, two babies had been successfully delivered, Louise Brown, 5½ lb, and a little boy, implanted at Oldham, but born in Scotland, who also weighed 5½ lb. Both survived and are thriving. The authors' comprehensive account of their research has been published recently by Hutchinson[144].

The revolutionary developments in human reproductive physiology of recent years have created problems far beyond the realms of biology and psychology.

We have seen that artificial insemination by the husband (AIH) has been practised successfully by Lazzaro Spallanzani (see p. 187) and John Hunter (p. 205), but goes back much further, perhaps into antiquity. Artificial insemination carried out deliberately by a known or unknown donor (AID) other than the husband was first carried out in 1884 by William Pancoast (of Jefferson Medical College, USA)[145]. It was bound to create problems immediately in the legal and social systems of the Western countries. There were the questions of inheritance of money, property and titles, not to mention the practical and ethical problems concerning the choice of the donor. According to the current law of the United Kingdom, such an offspring is illegitimate. In some States of the United States of America, legitimacy can be conferred on the child so conceived, and steps are afoot to reconsider the legal situation in Great Britain. In ancient Rome, where the law maintained that the father was never certain ('Pater semper incertus'), recognition of an offspring or adoption was sufficient to establish his or her legal rights; a much simpler procedure (thus Octavianus Augustus became the son and heir of Julius Caesar by adoption)!

The recent success of extracorporeal fertilization may create further such problems. It should now be possible to fertilize an ovum by a donor woman by the 'host-mother's' husband (or a donor-father), because the host-mother cannot produce suitable ova herself. Successful uterine implantation would result in pregnancy of the host-mother, and she could be delivered of a viable child. At present, the woman who carries through the pregnancy and gives birth to the child is regarded the mother. In fact, such a child may carry the genetic inheritance of a donor-woman (and even of a donor-father). As the technique of extracorporeal fertilization will improve, it could happen that a married woman is not regarded capable of a pregnancy for medical reasons (e.g. heart disease). She might, however, be capable of providing an ovum, fertilized in the test tube by her husband's sperm, which would then be implanted into the womb of another woman, carrying and developing the baby for the couple. The ethical and legal confusion of such possibilities may make the mind boggle[146].

Finally, there have been recent developments on the question of choosing the child's sex. This has been a problem older than the alchemists' stone[147]. This is not the place to discuss the numerous superstitions and theories of the last 3000 years as to how sex could be predetermined. It was believed that simultaneous orgasm will produce a male child, because the faster moving Y-bearing sperm will reach the ovum first; or that intercourse at the time of ovulation will achieve conception of a girl. The ancient Spartans adjusted the need for regulation of the proportion of sexes by the simple method of exposing the undesirable newborn infant (usually girls) to the climatic dangers of the Taygetos mountain.

Scientifically, the present possibilities of the dangerous attempts of regulating the sex of the offspring, are:

(1) Experiments of separating X-bearing and Y-bearing sperm, either because the latter is slightly lighter in weight, or on the basis of (sperm-) head size, surface charge or swimming ability. Although most such attempts have proved, so far, to be mainly ineffective, the use of albumin gradients can increase the proportion of Y-bearing sperm in a sample to 75%[148]. The total sperm count is, of course, considerably diminished by

this method and reduces the chances of fertilization to only 30%, but of those, 75% produce males.

(2) Selective termination of pregnancy, having determined the sex of the embryo by amniocentesis. Apart from the fact, however, that this procedure entails risk and can be performed at the fifteenth week of pregnancy at the earliest, the cost of this method is high. For those reasons, and on ethical grounds, it should be used only if there exists a risk of serious sex-linked disorder. There is, however, a recent report from China, indicating that the sex of the embryo can be determined during the first trimester, by passing a fine cannula through the cervix and aspirating cells from the chorionic villi[149]. The Chinese figures suggest that such preselection could lead to a preponderance of males in the population, achieved easier than by the old Spartan method, but with no less dangerous consequences!

Diabetes mellitus

In his Presidential Address to the Section of Endocrinology of the Royal Society of Medicine in London on 25 October 1978, Professor Raymond Hoffenberg of Birmingham (England), mentioned Bayliss' and Starling's experiments in 1902, which resulted in the discovery of 'secretin' (see also Chapter 17)[150], as "endocrinology's equivalent of man's first lunar footsteps". The creation of the concept of a hormone "as something synthesised, secreted, transported to and acting on a target cell", became the basis of endocrine thinking for the next 60 years. Hoffenberg stressed, however, that

> nothing is ever as simple as it first seems. And we know now that what is synthesised by a cell is not necessarily what is secreted by it; what is secreted by a cell, is not necessarily what reaches the target, and what reaches the target is not necessarily what acts on it.

He selected insulin as a model of a protein hormone (like PTH and glucagon), because it demonstrates prohormone synthesis and receptor interactions. Hoffenberg also discussed 'big' ACTH as a prohormone of the pituitary peptide ACTH, and the method of actions of thyroxine (T_4), which are mediated through its metabolites. He also used other examples "to survey some of the funny things that can happen to hormones on the way to their targets".

That address exemplified the new look at hormone action. To return to the subject of treatment of diabetes mellitus, it has been known for a long time that insulin, contrary to the original expectations, does not cure diabetes. It merely ensures, in many cases, a form of peaceful co-existence between man and the disease. Hans Christian Hagedorn (b. 1888), B. N. Jensen, N. B. Krarup and I. Woodstrup introduced protamine-zinc-insulin[151] in 1936, in order to delay the absorption rate (NPH = neutral protamine Hagedorn) and other forms which convert fast-acting insulins into intermediate-acting (NPH; Lente) or long-acting: protamine-zinc-insulin (PZI)[152], and ultralente. There are several newer types in use in all three categories. Moreover, the optimum dosage of insulin and its distribution in 24 hours varies greatly from one patient to another. Protamine-zinc-insulin was, however, not entirely satisfactory because of the delay in its action, making it necessary to use soluble insulin in addition to it. In 1952 Knud Hallas-Møller (b. 1914), K. Petersen and J. Schlichtkrull introduced the now generally used insulin-zinc-suspensions[153]. (Insulin semilente = amorphous; insulin lente = 30% amorphous, 70% crystalline; insulin ultralente = crystalline.) Many highly purified insulins were introduced in the 1970s; there are now 18 available in Britain. If they are suspended in a neutral phosphate buffer, they dissolve because the zinc is liberated and precipitated as zinc phosphate. The lente insulins are suspended in an acetate buffer. Ordinary insulin crystals suspended in water act similarly to ordinary dissolved insulin; crystals with increased zinc content have a marked prolongation of action. Ultralente is prolonged up to 36 hours; semilente up to 16 hours. Lente, which is the most commonly used, has an action radius of 18–24 hours, which enables the patient, in most cases, to have only one injection a day.

Particularly interesting and important during the last 40 years has become the development of the oral anti-diabetic substances. Celestino L. Ruiz (b. 1904), L. L. Silva and L. Libenson in the Argentine, described in 1930 their observation of the hypoglycaemic effect of certain sulphonamide derivatives[154]. It seems that their paper was overlooked, perhaps because its title indicated mainly a contribution to the chemical composition of insulin, and the study of the hypoglycaemic effect of some sulphurated substances was given as a subtitle. Actually, the discovery of oral blood-sugar-depressing substances dates back to the pre-insulin era. In 1914, F. D. Underhill and N. R. Blatherwick observed that in animals, removal of the parathyroids resulted not only in tetany, but also in a fall of blood-sugar level accompanied by the disappearance of glycogen from the liver[155]. Glucose cancelled the hypoglycaemia, but not the tetany. C. K. Watanabe was the first to connect the hypoglycaemia after parathyroidectomy with an increase of blood-guanidin[156], and attempted to produce hypoglycaemia by injections of guanidin into the rabbit. Such an injection first caused hyperglycaemia, followed by hypoglycaemia about seven hours later (after giving at least 150 mg/kg subcutaneously). This was accompanied by an increase in anorganic serum-phosphate and a (later) decrease in blood-calcium, which he regarded as the cause of muscular cramp following guanidin injection. In 1931 A. S. Minot prevented guanidin-induced hypoglycaemia by giving calcium[157]. G. A. Clark demonstrated in 1923 that the hypoglycaemic effect of guanidin was the more marked, the less glycogen there was in the liver[158]. He concluded that guanidin first stimulates the sympathetic nervous system, which leads to transient hyperglycaemia provided there is glycogen in the liver. It also stimulates the vagus, which results in stimulation of the secretion of insulin after the sympathetic nerve effect has passed.

Watanabe also studied the possibility of another mechanism of guanidin action. In the wake of these studies, E. Frank, M. Nothmann and A. Wagner attempted, in 1926, to modify the guanidin molecule in order to separate the hypoglycaemic and the toxic effects of guanidin[159]. Three groups of guanidin derivatives were studied by various authors: monoguanidins, diguanidins and biguanidins. The diguanidins were found to have the greatest hypoglycaemic effect, increasing with the number of methylgroups, until dekamethyl-diguanidin proved to be 150 times more effective than guanidin[160] (in 1928). This substance was introduced into the oral treatment of diabetes under the name of 'Synthalin' or 'Synthalin A', respectively. The same researchers, F. Bischoff, M. Sahyun and M. L. Long, developed dodeka-methyl-diguanidin or 'Synthalin B'. The biguanids, investigated extensively by E. Hesse and G. Taubmann[161], in 1929, were somewhat less active, but phenylethylbiguanid ('phenethyl') was introduced into the treatment of diabetes in the USA by G. Ungar and colleagues in 1957[162,163], under the name of 'Phenformin' (DBI; Dibotin), which became available for general use in November, 1959. It is, however, important to stress that hypoglycaemia caused by guanidin or guanidin-derivatives cannot be relieved by glucose administration, in contrast to insulin hypoglycaemia. This fact had already been noted by Watanabe, by Frank, Nothmann and Wagner, and for the biguanids by Hesse and Taubmann. The other biguanid compound used in treatment was dimethyl-biguanid (= 'Metformin'). Incidentally, Paludrine, used in malaria prophylaxis, is also a biguanid, which, however, has little hypoglycaemic effect. It appears that the blood-sugar-level in normal people is not influenced by biguanids. The anode action of the biguanids seems to be the increase of the ultilization of glucose by the tissues and inhibition of gluconeogenesis. On the other hand, the hypoglycaemic action and the toxic action in biguanids are not separated by a large margin.

As to the use of Synthalin for the treatment of human diabetes, it was specially recorded by F. Bertram[164,165]. It was eventually abandoned because of its toxic effect on the liver and the kidneys, although it was on the market in Germany until 1945.

The practical application of the use of thiodiazol derivatives as oral antidiabetic substances has a somewhat romantic history. We mentioned that in 1930 Ruiz et al. had already reported on the hypoglycaemic effect of orally administered 4–5-methyl-thioimidazole in rabbits. Yet, in 1928, Ferdinand Bertram (1894–1960) declared that "All attempts to replace the parenteral insulin therapy by oral methods of equal value can be regarded as having failed"[166]. Bertram was one of the most experienced diabetologues of his generation[164,167] (in Germany).

In 1941, Joseph Kimmig (b. 1909) synthesized a new sulphon-amide, VK 57, which was handed to the pharmaceutical company Rhône-Poulenc for clinical tests. At that time, an outbreak of typhoid occurred in Montpellier. M. J. Janbon, Professor of Medicine in Montpellier, was asked to give the new substance VK 57 (or IPTD = isopropyl-thiodiazole), a derivative of sulphonamide, a trial run at the Fever Unit. Surprisingly, serious side-effects were registered of cramps and coma, never before observed in sulphonamide therapy. Three patients died, although the drug seemed to be effective from the point of suppressing the infection. In some of the patients with the more serious side-effects, intravenous glucose was given, which resulted in a quicker recovery than usually seen after glucose. Janbon and his colleagues drew the correct conclusions. They observed that there was a dramatic fall in blood-sugar when other patients were given the drug, and they recorded these observations in two important papers[168,169]. Janbon also informed a young colleague, who worked in the Institute of Physiology of the University on pharmacodynamics, carrying out research on the action of new preparations of insulin since 1938. His name was Auguste Loubatières (b. 1912). Loubatières immediately grasped the importance of Janbon's observations and set up carefully planned experiments to study the pharmacological action of the new drug. He ascertained in a crucial experiment on 13 June, 1942, that a single, orally administered dose of IPTD (VK 57) produced a marked and long-lasting hypoglycaemia, which was quite different from that caused by insulin, as he could not produce the same effect in the pancreatectomized dog. He reported his observations in Montpellier (then still unoccupied by the Germans) by the end of October, 1942 at a meeting of French Psychiatrists and Neurologists[170]. Owing to the war situation, his communication to the Société de Biologie in Paris, analysing the mode of action of IPTD, could not be given until 14 October, 1944, and extended and summarized in a brilliant 'Thèse Doctorat' (= M.D. thesis) in 1946[171]. This was followed by a spate of important accounts of his and his group's researches during the next 20 years. (He became professor of medicine in Montpellier.) His experiments resulted in the conclusion that the mode of action of IPTD was not due to selective damage to the alpha-cells of the pancreatic islet-organ, but to a stimulation of the beta-cells. He summed up:

> Logically, it seems entirely possible that such medicaments which produce hypoglycaemia may be used for the treatment of forms of diabetes. Apart from the diabetes which is due to anatomical damage to the islets of Langerhans, there obviously exists another form, in which the island cells appear normal, but there is some disturbance in the insulin discharge, so that less insulin is liberated than is necessary to maintain the insulin level in the blood. For this form of diabetes the use of these and similar sulfonamides would definitely be indicated[172].

In those days, the complex story of pro-insulin and of receptor mechanisms was quite unknown. His work remained unknown in Germany during the early post-war years. Thus it happened, that independently of Loubatières, a young hospital assistant in Berlin, Dr. K. Joachim Fuchs, experienced the hypoglycaemic effect of oral sulphonamides on himself. While penicillin had taken first place among antibiotics, research had gone on in the field of depot sulphonamides with long-lasting effect. At the Augusta Victoria Hospital in Berlin-Schoeneberg, high doses of BZ 55, a simple sulphonamide of the butyl-carbamide series, was effective in patients with stubborn infections, but seemed to cause severe neurological side-effects in otherwise normal persons. Fuchs tried the preparation on himself. He experienced nervousness, perspiration, tremor, his handwriting became difficult, he dropped a test tube in the laboratory, at the same time he felt hungry and was euphoric. His symptoms disappeared as soon as he had eaten lunch. He suspected a hypoglycaemic reaction and reported his observation to his chief, Professor Hans Franke (1909–1955). They decided on a planned experiment with low doses on normal individuals, including themselves. They found that the blood-sugar level decreased, but – on low doses – without severe reactions. Next, they tested it on diabetics on a diet only, and on older patients, who had been controlled with small doses of insulin. It appeared that older patients with physical handicaps were particularly pleased to be able to do without injections of insulin. Franke and Fuchs published their observations in 1955[173], but Franke died before the publication. Messrs. Boehringer in Mannheim, whose product BZ 55 (carbutamide) had been, took up large scale clinical trials and developed their first oral antidiabetic from that substance, i.e. sulphonamides with the amino-group in the para-position on the benzene nucleus. Hoechst Farben had been (and still are) leading in the field of insulin manufacture in Western Germany, which became particularly important after Frederick Sanger (b. 1918) in Cambridge (England) managed to achieve the exact chemical structure formula of bovine insulin ($C_{254}.H_{577}.O_{75}.N_{65}.S_6$), after 15 years of intensive research! It contains 777 atoms forming 51 amino acids. These amino acids are arranged in two chains, one consisting of 30 and the other of 21 molecules, held together by two pairs of sulphur atoms. A shorter disulphide bridge connects the two amino acids in the shorter chain. For this, he received the Nobel Prize for chemistry in 1958[174].

The chemists of Hoechst also experimented with guanidins, amino acids and sulphonamides, attempting to obtain a suitable oral antidiabetic. They advanced from the sulphonamides to the chemically related sulphonureas. They discovered that the sulphonurea group was mainly responsible for lowering the blood-sugar, and not the amino-group in the para-position. Eventually, they found that if the amino-group is exchanged for a methyl-group, the antibacterial property of the compound disappeared, but the blood-sugar went down by 40% and took up to 90 hours to return to normal, on doses of 100 mg per kg body weight in animals. This compound was called 'D 860' (= N-p-toluyl-sulphonyl-N-butylurea). The mode of action seemed to be that sulphonylurea causes discharge of insulin from the beta-cells and *not* destruction of the alpha-cells. The final proof was that pancreatectomized dogs, which had developed diabetes, showed no change in the blood-sugar level after being given either sulphonurea or IPTD, all of which had already been shown by the work of Loubatières. There were, coincidentally, several reports by other observers on similar experiences, confirming and broadening the fundament on which the knowledge of oral antidiabetics rests. Of these, Johann Daniel Achelis (1898–1963) and K. Hardebeck of the research laboratories of Boehringer who carried out crucial animal experiments must be mentioned[175]; Elenor Bendtfeldt and Helmut Otto (b. 1925) recorded their observations on 82 patients treated with BZ 55[176], and Ferdinand Bertram, who had been so sceptical in 1928 (see p. 665), joined them[177]. Finally, Professor H. Kleinsorge of the Klinikum Mannheim of the University of Heidelberg reported that between 1951 and 1953, when he was at the Medical University Policlinic in Jena, he had tested Ca 1022 (carbutamid) for use in infectious diseases and found as side-effects hypoglycaemic shock, similar to those he had observed previously with a related substance D1 or Loranil[178]. He recorded results not only in animal experiments, but also in the case of selected diabetic patients. In non-selected diabetics, he found that the substance potentiated the action of insulin in a great number of them.

All that time, however, Loubatières and his team had continued their fundamental research, whereas the German workers seemed to concentrate on the practical clinical application. Loubatières called the actions of sulpha derivatives "beta-cytotrophic effects", implying that these compounds (1) stimulated the secretion of insulin, lowering the blood-sugar; they could, therefore, not act in the absence of the pancreas. (2) There were also detected some actual proliferative effects under certain conditions of the beta-cell. From these beginnings developed the principles on which oral antidiabetic therapy has become an established part of the diabetic field, the details of which cannot be discussed within the framework of this book. It may suffice to say that it is now recognized that diabetes mellitus is a multifactorial and multifaceted disease. Moreover, that age and obesity are of great importance in trying to define the type of diabetes in a patient, in addition to his immunological status.

It is interesting to note that the aforementioned compound 'D 860' (see p. 667), named 'Tolbutamid', became popular more quickly in the United States, where it was put on the market in September 1956, under the name of 'Rastinon' or 'Artosin', than in Germany. This preference to BZ 55 ('Carbutamid' or 'Oranil') seemed to be due to the fact that D 860 had no longer an antibacterial property like BZ 55.

At this stage it should be recorded that the hypoglycaemic effect of salicylates and salicylate derivatives in sugar diabetics was known long before 'aspirin' became popular in about 1899. In 1876, Wilhelm Ebstein (1856–1912) reported on the therapy of diabetes mellitus[179], especially on the use of sodium salicylate. (He had also described 'Ebstein's disease', hyaline degeneration and necrosis of the epithelial cells of the renal tubules, occasionally seen in diabetes mellitus[180].) He was a pupil of Frerichs, Virchow and Romberg and became Professor of Medicine in Goettingen. He also published an interesting study of medicine in the Old Testament (1901).

The effect of salicylic acid and of its sodium salt was confirmed by Maximilian Carl August Bartels (1843–1904) in 1878[181]; also by E. H. Grenhow[182] and especially by R. J. Williamson[183]. They described a reduction of the glycosuria and polyuria, increase in weight and an improvement of the general condition; but the treatment had to be carried on for several weeks with relatively large doses. The occurrence of side-effects and the ineffectiveness in severe cases of diabetes made doctors abandon this treatment before the insulin era. Interestingly enough, in the normal animal or in normal man, salicylates cause an increase in the blood-sugar level, at least in toxic doses[184], but A. Hecht and G. Goldner[185] found in 90 patients with salicylate intoxication only three with increased blood-sugar. They found a fall of blood-sugar in twelve out of thirteen non-diabetics (up to 20%), after 4–8 g of oral aspirin daily for 1–3 weeks; but salicylates act on the pituitary and suprarenal glands and produce an increased ACTH-secretion with increased corticoid production, and thus a 'stress-reaction', according to B. S. Hetzel and D. C. Hine[186]. J. Reid and colleagues studied the practical application of salicylates[187], which has not proved to be very exciting.

A great number of other substances has also been studied in the last 30 years, but without great practical importance. Of 8000 substances which the research chemists of Boehringer (Mannheim) and of Hoechst investigated between 1962 and 1977, 6000 were found to cause a fall in blood-sugar in the animal experiment. Of these only five reached the stage of clinical tests; four of them did not fulfil the expectations; only one substance qualified: HB 419 (glibenclamid). That was determined in 1969. It is assumed that a great number of further substances have been synthesized since that time. Finally, Dr. David S. Schade of the University of New Mexico School of Medicine explained to the American Diabetes Association conference in Dallas, Texas, in May 1979[188], that an excess of counter-regulatory ('stress') hormone is a pre-condition for severe hyperglycaemia or ketoacidosis (see p. 625). Infusion of cortisol and of growth hormone in physiological concentration into six diabetics produced no acute ketogenic, hyperglycaemic effects, but a marked delayed effect occurred with growth hormone 12 hours later, when the concentration of the hormone itself had returned to normal. S. R. Bloom, P. M. Daniel and colleagues showed that anxiety or stress, such as a sudden loud noise, produced a marked and rapid rise in plasma glucagon in the conscious primate. A similar rise occurred also when (painful) stresses were applied to anaesthetized animals[189]. Glucagon and catecholamines work by increasing cyclic AMP levels, producing results in minutes. Steroids and perhaps also growth hormone are taken up by cells and transported to the nuclei, where they induce the formation of a new RNA, which in turn causes new protein to form, creating the much delayed diabetogenic effect. The complexity of diabetes can be understood, when one considers that several mechanisms of blood-glucose regulation can be affected. Dysregulation of the effect of insulin-release from the pancreas on the uptake of glucose by the tissues due to receptor abnormalities (e.g. anti-receptor antibodies), is one of these mechanisms, whereas the lack of insulin-response to induced hyperglycaemia points to a pancreatic (islet-cell) origin of the disease, the true endocrine insufficiency of the beta-cells, as usually found in juvenile diabetes.

Hypoglycaemia. Hypoglycaemia, especially idiopathic hypoglycaemia of childhood (IHC) can be a frightening condition. It was first described by I. McQuarrie in 1954[190], and may be detected at birth, or before the age of two. Apart from excessive insulin secretion, there may be spontaneous hypoglycaemia with convulsions. Diazooxide, a non-diuretic anti-hypertensive drug of the benzothiadiazine group of compounds[191], was found by C. T. Dollery, B. L. Pentecost and N. A. Samaan in 1962, to cause marked hyperglycaemia in two patients treated for hypertension with diazooxide and hydrochlorothiazide[192]. A Drash and F. Wolff then used it successfully in the case of a child with severe leucine-sensitive hypoglycaemia and correctly concluded that it would have an important place in the acute treatment of hypoglycaemias[193].

Obesity. We said (on page 668), that "age and obesity are of great importance in trying to define the type of diabetes in a patient. . . ." This will, of necessity, lead us to a discussion of obesity. It is clear that most cases of obesity have to be regarded as genetic in origin, but the influence of physical (environmental) and psychological factors cannot be underrated. If there are compulsive alcoholics, dipsomaniacs, there are certainly also many compulsive eaters; in the present writer's (and many other authors') experience, this is sometimes connected with the phases of manic-depressive conditions (see also the alcohol-induced pseudo-Cushing's syndrome[194], p. 631).

Obesity can be one of the recognized signs of well-defined endocrine disorders, such as myxoedema of Cushing's syndrome. If obesity is defined as an excessive accumulation of (triglyceride) fat in the adipose organ, it is understood that the fat depots of the body, which constitute the normal 'adipose organ', normally have a dynamic metabolic function: their task is to store surplus carbohydrate, not immediately used after ingestion, and to mobilize free fatty acid when needed to be oxidized in the tissues of the periphery to provide energy. Excessive fat deposits, which cannot be mobilized readily when needed, have long been known to run in families and often in families of diabetics, and to be somehow connected with emotional and even psychiatric characteristics ("let me have men about me that are fat; sleek-headed men and such as sleep o'nights; Yond' Cassius has a lean and hungry look; he thinks too much; such men are dangerous." Shakespeare's *Julius Caesar*. i, ii, 191). Fat people are often an object of ridicule and exhibits at fairs and markets in Western societies, but this is not so in Arab or Eastern communities. To Sir Walter Scott's "Fair, fat and forty" (*St. Ronan's Well*, ch. 7), the doctors have added the word "fertile", for women, who may be prone to inflammation of the gallbladder and stone-formation therein.

Weight gain or loss in adults causes no change in the number of fat cells, but the cell size varies with the weight. Calorie balance and the metabolism of energy are often used in attempting to define obesity, though their study does not really bring us nearer to the aetiology in many cases, just as the control of feeding is not always the best means of treatment. Apart from those endocrine disorders which may show obesity as one of their symptoms, such as gluco-neogenesis in Cushing's syndrome, where calories are diverted into fat and lean body tissue is depleted, and where cortisol stimulates hunger, with the resulting typical distribution of fat, it has often been suggested that in genetically determined obesity, there is a storage failure of the body tissues, due to lack or diminished manufacture of a hypothetical fat mobilizing hormone (FMH), which prevents the utilization of stored fat from the adipose organ.

From January to March, 1938, the present writer carried out a series of experiments on the utilization of the so called 'brown fat' in rats. The existence of the usual amount of brown fat (intra-scapular) was established in well-fed, young, adult, healthy, male rats by direct inspection by means of a simple surgical incision. When these animals were starved for *ca.* 10 days, they remained quite fit, although losing weight, but the brown fat had usually disappeared or was considerably diminished. In similar animals, if the (sympathetic) nerve supply of the fat was cut, the brown fat changed into white fat tissue. If these animals were then starved, they succumbed much faster and more readily, but on post-mortem examination the white fat pad, which had changed from brown to white after the nerve supply had been severed, was still present. For reasons beyond my control, these experiments ceased and their results could not be published. Present-day investigations seem to indicate that such brown fat is capable of maintaining the body temperature in rats exposed to cold, which white fat cannot do[195].

Water and salt balance also play an important role in many forms of obesity. Herrman Zondek (1887–1979) in 1935, coined the term 'water–salt obesity'[196], which is caused by damage to the centres in the dienkephalon and the pituitary (cerebro-pituitary-peripheral obesity), and which is responsible for a certain number of cases of obesity. Such damage may also have been incurred by violence (blow to the head). Hypogonadism and, especially, castration may lead to generalized obesity: but – as Julius Tandler and S. Gross

671

showed[197] – eunuchoids or castrates may either be obese (and often tall as well) or tall and thin. From obesity with generalized distribution have to be distinguished the lipomatoses where there is an accumulation of localized fat with the extreme of the formation of one or more lipomas. A constitutional form of localized lipomas is the steatopegia of Hottentot women, the spectacular deposit of fat over the coccygeal region, which has become a racial characteristic.

The connection of obesity with diabetes mellitus, with hypertension, with an excessive strain – in some cases – on the heart and on locomotion, makes it an undesirable condition, although in some cultures female obesity is equated with beauty and in others (Japanese wrestlers), male obesity is equated with strength.

To sum up, excessive alimentary (overfeeding) obesity is perhaps less common than has been assumed in the past, and some obese people show a smaller increase in metabolic rate to stimuli such as cold, food and even thyroid hormone. On the other hand, Blaza and Garrow found recently that, comparing fat and lean people who are each maintaining weight and are put in a direct calorimeter for 24 hours, the fat ones produce more heat than the thin ones[259]. The description of the 'Pickwickian syndrome' after 'Fat Joe', Mr Wardle's servant in Charles Dickens *Pickwick Papers*, is of recent creation (1955). It is marked generalized obesity with short stature, somnolence, twitching, cyanosis, secondary polycythaemia, alveolar hypoventilation, right ventricular hypertrophy and failure[198]. The actual term 'Pickwickian syndrome' was coined by C. S. Burwell *et al.*[199], in 1956. When the present writer was a medical student, we were taught that 'Fat Joe' was a typical case of 'Froehlich's syndrome' (pituitary tumour without acromegaly, but excessive obesity, hypogonadism, headache, somnolence and vomiting) (see also p. 321).

Finally, a very recent study by a British research team at Guy's Hospital, London, produced surprise results from a large experimental population of 3500 subjects, drawn from three separate normal office populations, that the fattest people ate the least[200]. The conclusions drawn from these findings were that obese people have a 'low energy' throughput. Pre-existing studies demonstrated that metabolic overefficiency, rather than physical inactivity, was the cause of low-energy expenditure.

> The association of increased adiposity with low food energy consumption may indicate an underlying 'low energy throughput' state, and it may be the mechanisms of this, as well as the obesity, that are responsible for disease[200].

But recent speculation goes further than that. David Margules of the Psychology Department at Temple University in Philadelphia[201] has always been interested in the addictive element similar to that in some alcoholics in those patients with obesity, who are continuous, or more often, periodic over-eaters, comparable to dipsomaniacs. Human and animal (and even plant) biology developed when there were periods of food efficiency or even surfeit, followed by scarcity and famine. During the latter, prolonged survival was aided by reduced energy expenditure, by dampening down the activity of the sympathetic nervous system, of muscular action, sex drive, of full response to cold, pain and lack of oxygen and making use of stored water, salt and nutrients, such as, for example, in hibernation (see also p. 599). Today, in some parts of the world, is an era of excess calories; the problem is not to find enough food but to avoid a surfeit of it. Margules learned that certain strains of genetically obese mice have a pituitary ACTH level about fourteen times greater than normal. He also knew that release of ACTH from the pituitary is accompanied by simultaneous release of the 'endogenous opiate' β-endorphin, perhaps because the two are fragments of the same precursor molecule. This 'people's opiate', like morphine, has among its many functions (induction of analgesia, lowering cardiac output, reducing secretion of TSH, reducing emotional reactivity, stimulating release of antidiuretic hormone etc.) the reduction of the propulsive contractions of the gastrointestinal tract, but improving its capacity to extract fluid and nutrients, and constrict the anal sphincter. Thus, the overeating and storage of food during favourable periods will act to good purpose at the time of starvation. In an age of calorific excess, however, when the starvation never occurs, such endorphin-induced obesity serves no purpose. Margules, who had experimented with naloxone and found that small doses reversed the state of hibernation and shifted it towards arousal, also remarked that naloxone seemed to have certain actions countering the effects of morphia and the natural opiates. Although naloxone has not been found to be manufactured in the animal organism, Margules speculates that there is evidence to suggest that the same action might be played by a combination of calcitonin, melanocyte-stimulating hormone and fragments of ACTH or by any one of them. If the exogenous and endogenous opiates modulate pain thresholds, it is permissible to speculate that they are released, normally, when sufficient food has been taken for the immediate needs of the body, and diminish or abolish the sensation (the pangs) of hunger. Moreover, enkephalins are distributed not only in the brain but also throughout the gut. Arguing that living organisms strive to keep in balance, Margules suggested that to counteract the morphine/endorphin/endorphinergic system, we may assume the existence of a naloxone/endoloxone/endoloxonergic system. He would, accor-

673

dingly, like to double the divisions of the sympathetic and parasympathetic systems, with the sympathetic being under the inhibitory influence of the endorphinergic and the stimulation of the endoloxonergic system. In fact Margules and his group succeeded in proving experimentally that by giving a series of genetically obese mice naloxone, the animals ceased to overeat and their weight dropped to that of their non-obese littermates.

To this speculation, James and Rory McCloy have added a further alternative[202]. If Margules argued that the pituitary controls the rate of feeding by the production of β-endorphin which acts on receptors in the gut and increased food intake, their alternative hypothesis is that the normal episodic production during stress will have the opposite effect. It will reduce appetite

> by providing the food reward in the central nervous system through the enkephalinergic system of the gut without the presence of food. Loss of appetite in stress is a common experience and would have some survival value.

They explain the experiments on the obese mice by assuming that the excessive level of endorphins in the blood will act on the enkephalin receptors in the gut and produce a chronic state of tolerance in the enkephalin food-reward system.

> With the switch-off mechanism jammed, more food would be eaten leading to obesity. Addicted as they are they may never experience satiety. Dosed with naloxone, the circulating endorphin would be blocked.

Accordingly, with endorphins reducing eating except in continuous excess, there is no need to postulate a balancing endoloxone system to block them. The McCloys remarked that morphia addicts normally have poor appetites and are rarely obese as one could expect on Margules' hypothesis.

Treatment of diabetes insipidus

Diabetes insipidus (D.I.) is caused by a deficiency of antidiuretic hormone (ADH) secretion and/or release from the posterior pituitary. This is usually due to trauma, pituitary surgery, but inflammation, e.g. sarcoidosis, may also cause damage to the hypothalamus and the posterior lobe of the pituitary. Occasionally, but much more rarely, infarction or tumours produce the condition. D.I. was distinguished from diabetes mellitus (D.M.) by Johann Peter Frank (1745–1821) (see pp. 174 and 733–734) in 1794[203]. D.I. was related to the posterior lobe by Alfred Erich Frank (1884–1957)[204] in 1912. Nephrogenic

D.I., transmitted by females and appearing during infancy in males, was first described under that name by R. H. Williams and C. Henry in 1947[205], but the first description was really given by Dr. Samuel Gee in 1876 (see Chapter 16). The usual treatment of ADH deficiency is intramuscular administration of pitressin tannate in oil. The separation and isolation of vasopressin and oxytocin was achieved by Oliver Kamm (b. 1888) *et al.* in 1928[206]. The synthesis of vasopressin was achieved 25 years later, in 1953–1954, by Vincent du Vigneaud (b. 1901) and his colleagues[207]. The administration of diuretics like chlorothiazide may also reduce urine volume by 50%. Although the use of chlorothiazide was described by J. D. Crawford and G. C. Kennedy in 1959[208], the effect of injecting a mercurial diuretic (Salyrgan) in D.I. was first observed and described, but overlooked, as early as 1920, by Julius Bauer (1887–1979) and Berta Aschner (1894–1968)[209]!

Recently, synthetic lysine vasopressin has been used successfully, the patient giving himself a dose of spray into each nostril after passing urine.

Although the newly introduced method of transphenoidal micro-surgery has meant a great step forward in the treatment of some pituitary tumours (see also p. 655), especially in the case of micro-adenomas, as post-operative morbidity is very much reduced, occasionally transient D.I. does occur[210].

Calcitonin and the treatment of Paget's disease

Calcitonin (see also pp. 486–487) is a 32 amino-acid single-chain polypeptide with a disulphide loop at the amino-terminal. Its molecular weight is about 3000. In man, it is manufactured in the parafollicular or C-cells of the thyroid, which are interspersed between the follicles. Embryologically they stem from the 6th (ultimobranchial) pouch, but in fishes, amphibians and hens they form a distinct glandular body. It is released by an increase in the calcium level of the blood, but also by administration of magnesium or glucagon. Its function is the lowering of calcium and phosphate in the blood and the inhibition of osteolysis by inhibiting osteoclastic activity. Therapeutically its main use has been in Paget's disease of the bone, first described by Sir James Paget, Bart. (1814–1899) in a paper to the Medico-Chirurgical Society of London, in November, 1876[211]. It is a common disease of the bone of middle and advanced age and is still of unknown aetiology. There is usually a strong familial tendency and men are affected more often than women. It affects the bones in a patchy manner and is, therefore, not to be regarded as a metabolic disorder. It is slowly progressive, but can occasionally 'burn itself out'. Calcitonin therapy was introduced by Shai and his colleagues in 1971, using porcine calcitonin[212], and, at the same time, by Woodhouse and his group, by using human calcitonin[213], with good results. Salmon calcitonin has also been used, being 5 to 10 times more potent[214]. Calcitonin is used for short-term treatment of bone pain and for immobilization hypercalcaemia; for long-term, it is applied prophylactically, and in case of high output congestive failure, and in spinal compression. The skull may, however, react differently to calcitonin administration and the vault may become more sclerotic during treatment. The pain relief is marked after several months, extension is prevented and radiological regression may occur. Calcitonin has also been used to treat other bone diseases[215].

Sexual behaviour and the sex hormones

This heading, taken from the title of a leading article in *The Lancet*[216], may seem an unusual choice for the concluding section of this final chapter. It will be readily understood, however, when we consider how human sexuality and sex roles have always been of interest and how the development of modern endocrinology has been linked with this problem.

As so often, Aristotle appears to have first recorded intersexuality in birds[226]. He described cocks with female behaviour and hens that behaved and even began to look like cocks. In the Middle Ages it was reported that some cocks could lay eggs and in 1474 a cock was tried in Basel for having laid an egg and burned at the stake with the egg, as being possessed by the devil. Public opinion maintained that from such eggs a basilisk, a being part hen and part serpent, would develop; the glance of a basilisk could kill any living being and destroy all vegetation. At the command of Frederick III, Thomas Bartholin in Copenhagen dissected and investigated in 1654 an egg, allegedly laid by an aged cock[226].   The existence of mixed sexual characteristics in a bird was regarded an evil omen. The crowing of a white hen implied indication of death in the household, in Bohemia; that of a red hen meant fire and that of a black one predicted visitation by a thief.

We have seen this development in the experiments of John Hunter, in the classic (and forgotten) experiment of Arnold Adolph Berthold and in the much publicized and much criticized experiments of the legendary Charles Edouard Brown-Séquard, who recalled the ancient folk-lore that virility and feminity reside in the gonads.

Schaefer, Starling and their colleagues attempted to introduce a scientifically better defined line into the search for the fundamentals of endocrinology. Under their influence, and because biochemistry was only just beginning, this area of the vast field of endocrinology was looked upon with some suspicion in the 1920s. Professor Diana Long Hall has written an interesting paper on 'Biology, sex hormones and sexism in the 1920s', in which she points out that after the First War, both in Britain and in the United States, there developed a hostility to this 'frivolous' subject, almost amounting to revulsion[217]. George W. Corner (b. 1889), gynaecologist, endocrinologist of progesterone fame, and medical historian, described the early phase of medical sex endocrinology as the testing of "ill defined extracts on hysterical women and cachectic girls"[218]. The mix-up of biological progress, of educational, emotional and social influences created confusion, which made planned research into questions like 'What is human sexuality?' impossible. Swale Vincent in Britain and Herbert M. Evans in the United States were severely critical of Brown-Séquard and "the monkey gland men" who succeeded him. Julian Huxley (1887–1972) seemed convinced that the differences between the sexes are "so considerable that they can never permit of the simple equivalence of the sexes"[219]. Patrick Geddes and J. Arthur Thomson came to the conclusion that all sex differences are due to the greater "activity of the male organism"[220]. Sex determination was one of the most controversial issues, even after F. H. A. Marshall's classical review of 'The Physiology of Reproduction'[221]. Marshall, like Geddes and Thomson, and Walter Heape (and Oscar Riddle, for that matter) regarded the embryos of higher animals as initially bisexual, the sex characters being developed by physiological and environmental conditions. The discovery of sex chromosomes by Clarence Erwin McClung (1870–1946) in 1902[222], produced a basis for strictly scientific genetics, but confused the issue even more. For the geneticist, the problem was henceforth simplified: the male or female sex chromosome was present or absent and determined the sex of the organism.

The experimental physiologist, the animal breeder and the clinician found that sex characteristics were widely variable. The embryologists were able, however, to bridge the gap between genetics and physiology with a chemical (hormonal) factor. Frank R. Lillie's studies of the freemartin (see pp. 199–201), recently critically reviewed by R. V. Short (see pp. 201–203), indicated a link between the genetic mechanism and the sex characteristics by the hormones produced in the gonads and, later, in the adrenal cortex and other tissues. These ideas were supported by Eugen Steinach's (1861–1944) gonadal graft studies in guinea pigs and rats. In a castrated animal of the opposite sex, the other 'inappropriate' gonad would take and produce remarkable changes in sexual form and behaviour. His results, which amounted to a bioassay of sex hormones, indicated that the sex hormones are directional forces in the embryo and the adult[223]; they compete for the differentiation of the soma which can develop into the masculine or feminine form; they are opposite hormones and antagonistic. This convinced Lillie that the masculinization of the female freemartin was not caused by the superior potency of the male hormone, but by the timing of the release of the hormones, which coincided with the view at the time.

This complex situation has recently been confirmed by the studies of Sir Cyril Clarke and his group. The *Lancet* put it in a Leading Article as follows[257]:

> A mule, being the offspring of a species cross, is infertile – or so we have always been told. But that rule is apparently not without exceptions, and occasional female mules (but not males) are fertile. How strange, though, that a female mule if served by a stallion will produce a horse foal but if mated with a donkey will give birth to another mule. That biological oddity neatly illustrates what Sir Cyril Clarke, at an Institute of Biology symposium last month, called the "uncertainty principle" – the unexpected event which makes nonsense of so-called facts and renders long-established dogma suspect. (The mule puzzle, as Sir Cyril explained, seems to be turning out to be delightfully simple: mule ova probably retain only horse chromosomes, so that the mule mother is, so far as reproduction is concerned, technically a mare.)
>
> Sir Cyril's pessimistic theme – that our interpretation of biological facts is so changeable that it can seldom be used on a basis for rational choice – is, he showed, nowhere more apparent than in medicine, where advice to patients or to society is continually changing.

A further example of the 'uncertainty principle' is the very recent development in the field of genetics, which seems to amend, correct and extend the ideas of the Neo-Darwinist School and re-instate Lamarck's ideas of evolution, but annihilate Weismann's theories (see Chapter 15). A young Australian scientist, Ted Steele (b. 1949) postulated that evolution is unlikely to progress through random mutations with the fittest of them surviving[258]. It is difficult to fit in that a complex system like the eye, for example, should have evolved by chance mutations. On the historical side of the study of evolution, it may be conceded that there are some gaps in our records of progress, such as the emergence of birds from the reptiles. On the other hand, the slow progress of evolution which Neo-Darwinism, a blend of natural selection and modern genetics, implies, makes it surprising that no evidence should have been found of the intermediate stages of some of the most important steps. Moreover, there were, even before Steele, several facts which could not be explained on strictly Neo-Darwinian lines. For example, chemically induced brain-tumours in mice were treated. If those mice then proceeded to breed, there occurred a significantly high proportion of brain-tumours among the next generation. Similar observations existed in the plant world, e.g. in the case of flax.

Steele himself and Reg Groczynski (of Plymouth, England) (b. 1947) seem to have shown experimentally the "Inheritance of Acquired Immunological Tolerance to Foreign Histocompatibility Antigens in Mice". This experiment appeared so important that Sir Peter Medawar deemed it necessary to repeat it in his laboratory in London.

Mutations in the antibody-producing cells are entirely separate from mutations in the reproductive germ line. According to Neo-Darwinian ideas they will not be absorbed into the germ line; they will, therefore, disappear with the death of the individual that produced them. Steele, however, pointed out that there are, among other phenomena, some virus groups which possess a mechanism which enables them to incorporate mutation results into mammalian genes; for example, those discovered by Howard Temin of the University of Wisconsin, for which discovery he became a Nobel Laureate. Steele asserted that this phenomenon was not restricted to the immune system, but applied also to blood- and liver-cells, cells lining the gut and others. He proposed to explore these possibilities further with Jeffrey Pollard, of Queen Elizabeth College, London.

The subsequent extraction, isolation and synthesis of the gonadal hormones contributed to the change of scientific opinion in the 1930s. Lillie's colleagues, Carl Moore and Dorothy Price[224] introduced the idea of endocrine feedback (towards the pituitary); male and female hormone are not antagonistic or competing, but act in their own sphere. Herbert M. Evans found, however, that the "recent brilliant period of successful isolation and chemical characterization of the male and female sex hormones has now been succeeded by a period of confusion"[225]. The confusion arose from the fact that a close chemical relationship had been shown between all the sex hormones. They were all steroids and there was the possibility of conversion of one to the other (see also pp. 564–565); the urine of the stallion is especially rich in oestrone, which is not present in the urine of the gelding, and all females manufacture some androgens and all males some oestrogens.

Sexual behaviour can be influenced by the normal sex hormones to such an extent that it is difficult to decide whether the condition can be regarded as entirely pathological as it occurs in up to 40% of women between menarche and menopause in Britain and the United States. This was discussed under the name of "The Premenstrual Syndrome" by Raymond Greene and Katharina Dalton in 1953[263]; Dalton followed up the subject and published a number of papers and a monograph in 1964[264]. In brief, many women experience, seven to fourteen days before the onset of the menstruation, headache, sleep disturbance, 'crabbiness', tension, depression, lethargy, anxiety, irritability (even epileptic fits), rhinitis, soreness of the breasts, feeling bloated, nauseous, having backache, joint pains and, occasionally, subcutaneous haemorrhages. Fluid retention, oedema and increase in weight may be noted (tightness of clothing), oliguria and constipation. Rarer symptoms observed, were alcoholic excess, nymphomania, distortion phenomena and feelings of unreality, paraesthesiae of hands and feet, palpitations and asthma. Hypoglycaemia was described which could have accounted for a number of the other symptoms[271]. Dalton stressed the remarkable similarity of the premenstrual syndrome to toxaemia of pregnancy, and the increase of symptoms during pregnancy in those who later developed toxaemia; and, vice versa, the high incidence of the premenstrual syndrome in women who had previously suffered from toxaemia[264]. All these symptoms may be slight, but in some women severe enough to cause a temporary change in character and interference with clear thinking and working capacity, even in schoolgirls. These symptoms all disappear with the onset of the menstrual flow. Clare[265] found that ca. 75% of a General Practice sample of women complained of at least one premenstrual symptom. Sutherland and Stewart found[266] that 33% of university students and student nurses suffered symptoms of depression, irritability, lethargy and bloatedness. Coppen and Kessel recorded premenstrual irritability in 40% of married women[267]. The onset of the syndrome is either at puberty, or after the birth of the first, more rarely of subsequent, children, when the hormone balance is upset. Such hormonal imbalance, which occurs in the puerperium and may cause puerperal depression, is often reminiscent of the premenstrual syndrome. Hormonal imbalance was already suspected by Frank, who described the syndrome in 1931[268]. Although the premenstrual syndrome may disappear with the menopause, Katharina Dalton collected evidence that untreated sufferers from it may develop menopausal depression, hypertension and glaucoma, especially if there is a family history of glaucoma; but an unexplained fact appeared to be that the menopause, including artificial menopause (i.e., hysterectomy or hysterectomy and oophorectomy or castration), sometimes six to twelve months later, did not necessarily prevent recurrence of cyclical symptoms in women who had suffered from the premenstrual syndrome previously. Dalton considered it possible that endocrine re-adjustment, perhaps involving the adrenal cortex, was responsible for the cyclical nature of the recurrent symptoms. She stressed, therefore, that the name of "Premenstrual Syndrome" was perhaps an unsuitable choice. Alcoholic excesses and tendency to shoplifting were observed to increase in post-menopausal women who had been suffering from the premenstrual syndrome before. In such patients progesterone treatment proved also effective[264].

Curiously enough, among prostitutes, the premenstrual syndrome seemed to occur in only 19% and Greenblatt noted a low incidence among professional dancers[272].

Apart from the actual individual suffering, the premenstrual syndrome has considerable social significance in its effect on the family, the children, the husband, on society and on the work performance of the working woman. The premenstrual syndrome and dysmenorrhoea appeared to be two distinct and different entities. Dysmenorrhoea pain begins on the first day of the period.

A direct relationship has been demonstrated between reduced plasma progesterone levels and the occurrence of the premenstrual syndrome[269], whereas plasma oestrogen levels may be raised prior to menstruation[270]. Progesterone levels in target organs may, however, differ from the plasma levels. Diuretics and progesterone have been used as treatment of the condition. Dalton stressed that progesterone, with its aldosterone-antagonistic action, is more effective than synthetic progestogens, which, however, have the advantage of oral administration. The negative and positive feedback actions of progesterone concerning release or – less effectively – inhibition of gonadotrophins have to be considered.

Men do not seem to suffer from periodic hormonal variations.

The perimenopausal and postmenopausal time-periods in women and their hormonal balance – or imbalance – have been the subject of intensive study in the past decade, but it is outside the scope of this book to discuss them in detail.

A more satisfactory discussion on the subject of the definition of human sex was presented by the studies of Charles Nathaniel Armstrong (b. 1897) of Newcastle and A. J. Marshall[226], which was summarized in the book *Intersexuality in Vertebrates including Man*, which they edited. According to them, biological sex is determined by (1) chromosomal sex; (2) gonadal sex; (3) apparent (phenotype) sex; (4) psychological sex. Regarding chromosomal sex, normally, the indifferent gonad would develop into a testis when a Y-chromosome was present, and into an ovary when there was no Y-chromosome. The method of the action of the Y-chromosome is still not definitely established, but it is most likely that it is the presence of the H–Y antigen, a cell surface component, which causes an indifferent gonad to develop testes in XY mammals. The H–Y antigen, a weak transplantation antigen discovered by E. J. Eichwald and C. R. Slimser in 1955[227], has its biological activities in a small peptide chain (molecular weight *ca*. 20 000); it is ubiquitous and highly conserved during evolution, cross-reacting throughout the higher vertebrates down to the fishes and amphibia. It seems to control gonadal determination in the heterogametic sex. Each society will add to the above points its own environmental, social and, indeed, legal definitions and restrictions, which will have to take into account problems like family structure, upbringing, work, wages, status in the community, retirement, pensions, inheritance (of property, title, estates), and a definition of marriage. The doctors assign (for example, at birth) gender rather than sex. Diana Long-Hall, in her above-quoted paper, relates the amusing example of the third-century Greek gossip-writer Athanaeus, "whoever heard of a woman cook?"[228]. One of the social variables is, of course, marriage, the definition of which differs greatly in various communities. It appears that from a legal point of view, at least in Britain, the main criteria establishing sex have to be biological. Psychological sex is regarded as a determining factor only in physically ambiguous cases. In 1964 Armstrong presented the concept of the 'sexual spectrum' based on all the above-named criteria of biological sex. Clustered at one end there is 'man', determined positively by all four factors: at the other end is 'woman'; the spectrum representing a curve with bimodal distribution, the two poles forming the majority in roughly equal proportions. Between these poles, the spectrum permits a continuum, in which individuals may display mixed characteristics, some of which would be called 'female' and some 'male'. Thus the existence of intersexuality and of transsexuals can be adequately covered.

Hormonal (neuro-humoral, immunological and receptor) influences play a particular role at the time of puberty and of the climacteric, in both sexes and during pregnancy in woman and in the foetus. It was not thought that the *direction* of sexual orientation is influenced in the human by the sex hormones during puberty or in adult life, but most recent investigations seem to indicate that prenatal and early postnatal exposure to hormones has an influence on adult human behaviour[216], and so have the rise of hormonal concentrations of puberty[229].

There seems little information, at present, on the metabolism of sex hormones in the human brain. In animals, it has been long known that the brain becomes sexually differentiated through the influence of sex hormones during critical early periods of development[230].

Moreover, sex centres have been identified in the rat hypothalamus. These centres determine the pattern of gonadotrophin secretion, which is cyclic in the female and continuous or 'tonic' in the male (and in some females)[231]. In the medial basal hypothalamus, a gonadotrophin-releasing hormone is secreted[232] under the influence of neurotransmitters[233]. It is transported by the hypothalamo-pituitary portal vessels to the anterior pituitary, where it stimulates gonadotrophin secretion. On that secretion the sex hormones exert a negative, inhibitory, or positive, stimulating, feedback effect, which depends on the sex hormone level during the critical period in the phase of differentiation of the brain, and during the postpubertal functional period as well[234]! There is also some evidence that the steroid sex hormones continue to modify the structure of the hypothalamus until puberty, when the final adult form is achieved[235]. It is possible that excessive levels of sex steroids could affect hypothalamic structure even in adult life, resulting in disruption of specific pathways. This has been suspected in rats associated with multicystic ovaries and persistent oestrus[236].

Is homosexuality due to abnormal hormone concentrations in the perinatal period? G. Doerner and G. Hinz found that in female rats, excessively high levels of androgen or oestrogen during the hypothalamic differentiation period resulted in anovulatory sterility, and/or a neuroendocrine predisposition to female hypo-, bi- or homosexuality[237]. A complete masculinization of sexual behaviour in female rats was observed after combined pre- and postnatal androgen treatment[238]. G. Doerner and colleagues also observed a slight increase in plasma testosterone level in lesbian women. Moreover, a significant increase was found in 9 out of 21 lesbian women who showed signs of virilism[239]. Unlike women, men do not normally discharge luteinizing hormone (LH) in response to oestrogens; Doerner et al. reported, however, a positive oestrogen feedback in LH secretion in some homosexual males[240]. They also found abnormally low levels of testosterone. They put forward the theory that the 'female' pattern of gonadotrophin-release may be due to exposure to abnormally low levels of testosterone in perinatal life; but ejaculates of homosexual men were found to be normal in one study[241]. Doerner suggests the identification of individuals who have low androgen levels at birth; he would like to treat them prophylactically with androgen to ensure heterosexual orientation in later life.

For men and women with severe gender identity problems, which concern the psychological constitution of sex only, i.e. when chromosomal, gonadal, phenotypical and chemical (hormonal) constitution are positively determined in one direction, male or female, but who wish to be a man when born as a woman, and vice versa: for those D. Cauldwell coined, in 1949, the term 'transsexual'[242], and their increasing number in the last 25 years has caused a number of problems for the medical profession, especially for the psychiatrists, endocrinologists, surgeons and plastic surgeons. Strangely enough, although some, particularly biologically male transsexuals, have transformed themselves by means of surgery and the use of hormones into an apparently female phenotype and live with a male consort, some psychiatrists have the impression that these patients are not psychologically homosexuals. These patients suffer from severe intrapersonal conflicts, quite different from the problems of the homosexual men or lesbian women[243]. Applying the concept of the sexual spectrum, it has been suggested that marriage (in Britain) can be contracted by a man and a woman at the extreme ends of the spectrum. The man must wish to have and must be capable of performing sexual intercourse with a woman, who – on her part – must wish to have and be capable of performing intercourse with a man. The crucial question is whether a transsexual (biological) man who has had his gonads removed and has obtained a functional vagina by plastic surgery and who is taking female hormones, can be regarded capable of performing sexual intercourse as a woman. Although the terminology is new, the condition was known in antiquity. Teiresias, the Theban, in Greek mythology was transformed for seven years (according to the reference in Ovid's *Metamorphoses*) into a woman for killing the female of a pair of snakes. Later, Hera and Zeus asked his opinion whether a man or a woman derives greater pleasure from love. He supported the view of Zeus. Because of that, Hera struck him with blindness, but Zeus granted him long life and the gift of prophecy.

Richard von Krafft-Ebing (1840–1902), the celebrated German psychiatrist, in his 'Psychopathia sexualis'[244], the standard work on the subject in his times, discussed transvestitism, of which he had made a careful study. He called it 'dress-fetishism' and regarded it as the first stage in the onset of 'metamorphosis sexualis paranoica'. He described four categories: (1) Obsession for wearing women's clothes. (2) The passive homosexual's desire to be accepted as a woman. (3) Heterosexuals with some signs of (pseudo-)hermaphroditism, who dress as women for that reason. (4). People with a delusion that a sex change had taken place. Curiously, most of Krafft-Ebing's observations referred to men transvestites or transsexuals, although women are by no means an exception, but perhaps less spectacular and occur in a smaller number.

Before 1949, most transsexuals were called 'Transvestites', because they preferred to wear the clothes of the opposite sex; for this a special permit had to be obtained from the police.

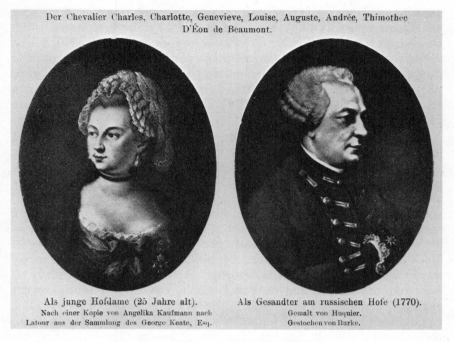

Der Chevalier Charles, Charlotte, Genevieve, Louise, Auguste, Andrée, Thimothée
D'Éon de Beaumont.

Als junge Hofdame (25 Jahre alt).
Nach einer Kopie von Angelika Kaufmann nach
Latour aus der Sammlung des George Keate, Esq.

Als Gesandter am russischen Hofe (1770).
Gemalt von Huquier.
Gestochen von Burke.

Figure 74 Le Chevalier d'Eon

In the 18th century, the chevalier d'Éon achieved a certain
reputation because he preferred female attire and could pass easily as
a woman. He used this ability also for his spying activities.

The other famous French transvestite was François Timoléon de
Choisy (1644–1724), who – in spite of a somewhat chequered life –
died as Abbé de Choisy and wrote a 'History of the Church'.

Of British transvestites, 'James Barry' (1799–1865) is of particular
interest. She studied medicine in Edinburgh, wrote a thesis at the age
of 12, enlisted in the Army in 1813 and rose to a very senior rank as a
Colonial Medical Officer, having been present at many actions on
active service; yet, she managed to keep the secret of her sex until her
death in London.

Today, 'unisex' hairstyles and clothes have made life for transsexuals much easier in that respect.

The concept of the 'sexual spectrum' has been of great help in
classifying the intermediate forms (intersexuality) in vertebrates and
in defining the disorders arising from them. Disturbances may occur
due to abnormalities in any part of the biological sex. The normal
chromosomal constitution of the fertilized ovum is in case of a male

46(XY), and 46(XX) in case of female. A variety of karyotypes or sex chromosomes of an abnormal zygote have been detected, such as, XO, XXX, XXXX, XXXXX, XXY, XXXY, XXXXY, XXYY and XYY, with concomitant abnormal formations of the gonads (except in XYY, where there is a fertile testis with a male phenotype). The XO–XXXXX have usually sterile ovaries in a female phenotype; the XXY–XXYY display sterile testes in a male phenotype[245].

Foetal chromosomal anomalies can now be discovered during early pregnancy and are sometimes so serious that there seems to be justification for abortion in some cases. Others are much more problematical. An example for this can be the sex chromosome aneuploidy 47XYY. It has been alleged that such a man is often tall, mentally retarded, and may be a violent criminal. But chromosome surveys in prisons, detention centres, borstals and psychiatric hospitals in Britain have not shown any great excess of XYY males[246,247]. Yet there is evidence that there is a higher frequency of XYY males in special hospitals and that abnormal behaviour, when it occurs, is not due to upbringing or other social environments. A recent review[248] ends with the question: "But the dilemma remains: what is to be done with the XYY fetus?" This reminds me of a passage from the detective story by the late Dorothy L. Sayers, *The Unpleasantness at the Bellona Club* (Mrs Rushworth is speaking):

'Are you devoted to young criminals by any chance?' Wimsey said that they presented a very perplexing problem. 'How very true. So perplexing. And just to think that we have been quite wrong about them all these thousands of years. Flogging and bread and water, you know, and Holy Communion, when what they really needed was a little bit of rabbit gland or something to make them just as good as gold. ... And all those poor freaks in sideshows too – dwarfs and giants you know – all pineal and pituitary, and they come right again. Though I daresay they make a great deal more money as they are, which throws such a distressing light on unemployment, does it not?' Wimsey said that everything had the defects of its qualities.

In 1949, an important discovery was described by Murray Llwellyn Barr (b. 1908) and Ewart George Bertram (b. 1908): a morphological distinction between neurones of the male and female, and the behaviour of the nucleolar satellite during accelerated nucleo-protein synthesis, which made it possible to determine the genetic sex of an individual depending on the presence of a Barr body[249], i.e. a chromatin mass on the inner surface of the nuclear membrane of cells with resting nuclei. It was the beginning of intensive chromosome studies, which Professor Paolo Polani of Guy's Hospital, London, and his team developed to great perfection.

Individuals, in whom many cells, e.g. from a smear of the oral mucous membrane, contain Barr bodies, are called chromatin positive. Normal males are chromatin negative, although not all chromative negative persons are necessarily male. Turner's and Klinefelter's syndromes, mentioned on p. 488, fall into the category of chromosomal sexual disturbances, although they do not form a uniform picture. In 1964 S. Blatch, for example, recorded ten patients with Klinefelter's syndrome with an XXXXY variant[250]. It is, however, not possible to discuss the many abnormal varieties occurring along the sexual spectrum within the framework of this book.

We have come to the end of our narrative, although there are still many gaps which should be filled. Perhaps that will be done in future editions. *Ave atque vale!*

REFERENCES

1. Harrington, M.: Occupational endocrinology – the new sub-specialty. World Medicine, 49–50, 3rd May 1978.
2. Medvei, V. C.: Hot baths and human fertility. Lancet **I**, 833, 1945.
3. Bauer, J., Gutman, G.: The effect of diathermy on testicular function. Urol. Cutaneous Rev. **44**, 1–2, 1940.
4. Chevreul, M. E.: Recherches chimiques sur plusieurs corps gras, et particulièrement sur leur combinations avec les calculs. Cinquième mémoire. Ann. Chim (Paris) **95**, 5–50, 1815.
5. Chevreul, M. E.: Note sur le sucre de diabètes. Ann. Chim. (Paris), **95**, 319–320, 1815.
6. Doisy, E. A., Eler, C. D., Thayer, S. A.: The preparation of the crystalline ovarian hormone from the urine of pregnant women. J. Biol. Chem. **86**, 499–509, 1930.
7. Marrian, G. F.: The chemistry of oestrin. III. An improved method of preparation and the isolation of active crystalline material. Biochem. J. **24**, 435–445, 1930.
8. Butenandt, A. F. J.: Ueber die chemische Untersuchung der Sexual-hormone. Z. Angew. Chem. **44**, 905–908, 1931.
9. Ruzicka, L., Goldberg, M. W., Meyer, J., Brüngger, H., Eichenberger, E.: Ueber die Synthese des Testikelhormons (Androsteron) und Stereoisomerer desselben durch Abbau hydrierter Sterine. Helv. Chim. Acta **17**, 1395–1406, 1934.
10. MacCorquodale, D. W., Thayer, S. A., Doisy, E. A.: Isolation of the principal oestrogenic substance of liquor folliculi. J. Biol. Chem. **115**, 435–448, 1936.
11. Butenandt, A. F. J.: Neuere Ergebnisse auf dem Gebiet der Sexual-hormone. Wien. Klin. Wochenschr. **47**, 897–901, 934–936, 1934.
12. David, K., Dingemanse, E., Freud, J., Laqueur, E.: Ueber krystallinisches maennliches Hormon aus Hoden (Testosteron), wirksamer als aus Harn oder aus Cholesterin bereitetes Androsteron. Hoppe-Seyl. Z. Physiol. Chem. **233**, 281–282, 1935.

13. Kendall, E. C., Mason, H. L., Myers, C. S., Allers, W. D.: A physiologic and chemical investigation of the suprarenal cortex. J. Biol. Chem. **114,** lvii–lviii, 1936.
14. Steiger, M., Reichstein, T.: XII. Concerning the constituents of the adrenal cortex. Deoxycorticosterone. Helv. Chim. Acta **20,** 1164–1179, 1937.
15. Samuels, L. T., Henschel, A. F., Keys, A.: Influence of methyltestosterone on muscular work and creatine metabolism in normal young men. J. Clin. Endocrinol. **2,** 649, 1942.
16. Clauberg, C., Üstün, Z.: Zentralbl. Gynaekol. **62,** 1745, 1938.
17. Inhoffen, H. H., Hohlweg, W.: Neue per os wirksame weibliche Keim-druesenhormon Derivate. Naturwissenschaften **26,** 96, 1938.
18. Dodds, Sir Edward Charles, Goldberg, L., Lawson, W., Robinson, R.: The oestrogenic activity of certain synthetic compounds. Nature (Lond.) **141,** 247–248, 1938.
19. Astwood, E. B.: Treatment of hyperthyroidism with thiourea. J. Am. Med. Assoc. **122,** 78–81, 1943.
20. Chesney, A. M., Clawson, T. A., Webster, B. P.: Endocrine goiter in rabbits: I. Incidence and characteristics. Bull. Johns Hopkins Hosp. **43,** 261–277, 1928.
21. Ibid.: p. 278.
22. Webster, B. P., Chesney, A. M.: Bull. Johns Hopkins Hosp. **43,** 291, 1928.
23. Marine, D., Baumann, E. J., Cipra, A.: Proc. Soc. Exp. Biol. Med. **26,** 822, 1928/29.
24. Marine, D., Baumann, E. J., Spence, A. W., Cipra, A.: Proc. Soc. Exp. Biol. Med. **29,** 792, 1932.
25. Hertz, S., Roberts, A.: Application of radioactive iodine in therapy of Graves' disease: J. Clin. Invest. **21,** 624, 1942.
26. Plummer, H. S., Boothby, W M.: The value of iodine in exophthalmic goiter. J. Iowa Med. Soc. **14,** 66–73, 1924.
27. Taylor, Selwyn: Personal Communication, July, 1979.
28. Armstrong, C. N.: History of Endocrinology in Newcastle-upon-Tyne. Slide/Tape, Univ. Newcastle, 1979.
29. Riccabona, G., Inst. for Nuclear Med. Univ. Innsbruck, Austria. Personal Communication. July, 1979.
30. Medvei, V. C.: The assessment of the treatment of toxic goitre by means of live sick records and working capacity. Trans. Assoc. Ind. Med. Off. (Lond.) **10,** 136–137, 1961.
31. Medvei, V. C., Jones, A., Williams, I., Besser, G. M.: Long-term follow-up of hyperthyroid patients treated with radioiodine. *In Preparation.*
32. Smith, R. N., Wilson, G. M.: Lancet **2,** 1187, 1967.
33. Jones, R. G., Kornfeld, E. C., McLaughlin, K. C., Anderson, R. C.: J. Am. Chem. Soc. **71,** 4000, 1949.
34. Lawson, A., Rimington, C., Searle, C. E.: Lancet **2,** 619–621, 1951.
35. Lawson, A., Barry, G.: Lancet **2,** 621, 1951.
36. Doniach, Deborah: Lancet **1,** 873, 1953.
37. Shanks, R. B., Hadden, D. R., Lowe, D. C., McDevitt, D. G., Montgom-ery, D. A. D.: Lancet **1,** 993, 1969.
38. Fourman, P., Davis, R. H., Rawnsley, K., Jones, K. H., Morgan, D. B.: Lancet **2,** 914–915, 1967.
39. Thomas, I. D., Hart, J. K.: Retrobulbar repository corticosteroid therapy in thyroid ophthalmopathy. Med. J. Aust. **2,** 484–487, 1974.
40. Hill, S. R., Jr., Reiss, R S., Forsham, P. H., Thorn, G.: J. Clin. Endocrinol. **10,** pp. 1, 375, 1950.

41. Hoffenberg, R., Jackson, W. P. U.: Lancet 1, 693, 1958.
42. Jones, A.: Br. J. Radiol. 24, 637, 1951.
43. Boyle, I. T., Greig, W. R., Thomson, J. A., Winning, G., McGirr, E. M.: Proc. R. Soc. Med. 62, 19, 1969.
44. Raiti, S., Newns, G. S.: Arch. Dis Childh. 46, 692, 1971.
45. Klein, A. H., Foley, T. P., Larsen, P. R., Augustin, A. V., Hopwood, N. I.: Neonatal thyroid function in congenital hypothyroidism. J. Paediat. 89, 545–549, 1976.
46. Beaupré, M.: Dissertation sur les crétins. 1845. Cited from the Encyclopaedia Britannica, 11th ed. (1910). London, New York.
47. Dussault, J. H., Morisette, J., Letarte, J., Guyda, H., Laberge, C.: Modification of a screening program for neonatal hypothyroidism. J. Pediat. 92, 274–277, 1978.
48. Illig, R., Rodriguez de Vera Roda, C.: Schweiz. Med. Wochenschr., 106, 1676–1681, 1976.
49. Borrows, E. T., Clayton, J. C., Hems, B. A.: J. Chem. Soc., Suppl. I, 189, 1949.
50. Lerman, J.: J. Clin. Endocrinol. 13, 1341, 1953.
51. Smith, R. N., Taylor, S. A., Massey, J. C.: Controlled clinical trial of combined triiodothyronine and thyroxine in the treatment of hypothyroidism. Brit. Med. J. 1, 145, 1970.
52. Mitchell, J. R. A., Surridge, D. H. C., Willison, R. G.: Br. Med. J. II, 932, 1959.
53. Wintersteiner, O. P., Pfiffner, J.: Chemical studies on the adrenal cortex. II. Isolation of several physiologically inactive crystalline compounds from active extracts. J. Biol. Chem. 111, 599–612, 1935.
54. Wintersteiner, O. P., Pfiffner, J.: Chemical studies on the adrenal cortex. III. Isolation of two new physiologically inactive compounds. J. Biol. Chem. 116, 291–305, 1936.
55. Sarett, L. M.: J. Biol. Chem. 162, 601, 1946.
56. Hench, P. S., Slocumb, C. H., Barnes, A. R., Smith, H. L., Polley, H. F., Kendall, E. C.: The effects of the adrenal cortical hormone 17-hydroxy-11-dehydrocorticosterone (compound E) on the acute phase of the rheumatic fever: preliminary report. Proc. Mayo. Clin. 24, 277–297, 1949.
57. Thorn, G. W., Forsham, P. H.: Rec. Prog. Horm. Res. 4, 229, 1949.
58. Thorn, G. W., Jenkins, D.: Schweiz. Med. Wochenschr. 82, 697, 1952.
59. Spence, A. W.: Proc. R. Soc. Med. 46, 575, 1953.
60. Wendler, N. L., Graber, R. P., Jones, R. E., Tischler, M.: J. Am. Chem. Soc. 72, 5, 793, 1950.
61. Weitzman, E. D., Fukushima, D., Nageire, C. et al.: 24 hour pattern of the episodic secretion of cortisol in normal subjects. J. Clin. Endocrinol. Metab. 33, 14, 1971.
62. Grundy, H. M., Simpson, S. A., Tait, J. F.: Isolation of a highly active mineralocorticoid from beef adrenal extract. Nature (Lond.) 169, 795–796, 1952.
63. Simpson, S. A., Tait, J. F., Wettstein, A., Neher, R., Euw, J. von., Schindler, O., Reichstein, T.: Experientia, 10, 132, 1954.
64. Mach, R. S., Fabre, J., Duckert, A., Borth, R., Ducummun, P.: Schweiz. Med. Wochenschr. 84, 407, 1954.
65. Fried, J., Sabo, E. F.: J. Am. Chem. Soc. 76, 1455, 1954.
66. Liddle, G. W., Pechet, M. M., Bartter, F. C.: Science 120, 496, 1954.
67. Goldfien, A., Laidlaw, J. C., Haydar, N. A., Renold, A. E., Thorn, G. W.: N. Engl. J. Med. 252, 415, 1955.

68. Garrod, O., Nabarro, J. D. N., Pawan, G. L. S., Walker, G.: Lancet **II**, 367, 1955.
69. Childs, B., Grumbach, M. M., Van Wyck, J. J.: Virilizing adrenal hyperplasia: A genetic and hormonal study. J. Clin. Invest. **35**, 213, 1956.
70. Wilkins, L., Lewis, R. A., Klein, R., Rosenberg, E.: Bull. Johns Hopkins Hosp. **86**, 249, 1950.
71. Wilkins, L., Gardner, L. I., Crigler, J. F., Jr., Silverman, S. H., Migeon, C. J.: J. Clin. Endocrinol. **12**, 257, 277, 1952.
72. Mason, A. S., Morris, C. J. O. R.: Lancet **I**, 116, 1953.
73. Jailer, J. W.: Bull. N. Y. Acad. Med. **29**, 377, 1953.
74. Dorfman, R. I.: Fifth Macy Conference on Adrenal Cortex, 27, 1954.
75. Wilkins, L., Bongiovanni, A. M., Clayton, G. W., Grumbach, M. M., Van Wyk, J.: CIBA Colloquia on Endocrinology, **8**, 460, London, Churchill Livingstone, 1955.
76. Bongiovanni, A. M.: Unusual steroid pattern in congenital adrenal hyperplasia: Deficiency of 3-beta-hydroxydehydrogenase. J. Clin. Endocrinol. Metab. **21**, 860, 1961.
77. Spence, A. W.: Advances in endocrine treatment, 1946–1971. Br. J. Clin. Practice: **25**, 435–448, 1971.
78. Soffer, L. J.: Diseases of the Adrenals. 251–254, London. Kimpton, 1946.
79. Sprague, G. R.: Proc. R. Soc. Med. **46**, 1070, 1953.
80. Lee, P. A., Weldon, V. V., Migeon, C. J.: Short stature as the only clinical sign of Cushing's Syndrome. J. Paediat. **86**, 89, 1975.
81. Nelson, D. H., Meakin, J. W., Thorn, G. W.: ACTH producing pituitary tumours following adrenalectomy for Cushing's Syndrome. Ann. Int. Med. **52**, 560, 1960.
82. Hopwood, N. I., Kenny, F. M.: Increased evidence of post-adrenalectomy Nelson's Syndrome in pediatric vs. adult Cushing's disease. Nationwide study. Pediat. Res. **9**, 290, 1975.
83. Orth, D. N., Liddle, G. W.: Results of treatment in 108 patients with Cushing's Syndrome. N. Engl. J. Med. **285**, 243, 1971.
84. Liddle, G. W.: Does the hypothalamus play a role in the aetiology of Cushing's Disease? In: Blueprints for the Solution of Three Endocrinological Enigmas. Sir Henry Dale Lecture for 1973. J. Endocrinol. **59**, No. 2. Proc. Soc. Endocrinol. pp. III–IX, Nov. 1973.
85. Jeffcoate, W. J., Rees, Lesley, H., Tomlin, Susan, Jones, A. E., Edwards, C. R. W., Besser, G. M.: Metyrapone in long-term management of Cushing's disease. Br. Med. J. **II**, 215–217, 1977.
86. Nabarro, J. D. N.: Proc. R. Soc. Med. **50**, 768, 1957.
87. Spence, A. W.: Proc. R. Soc. Med. **50**, 768, 1957.
88. Bishop, P. M. F., Glover, F. H., de Mowbray, R. R., Thorne, M. G.: Lancet **II**, 1137, 1954.
89. Temple, T. E., Jones, D. J., Liddle, G. W., Dexter, R. N.: Treatment of Cushing's Disease: Correction of hypercortisolism by the *ortho-para*-isomer of dichlordiphenyldichloroethane (o,p′-DDD) and aminoglutemide without induction of aldosterone deficiency. N. Engl. J. Med. **281**, 801, 1969.
90. Conn, J. W.: Primary aldosteronism, a new clinical syndrome. J. Lab. Clin. Med. **45**, 6–17, 1955.
91. Mader, I. J., Isery, L. T.: J. Lab. Clin. Med. **44**, 895, 1954.
92. Evans, B. M., Milne, M. D.: Potassium losing nephritis presenting as a case of periodic paralysis. Br. Med. J. **II**, 1067, 1954.
93. Cope, C. L.: Adrenal Steroids and Disease, p. 465. London, Pitman, 1964.
94. Conn, J. W.: J. Am. Med. Assoc. **172**, 1650, 1960.

95. Van Buchem, F. S. P., Doorenbos, H., Ellings, H. S.: Lancet **2**, 335, 1956.
96. Liddle, G. W., Bledsoe, T., Coppage, W. S.: A familial renal disorder, simulating primary aldosteronism, but with negligible aldosterone secretion. Trans. Assoc. Am. Phys. **76**, 199, 1963.
97. Bartter, F. C., Pronove, P., Gill, J. R., MacCardle, R. C.: Hyperplasia of the juxtaglomerular complex with hyperaldosteronism and hypokalemic alkalosis. Am. J. Med. **33**, 811, 1962.
98. Liddle, G. W.: Specific and non-specific inhibition of mineralocorticoid activity. Metabolism **10**, 1021, 1961.
99. Herzog, H. L., Nobile, A., Tolksdorf, S., Charney, W., Herschberg, E. B., Perlman, P. L., Pechet, M. M.: Science **121**, 176, 1955.
100. Arth, G. E., Fried, J., Johnston, D. B. R., Hoff, D. R., Sarrett, L. G., Silber, R. H., Stoerk, H. C., Winter, C. A.: J. Am. Chem. Soc. **80**, 3161, 1958.
101. Liddle, G. W.: Tests of pituitary–adrenal suppressibility in the diagnosis of Cushing's Syndrome. J. Clin. Endocrinol. Metab. **20**, 1537, 1960.
102. Pal, Jacob: Gefaesskrisen. Leipzig, S. Hirzel, 1905.
103. Bernal, Pierre: Crises Hypertensives. Paris, G. Doin, 1934.
104. Orth, J.: Ueber eine Geschwulst d. Nebennierenmarks. Sitzungsber. Preuss. Akad. Wiss., 34, 1914.
105. Labbé, E. M., Tinel, J., Doumer, E.: Crises solaires et hypertension paroxystiques en rapport avec une tumeur surrénale. Bull. Soc. Méd. Hôp. Paris. 3 sér., **46**, 982–990, 1922.
106. Vaquez, L. H., Donzelot, E., Géraudel, E.: Presse Méd. 169, 1929.
107. Mayo, Chas.: J. Am. Med. Assoc. **89**, 1047, 1927.
108. Oberling, Ch., Jung, G.: Bull. Mém. Soc. Méd. Hôp. Paris **43**, 366, 1927.
109. Shipley, A. M.: Ann. Surg. **90**, 742, 1929.
110. Bauer, J., Lériche, R.: Zur Klinik und Therapie des Paraganglioms: Adrenalogene Hochdruckkrisen: Wien. Klin. Wochenschr., No. 41, 1–14, 1934.
111. Holton, P.: J. Physiol. **108**, 525, 1949.
112. Goldenberg, M., Faber, M., Alston, E. J., Chargaff, E. C.: Science **109**, 534, 1949.
113. Euler, U. S. von: A specific sympathomimetic ergone in adrenergic nerve fibres (sympathin) and its relations to adrenaline and nor-adrenaline. Acta Physiol. Scand. **12**, 73–97, 1946.
114. Meier, R.: Farmacoter. Acta **44**, 84, 1948.
114a. Brown, M. J., Lewis, P. J., Dollery, C. T.: Diagnosis of small phaeochromocytomas. Lancet **1**, 1185-1186, 1980.
115. Sjoerdsma, A., Udenfried, S.: Blockage of endogeneous norepinephrine-synthesis by α-methyl-tyrosine, an inhibitor of tyrosine hydroxylase. J. Pharmacol. Exp. Ther. **147**, 86, 1965.
116. Carman, C. T., Brashear, R. E.: Phaeochromocytoma as an inherited abnormality. N. Engl. J. Med. **263**, 419, 1960.
117. Sipple, J. H.: The association of phaeochromocytoma with carcinoma of the thyroid gland. Am. J. Med. **31**, 163, 1960.
118. Steiner, A. L., Goodman, A. D., Powers, S. R.: Study of a kindred with phaeochromocytoma, medullary thyroid carcinoma, hyperparathyroidism and Cushing's Disease: Multiple endocrine neoplasia, type 2. Medicine, **47**, 371, 1968.
119. Raben, M. S.: Rec. Progr. Horm. Res. **15**, 71, 1959.
120. Talwar, G. P., Pandian, M. R., Kumar, N. *et al.*: Mechanism of action of pituitary growth hormone. Rec. Progr. Horm. Res. **31**, 141, 1975.
121. Raben, M. S.: J. Clin. Endocrinol. Metab. **18**, 901, 1958.

122. Tanner, J. M., Whitehouse, R. H.: Br. Med. J. **II,** 69, 1967.
123. Brook, C. G. D.: 24. Short Stature. In: Hormone Receptors and their Diseases. Symposium held at the Roy. Soc. Med. (Lond.) on 27 and 28 February, 1979.
124. Salmon, W. D. Jr., Daughaday, W. H.: A hormonally controlled serum factor which stimulates sulfate incorporation by cartilage (in hypophysectomized rats) *in vitro*. J. Lab. Clin. Med. **49,** 825, 1957.
125. Van Wyck, J. J., Underwood, L. E., Hintz, R. L. *et al.*: The somatomedins: A family of insulin like hormones under growth hormone control. Rec. Progr. Horm. Res. **30,** 259, 1974.
126. Besser, G. M., Wass, J. A. H., Thorner, M. O.: Acromegaly – Results of long term treatment with bromocriptine. Acta Endocrinol., Suppl. 216, **88,** 187–198, 1978.
127. Besser, G. M., Wass, J. A. H.: Medical management of acromegaly with bromocriptine. Effect of continuous treatment for over three years. Med. J. Aust., Special Suppl., 41–33, 4 November 1978.
128. Liuzzi, A., Chiodini, P. G., Botalla, L., Cremascoli, G., Mueller, E. E., Silvestrini, F.: Decreased plasma growth hormone (GH) levels in acromegalics following CB 154 (2-bromo-α-ergokryptine) administration. J. Clin. Endocrinol. Metab. **38,** 910, 1974.
129. Holtkamp, D. E., Greslin, J. G., Root, C. A., Lerner, L. J.: Proc. Soc. Exp. Biol. N.Y. **105,** 197, 1960.
130. Segal, S. J., Nelson, W. D.: Anat. Res. **139,** 273, 1961.
131. Greenblatt, R. B. G., Barfield, W. E., Jungck, E. C., Ray, A. W.: J. Am. Med. Assoc. **178,** 101, 1961.
132. Charles, D.: Lancet **II,** 278, 1962.
133. Paulsen, C. A., Herrmann, W. I.: 44th Meeting of the Endocrine Society in Chicago, June 1962.
134. Bishop, P. M. F.: Proc. R. Soc. Med. **58,** 905, 1965.
135. Gemzell, C. A., Diczfalusi, E., Tillinger, G.: J. Clin. Endocrinol. **18,** 1333, 1958.
136. Gemzell, C. A., Diczfalusi, E., Tillinger, G.: CIBA Colloquia on Endocrinology, **13,** 191, 1960.
137. Crooke, A. C. *et al.*: Br. J. Hosp. Med. **4,** 87, 1970.
138. Mortimer, C. H., McNeilly, A. S., Fisher, R. A. *et al.*: Gonadotrophin-releasing hormone therapy in hypogonadal males with hypothalamic or pituitary dysfunction. Br. Med. J. **1,** 617, 1974.
139. Besser, G. M., Parke, L., Edwards, C. R. W., Forsyth, L. A., McNeilly, A. S. Galactorrhoea successfully treated with reduction of plasma prolactin level by 2-bromo-α-ergocryptine. Br. Med. J. **II,** 669–672, 1972.
140. Franks, S., Murray, M. A. F., Jequier, A. M., Steele, S. J., Nabarro, J. D. N., Jacobs, H. S.: Clin. Endocrinol., **4,** 597, 1975.
141. Besser, G. M., Thorner, M. O., Wass, J. A.: Hyperprolactinaemia–hypogonadism syndrome: medical treatment. Excerpta Med. Int. Congress Series No. 403. Proc. Vth Internat. Congress Endocrinol, Hamburg., Vol. 2, 353–357, July, 1976.
142. Hippocrates: Aphorisms, Section V, No. 39 [on p. 225 in: Hippocratic Writings (ed. Lloyd, G. E. R., Translated by Chadwick, J. and Mann, W. N. *et al*. Pelican Classics, ISBN 014. Penguin Books, 1978].
143. McNeilly, A. S.: Prolactin Receptors. Presentation No. 19 in: Hormone Receptors and their Disease. Symposium held at the Roy. Soc. Med. (Lond.) on 27 and 28 Feb., 1979.
144. By a Special Correspondent: Comment: Pregnancies following implantation

of human embryos grown in culture. Br. J. Sexual Med. **6**, (46), 3–9, March, 1979.

145. Philipp, Elliot E.: Personal Communication.

146. McCall Smith, A.: Laws for Biology. World Med. **15**, (9), 28–32; 9 Feb. 1980.

147. Choosing the baby's sex. Leading Article. Br. Med. J. **I**, 272–273, 1980.

148. Dmowski, W. P., Gaynor, L., Rao, R., Lawrence, M., Scommegna, A.: Use of albumin gradients for X and Y sperm separation and clinical experience with male sex preselection. Fertil. Steril. **31**, 52–57, 1979.

149. Departments of Obstetrics and Gynaecology, Tietung Hospital of Anshan Iron and Steel Company, Anshan: Fetal sex prediction by sex chromatin of chorionic villi cells during early pregnancy. Chinese Med. J. **1**, 117–26, 1975.

150. Hoffenberg, R.: Peripheral metabolism of hormones: Clinical implications. J. R. Soc. Med. **72**, 400–408, 1979.

151. Hagedorn, H. C., Jensen, B. N., Krarup, N. B., Woodstrup, I.: J. Am. Med. Assoc. **106**, 177–180, 1936.

152. Lawrence, R. D., Oakley, W.: Br. Med. J. **I**, 422, 1944.

153. Hallas-Møller, K., Jersill, M., Petersen, K., Schlichtkrull, J.: Science **116**, 394–398, 1952.

154. Ruiz, C. L., Silva, L. L., Libenson, L.: Contribución al estudio sobre la composición quimica de la insulina. *Estudio de algunos cuerpos sintéticos solfurados con acción hypoglucemiante.* Rev. Soc. argent. Biol., **6**, 134–41, 1930 (= contribution to the study of the chemical composition of insulin. Study of some synthetic sulphurated substances with hypoglycaemic action.)

155. Underhill, F. D., Blatherwick, N. R.: Studies in carbohydrate metabolism: VI. The influence of thyreo-parathyroidectomy upon the sugar content of the blood and the glycogen content of the liver. J. Biol. Chem. **18**, 87, 1914.

156. Watanabe, C. K.: Studies in the metabolic changes induced by the administration of guanidine bases.: I. Influence of injected guanidine hydrochloride upon bloodsugar content. J. Biol. Chem. **33**, 253, 1918.

157. Minot, A. S.: The mechanism of the hypoglycaemia induced by guanidine and carbon-tetrachloride poisoning and its relief by calcium medication. J. Pharmacol. Exp. Ther. **43**, 295, 1931.

158. Clark, G. A.: Interrelation of parathyroids, suprarenals and pancreas. J. Physiol. **58**, 294, 1923/24.

159. Frank, E., Nothmann, M., Wagner, A.: Ueber synthetisch dargestellte Koerper mit insulinartiger Wirkung auf den normalen und den diabetischen Organismus (= concerning synthetic substances with insulin-like effect on the normal and on the diabetic organism): Klin. Wochenschr., 2100–2107, 1926.

160. Bischoff, F., Sahyun, M., Long, M. L.: Guanidine structure and hypoglycaemia. J. Biol. Chem. **81**, 325, 1928.

161. Hesse E., Taubmann, G.: Die Wirkung des Biguanids und seiner Derivate auf den Zuckerstoffwechsel. Naunyn-Schmiedebergs Arch. exp. Pathol. Pharmak. **142**, 290, 1929.

162. Ungar, G., Freedman, L., Shapiro, S. L.: Pharmacological studies of a new hypoglycaemic drug. Proc. Soc. Exp. Biol. (N.Y.), **95**, 190, 1957.

163. Ungar, G.: Pharmacology and toxicology of phenylethylbiguanide (DBI). Symposium on a New Hypoglycaemic Agent, Phenformin (DBI). Houston, Texas, 1959.

164. Bertram, F.: Zum Wirkungsmechanismus des Synthalins (= on the mechanism of action of synthalin). Dtsch. Arch. Klin. Med. **158**, 76, 1928.

165. Bertram, F.: Indikationen und Ergebnisse der oralen Diabetesbehandlung IV., Dtsch. Med. Wochenschr. 1260–1261, 1958.

166. Bertram, F.: Cit. After H. Schadewaldt: In: Die Entdeckung der oralen Antidiabetika (= the discovery of the oral antidiabetics): Dtsch. Med. Wochenschr. 2653, 1965.
167. Bertram, F.: The treatment of diabetes mellitus with small doses of guanidin derivatives. Med. Klin. 1229, 1928.
168. Janbon, M., Chaptal, J., Uedel, A., Schaap, J.: Accidents hypoglycémiques graves par un sulfamido-thiodiazole (le VK 57 ou 2254, R.P.). Communications Soc. Sci. méd. biol. Montpellier. pp. 222–250; 1942 and: Montpellier Méd. **85,** 441, 1942.
169. Janbon, M., Lazerges, P., Metropolitanski, J. H.: Étude du métabolisme du sulfaisopropyl-thiodiazol chez le sujet sain et en cours de traitement comportement de la glycémie. Communications Soc. Sci. Méd. Biol. Montpellier, 212–221, 1942; and Montpellier Méd. **85,** 489, 1942.
170. Loubatières, A. *et al.*: Étude expérimentale chez le chien des accidents nerveux irréversibles consecutifs à l'hypoglycémie prolonguée par le sulfaisopropyl-thiodiazol. Comm. 43ᵉ Congr. médecine aliénistes et neurologistes de France et des pays de langue française, Montpellier, 415. Paris, Masson, 1942.
171. Loubatières, A.: Thèse Doctorat (= MD thesis), Sci. naturelles, No. 86, Montpellier; 1946. Montpellier. Edit. Causse, Graille et Castelnau, 1956.
172. Baeumler, E.: In Search of the Magic Bullet, p. 109. Thames & Hudson, 1965.
173. Franke, H., Fuchs, K. J.: Ein neues antidiabetisches Prinzip. Ergebnisse klinischer Untersuchungen. Dtsch. Med. Wochenschr. **80,** 1449, 1955.
174. Ryle, A. P., Sanger, F., Smith, L. F., Kitai, R.: The disulphide bonds of insulin. Biochem. J. **60,** 541–556, 1955.
175. Achelis, J. D., Hardebeck, K.: Ueber eine neue, blutzuckersenkende Substanz (= a new bloodsugar-lowering substance), Dtsch. Med. Wochenschr. **80,** 1452–1455, 1955.
176. Bendtfeldt, Elenor, Otto, H.: Schwere hypoglykaemische Reaktion im Verlauf der peroralen Diabetesbehandlung mit BZ55 (= severe hypoglycaemic reaction during peroral treatment of diabetes with BZ55). Muench. Med. Wochenschr. 1136–1137, 1956.
177. Bertram, F., Bendtfeldt, E., Otto, H.: Ueber ein wirksames perorales Antidiabeticum (BZ55). Dtsch. Med. Wochenschr. **80,** 1455–1460, 1955.
178. Kleinsorge, H.: Bemerkung zu den Arbeiten ueber N_1-sulfanilyl-N_2-*n*-butylcarbamid als perorales Antidiabeticum. Dtsch. Med. Wochenschr. **81,** 750, 1956.
179. Ebstein, W.: Zur Therapie des Diabetes mellitus, insbesondere ueber die Anwendung des slicyl-sauren Natrons bei demselben (= on the treatment of diabetes mellitus, esp. on the use of salicylic-acid sodium). Berlin. Klin. Wochenschr. **13,** 337–340, 1876.
180. Ebstein, W.: Dtsch. Arch. Klin. Med. **28,** 143–242, 1881.
181. Bartels, M. C. A.: Ueber die therapeutische Verwertung der Salicylsaeure und ihres Natronsalzes in der inneren Medizin. Dtsch. Med. Wochenschr. 435–437, 1878.
182. Greenhow, E. H.: Med. Times **I,** 597, 1880.
183. Williamson, R. J.: On the treatment of glycosuria and diabetes mellitus with sodium salicylate. Brit. Med. J. **I,** 760–762, 1901.
184. Schadt, D. C., Purnell, D. C.: Salicylate intoxication in an adult. Am. Med. Assoc. Arch. Int. Med. **102,** 203–206, 1958.
185. Hecht, A., Goldner, G.: Reappraisal of the hypoglycaemic action of acetylsalicylate. Metabolism **8,** 418–428, 1958.
186. Hetzel, B. S., Hine, D. C.: The effect of salicylates on the pituitary and suprarenal glands. Lancet **2,** 94, 1961.

187. Reid, J., Dougale, A. J., Andrews, M. M.: Aspirin and diabetes. Br. Med. J. **II,** 1071–1074, 1957.
188. Schade, S. D. Diabetes Outlook **14** (4), 1, 8, 1979.
189. Bloom, S. R., Daniel, P. M., Johnston, D. I., Ogawa, O, Pratt O. E.: Release of glucagon, induced by stress. Q. J. Exp. Physiol. **58,** 99–108, 1973.
190. McQuarrie, I.: Idiopathic spontaneously occurring hypoglycaemia in infants: Clinical significance of problem and treatment. Am. J. Dis. Childh. **87,** 399, 1954.
191. Rubin, A. A., Franklin, E. R., Taylor, R. M., Rosenkilde, N.: J. Pharmacol. Exp. Ther. **10,** 184, 1962.
192. Dollery, C. T., Pentecost, B. L., Samaan, N. A.: Lancet **II,** 735, 1962.
193. Drash, A., Wolff, F.: Metabolism **13,** 487, 1964.
194. Rees, L. H., Besser, G. M., Jeffcoate, W. J., Goldie, D. J., Marks, V.: Alcohol induced pseudo-Cushing's Syndrome. Lancet **I,** 726–728, 1977.
195. Rothwell Nancy J., Stock M. J.: A role for brown adipose tissue in diet induced thermogenesis. Nature (London) **281,** 31–35, 1979.
196. Zondek, Herrman: Diseases of the Endocrine Glands. 2nd English ed., pp. 261–264. London, Arnold, 1944.
197. Tandler, J., Gross, S.: Wien. Klin. Wochenschr. **20,** 1596, 1907.
198. Sicker, H. O., Estes, E. H., Kelser, G. A., McIntosh, D.: Am. J. Clin. Invest. **34,** 916, 1955.
199. Burwell, C. S., Robin, E. D., Whaley, R. D., Bickelmann, A. G.: Am. J. Med. **21,** 811, 1956.
200. Keen, H., Thomas, Briony J., Jarrett, R. J., Fuller, J. H.: Nutrient intake, adiposity and diabetes. Br. Med. J. **I,** 655–658, 1979.
201. Watts, G.: Endorphins we have: endoloxones may take a little longer. World Med. **14** (19), 21–22, 1979.
202. McCloy, J. and McCloy, R. F.: Enkephalins, hunger and obesity. Lancet **2,** 156, 1979.
203. Frank, J. P.: De curandis hominum morbis epitome. Liber V. 38–67. Mannheim, C. F. Schwann and C. G. Goetz, 1794.
204. Frank, A. E.: Ueber Beziehungen der Hypophyse zum Diabetes insipidus (= the Relations of the pituitary to Diabetes Insipidus). Berl. Klin. Wochenschr., **49,** 393–397, 1912.
205. Williams, R. H., Henry, C.: Ann. Int. Med. **27,** 84, 1947.
206. Kamm, O., Aldrich, T. B., Grote, I. W., Rowe, L. W., Bugbee, E. P.: The active principles of the posterior lobe of the pituitary gland. I. The demonstration of the presence of two active principles. II. The separation of the two principles and their concentration in the form of potent solid preparations. J. Am. Chem. Soc., **66,** 573–601, 1928.
207. Du Vigneaud, V., Gish, D. T., Katsoyannis, P. G.: A synthetic preparation possessing biological properties associated with arginin-vasopressin. J. Am. Chem. Soc. **76,** 4751–4752, 1954.
208. Crawford, J. D., Kennedy, G. C.: Nature (London) **183,** 891, 1959.
209. Bauer, J., Aschner, Berta: Wien. Arch. Int. Med. **I,** 297, 1920.
210. Cowden, E. A., Thomson, J. A., Doyle, D., Ratcliffe, J. G., MacPherson, P., Teasdale, G. M., Tests of prolactin-secretion in diagnosis of prolactinomas. Lancet **I,** 1155–1158, 1979.
211. Paget, Sir James: On a form of chronic inflammation of bones (osteitis deformans). Med.-Chir. Trans. **60,** 37–64, 1877.
212. Shai, F., Baker, R. K., Wallach, S.: The clinical and metabolic effects of porcine calcitonin on Paget's disease of bone. J. Clin. Invest. **50,** 1927, 1971.

213. Woodhouse, N. J. Y., MacIntyre, I., Joplin, G. F., Doyle, F. H.: Human calcitonin in the treatment of Paget's bone disease. Lancet I, 1139, 1971.
214. De Rose, J., Singer, F. R., Avramides, A., Flores, A., Dziadiw, R., Baker, R. K., Wallach, S.: Response of Paget's disease to porcine and salmon calcitonin. Am. J. Med. 56, 858, 1974.
215. Kanis, J. A. (Ed.) Bone Disease and Calcitonin. To commemorate the centenary of the original description of osteitis deformans. Proceedings of a Symposium in Jersey, 2–4 December, 1976. Eastbourne (Eng.). Armour Pharmaceutical Co., 1976.
216. Sexual behaviour and sex hormones. Leading article, Lancet 2, 17–18, 1979.
217. Long Hall, Diana: Biology, sex hormones and sexism in the 1920s. Philos. Forum, 5, 81–96, 1973–1974.
218. Corner, G. W.: The Early History of the Oestrogenic Hormones. Sir Henry Dale Lecture for 1965. Proc. Soc. Endocrinol. pp. III–XVII, 1965. In: J. Endocrinol. 1965.
219. Huxley, J.: Cit. after Long Hall, Diana, p. 81, as 217.
220. Geddes, P., Thomson, J. A.: The Evolution of Sex. London, Walter Scott, 1889.
221. Marshall, F. H. A.: The Physiology of Reproduction. London, Longmans Green, 1910.
222. McClung, C. E.: The accessory chromosome; sex determination. Biol. Bull. 3, 43–84, 1902.
223. Steinach, E.: Antagonistiche Wirkungen der Keimdruesen Hormone. Biologia Generalis 2, 815–834, 1926.
224. Moore, C. R., Price, Dorothy: Gonad hormone functions and the reciprocal influence between gonads and hypophysis, with its bearing on the problem of sex hormone antagonism. Am. J. Anat. 50, 13, 1932.
225. Evans, H. M.: Present position of our knowledge of anterior pituitary function. J. Am. Med. Assoc. 101, 425–432, 1933.
226. Armstrong, C. N., Marshall, A. J. (Eds.) Intersexuality in Vertebrates including Man. London and New York, Academic Press, 1964.
227. Eichwald, E. J., Slimser, C. R.: Transplantation Bull. 2, 148, 1955.
228. Huxley, J.: The concept of race in the light of modern genetics. p. 111 in The Uniqueness of Man. London., Chatto & Windus, 1941.
229. Imperato-McGinley, J., Peterson, R. E., Gautier, T., Sturla, E.: Androgens and the evolution of the male gender identity among male pseudohermaphrodites with 5α-reductase deficiency. N. Engl. J. Med. 300, 1233–1237, 1979.
230. Phoenix, C. H., Goy, R. W., Gerall, A. A., Young, W.C.: Organising action of prenatally administered testosterone propionate on tissues mediating mating behaviour in the female guinea-pig. Endocrinology 65, 369–382, 1959.
231. Barraclough, C. A., Gorski, R. A.: Evidence that the hypothalamus is responsible for androgen-induced sterility in the female rat. Endocrinology 101, 1716–1725, 1961.
232. Schally, A. V., Kastin, A. J., Arimura, A.: Hypothalamic follicle stimulating hormone (FSH)- and luteinizing hormone (LH)-regulating hormone: Structure, phsyiology, and clinical studies. Fertil. Steril. 22, 703–721, 1921.
233. Sawyer, Ch. H.: Some recent developments in brain–pituitary–ovarian physiology. Neuroendocrinology 17, 97–124, 1975.
234. Doerner, G.: Hormones and Brain Differentiation. Amsterdam, Oxford & New York, Elsevier, 1976.
235. Hatsumoto, A., Arai, Y.: Precocious puberty and synaptogenesis in the hypothalamic arcuate nucleus, in pregnant mare serum gonadotrophin (PMSG) treated immature female rats. Brain Res. 129, 375–378, 1977.

236. Brewer, J. R., Naftolin, F., Martin, J., Sonnenschein, C.: Effects of a single injection of oestradiol valerate on the hypothalamic arcuate nucleus and on reproductive function in the female rat. Endocrinology **103,** 501–512, 1978.

237. Doerner, G., Hinz, G.: Neuroendokrin bedingte Praedisposition f. weibliche Homosexualitaet bei erhaltener zyklischen Ovarialfunktion. Endokrinologie **59,** 48–52, 1972.

238. Doerner, G.: Hormonal induction and prevention of female homosexuality. J. Endocrinol. **42,** 163–164, 1968.

239. Doerner, G.: Hormones and sexual differentiation of the brain, p. 88. In Sex, Hormones and Behaviour (eds. Porter, Ruth and Whelan, Julie) CIBA Foundation Symposium 62 (new series), pp. 81–112. Amsterdam, Excerpta Medica, 1979.

240. Doerner, G., Rohde, W., Stahl, F., Krell, L., Masius, W.: Neuroendocrine condition, a predisposition for homosexuality in men. Arch. Sex. Behav. **4,** 1–8, 1975.

241. Doerr, P., Kockott, G., Voigt, H. J., Pirke, K. M., Dittmar, F.: Plasma testosterone, estradiol, and semen analysis in male homosexuals. Arch. Gen. Psychiat. **29,** 829–833, 1973.

242. Cauldwell, D.: Psychopathia transsexualis. Sexology **16,** 274–280, 1949.

243. McCauley, E. A., Ehrhardt, A. A.: Role expectations and definitions: a comparison of female transsexuals and lesbians. J. Homosexual. **3,** 137–147, 1978.

244. Krafft-Ebing, R. von: Psychopathia sexualis. Stuttgart, Enke, 1886.

245. Brown, W. M., Harnden, D. G., Jacobs, A., McLean, N., Mantle, D. J.: Abnormalities of the sex-chromosome complement in man. Med. Res. Council, Special Report Series No. 305, London, H.M.S.O., 1964.

246. Hook, E. B.: Science **179,** 139, 1973.

247. Hook, E. B.: In Genetics and the Law (eds. Milunsky, A. and Annas, G. J.) p. 73. New York, Plenum, 1976.

248. What is to be done with the XYY fetus? Leading article, Br. Med. J. **I,** 1519–1520, 1979.

249. Barr, M. L., Bertram, E. G.: A morphological distinction between neurones of the male and female, and the behaviour of the nucleolar satellite during accelerated nucleo-protein synthesis. Nature (London) **163,** 676–677, 1949.

250. Blatch, S., Coles, H. M. T.: Klinefelter Syndrome (XXXXY) variant. Proc. R. Soc. Med. **57,** 842, 1964.

251. Willis, Thomas: Cerebri anatome: cui accessit nervorum descriptio et usus. Londini, J. Flesher, 1664.

252. Morgagni, Giovanni, B.: De Sedibus, et causis morborum per anatomen indagatis libri quinque. Venetiis, typog. Remondiniana, 1761. In: Liber, I, art. 21.

253. Miller, C.: Transactions of the Medico-Chirurgical Society of Edinburgh, **2,** 243–248, 1826.

254. Tillaux, P. J.: Traité d'Anatomie Topographique. p. 56. Paris, 1877 (cit. St. Clair Thompson).

255. Thompson, St. Clair: The Cerebrospinal Fluid: Its Spontaneous Escape from the Nose. London, Cassell, 1899.

256. Cole, I. E. and Keene, M.: Cerebrospinal fluid rhinorrhoea in pituitary tumours. J. Roy. Soc. Med., **73,** No. 4, 244–254, 1980.

257. The uncertainty principle, Leading Article, Lancet **2,** 784, 1980.

258. Steele, E. J.: Somatic Selection and Adaptive Evolution. London, Croom Helm, 1980.

259. Blaza, S. E., Garrow, J. S.: The thermogenic response to comfortable

temperature extremes, in lean and obese subjects. Proc. Nutr. Soc. **39,** 85A, 1980.

260. Vaughan, N. J. A., Slater, J. D. H., Lightman, S. L., Jowett, T. P., Wiggins, R. C., Ma, J. T. C., Payne, Nadia, N.: The Diagnosis of Primary Hyper-aldosteronism. Lancet **1,** pp. 120–125, 1981.
261. Berdez, A.: Arch. de Méd. Expér. et d'Anat. Path. Paris **4,** 142, 1892.
262. Manasse, P.: Virchow's Arch. **145,** 127, 1893.
263. Greene, R., Dalton, K.: Br. Med. J. **1,** 1007–1009, 1953.
264. Dalton, K.: The Premenstrual Syndrome. London. Wm. Heinemann, 1964.
265. Clare, A. W.: Symposium: Recent Research on Premenstrual Syndrome. Curr. Med. Res. Opin. **4,** Suppl. 4, 23, 1977.
266. Sutherland, J., Stewart, I.: Lancet **I,** 1180, 1965.
267. Coppen, A., Kessel, N.: Br. J. Psych. **109,** 390.
268. Frank, R. T.: Arch. Neurol. Psychiatr. **26,** 1053, 1931.
269. Munday, M.: Symposium: Recent research on Premenstrual Syndrome: Curr. Med. Res. Op. **4,** Suppl. 4, 16, 1977.
270. Bachstrom, T., Cartensen, H.: J. Steroid. Biochem. **5,** 257, 1974.
271. Billig, H. E., Spaulding, C. A.: Industr. Med. **16,** 336, 1947.
272. Greenblatt, R. B.: J. Am. Med. Ass. **115,** 120, 1940.

BIOGRAPHIES

ADAMS, Joseph   1756–1818

Joseph Adams was born in London in 1756, the son of an apothecary, to whom he was later apprenticed. This was at about the time when the apothecaries succeeded in their struggle against the Royal College of Physicians and began to gain recognition as being concerned in first medical care of patients.

Adams attended lectures by Pitcairn and Potts. William Pitcairn (1710–1798) had been a student of Boerhave in Leyden in 1734 and graduated M.D. in Rheims, and D.M. in Oxford in 1749. He was physician at St. Bartholomew's Hospital in London from 1750 to 1780 and President of the Royal College of Physicians from 1775 to 1785. His nephew, David Pitcairn (1749–1809), studied at Edinburgh and Cambridge, and also became a physician at Bart's from 1780 to 1793. Percival Pott (1714–1788) was the celebrated surgeon at Bart's from 1749 to 1787. Adams later became a pupil of John Hunter at St. George's Hospital in London; Hunter's method of experimental research and concise reporting made a profound impression on him.

Adams practised as an apothecary for some time, without much enthusiasm. In 1795 he published his first book, *Observations on Morbid Poisons, Phagedena and Cancer* (London, J. Callow). In 1796, he became an M.D. at Aberdeen (in absentia), following which he went to Madeira, where he practised medicine for 8 years. He and his wife also ran a sanitarium there, mainly for invalids from England, at the cost of half a guinea a day.

In 1801 Adams published *A Treatise on the Cancerous Breast* (London, J. Callow). His election as Physician to the Hospitals for Smallpox, Inoculation and Vaccination in 1805 meant that the statutes of the College of Physicians and of the Hospital had to be waived, to allow a member of the Society for Apothecaries to be appointed. In 1809, Sir Lucas Popys,

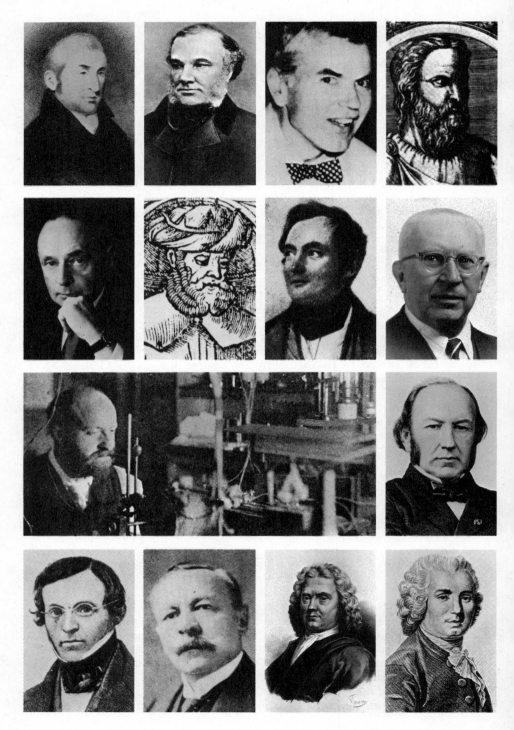

President of the Royal College of Physicians of London, granted special permission for Adams' admission as a Licentiate of the College without examination, which was a great honour. Adams also became Secretary, and eventually, President of the Medical Society of London.

In 1807 he published a paper confirming the value of vaccination. In 1809 he wrote *An Inquiry into the Laws of Epidemics* (London, Johnson & Callow) in which he put forward some quite modern ideas.

His main claim to fame appeared, however, in 1814, with the publication of his 41 page book: *A Treatise on the Supposed Hereditary Properties of Disease* . . ., which was discussed in greater detail in Section I, Chapter 15. It was certainly a remarkable achievement for a man who had never carried out experimental research, or had mathematical training (unlike Gregor Mendel) but it was based on sound clinical experience and clear thinking, which he had been taught by John Hunter. A year later, in 1815, the book was re-issued under a different title: *A Philosophical Treatise on the Hereditary Peculiarities of the Human Race and with Notes Illustrative of the Subject, Particularly in Gout, Scrofula and Madness. The Second Edition with an Appendix, On the Goitres and Cretins of the Alps and Pyrenees* (London, J. Callow). Although Adams was held in high esteem by his contemporaries, his common-sense conclusions were not always appreciated, and his disease examples were not always correct. His publication was forgotten until it was disinterred by Arno G. Motulsky, when he was working at the Galton Laboratory of University College in London at the end of the 1950s (AMA Arch. Int. Med. **104,** 490–496, 1959).

Adams died in 1818 at the age of 66, leaving no children. On his tombstone was written: 'Vir justus et bonus'.

ADDISON, Thomas   1795–1860

Thomas Addison was born in April 1795 at Long Benton, near Newcastle-upon-Tyne, the younger son of Joseph Addison, a grocer. He was educated at Newcastle Grammar School and in 1815 graduated M.D. Edinburgh with a thesis 'De Syphilide et Hydrargyro'.

For a time Addison was a house surgeon at Lock Hospital, London and in 1819 he was appointed physician to Carey Street Dispensary. He became an expert in dermatology. However, anxious to avoid being thought an expert in the field, it was not until much later that he published descriptions of vitiligoidea tuberosa with W. W. Gull in 1851, the first account of xanthoma diabeticorum, and of Addison's keloid in 1819.

Figure 75 (left to right) Top row: Joseph Adams; Thomas Addison*; Fuller Albright†; Aretaeus the Cappadocian. 2nd row: Charles Nathaniel Armstrong; Avicenna; Carl Adolf von Basedow‡; Julius Bauer. 3rd row: Sir William Maddock Bayliss; Claude Bernard. Bottom row: Arnold Adolph Berthold‡; Artur Biedl‡; Herman Boerhaave; Théophile de Bordeu†. (*by kind permission of Department of Medical Illustration, St Bartholomew's Hospital, London EC1; †by kind permission of Royal Society of Medicine, London; ‡from Ciba Monograph No. 10, by kindness of Ciba-Geigy Ltd.)

In December 1819 Addison became licentiate of The Royal College of Physicians in London, and a Fellow in July 1838. He entered Guy's Hospital as a pupil in 1820 and in 1824 was elected assistant physician, becoming full physician in 1837, and joint lecturer with Richard Bright on medicine. The first volume of *Elements of the Practice of Medicine* by Bright and Addison appeared in 1836. A devoted clinical scientist, Addison was an admirable lecturer, teacher and careful clinician. His original observations were numerous and his name was attached to the disease of the suprarenals, to the 'true' keloid and to pernicious anaemia. He advanced knowledge in pulmonary tuberculosis and fatty changes in the liver, and was the first in England to appreciate Laennec's method of auscultation and to use electricity for treatment.

Always of a melancholic and nervous temperament, Addison was subjected to such appalling attacks of depression that in early life he had intended suicide. In 1860, mental disorder necessitated his retirement from practice, he became suicidal and on 29 June 1860 threw himself out of a window in Brighton (England).

ALLEN, Edgar   1892–1943

Edgar Allen was born in Canon City, Colorado, U.S.A. He graduated Ph.D. at Brown University in 1913 and proceeded Ph.D. in 1921. In 1923, he became Professor of Anatomy at the University of Missouri. His meeting and collaboration with Edward Doisy was discussed in Chapter 18. After demonstrating with Doisy the effect of liquor folliculi in 1923, Allen showed four years later that the onset of menstruation in the monkey *Macacus rhesus* occurs when oestrogen ceases to act on the endometrium (withdrawal effect) (*Contrib. Embryol. Carnegie Inst.* **19**, 1–44, 1927), and that in the spayed monkey oestrus could be produced by injection of oestrin.

In 1933, Allen moved to Yale University School of Medicine as Professor of Anatomy. He remained there until he died in 1943 at the early age of 51.

ARETAEUS, The Cappadocian
81–138(?) AD

Aretaeus lived under Domitian and Hadrian and was a representative of the pneumatic school. As a clinician he ranks near to Hippocrates in his accuracy of descriptions of disease. He gave the first detailed account of diabetes, to which he gave its name ($\delta\iota\alpha\beta\alpha\acute{\iota}\nu\omega$ = to go through), and among the symptoms he stressed the importance of thirst (polydipsia). Both were taken over from him by Galen. Like other authors, he noticed that diabetes may occur following an acute disease, injury or emotional shock. "The cause of it may be, that one of the acute diseases may have left in the past some malignity lurking. It is not improbable that something pernicious, derived from the other diseases, which attack the bladder and kidneys, may sometimes prove the cause of this affection."

ASCHNER, Bernhard 1883–1960

Bernhard Aschner was born in January, 1883 in Vienna, where he studied medicine, qualifying in 1907. His medical progress was unusual. He was a demonstrator in anatomy to Professor Emil Zuckerkandl (1849–1910), and intent on a career in surgery, he later became surgical trainee under Anton von Eiselsberg. There encouraged by Eiselsberg, he soon became involved in scientific studies, jointly with Richard Paltauf (1858–1924), Professor of Experimental Pathology, and his first assistant, Artur Biedl.

Between 1908 and 1912, Aschner made two original experimental observations, which have become medical classics. He described the oculo-cardiac reflex (Aschner's phenomenon), the bradycardia produced by pressure on the eyeballs in children and in adults with vagotonia. The other outstanding result, was his success in achieving long-term survivals in hypophysectomized dogs, which enabled him to study the function of the pituitary (see Chapter 16). Cushing acknowledged his indebtedness to Aschner, from whom he learned a modification of his technique. Thus he became one of the Founding Fathers of modern endocrinology.

Aschner then entered the gynaecological clinic of Friedrich Schauta (1849–1919) in Vienna. From 1912 to 1914 he was assistant at the clinic of obstetrics and gynæcology of Johann Veit (1852–1917) in Halle in Germany. Between 1914 and 1918 he was in charge of an Austrian army surgical unit in the Tyrol, and was decorated with the Knight's cross of the Order of Francis Joseph. In 1913, he became 'Privat-Docent' in Halle, and after his army service, Privat-Docent in gynaecology at the University of Vienna. In, 1918, he published *The Endocrine Disorders of the Female* and in 1924 *Female Constitution and its Relations to Obstetrics and Gynaecology*. His contribution to Halban and Seitz's monumental *Handbook of Gynaecology* was 'Relationships of the endocrine glands to the female genital organs'. Aschner was fascinated by the therapeutic possibilities of celebrated physicians of the past and of folk medicine, and in 1928 published his first book on constitutional therapy under the title *Crisis in Medicine*, later continued in English as *Constitutional Therapy*. In 1931, he published his book *Clinic and Therapy of Menstrual Disorders*. This interest brought him into the ranks of medical historians. He translated the works of Paracelsus, whom he admired, into modern German; they were published in four volumes, with critical and analytical commentaries and a biography. It became the standard work on the subject.

Hitler's occupation of Austria forced Aschner to emigrate and he settled in New York. He developed a large private practice and was in charge of the arthritis clinics of the Stuyvesant and Lebanon Hospitals. In 1946, he published *Treatment of Arthritis and Rheumatism in General Practice*, which followed his book *The Art of the Healer* (1942).

Aschner was convinced that so called scientific medicine does not have all the answers and that empirical therapeutic procedures should be tested and used. There is no better drug than digitalis, he would say, and he was interested in acupuncture, rightly so, as we now realize. Aschner died in New York in March, 1960.

BAER, Carl Ernst Ritter von, Edler von Huthorn   1792–1876

Carl Ernst Ritter von Baer was born on his father's estate at Piep, near Jerwen, Estonia, in February, 1792. One of his ancestors, Andreas Baer, had emigrated from Westphalia to Reval, Livonia, in the mid-16th century. His father was Magnus Johann von Baer, an Estonian landholder, trained as a lawyer, and served as a district official (Landrat) and as an official of the Estonian knighthood, of which the family had gained membership in the mid-18th century. Carl was one of 10 children (including three sons), who was brought up partly by his father's childless brother Carl, a military gentleman. On his uncle's neighbouring estate he became interested in plants.

Baer's first education was by tutors at home; he next attended a cathedral school for the nobility in Reval. He decided against a military career and entered the University of Dorpat, founded six years before, as a medical student. He proceeded M.D. Dorpat in 1814. He continued his studies in 1814–1815 in Berlin and Vienna and in Berlin again in 1816–1817. In 1815, he went to Wuerzburg, where he studied comparative anatomy under Ignaz Doellinger. In 1817, he went as Prosector in Anatomy to Karl Friedrich Burdach (1776–1847), formerly his Professor of Physiology in Dorpat, then Professor at Koenigsberg. In 1819, he became Professor Extraordinary in Anatomy and in 1826, Ordinary Professor of Zoology. When in Koenigsberg, he taught anatomy, zoology and anthropology. He founded a zoological museum there and several times acted as Director of the Botanical Gardens. He became Dean of the Medical Faculty and Rector of the University. He married Auguste von Medem at Koenigsberg in 1820.

Most of Baer's contributions to embryology were made between 1819 and 1834, when he was in Koenigsberg. He made a number of specific discoveries in vertebrate morphogenesis, relating to the development of particular organs and organ-systems, and was the first to discover and describe the notochord. He was among the first to recognize that the neural folds represent the rudiment of the central nervous system and that they form a tube, although he did not understand the precise mechanism by which the folds form the substance of the brain and the spinal cord. He was the first to describe the five primary brain vesicles. He was responsible for the introduction of the term 'spermatozoa' for what were then known as animalcules in the seminal fluid, but he thought them to be parasites.

In 1826, he discovered the egg of the mammal in the ovary (see also Chapter 15). Thus was resolved a search which had started as early as the 17th century (Fabricius ab Aquapendente, Chapter 12; Buffon, Chapter 14; Wm. Harvey, Chapter 14). Harvey had unsuccessfully attempted to find eggs in the uterus of the deer; others, after Harvey, had mistaken ovarian follicles for mammalian eggs. Baer first found a true egg in Burdach's house dog, a bitch sacrificed for the investigation. Subsequently, he found eggs in a number of other mammals. Thus he concluded that "every mammal which springs from the coition of male and female, is developed from an ovum, and none from a single formative liquid" (De ovi mammalium at hominis genesi, O'Malley translation, p. 149). Equally important were von Baer's careful descriptions and thoughtful interpretations of the whole course of vertebrate development.

Baer's great contribution lay in his ability to envisage the living organism as a being that undergoes observable change during its lifetime. He described the development of vertebrates from the moment of conception to birth (or hatching). He stressed that development is epigenetic, that it proceeds from the seemingly homogeneous to the obviously heterogeneous stage, or from the general to the special. This finished the assumption of any preformation theory. He showed that embryos resemble one another more than the fully-developed adult individuals, in contrast to the theory of Johann Friedrich Meckel that embryos resemble the adult stage of other species. Nor did he agree with Darwin (*Origin of Species*, 1859) that all organisms could have evolved from one single, or a very few, progenitors.

Although a corresponding member since 1826, he declined an invitation to work at the Academy of Sciences in St. Petersburg two years later. After his brother's death in 1834, von Baer moved with his family to St. Petersburgh as a full member of the Academy in zoology, and remained there for the rest of his working life. From 1846 to 1852, he was Professor for Comparative Anatomy and Physiology at the medico-chirurgical Academy there. Retiring in 1862, he continued to work until 1867 when he returned to Dorpat, where he died in 1876.

Over 25 years he undertook extensive scientific travels to Lapland, the North Cape, the Caspian Sea, the Caucasus, the Sea of Azow, Kazan, to the Continent and to England. He also worked in anthropology and geography. Von Baer was a great wit and had many social accomplishments. Among the many honours during his lifetime, an island in the North was named after him. He was a patriotic Russian, interested in Russian geography and ethnography. He became a Fellow of the Royal Society (London) and was elected to the Académie in Paris.

BANTING, Sir Frederick Grant   1891–1941

Fredrick Grant Banting was born near Alliston, Ontario, Canada. He completed his medical training, at the University of Toronto, in 1916 and joined the Canadian Army Medical Corps, in which he served from 1917 to 1919, mainly overseas. After his return, he spent a year doing orthopaedic surgery at the Sick Children's Hospital in Toronto. From there he went to London, Ontario, to set up in mainly orthopaedic practice. In order to earn some much needed extra money, Banting took up a part-time post as Demonstrator in the Department of Physiology there, in July 1920 (see also Chapter 19). We have already described how, through these duties, he came across Moses Barron's paper which was the stimulus for his attempt to isolate insulin. In spring 1921 he returned to Toronto to start research at the Department of Physiology of Professor J. J. R. Macleod. The rest of the story is well known.

After the award of the Nobel Prize in Medicine to Banting and Macleod in 1923, Banting was appointed Professor of Medical Research at the University of Toronto in the same year and was also given an annuity for life by the Canadian Parliament. In 1930, the Banting Institute for Medical Research was founded at the University of Toronto. In 1934, Banting received a knighthood. When war broke out, he joined the army again. In 1941, on a wartime mission, he was involved in an aircrash in Newfoundland and died of exposure and injuries.

BASEDOW, Carl Adolf von   1799–1854

Carl Adolf von Basedow was born at Dessau in March, 1799. His medical education took place at the University of Halle. He then spent two years in Paris at the Charité and the Hôtel-de-Dieu, returning to Germany in 1822 to settle in Merseburg near Leipzig.

Von Basedow's celebrated paper, 'Exophthalmos durch Hypertrophie des Zell-gewebes in der Augenhoehle' (exophthalmos through hypertrophy of the cellular tissue in the orbit; Wochenschr. Heilk **6**, 197–204, 220–228, 1840), reviewed the available literature, mentioning that the *Traité des maladies des yeux* (1722) by C. Saint Yves (1667–1733) was original and marked a considerable advance. Estimates of his paper were varied, and it was not well received in his own country.

He died on 11 April 1854 of a septic infection, contracted at the necropsy of a patient with typhoid fever.

BAUER, Julius   1887–1979

Julius Bauer was born in Nachod in Bohemia, the son of a lawyer. After a humanistic education, he moved to Vienna in 1905, to study medicine, intending to take up psychiatry. He also attended lectures by Jodl on psychology and by Wirtinger on higher mathematics. He was keen on 'rerum cognoscere causas' (= to learn the causes of things). He was introduced into research by the neurologists Heinrich Obersteiner and Otto Marburg, and proceeded M.D. in November, 1910. His first teacher in internal medicine was Leopold Schroetter von Kristelli, a pupil of Joseph Skoda. He became a house physician to Edmund von Neusser, by that time already a sick man, but the spirit of his teaching left a permanent impression on the young doctor. He became conscious of the importance of under-standing the physical and psychological inborn individual differences which influence disease. From this concept arose the term 'constitution' which became Bauer's main interest. From 1910 to 1914, he worked with Rudolf Schmidt (a pupil of Neusser) as his assistant in Innsbruck (Tyrol). He spent a term in Paris (on a scholarship), where he came under the influence of George F. C. Widal (1862–1929), Pierre Marie, Déjerine, Babinski and E. Metschnikoff (1845–1916). On his return, he became assistant to Julius Mannaberg, a pupil of C. W. Hermann Nothnagel (1841–1905) at the Policlinic, where he remained until 1938, when Hitler's arrival forced him to emigrate to the United States.

In 1917 his book *Constitution and Disease* was published (published in English in 1943), which became a classic. The original title was *Constitution-al Disposition to Internal Diseases*, and it was based on the critical analysis of disease from Bauer's own medical experience and from the careful study of an enormous volume of literature of over 3000 medical publications. Within two years he proceeded to 'Privat-Docent' (University (senior) lecturer); in 1925, he was granted the title of Professor. His work was closely connected with the developing field of endocrinology, and in 1927, he published his monograph on 'Internal Secretion, its physiology, pathology and clinic'. He was, of course, much involved in the study of genetics in medicine, on which he also published his lectures; when the new 'Society for Endocrinol-ogy' was formed he persuaded the Council to add to the name of the society 'and Genetics'. In 1928, he became chief of the 3rd medical unit and in 1931, the 1st and 3rd medical units were joined under his guidance. In the meantime, there were frequent visits to the United States, where he gave the main lecture to the American College of Physicians in New Orleans in 1928. Bauer's department in Vienna became a centre of post-graduate study for many visitors from all over Europe, and especially from the United States, focused on the American Medical Association in Vienna. His pupils and assistants spread the gospel that medicine does not consist merely of classified facts, but that the understanding of the constitutional, genetic and endocrine background is equally important. Bauer used to stress that there is no such specialty as 'Psychosomatic Medicine', because all medicine is, fundamentally, psychosomatic. He was also one of the first to postulate that the apparent multiplicity of hormones in a small organ like the pituitary is, in reality, perhaps the variety of response to a few hormones by the various target organs. He was particularly determined to replace the idea of 'disease entities' and of 'cases' by the 'sick human being'.

In 1933, Bauer was asked to organize, as President, the First International Endocrine Congress, to be held in Marienbad, Czechoslovakia, in the summer of 1934. Just a month before it was due, Germany managed to stop it, because Bauer had been openly critical in an article in the Swiss medical journal, of Hitler's national-socialist medicine, especially of the proposed 'disposal' of mentally defective patients in hospitals.

After leaving Vienna, at the age of 51, and a short sojourn in Paris, Bauer went to New Orleans as Professor of Clinical Medicine. After a few years he joined, in the same capacity, the College of Medical Evangelists in Los Angeles, California. There he continued his teaching and writing, long after his retirement. He died there on 8 May 1979, in his 92nd year.

BAYLISS, Sir William Maddock   1860–1924

William Maddock Bayliss was born at Wolverhampton (England) on 2 May, 1860, the only son of Moses Bayliss, manufacturer of ironware, and his wife Jane Maddock. He retained a lifelong interest in the family firm of which he was a director, and was especially concerned with the condition of the employees. He was educated at Mowbray House School at Wolverhampton and later apprenticed to Wolverhampton Hospital, but he never finished his medical training. In 1881, he entered University College in London and came under the influence of Sir Edwin Lankester and Sir John Scott Burdon-Sanderson. When the latter went to Oxford as the first Waynflete Professor of Physiology, Bayliss followed him, entering Wadham College in 1885. In 1888, he obtained a first class in the School of Natural Science (Physiology), and in the same year returned to University College, London, where he remained for the rest of his life. It was there that in 1912 a professorship of general physiology was specially created for him. He also formed a close association with the Physiological Society, beginning in March, 1885, when the Society was small and mainly social. He was their Secretary from 1900 to 1922 and Treasurer from 1922 until his death.

During his life Bayliss produced an impressive amount of research, which began even before he went to Oxford in 1885. Much of it was carried out in collaboration with Rose Bradford, such as the study of electric currents developed in the salivary glands. In 1891 began his collaboration with Ernest H. Starling which was to last the rest of his life. First came the study of the electric currents of the mammalian heart. In 1894 the classic paper on venous and capillary pressures was published. In 1898–99 followed the papers on the innervation of the intestine, and; in 1902, the discovery of secretin (see Section I).

Bayliss, whose administrative and teaching duties were less strenuous than those of Starling, found time to continue his other studies, mainly on the vascular system. From 1900 onwards, he became increasingly interested in the chemical and physical sides of physiology and enzyme actions. This was borne out by the publication in 1915 of his magnum opus, the monumental *Principles of General Physiology*, which bore the stamp of his personal contribution. It went into four editions, the last of which appeared soon after his death. In 1908, he had published *The Nature of Enzyme Action*, and in 1923 *The Vaso-motor System*. During the 1914–18 war, his work resulted in the large-scale use of saline injections for the amelioration of surgical shock.

He received many honours: in 1903, he became a Fellow of the Royal Society and from 1913 to 1915 he was a member of their Council. In 1904 he was Croonian Lecturer of the Royal College of Physicians; in 1911, he was Royal Medallist; in 1911, he was awarded the Copley Medal, and in 1917, he received the Baly Medal of the Royal College of Physicians of London. In 1922, he was knighted.

In 1893, Bayliss married Gertrude Ellen Starling, sister of Ernest H. Starling. Barcroft wrote of him: 'Bayliss' honesty and generosity of outlook, the simplicity and nobility of his mind, his faculty of getting to the bottom of a problem, coupled with his great erudition, made intercourse with him at once a pleasure and an education.' He died at Hampstead on 27 August 1924.

BERNARD, Claude   1813–1878

Born in St. Julien (Rhône) in 1813, Claude Bernard was educated at Villefranche. He spent two years as assistant to a dispensing chemist and, disgusted with the quackery, then attempted a literary career. In 1834 he went to Paris with *Arthur de Bretagne*, a play he had written about Charles VI. However, his Professor at the Sorbonne encouraged him to study medicine. In 1841 he was appointed as assistant to François Magendie (1783–1855), the leader of French physiology at the Collège de France, and took his doctorate in 1843.

Bernard has been called the 'founder of experimental medicine'. His works and lectures dealt with experimental physiology in application to medicine (1855), the effects of poisons (1857), the physiology and pathology of the nervous system (1858) and of the body fluids (1859), experimental pathology (1872), anaesthetics and asphyxia (1875), diabetes and animal glycogenesis (1877), and operative physiology (1879). His *Introduction à l'Etude de la Médecine Expérimentale* (1865) is a philosophic guide to research and often reprinted. It is said that this won him a seat in the Académie Francaise. He became full professor at the Collège de France in 1855 and taught many distinguished research pupils and workers. He was elected a member of the Académie Francaise in 1868 and was made a Senator in 1867 by Napoleon III. In February 1878, he died a lonely death from acute nephritis as his wife and two daughters lived away from him because they felt distaste for his life's work.

Bernard was given a public funeral at the expense of the State, with much pomp and ceremony, a tribute previously only paid to princes, statesmen and soldiers.

BERTHOLD, Arnold Adolph   1803–1861

Arnold Adolph Berthold was born in February, 1803 at Soest in Westphalia. He studied medicine at Goettingen and proceeded M.D. with a thesis 'De cauteri actuali seu de igne ut medicamento', in 1823. He visited several other universities (including Berlin 1824–25, where he studied clinical medicine), before going to Paris to study zoology and comparative anatomy. In 1825, he became Privat-Docent and general practitioner in Goettingen; his thesis of 'habilitation' was: 'Ueber das Wesen der Wasserscheue' (= on the nature of hydrophobia). He lectured on physiology, zoology and comparative anatomy. In 1829 he published the *Lehrbuch der Physiologie des Menschen* (Textbook of Human Physiology), of which three editions were published by 1848. In 1835 he became Professor Extraordinary; in 1836, Ordinary Professor of Medicine at Goettingen, with the task of joint supervision of the division of zoology and zootomy of the museum. Among his numerous papers covering a wide range of medical subjects, were (apart from his celebrated transplant experiments): 'On lateral hermaphroditism observed in man' (1844), 'Poisoning by steam from coal', 'Coffee as treatment of antimony-poisoning' and 'Treatment of cholera'.

He died at Goettingen in February, 1861.

BEST, Charles Herbert 1899–1978

C. H. Best was born of Canadian parents in West Pembroke, Maine, U.S.A., where his father practised as a physician. He entered the University of Toronto in 1916 before enlisting and serving in the war until 1918. On return he resumed his studies and graduated in physiology and biochemistry in July 1921. He began his career as an unpaid research worker in Professor MacLeod's laboratory, living on savings from his discharge gratuity in 1919 and later by borrowing from Banting. Directed by MacLeod to assist Banting with the latter's experiments on isolating the islet hormone (jointly with Dr. Noble), Banting and he succeeded in doing so during the summer of 1921.

Banting and MacLeod received the Nobel prize in 1923, which Banting shared with Best.

In 1925 Best went to work in Sir Henry Dale's Laboratory at the Medical

Research Council in London, where he participated in research on histamine. He continued this work on his return to Toronto and later participated in obtaining heparin in crystalline form. When war broke out in 1939, he and his colleagues organized the Canadian dried serum project. From 1941 to 1946 he was director of the medical research division of the Royal Canadian Navy, which division he had helped to form. After Banting's death in 1941, Best became Director of the Banting and Best Department of Medical Research in the University of Toronto and honorary consultant to the Connaught Laboratories for the supply of insulin. A new Chas. H. Best Institute to house the department of physiology was soon added. He remained there until his retirement in 1967. He was also a member of the National Research Council of Canada and of the Internal Health Division of the Rockefeller Foundation. One of his best-known books became: *The Physiological Basis of Medical Practice* (7th ed: 1961), and *Selected papers by Chas. H. Best* was published in 1964. In 1949 he was made honorary president of the International Diabetes Federation. He was elected F.R.S. in 1938, C.B.E. 1944, Companion of the Order of Canada, 1967, C.H. in 1971 for his service to medical research.

Best's recreations were riding and golf. He married Margaret Hooper Mahon and they had two sons.

BIEDL, Artur   1869–1933

Artur Biedl was born in October, 1869 at Osztern (then in Hungary) and studied in Vienna from 1886 to 1892. In 1893 he became assistant to S. Stricker (1834–1898), proceeded to Privat-Docent in 1896 and to Professor Extraordinary in 1901, having received the title 'Professor' in 1899. In 1914, he became Professor to the Chair of General and Experimental Pathology at the German University in Prague (then Austria).

His first research studies concerned the nervous system, the excretion of micro-organisms, experimental diabetes, cerebral oedema, the detoxificating function of the liver, the lymphatic system and the pathology of arteriosclerosis. From 1895 onwards, he became interested in the glands of internal secretion, to begin with the physiology of the adrenals. 1903 saw the publication of a short monograph *Internal Secretion*, which was eventually expanded into the two massive volumes (1910), which became internationally known and translated into English in 1913. With Aschner he also edited the newly founded journal *Endokrinologie*. In 1922, he published the monograph on the pituitary. In the same year, he presented three patients with a rare syndrome of mental deficiency, diminished basal metabolic rate and disturbance of digestion without evidence of increased cerebral pressure or brain tumour or pituitary changes; this condition was named Biedl's disease.

Biedl was a lively, highly intelligent man. The favourite pupil of Stricker, promoted Privat-Docent at 27 and professor (by title) at 29, he was an excellent and popular teacher; he rightly hoped to succeed his teacher to the Chair of Experimental Pathology. To his deep disappointment, he was twice passed over, first by Knoll, who died within two years, and then by Paltauf, whose first assistant he remained until 1914, when he succeeded H. E. Hering in Prague.

His last years were saddened by a painful illness and deep mental depression. He died in 1933, in his 64th year. He was one of the pioneers of clinical and experimental endocrinology on the Continent, with great international reputation. Among his pupils were Bernhard Aschner, Hans Selye and Max Reiss.

BISHOP, Peter Maxwell Farrow   1905–1979

Peter M. F. Bishop was the son of a doctor, educated in Berlin, at Charterhouse and at Trinity College, Oxford, before proceeding to Guy's Hospital in London. As a young man, he was a popular member of the residents' plays at Guy's, later Warden of the Residents College and Deputy-Superintendent. He began as a physiologist and then became an endocrinologist with a special interest in reproductive endocrinology. As endocrinologist to the Chelsea Hospital for Women, he founded there an infertility clinic of international fame; he also became endocrinologist to the obstetrics department of the Royal Postgraduate Medical School. In 1964, he was Sims' travelling professor; he also became senior consultant to the Family Planning Association and Master of the Society of Apothecaries. Bishop was one of the pioneers in female reproductive endocrinology, investigating the actions of numerous oestrogens. He organized the first clinical trials of stilboestrol for the Medical Research Council; he warned of the effects of long-term administration in too high a dosage.

Bishop's last years were overshadowed by the suffering from a compression of the spinal cord, which confined him to a wheelchair.

BOERHAVE, Herman   1668–1738

Herman Boerhave was born in 1668, the son of a protestant clergyman at Voorhout, near Leyden in Holland. He did not follow in his father's footsteps, but turned to natural science and medicine. At the age of 32, be became lecturer in medicine at Leyden and eight years later, Professor of Botany at the same university. When he reached his 50th year, he had added to it the professorships of medicine and chemistry. He was a systematic and untiring worker, but a painful joint affection in 1722 and a serious chest complaint in 1727 left their mark, and in 1729 he had to give up his professorships in chemistry and botany, but kept the chair of medicine until he died.

Boerhave was a popular teacher and had a great number of pupils, many of them from abroad, who remained in correspondence with him for many years afterwards. While still in good health, he would get up at dawn, start work in clogs at the botanical gardens, then give his first lecture at 7 a.m. Next, he saw private patients; through his pupils, he had many consultations from abroad. He then went to the Cecilia Hospital, to teach at the bedside. After a short luncheon break, there were more lectures and private consultations until dinner time. Such a timetable did not permit active research or the publication of new and original papers, but his teaching was firmly based on observation and practical experiment and avoided idle speculation. He taught botany 'in the garden'. For the teaching of chemistry and medicine, he published textbooks which became the standard ones not in Holland but in universities in many other countries. His most celebrated work was the *Institutiones medicae in usus annuae exercitationes domesticos digestae* (Lugduni Batavorum, J. van der Linden, 1708). It consisted of five parts: physiology, pathology, diagnostic, hygiene and therapeutics, and it achieved over 100 editions; the last complete edition being in Spanish in 1798.

His other famous work was the *Aphorismi de cognoscendis et curandis morbis* (= aphorisms on the diagnosis and treatment of diseases). *Lugduni Batavorum* (Leyden, J. van der Linden, 1709) (English translation in 1715), which reached 130 editions in 30 years! His pupil, Gerard L. B. van Swieten (1700–1772), inspired by Boerhave's Commentaria, wrote six hefty volumes of *Commentaria in Herman Boerhave aphorismos et de cognoscendis et curandis morbis* (Lugduni Batavorum, J. and H. Verbeck, 1742–1776), which also reached repeated editions. Van Swieten, one of the personal physicians to Maria Theresa (1740–1780), was one of the founders of the first Vienna medical school (see Section I) introducing Boerhave's bedside teaching method there. Boerhave also wrote a treatise on *Methodus discendi medicinam* (= method of teaching medicine; London, 1726). When he discovered that some of his students had published their notes on his lectures on chemistry abroad under his name, he felt compelled to write a compact volume *Elementa Chemiae*, which was first printed in 1732 and became the standard textbook on the subject at several universities.

Boerhave showed some interest in the idea of the alchemists and between 1718 and 1734, he attempted to convert mercury into gold, but his experiment did not succeed. Although he had among his patients several crowned heads, he could not be persuaded to travel from Leyden to their courts. He treated poor people free of charge. He never went further than 60–70 miles from Leyden, on one occasion in order to obtain his degree at a small university, as he could not afford the cost of the expensive dinner which students at Leyden had to offer to the Faculty when obtaining their degree. His motto was "simplex sigillum veri" (= simplicity is the proof of truth). Albrecht von Haller called him: "Magnus ille medicorum universae Europae praeceptor" (= that great teacher of medical men all over Europe).

BORDEU, Théophile de   1722–1776

Born 1722 at Iseste, Théophile de Bordeu was the elder son of a medical man *and* lawyer and director of the spas of Aquitaine; he was educated at Pau and the University of Montpellier, and was a brilliant student. He obtained his doctorate in 1743 and published *Chylificationis Historia*. He moved to Paris in 1746 for further study, but later returned to Pau as director of the spas of Aquitaine and wrote articles on the mineral waters of Béarn (1746–8) and on the articulations on the bones of the face. In 1752, he finally settled in Paris, where he published his *Recherches Anatomiques sur les Différentes Positions des Glandes et sur leur Action*. This received a mixed reception, but did contain, however, a remarkable analysis of a modern version of the ideas of Hippocrates of some of the glands which later became known as endocrine organs.

In attacking the doctrines of the mechanistic chemical school he became one of the founders of the vitalistic school of Montpellier.

In 1753 he was awarded the prize of the Académie de Chirurgie for a thesis on tuberculous glands. After 1754 he practised in Paris, where he published investigations on the pulse in 1756 and became a physician at the Court of Louis XV. The jealousy of rivals led to the accusation in 1761 that he charged fees dishonestly for professional attention. He wrote a number of other papers including one in which he advised inoculation against smallpox.

In 1775 he published his last work on chronic diseases, which was the most important one for the purpose of this book. In its last section on the medical analysis of the blood, it contains the suggestion that all the organs of the body discharge their secretions into the blood.

Harassed by gout and financial difficulties, de Bordeu felt lonely and became depressed. He was a bachelor and without the support of a family. He died suddenly on 24 November 1776 from a stroke; remarkably, he had predicted the actual date of his death.

Max Neuburger of Vienna re-discovered de Bordeu's writings and claimed him, in 1903, as the Father of Endocrinology.

BRAMWELL, Sir Byrom   1847–1931

Byrom Bramwell was born in 1847 in North Shields, England, where his father and grandfather were general practitioners. After a brilliant medical course in Edinburgh, he practised for four years with his father, following a spell as house surgeon at the Royal Infirmary. In 1871 he was appointed lecturer in medical jurisprudence and pathology in the University of Durham. In 1874, he was appointed physician and pathologist to the Royal Infirmary, proceeding in 1877 to M.D. at Edinburgh. On leaving Newcastle in 1879, he became an extra-mural teacher of medicine in Edinburgh.

714

Later, he became pathologist (1882–1885), assistant physician (1885) and physician to the Royal Infirmary (1897). He was, in 1900, an unsuccessful candidate for the chair of medicine.

His scientific output covered a wide field in medicine, from nervous disorders of the spinal cord, intracranial tumours, aphasia to anaemia and diseases of the blood-forming organs. In 1888 he suggested that obesity, polyuria and glycosuria in some pituitary tumours are, in fact, caused by disturbance of the neighbouring brain tissue (hypothalamus) rather than of the pituitary. He had an extensive consulting practice. He was President of the Royal College of Physicians in Edinburgh and president of the Association of Physicians of Great Britain and Ireland.

As well as about half a dozen books, Bramwell also wrote the three volume work *An Atlas of Clinical Medicine* (1892–1896) and published some 160 papers. He died in 1931.

BRIGHT, Richard   1789–1858

Richard Bright was born in 1789. He studied medicine at Edinburgh and Guy's Hospital in London, becoming M.D. Edinburgh in 1812. He then studied at Peterhouse, Cambridge. He travelled on the Continent from 1818 to 1820. In 1824 he was appointed physician to Guy's Hospital, where he remained until 1843, when he became consulting physician. He assisted Addison in *Elements of the Practice of Medicine* (1839). In 1827, he published the first volume of *Reports of Medical Cases*, which contained his discovery of Bright's disease; the second volume was published in 1831. He also contributed to *Guy's Hospital Reports*, first published in 1836.

Bright was elected a Fellow of the Royal College of Physicians in 1832, Goulstonian Lecturer 1833 and member of Council 1838 and 1843, Lumleian Lecturer 1837, Censor in 1836 and 1839. He became Fellow of the Royal Society in 1821, physician extraordinary to Queen Victoria in 1837. In his 'Cases and observations connected with disease of the pancreas and duodenum' *(Med.-Chir. Trans.* **18,** 1–56, 1832), he also discussed the pancreas in diabetes mellitus, in which he reported on morbid changes in some patients. He did not know, of course, of the islet organ nor of a direct causative link between the pancreas and diabetes. He died in 1858, aged 69.

BROWN-SÉQUARD, Charles Edward
1817–1894

Charles E. Brown-Séquard was born in Mauritius in 1817, son of an American merchant navy Captain and a mother of French descent. He was keen to follow a literary career and went to France with his mother in 1838.

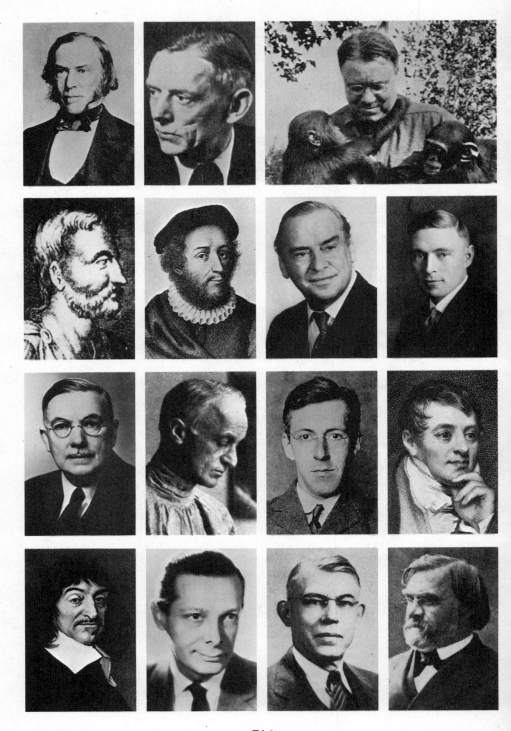

His writings were adversely criticized by Charles Nodier and he decided to turn to medicine. His studies were interrupted by illness and the death of his mother. He obtained his doctorate in Paris in 1846 with a thesis on experimental research on the physiology of the spinal cord. This was a subject that he later investigated and his name has always been associated with it. He founded, with others, the Société de Biologie. When Napoleon III ascended the throne in 1852. Brown-Séquard left for America, returning to Paris in 1855. In a small laboratory with others, he carried out experiments on the nervous system and adrenals. He came to England in 1858, started a practice and was appointed Physician to the National Hospital, Queen's Square in London, and was made a F.R.C.P. After more wanderings he was appointed Professor of Medicine at the Collège de France in 1878. His attempts at using testicular extract to prevent the deterioration of the organism of old age were criticized in many circles. In 1869, he suggested that injections of sperm into the blood circulation of old men would improve their physical and mental powers. Six years later he attempted testicular grafts in guinea-pigs without success. Finally at the age of 72, he gave himself sub-cutaneous injections of a watery mixture, made of the juice of the testicles and the blood of the spermatic vein, and claimed he gained great benefit from them.

His advocacy of giving these testicular extracts to patients suffering from a variety of conditions, for example tabes, was unfortunately exploited by professional and not so professional followers in Britain and U.S.A.

Brown-Séquard wrote several hundred papers. He was not interested in money and often refused enormous fees offered to him, if he believed that he could be of no help.

Just before giving himself his organ extract injections he had suffered from prostatic discomfort but he recovered, as he maintained, through his organo-therapy. Some time later he had whooping cough.

The death of his third wife (English) who was the widow of the painter Doherty, in 1894 upset him considerably. In March 1894 he had a cerebral attack which he described critically in a letter to his friend Dr. Waterhouse. He died on 1 April 1894.

Figure 76 (left to right) Top row: Charles Edouard Brown-Séquard; Adolf Butenandt*; Walter B. Cannon with two of the Yerkes chimpanzees, Chim and Panzee. 2nd row: Celsus; Guy de Chauliac†; Ian Chester Jones; James Bertrand Collip. 3rd row: George Washington Corner†; Harvey W. Cushing‡; Sir Henry Hallett Dale; Sir Humphrey Davy†. Bottom row: René Descartes†; Egon Diczfalusy; Edward A. Doisy*; Alexander Ecker*. (*from Ciba Monograph No. 10, by kindness of Ciba-Geigy Ltd.; †by kind permission of Royal Society of Medicine, London; ‡by kind permission of Department of Medical Illustration, St. Bartholomew's Hospital, London EC1)

BUTENANDT, Adolf Friedrich Johann 1903–

Adolf F. J. Butenandt was born in Wesermuende and studied medicine in Goettingen. He became a pupil of Adolf Windaus (1876–1959), who shared the Nobel Prize in 1928 for his work on Vitamin D and steroid chemistry. At his recommendation, Butenandt moved to Mssrs. Schering to work on the elucidation of the female sex hormones. In 1929, he succeeded in isolating oestrone from pregnancy urine, independently of the American researchers. In 1930, he identified the corpus luteum hormone and the male sex hormone as members of the steroid group. In 1939, he shared the Nobel Prize for chemistry with Leopold Ruzicka.

From 1933 to 1936, he worked at Danzig; in 1936, he moved to the Kaiser Wilhelm Institute for Biochemistry at Berlin-Dahlem. There he developed a close co-operation with the Director of the Institute for Biology, who was a zoologist in the study of the chemical guide substances in insects, omnochtomes (pigments). Later he moved to Tuebingen, where the Kaiser Wilhelm Institute was re-named in 1949 'Max Planck Institute', and in 1956, he moved with the Institute to Munich, where the insect hormone ecdysone was discovered and isolated as the first insect hormone in crystalline form (see Chapter 22). Later, his team isolated and then synthesized bombykol, the scent produced by female silkworms which attracts the male. In 1960, on his election to President of the Max Planck Society, he retired from active research, in a similar manner and for similar reasons as Sir Charles Harington, when he became Director of the National Institute for Medical Research.

CHAULIAC, Guy de   1300–1368 (?1370)

Guy de Chauliac was born in the Auvergne, France. He took Holy Orders and studied medicine at Toulouse, Montpellier and Paris, having had a course in anatomy at Bologna under Niccolò Bertuccio. Being one of the best educated surgeons of his time, he eventually settled in Avignon, where he also became 'commensal chaplain' to several popes. As well as being learned, he was a gentleman with high ideals; he remained at his post during the plague epidemics of 1348 and 1360, healing the sick. As a surgeon, he was fully aware of the importance of anatomy. He undertook cataract and hernia operations, normally carried out by the quacks of the market place.

In his writings, he believed in cutting out malignant new growth at an early stage with the knife or, if necessary, by cautery, which he also seems to have used in anthrax and caries. Fractures of the femur he suspended in a sling bandage or by means of weight and pulley. He used Theodoric's soporific inhalations when operating, which was a forerunner of anaesthesia. Concerning large goitres, he recommended removal of the diseased gland by surgery.

His wound treatment was less commendable, as he believed in interference by the surgeon (compare Ambroise Paré). His most important work was the *Inventarium et Collectorium* (Chirurgia Magna) written in 1363 and translated into French in 1478: *La pratique et chirurgie du maistre Guidon de Chauliac* (Lyon, Barthelemy Buyer), which saw many editions, and the abridged version of which (*Les fleurs du grand Guidon*) became the surgical vademecum for many centuries. This contained about 3300 quotations, 1400 from Arab writers and 1100 from ancient authors.

From de Chauliac's description of the outbreaks of plague in 1348 and 1360, it is clear that he suspected the contagious nature of the disease, which, like many of his contemporaries, he blamed on the Jews, or on certain conjunctions of the planets. In Avignon, where he was personal physician to Pope Clement VI (1342–52), Innocent VI (1352–62) and Urban V (1362–70), he also met the Italian poet Petrarca (Petrarch).

COLLIP, James Bertrand   1892–1965

James B. Collip was born in November, 1892 in Belleville, Ontario, Canada. He studied Physiology and Biochemistry in Toronto under Macallum and graduated there in 1908, proceeding M.A. in 1913 and Ph.D. in 1916 (in Biochemistry). From 1915 to 1928 he worked at the University of Alberta in Edmonton, where he isolated parathormone in 1925 and established a blood-calcium assay.

In 1921 (to 1922), he was on sabbatical leave in Toronto, when McLeod recruited him to his team to help in the purification of insulin.

In 1928, he was called to Toronto to succeed McCallum at McGill University. In the subsequent years he studied and described several placental and anterior pituitary-like hormones.

Between 1938 and 1958 he was also a member of the National Research Council of Canada, a Medical Liaison Officer with Washington. During the war, he served first as Lt.-Colonel and after 1944 as Colonel in the Royal Canadian Medical Corps, being created a C.B.E. in 1943. Later, he moved to the University of Western Ontario in London, Ontario, where he was Dean of the Faculty of Medicine and Head of the Department for Medical Research. He was elected a Foreign Member of the Royal Society of London (England), among many other honours.

Collip was a modest and shy man, much loved by his friends and fellow workers. He was a keen car driver and died of a stroke at the age of 72 in London (Ontario), after a strenuous drive home from a meeting at Vancouver.

CONSTANTINUS, Africanus
ca. 1020–1087

Constantinus was born at Carthage. He studied by travelling extensively in the Middle East and acquired not only a great medical knowledge, but also a knowledge of many of the languages. On his return to Carthage he was persecuted as a magician and had to flee. He lived for some time at Salerno at the High (Middle) Salerno period (1072–1224 according to Sudhoff), from where he went to Monte Cassino, where he carried out most of his important literary work and where he eventually died. His writings consisted mainly of translations into (moderate) Latin of Arab versions of the *Liber Regius* (= The Royal Book) of Haly Abbas, the Dietetics, Elements, Fevers and Wines of Isaac Judaeus, of Arabic versions of writings of Hippocrates and some of Galen. The *Golden Book* (Liber aureus) was probably written by one of his Saracen pupils.

This Latinized presentation of the Arabic culture and medical thought had great influence upon Western medicine up to the 17th century, according to Sudhoff. Constantinus' poor Latin rendering was later corrected and improved upon by his pupil Atto.

COOPER, Sir Astley Paston, Bart.
1768–1841

Astley P. Cooper was born in Norfolk, the son of a rector. He entered Guy's Hospital at the age of 16 as an apprentice to his uncle William Cooper. He then went to St. Thomas's to Henry Cline. At the age of 21, he was made Demonstrator of Anatomy at the United Hospitals' School at St. Thomas's. In 1791, he became joint lecturer with Cline. He was appointed surgeon when his uncle, William Cooper, retired in 1800. In 1802, he became a Fellow of the Royal Society and was awarded the Copley Medal for his paper 'On the Membrana Tympany of the Ear'. In 1804, he produced a beautifully illustrated book on hernia, at great expense.

Astley Cooper had an exceptional knowledge of anatomy and was a very skilful surgeon. He was a very good looking man with a charming manner and had a very successful practice. After operating on King George IV for a sebaceous cyst, he was awarded a baronetcy in 1821. In 1825, he resigned from Guy's, but he remained as a consulting surgeon, a position specially created for him. He was twice President of the Royal College of Surgeons. He published many important monographs on surgical subjects, especially on the thyroid, the thymus and the testes (see Section I). He was also one of the pioneers of surgical treatment of arterial aneurysms. In his monograph on the anatomy and surgical treatment of abdominal hernia (1804–1807) he described 'Cooper's ligament' and 'Cooper's hernia' (i.e. hernia femoralis fasciae superficialis). In 1829, he published *Illustrations of the Diseases of the Breast*, which included one of the earliest descriptions of hyperplastic cystic disease of the breast, which he called 'hydatid disease'. He died in 1841.

CORNER, George Washington 1889–

Born in December, 1889, G. W. Corner studied medicine at the Johns Hopkins Medical School, Baltimore. After holding junior posts in anatomy at the University of California and at the Johns Hopkins, he became Professor of Anatomy at the University of Rochester, 1923–1940. From 1940 to 1955, he was Director of the Department of Embryology, Carnegie Institution of Washington, Baltimore. Between 1956 and 1960, he was Historian at the Rockefeller Institute, New York, and afterwards, Executive Officer of the American Philosophical Society, a post which he still occupied in 1969, when 80 years of age.

In the citation on the occasion of his tenth honorary degree, that of Doctor of Letters of the University of Pennsylvania, in May 1965, it was said: "He has shown an astonishing facility in the mastery of several métiers; a renowned scientist, he is also an accompanied humanist. His contributions to the understanding of the ovulatory cycle in primates and of the corpora lutea led to the discovery in his laboratory of the hormone progesterone". As to his humanistic interests, he himself has attributed them to the excellent education he received at his university. He wrote: "I did not 'major' in biology, because the Johns Hopkins University carefully avoided undergraduate 'majoring', by requiring the students to follow prescribed 'groups' of studies. I received excellent instruction in English and French literature, in Latin (including Horace, Plautus, Terence and Livy) and in logic and ethics. The Johns Hopkins Medical School was (in my day) by no means . . . devoid of cultural interest . . . It was at the Medical School that history really began to interest me". (See also Chapters 18 and 20.

Corner published his first medical historical paper on mithridaticum and theriac in 1915, in volume 26 of the *Johns Hopkins Medical Bulletin*. It was in the same year that his first paper was issued from the Carnegie Institution of Washington, on the corpus luteum. A short treatise on 'Anatomists in the search of the soul' (*Annals of Medical History*, 1919) was followed by the first book in 1927, *Anatomical Texts of the Earlier Middle Ages. A study in the transmission of culture*, with revised Latin text of Anatomia Cophonis and translations of four texts.

Among other papers, he wrote in 1930 on the discovery of the mammalian ovum and, in 1931 on medicine in Salerno in the 12th century, to the latter theme he returned in 1937, after giving the Thomas Vicary Lecture at the Royal College of Surgeons of England on 10 December 1936 on 'Salernitan Surgery in the 12th century'. In 1943, a volume of essays in biology was published to honour Herbert M. Evans. Corner entered a translation of Regner de Graaf's treatise on the female testes or ovaries.

Between 1948 and 1950 he wrote several papers on Benjamin Rush (1743–1813), friend of Benjamin Franklin and one of the foremost American clinicians of his time, who worked in Philadelphia. Rush had written with equal facility on mental disorders, on yellow fever and on military sanitation, of all of which he had personal experience. Corner translated William Shippen Jr.'s Edinburgh Dissertation of 1761 'De placenta cum uteri nexu'. In 1953, he wrote two papers on Benjamin Franklin's illnesses, and contributed to a 'Festschrift' for Charles Singer in 1953 'The Adventures of Dr. Kave in Search of an Open Polar Sea'.

When Richard A. Shryock wrote his paper 'George W. Corner as historian and humanist' for the *American Journal of Anatomy*, Corner's papers had increased in number. 'The History of the Rockefeller Institute 1901–1953' was dated 1964, but was in fact, published in 1965. It had 600 pages. A few months before, his book appeared: *Two Centuries of Medicine; A History of the School of Medicine, University of Pennsylvania*, which was hailed as meticulous yet readable, the author being "able to view events with broad and dispassionate perspective" (Elizabeth H. Thomson).

Corner is a contributor to the *Dictionary of American Biography*. Above all, his autobiography: *Anatomist at Large* (New York, Basic Books, 1958), is as delightful as informative on the life and times of George W. Corner, and also includes selected essays.

Dr. Corner is a Foreign Member of the Royal Society (London) and is listed in the 1979 Yearbook of the Society. I would like to extend my warmest wishes on the occasion of his 90th birthday on 12 December 1979.

DALE, Sir Henry Hallett   1875–1968

Henry H. Dale was educated at Leys School, proceeding to Trinity College, Cambridge as a scholar in 1894. Four years later, he was made Coutts–Trotter student and began his first research, under J. N. Langley, on a problem of neuro-anatomy and movements of the infusoria. In 1900, he moved to St. Bartholomew's Hospital, London, influenced by Gee, who told him that the medicine he would learn at Bart's would be based on clinical observation only. Gee hoped that Dale would live to see a true science of medicine. Dale qualified in 1903, and a scholarship enabled him to return to the laboratory (Starling's at University College). In 1904, he was appointed, on Starling's recommendation, Director of the Wellcome Physiological Research Laboratories, then at Herne Hill, where he remained for ten years (during which time he was elected Fellow of the Royal Society). He then became the first director of the National Institute for Medical Research.

In 1938, Dale shared the Nobel Prize with O. Loewi. The concepts were: the nerve-impulse travels along the nerve fibres as a wave of electrical excitation; when the impulse reaches the nerve-endings it changes to a chemical process and discharges pharmacologically-active agents, such as acetylcholine and noradrenaline, which in turn activated the next excitable structure. The new theory was founded on Loewi's crucial experiments, "but Dale gave them life and substance". He divided the actions of acetylcholine into muscarine and nicotine actions. An early clinical application of this concept was the clinical use of tubocurarine, which blocks the effect of acetylcholine at the neuro-muscular junction. The muscle relaxants have since become an indispensable aid to surgery. One of the most important applications of the theory has been the use of drugs to control hypertension, including the use of ganglion blockers. Dale seemed to be surprised at the great usefulness of his experimental work.

Dale made important contributions in many fields. His method of approach was to tackle a subject exhaustively and then to present his results in one or two large-scale papers. Thus, in a paper with Barger he covered the sympathicomimetic amines, thus determining direction of work for years. In a paper on ergot, he described the phenomenon which became the basis of all subsequent work on the alpha and beta actions of adrenaline. This has recently led to the introduction of beta-blockers, such as propranolol, for the treatment of cardiac irregularity. He laid the groundwork for the histamine theory of anaphylaxis. His classical experiments on the cellular theory, according to which the anaphylatic antibody must in the first instance become fixed to cells, has formed the basis of all later development.

Dale was a skilful and, indeed, passionate experimenter. In 1939, at the outbreak of war, he retired from experimental work, to undertake national and international responsibilities. He became secretary and president of the Royal Society. In 1945, he retired from the Medical Research Council, but his energy remained unabated. Since 1936 he was chairman of the dormant Wellcome Trust until 1960. After the war he revived it with unusual energy.

Dale was the most human of human beings, with a rich capacity for enjoyment, a keen sense of humour, and a wonderful aptitude for recounting in an interesting and amusing way the many encounters and experiences of his long life. He was a great admirer of Ehrlich and gave an endearing talk on him over the wireless during the 1939–45 war, expressing the hope and confidence that there would come a day when there would be again a Paul Ehrlich Strasse in Frankfurt. He warned on the dangers of an atomic war: "Nothing it seems but a general resurgence of human ideas can halt the world now on the ever more precipitous slope".

DESCARTES, René   1596–1650

René Descartes was born at Chatellevault in March 1596 in Poitou, where his grandfather practised medicine. The medical atmosphere in which he grew up influenced his future. He suffered from poor health. He was educated at La Flêche at Anjou by the Jesuits, going on to work at mathematics at Poitiers and Paris, and in 1617 volunteered for the army of Prince Maurice of Orange. While on a campaign at Breda he saw a notice of a challenge to solve a mathematical problem. He did so and gave the answer to Isaac Beckman and was introduced to other mathematicians. From 1628 to 1649 Descartes lived mainly in Holland. He went to Stockholm in 1649 where he founded an Academy of Science, and died there of pneumonia in 1650.

Although his fame is based mainly on his philosophical works, Descartes's teaching has influenced the development of medicine profoundly. He was particularly concerned with methodology to find the correct method for obtaining true knowledge, which was underlined by his work in mathematics and physics. In 1637, he published the *Discours de la méthode*, the cornerstone of his achievements. In his opinion, science was a tree, with metaphysics representing the root, physics the trunk and mechanics, medicine and morals its three main branches. His particular interest was in anatomy and physiology, the latter closely linked with psychology, as a forerunner of the experimental psychology of Wilhelm Wundt (1832–1920) in the 19th century. The problems stated in his work *De Homine Liber* (the Book on Man), published in 1662, had great influence on research in physiology; in the opinion of Sir Michael Foster, Descartes's views, when translated into modern terminology, appear akin to those voiced today. He seems, for example, to have anticipated in 1649 the concept of reflex action. There was more than simple justification to regard him as one of the "médecins amateurs" (A. Cabanès, 1932).

DOBSON, Matthew   1732–1784

Matthew Dobson was a Yorkshireman (England), the son of a non-conformist minister. He refused to follow in his father's footsteps and studied medicine in Edinburgh, where he qualified in 1756. In about 1762, he settled in Liverpool, becoming physician to the Liverpool Infirmary in 1770. In 1780, he relinquished his position because of ill-health and moved to Bath, where he died in 1784, aged only 52.

In 1774, he carried out his now famous experiments (I–VI) on the urine in diabetes, which were published in 1776 (Experiments and observations on the urine in diabetes. *Med. Obs. Inq.* **5**, 298–316, 1776). In them he proved that the sweetish taste of diabetic urine was produced by sugar, an observation following on Willis's discovery of the sweetness of diabetic urine. He also discovered that the blood of diabetics had a sweet taste, i.e. hyperglycaemia. He communicated the results of his experiments in a letter to John Fothergill (1712–1780) (see Chapter 19), who first described sick headache (migraine) in 1777 and facial neuralgia in 1776, but also left an interesting account of the weather and diseases of London (1783). Dobson's doctoral

thesis in 1756 was on: 'De menstruis'. He was elected a Fellow of the Royal
Society (London).

DODDS, Sir Edward Charles, Bart.
1899–1973

Edward Charles Dodds was born in Liverpool in October, 1899, son of Ralph
E. Dodds. When still very young, he moved with his parents to Darlington,
Yorkshire, where his father was in the retail footwear business. In 1910 or
1911 the family moved again, to London, where they first settled in Maida
Vale.

In January, 1911, Dodds entered Harrow County School for Boys, which
had good science teaching and excellent laboratories. Known as 'Tommy',
Dodds showed outstanding ability.

His mother (née Pack) was of a thriving London family; her brother,
George Pack, was a dentist in Harley Street and another brother, Edward,
owned a successful tailoring shop in Oxford Street, and was the 'wealthy
uncle'. He wanted Edward Dodds to enter his firm, but Dodds followed his
parents' wishes, and took up medicine.

In 1916 Dodds entered the Medical School of Middlesex Hospital in
London, and won the class prize in chemistry, and a certificate for Physics
in 1916–17. Called up for military service in July, 1917, he contracted
pneumonia on a long route march. After 18 months of service he was
discharged on grounds of ill health. In 1923 he married Constance Elizabeth
Jordan of Darlington, whose parents were well-known local business people.

Failure of his father's business caused him serious financial trouble. He
became a demonstrator to Dr. A. M. Kellas, who taught chemistry and
physics (with one assistant); he also undertook private coaching of students.

In 1919, Dr. Swale Vincent was appointed the first Professor of Physiology on his return from Winnipeg; he had made a name for himself through
his work on the endocrine glands. Dodds, who had obtained distinction in
physiology and pharmacology in March, 1919, was appointed assistant to
the new professor. The first Director of the Bland Sutton Institute for
Pathology at the Middlesex Hospital, Dr. Carl H. Browning, F.R.S. (who
died in 1970 aged 90), in 1919 appointed, Dr. E. L. Kennaway to be his first
assistant in Chemical Pathology and provided him with 2–3 rooms in his
new institute. (He became later Sir Ernest Kennaway, F.R.S., leader in
cancer research and discoverer of the first pure chemical carcinogens and
Director of Research at the Royal Marsden Hospital.) Dodds, still a medical
student, was appointed to Kennaway in 1920, and succeeded him in the
following year as 'Demonstrator in Biochemistry' as C. E. Dodds,
M.R.C.S., L.R.C.P. he passed his Primary F.R.C.S. in 1919, then obtained
an M.B., B.S. (Honours) London, proceeded Ph.D. in January, 1925,
M.D. London in July, 1925, M.R.C.P. London in 1927.

Dodds had a photographic memory (including the footnotes) and an ability for rapid reading. Mr. Samuel Augustine Courtauld, of Huguenot descent, was persuaded by the Dean of the Middlesex Medical School, Alfred Webb-Johnson, to endow a professorship on Dodds, in 1925, the Courtauld Chair of Biochemistry, and to provide funds for a New Institute of Biochemistry, which was finished in 1928 and of which Dodds became the first Director. Thus, Dodds was professor from the age of 25 to the age of 65! The graduate staff of the Institute rose during that time from the original 6 to 42.

Dodds' views on his reform of teaching of his subject were expressed in his paper 'The teaching of chemistry' (*Br. Med. J.* **2,** 505–508, 1949). One of his friends, Mr. Philip Hill, left in his estate in 1946 provision for a professorship in experimental biochemistry (first holder: F. Dickens, F.R.S.).

The necessity for blood analysis, especially after insulin, made large scale investigations essential. This could be achieved by adopting the colorimetric methods developed by Otto Folin in the United States. Because of this, Dodds and Dr. George Beaumont published in 1924 a book: *Recent Advances in Medicine*, new editions of which have been continued to the present time. It had a profound influence in Britain and abroad. During the illness of King George V, Lord Dawson of Penn called in Dodds for biochemical investigations, for which services he was awarded the decoration M.V.O. (Member of the Royal Victorian Order) in 1929.

In 1932 Dodds carried out an extended tour of the clinics and laboratories of North America (on Mr. Courtauld's generous cheque), on which he reported in the *Middlesex Hospital Journal*. Dodds then added a small ward to the Courtauld Institute with a sister in charge and proper nursing facilities. "In 1921, the total number of requests for analysis received by the Courtauld Institute amounted to 1060; in 1969, the figure was 200 000; by 1973 it reached 333 000 per annum!" In 1958, Dodds introduced the American machine known as the autoanalyser, which deals with 80% of the routine work. As an administrator, he had the ability to decentralize.

His personal researches were originally respiratory studies, influenced by Dr. Kellas and by J. S. Haldane of Oxford. Simultaneously, he participated with Dr. Izod Bennett in extensive studies of gastric secretion by means of the fractional test-meal (Bennett had worked with Ryle at Guy's); the results were published between 1921 and 1925. With Dr. J. D. Robertson, he also studied the role of lactic acid in gastric carcinoma (published in 1931). From 1923, he became involved in insulin research, together with F. Dickens. They published 'The chemical and physiological properties of the internal secretions' in 1925. During 1923 and 1930 they were interested in the purification of crude ovarian and placental extracts. In 1930, H. Allan, C. E. Dodds and F. Dickens developed a satisfactory assay method: 'Observations on the standardization of the water-soluble oestrus-producing hormone' (*J. Physiol.* **68,** 348–362, 1930).

From 1932, Dodds began his 'chapter of discoveries', based on the idea that there might be "modifications of basic structures which might still possess the same characteristic (oestrogenic) activity". Eventually, a collaboration between Kennaway, J. W. (now Sir James) Cook, F.R.S. and Dodds brought about the discovery of stilboestrol, the name of which was introduced by Dodds, L. Goldberg, W. Lawson and (later Sir) Robert Robinson in 1938: 'Oestrogenic activity of certain synthetic compounds' (*Nature, London* **141,** 247–248, 1938). Another substance, hexoestrol, which lacked the double bond present in (diethyl-) stilboestrol, was next presented as an artificial oestrogen. The clinical uses of these preparations need not be described at this point. Dodds had certainly made his mark in endocrine research.

Dodds also had interest in cancer research and was for many years Chairman of the Scientific Advisory Committee of the British Empire Cancer Campaign. He also showed great interest in Addison's disease. He delivered the first Addison's Lecture at Guy's in 1946 and the Centenary one in 1960. The discovery of aldosterone by Mrs. Simpson (now Mrs. Tait) occurred at the Courtauld Institute in 1952.

Dodds was a great traveller and became an honoured member of many international institutions. He became an Apothecary in 1934 and Master of the Worshipful Society of Apothecaries (London) in August, 1947. He was elected President of the Royal College of Physicians in London in 1962, and created a baronet in 1964. His coat of arms is the first in heraldry to contain a chemical formula, that of stilboestrol, to be seen in a stained glass window in the Great Hall of the Society of Apothecaries. He died in 1973, aged 74.

DOISY, Edward Adelbert   1893–

Edward A. Doisy was born in Hume, Illinois. He obtained his B.A. degree at the University of Illinois in 1914 and became Ph.D. Harvard in 1920. In 1923, he was appointed Professor of Biochemistry at the St. Louis University School of Medicine. In 1923 his celebrated collaboration with Edgar Allen occurred (see Allen), when they proved that the liquor folliculi of the ovaries and follicle cells exert an influence upon the oestrus through a hormone, thus giving the impetus to the prolonged research, which was eventually successful in unravelling the complex hormonal mechanism of the oestrous cycle and of pregnancy.

In 1943, Doisy shared the Nobel Prize with Carl Pieter Henrik Dam (b. 1895) for the isolation of Vitamin K from alfalfa.

In 1936, he delivered the Porter Lectures at the University of Kansas School of Medicine on 'Sex Hormones', in which he defined the "Four stages of endocrinology" (see Introduction).

ECKER, Alexander   1816–1887

Alexander Ecker was born in Freiburg in July, 1816, the son of Johann Matthias Alexander Ecker, who was Professor of Surgery in Freiburg and a

727

noted military surgeon (in the Imperial Austrian Army). He had classical training in Greek, studied in Freiburg and Heidelberg, qualifying in 1837, and proceeded Privat-Docent in Freiburg in 1839. He became Prosector and Docent in Heidelberg in 1841. In 1844, he moved as Ordinary Professor of Physiology and Anatomy to Basle and in 1850 in Freiburg.

He was the author of many scientific papers and monographs. He wrote on the movements of the brain and the spinal cord in 1843 ('Physiologische Untersuchungen ueber die Bewegungen des Gehirns und des Ruecken-markes'). In 1849, he contributed a chapter to L. Wagner's *Dictionary of Physiology* on 'The Blood vessel-glands', the name for the endocrine glands which even Falta used in 1913 and which is still officially recognized as an alternative ('Blutgefaessdruesen' fuer L. Wagner's Handwoerterbuch der Physiologie). In 1846, he had published a monograph on the finer structure of the suprarenals ('Der feinere Bau der Nebennieren', Braunschweig, 1846). At a much later stage he also published anthropological studies and an interesting autobiography in 1883.

He was a good representative of the celebrated group of German scientists of his time, who had a broad humanistic background and made such exceptional contributions to the progress of scientific research.

EISELSBERG, Anton Freiherr von
1860–1939

Anton von Eiselsberg was born in 1860, on the family estate of the Barons von Eiselsberg near Wels in Austria. After attending a monastic grammar school of the Benedictines, he studied medicine in Vienna, Würzburg, Zurich and Paris, qualifying in Vienna. He then became a surgical trainee under Billroth. In 1884, he was sent to Robert Koch (of Koch bacillus fame) in Berlin, to study bacteriological problems of anti- and asepsis. In 1887, he became Billroth's assistant, proceeding to Privat-Docent in 1890. His main thesis on that occasion was: 'On tetany following goitre surgery'. Three years later, he became Professor of Surgery at Utrecht, aged 33. In 1896, he became Professor of Surgery in Koenigsberg, and in 1901, he succeeded Billroth's colleague, Eduard Albert in Vienna. In 1909, he founded, together with his colleague, Julius von Hochenegg and the ophthalmologist Ernst Fuchs, the Accidents Departments within the surgical university

---

Figure 77 (left to right) Top row: Anton von Eiselsberg*; Herbert M. Evans†; Ch. F. Fritzsche†; Fielding Hudson Garrison‡. 2nd row: Regnier de Graaf; A. von Graefe‡; Robert James Graves°; Sir William W. Gull, Bart.‡. 3rd row: Ludwig Haberlandt*; Anton de Haen*; Josef Halban*. Bottom row: Albrecht von Haller; Sir Charles Robert Harington†; G. W. Harris; William Harvey[1]. (*by kind permission of the Institute for the History of Medicine, University of Vienna, Austria; †from Ciba Monograph No. 10, by kindness of Ciba-Geigy Ltd.; ‡by kind permission of Royal Society of Medicine, London; °by kind permission of Department of Medical Illustration, St. Bartholomew's Hospital, London EC1; [1]copyright National Portrait Gallery, London)

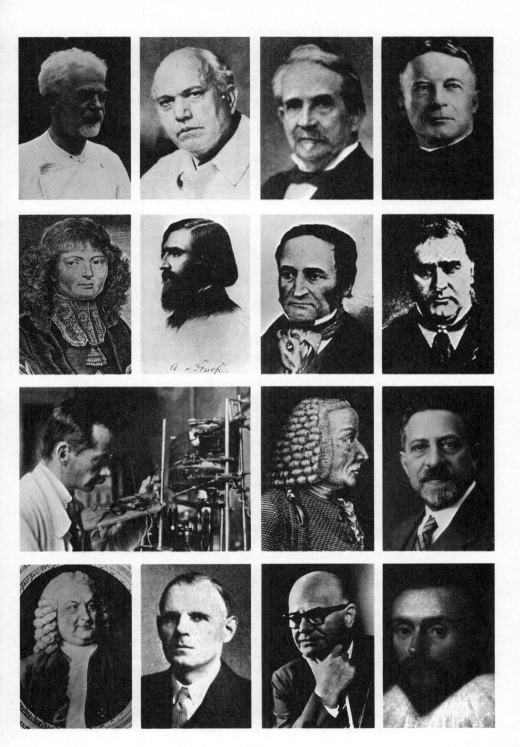

clinics. A friend of Billroth, Jaromir Mundy, had been the founder, in 1886, of the voluntary society for medical succour in accidents and emergencies, with its ambulances, trained personnel and doctors, in Vienna.

Eiselsberg's main fields of interest were thyroid surgery (supported by experimental physiological studies), abdominal surgery, and neuro-surgery. During the 1914–18 war, he organized 'surgical groups', which he continually visited and supervised personally, at the battle-fronts as well as at major surgical centres. There he laid the foundations for the development of independent units for facial, orthopaedic and neuro-surgery.

Many of his pupils (11) became professors of surgical chairs at universities, many more, heads of specialized surgical departments. He retired in September, 1931, still retaining great interest in and influence on the development of surgery. He died on 25 October, 1939, the victim of a railway accident.

ERDHEIM, Jacob   1874–1937

Jacob Erdheim was born in May, 1874 in Boryslaw, Galicia (then Austria). He went to grammar school in Drohobycz, and began his medical studies in Vienna in 1894, proceeding M.D. in 1900. He joined the Institute of morbid anatomy of Anton Weichselbaum (1845–1920), discoverer of the mening-ococcus, and of many other morbid conditions. Assistant in 1908, Privat-Docent in 1913, professor extraordinary in the same year, he became director of the Institute of Morbid Anatomy of the City (of Vienna) Hospital in Lainz in 1924, where he remained until his death. He was, to use a modern term, a 'workaholic', a bachelor who lived at the hospital and slept usually only from 1 to 4 a.m. He was a meticulous, very able, enthusiastic worker, a brilliant teacher, a convincing orator, with a superb style in writing, deeply honest, modest and self-effacing. His pupils came from far and wide (Albright spent a happy and productive year with him), and adored him. His scientific output was enormous, original, solidly founded and of the highest standard. It is impossible to give the extent of it in a thumbnail-sketch biography; for us, the most important contributions were his studies of pituitary tumours, the description of craniopharyngiomas (Erdheim's tumours), pituitary dwarfism, pregnancy changes in the pituit-ary, his work on the parathyroids, on the cartilage system and on its changes in acromegaly, and on bone disorders, especially Paget's disease. Erdheim's last important work, a study of the fingerjoints and Heberden's nodes, a typescript of 700 pages and 200 illustrations, was never published. It was found and destroyed during the Second World War during the course of the systematic destruction of Jewish property (except for valuables of a material nature).

During the 1914–18 war, although not in uniform (for medical reasons), he carried out duties to combat an epidemic of typhus in Serbia in 1915/16 with great energy and success; he also managed to deal with an outbreak of scurvy in a certain army group. He became known, near the frontline, a pathetic civilian figure, carrying out post-mortem examinations knee-deep in snow and under artillery bombardment. Another major field of research became the study of rickets. His brother, Sigmund, was a professor of surgery at the Policlinic in Vienna. Erdheim died suddenly of a heart attack in April, 1937.

FALLOPPIO (FALLOPIUS), Gabriele 1523–1562

Gabriele Falloppio was born in 1523 in Modena, going through great financial hardship as a medical student. He became one of the favourite pupils of Vesalius for whom he showed great veneration. In 1548 he became Professor of Anatomy in Ferrara, and shortly afterwards in Pisa. In 1551 he was appointed Professor of Anatomy and Botany in Padova.

He wrote many good treatises on anatomy, the best on the skeletal system and the development of the bones. He also gave a good account of the organ of hearing. His celebrated *Observationes anatomicae* appeared in Venice in 1561, a year before his untimely death at the age of 39. One of his writings: 'Lectiones de partis similaribus – et sceletorum explicationes' was published at Nuremberg in 1575. His second, most celebrated, book was *De morbo Gallico*, dealing with syphilis and its treatment (he was opposed to the use of mercury); he also distinguished between venereal and non-venereal condylomata. Falloppio died two years before Vesalius.

FALTA, Wilhelm 1875–1950

Wilhelm Falta was born in Karlsbad (Bohemia) in 1875. He eventually became assistant to von Noorden (of diabetes fame) in Vienna, where his main interest in endocrine and metabolic disorders developed. As head of a medical department of the Empress Elizabeth Hospital in Vienna, he established special laboratory facilities for the study and treatment of diabetes mellitus, which had international reputation. He also wrote a textbook of endocrinology, which appeared in 1913, soon after Biedl's and which also became one of the standard works on the subject and was translated into English in 1915. *The Diseases of the Bloodglands* was the first attempt at a systematic treatment of endocrine disorders. Falta's researches into the pathology of diabetes mellitus were of fundamental importance. He proceeded to Privat-Docent and Professor of Medicine Extraordinary in due course and was shortlisted for the succession of Wenkebach. He died in Vienna in July, 1950, in his 76th year.

FELLNER, Otfried Otto   1873–19??

Otto O. Fellner was born in September, 1873 in Vienna, the son of a doctor. He was educated at the celebrated 'Academic Gymnasium' and at the University of Vienna, where he qualified in 1898. As a medical student, he was interested in the obstetric and gynaecological lectures of Rudolf Chrobak (1843–1910), whose assistant Emil Knauer (1867–1935) had just undertaken experimental ovarian transplants in rabbits. The next summer (1896), Fellner attended the lectures of Friedrich Schauta (1849–1919), where Joseph Halban (1870–1937) was soon to carry out his ovarian transplants and demonstrate the endocrine function of the ovary. After qualifying, he took up gynaecology and was for four years surgical trainee (resident intern) at Schauta's clinic. He did not achieve an assistantship, but went into private medicine. At the same time, he carried out his own private studies in the field of reproductive endocrinology, mainly at the Institute for General and Experimental Pathology of the University of Vienna, where Artur Biedl became his guide and mentor. After Biedl's departure to Prague in 1914, Fellner carried on at the Institute, and as late as 1935, published papers from there. Before confirming Ludwig Haberlandt's (1885–1932) work, Fellner made considerable fundamental contributions to the concept of hormonal contraception, from 1913 onwards, and to gonadal and placental endocrine function. He was also one of the first to observe the effects of X-ray radiation on the ovaries, and the histological changes of the ovaries during pregnancy. His co-operation and, later, controversy with Haberlandt, became well known to a limited circle of people at the time. Working privately as a specialized gynaecologist, Fellner's work was conveniently overlooked by the University of Vienna, from which he never received any recognition. It was largely forgotten and is still widely unknown, although George W. Corner discussed some of his work (Fellner was one of the first to use organic solvents and thus obtain potent ovarian and placental extracts), and H. H. Simmer wrote an important paper on Fellner's work (see Chapter 19). Fellner was Jewish and seems to have disappeared without trace in Hitler's Teutonic holocaust.

FRÄNKEL, Ludwig   1870–1950

Ludwig Fränkel was born Louis Fränkel in April, 1870, the son of a Jewish malt factory owner, in Leobschuetz, Prussian-Silesia. He had a brother and a sister who were both killed during Hitler's rule. He had a humanistic grammar school education in Leobschuetz, before studying medicine at Wurzburg, Berlin, Greifswald, Munich and Freiburg im Breisgau. He qualified in Freiburg in 1893, after receiving his M.D. Berlin a year earlier (1892) for his thesis on the treatment of ankylosis of the elbow joint. His uncle, Ernst Fränkel (1844–1921) had become a Privat-Docent in Breslau in

732

1873 and received the title Professor in 1893. Ernst Fränkel had an extensive practice, mainly of obstetrics and gynaecology, and taught students at home and in his own private hospital, where he also had an experimental laboratory. Although he originally discouraged his nephew from pursuing academic medicine, he allowed him to work in his laboratory. He also influenced him to take up the practice of gynaecology and obstetrics, and, at 26, Louis (Ludwig) joined his uncle's private hospital, of which he later became chief. When Fränkel began his experiments on the function of the ovary which led to the crucial investigation in May and June, 1900, with the then medical student Franz Cohn, he was already well trained in obstetrics and gynaecology, having studied under Hegar in Freiburg, Saenger in Leipzig and Kuestner in Breslau. He was, however, particularly influenced by Gustav Born (1851–1900), the brilliant experimental embryologist in Breslau, whose theories he intended to prove.

The University of Breslau recognized his scientific achievements by making him a Privat-Docent in 1905 and granting him the title of Professor in 1909, a rare occurrence there in the case of an academic outsider and a Jew to wit. In 1921, he proceeded Professor Extraordinary, and in 1923, when Otto Ernst Kuestner (1850–1931) resigned, he succeeded him to the chair of obstetrics and gynaecology. He founded, in this capacity, a clinical school. In 1930, when he was 60, German gynaecologists and his students dedicated an issue of the *Archiv fuer Gynaecologie* to Fränkel (= Festschrift); but in 1933, he was no longer allowed to speak at the Annual Congress of the German Society of Gynaecology: "Though we esteem these persons", the president said, "and value their contributions highly, . . . they are regrettable victims of hardship, which has become necessary for the recuperation of the German people" (W. Stoeckel). Fränkel also lost his position as professor. In 1936, he left Germany and in 1937, he was offered a position as lecturer and consultant in Montevideo (Uruguay). He again engaged in active research and founded a school. On his 70th birthday, he was honoured with a 'Festschrift' in Spanish. This was followed by another on his 80th birthday, also in Montevideo, and soon after he was elected an Honorary Professor of the University of Montevideo. In 1951, just before his death, the German Gynaecological Society made him an honorary member. He died in July, 1951 while travelling in Europe, in Bad Ischl, Austria. His last paper was received for publication five days after his death. It was the study of the corpus luteum of the armadillo.

FRANK, Johann Peter   1745–1821

Johann Peter Frank hailed from Rotalben (Palatinate) and Garrison refers to him as "A rare and happy mixture of German thoroughness with French intelligence". This reminds me of a favourite dictum of the late Eric Benjamin Strauss, D.M. Oxon, F.R.C.P., Psychiatrist to St. Bartholomew's Hospital, London (England) from 1938 to 1959: "How splendid it would be, to have a standard textbook of psychiatry written by a combined effort of Gallic wit and elegance, German thoroughness and British lucidity, brevity and self-effacing criticism!"

Frank worked his way up from poverty by his own ability and industry, to lay the foundation of modern public hygiene, culminating in his nine volume work *System einer vollstaendigen medicinischen Policey* (= System of a complete medical Police; Mannheim, Tuebingen, Wien: Schwann, 1779–1827). It dealt with water supply, sewerage, sexual hygiene, taxation of bachelors, school-meals, school-hygiene, the idea of a scientific 'medical police', in a word, preventive medicine from the cradle to the grave, long before Josef von Pettenkofer (1818–1901) in the mid-19th century. Frank also wrote important studies on the spinal cord: 'De vertebralis columnae in morbis dignitate' (in *Delect. opusc. Med. Ticini* **11,** 1–50, 1792) and on therapeutics: *De curandis hominum morbis epitome* (7 volumes, Mannheimi, Tubingae, Viennae, Taurini; C. F. Schwann and C. G. Goetz, 1792–1825). In volume V of the last work (pp. 38–67) he first defined diabetes insipidus.

He had originally studied philosophy in Metz in 1761 and at Pont-à-Mousson in 1762, where he became Ph.D. in 1763. In 1765 he began the study of medicine in Heidelberg, Strasbourg, and Heidelberg again, where he proceeded M.D. in 1766. He went into practice in Bitsch, in France, after first passing a medical examination in Pont-à-Mousso. In 1767, he moved to Baden-Baden, in 1769 to Rastatt where he became 'Garnisons- und Stadtarzt'. In 1772 he went to Speier as personal physician to the Prince-bishop. He became Lecturer in Anatomy and Surgery at Bruchsal, where he founded an institute for the training of midwives. There he remained for 9 years. In 1784 he went to Goettingen as Professor of Medicine, but could not tolerate the climate. In 1786, he moved to Pavia as successor to S. A. Tissot (1728–1797), where he was also Director of the Hospital and Director General of Medicine in Lombardy and Protophysicus. In 1788 he became Superintendent of all hospitals in Lombardy and Mantua, and designed a new syllabus of medical education for the universities. In 1795 he turned up in Vienna, Austria, as organizer of army medicine. He also became Director of the Allgemeines Krankenhaus (= General Hospital) and Clinical Professor at the very high salary of 5000 guilders per annum. There he founded the Pathologisch–anatomisches Museum, created the post of Prosector in Pathology at the Allgemeines Krankenhaus (first holder: Alois Rudolph Vetter (1765–1806)). In Vienna, he encountered the hostility of the powerful clergy, because he was against the celibacy. He also suffered from the professional jealousy and envy of his colleagues. In 1804, he moved, therefore, as Professor of Clinical Medicine to Wilna, with his son Joseph, who became Professor of Pathology, but only ten months later he accepted a call to St. Petersburg as personal physician to the Emperor Alexander and Professor at the medico-surgical Academy, there. In 1808, he retired with a pension of 3000 roubles and returned to Vienna, where Napoleon consulted him in 1809. Napoleon called him to Paris as his personal physician, but the plan was not successful, because of the resistance of the doctors in Paris. Next, he moved to Freiburg, but returned to Vienna in 1811. There he was engaged mainly in literary work and 'Nobelpraxis' (= private practice among the nobility). He died in April, 1821, much mourned by the population. He was a great clinician and, in spite of his restlessness, a man with a very broad knowledge of medicine and of people.

GALENOS   130–200 AD

Galenos was born at Pergamus, the son of an architect. His youth and old age were peripatetic. Garrison, in fact, says (p. 112): "His life was one long 'Wanderjahr'" (but see also the biography of Johann Peter Frank).

He started practice in Rome in 164 AD, soon rising to the top of the medical profession. After a comparatively short time he gave up his practice, however, and returned to his studies, travels and teaching. He was a highly skilled practitioner, but his successes were more often flashes of brilliance, rather than the result of a systematic and methodical approach. Similarly, his methods of treatment were not often along singular, logical lines of consideration, but more often polypharmacy, "the memory of which survives in our language in the term 'galenicals' as applied to vegetable simples" (Garrison: An Introduction to the History of Medicine; 4th ed. Reprinted. p. 112, Philadelphia and London. W. B. Saunders Co., 1929).

He was the most prolific medical author of ancient times and his writings are encyclopaedic. His anatomical descriptions were based mainly on dissection of animals (apes and swine), the neurology being the best part of his studies. He knew seven pairs of the twelve cerebral nerves; he discerned the pia from the dura mater, the third and fourth ventricles, the aquaeductus Sylvii ('iter'), the corpora quadrigemina, calamus, hypophysis and infundibulum. He was a good experimental neurologist and physiologist. Reference to endocrine considerations was made in Chapter 7 of the first section of this book.

Unfortunately, he indulged in strange hypotheses, based on his idea that everything in nature reflects some basic design and the goodness of the Creator. It was "a skilful and well-instructed special pleading for the cause of design in nature" (M. Neuburger).

GARRISON, Fielding Hudson   1870–1935

F. H. Garrison was born in Washington, D.C., the son of a civil servant from Virginia. He became one of the first students at the Johns Hopkins University, where he obtained his B.A. in 1890.

In 1891, he entered the Surgeon-General's Library under John Shaw Billings (1838–1913), its founder, who, incidentally, had also helped to design the Johns Hopkins Hospital, Baltimore. At the same time, Garrison also continued to study medicine and qualified as a doctor. He became an army medical librarian and was commissioned in the U.S. Army Medical Corps, in which capacity he had to serve in Manila from 1922 to 1924, the only time he left the library until his retirement in 1930. In 1918, he had been promoted Lt.-colonel. He retired with the rank of Colonel.

After his retirement, he became Director of the Library of the Johns Hopkins Medical School in Baltimore and Lecturer in the History of Medicine. He was a great lover of mathematics and of music. He died in April 1935 of carcinoma of the colon.

Garrison gained international reputation through his many medical historical studies and publications, but especially through his magnum opus: *An Introduction to the History of Medicine*, published in Philadelphia and London by W. B. Saunders Co., the fourth edition of which was published in 1929, and reprinted many times. On Sir William Osler's suggestion, Garrison compiled a bibliography of the most important contributions to the literature of medicine and its associated sciences. This first appeared in the Index-Catalogue of the Library of the Surgeon-General's Office, Washington, 1912, 2nd Series, XVII, pp. 89–178, from which, eventually, emerged the now celebrated *A Medical Bibliography* (Garrison and Morton), "An annotated check-list of texts illustrating the history of medicine", by Leslie T. Morton, F.L.A., Librarian, National Institute for Medical Research, London, 3rd edition (2nd impression), London. André Deutsch; Sept. 1976. He also wrote an excellent biography of John Shaw Billings after the latter's death. In 1924 his contribution to *Endocrinology and Metabolism presented in their Scientific and Practical Clinical Aspects by Ninety-eight Contributors*, edited by L. F. Barker (5 Vols., New York, Appleton, 1922–24) was 'History of Endocrine Doctrine' (Vol. 1, pp. 45–78).

GEE, Samuel   1839–1911

Samuel Gee was born in London in September, 1839, the son of William Gee and his wife Lydia Sutton. Educated at University College School in London, 1852–54, he studied medicine at University College Hospital, where he qualified in 1861 and proceeded M.D. in 1865. He was elected a Fellow of the Royal College of Physicians in 1870. He was a house-surgeon at the Hospital for Sick Children, Great Ormond Street in London, in 1865, and in 1878, he was elected physician to St. Bartholomew's Hospital in London, where he became consulting physician in 1904, but continued to work until his death. He was also physician to the Hospital for Sick Children in Great Ormond Street and became an authority on children's diseases. He was Goulstonian Lecturer, Bradshaw Lecturer and Lumleian Lecturer of the Royal College of Physicians. His numerous papers on medical subjects have all retained permanent value. Many appeared in *St. Bartholomew's Hospital Reports*. They are all succinct, clearly and simply presented, strictly factual and display a very high standard of clinical observation. The one quoted in Chapter 16, perhaps the first description of familial nephrogenic diabetes insipidus, is an observation recorded in a two page note! In 1870, he wrote on *Auscultation and Percussion together with other Methods of Physical Examination of the Chest*, which saw many editions during fifty years. His only other book was *Medical Lectures and Aphorisms* in 1902. His many observations and descriptions justly deserve to be called scientific discoveries.

He was Librarian to the Royal Medical and Chirurgical Society and had a wide knowledge of books on medicine. He also had an extensive medical practice, and his Gee's linctus (Linctus Scillae Opiatus) is still in use. Samuel Gee died suddenly of a heart attack in Keswick in August, 1911, and his ashes were deposited at Kensal Green Cemetery in London.

GLEY, Eugène   1857–1930

Eugène Gley was born in January, 1857 at Epinal in France and studied at Nancy, qualifying in 1881. In 1883, he became Praeparator of Practical Physiology in Paris and in 1889, Professeur Agrégé at the Faculty in Paris. In 1893, he became Assistant at the Museum (Musée) d'Histoire Naturelle; in 1908, he obtained the chair of General Biology at the Collège de France. He died in October, 1930 in Paris.

Gley carried out research in the field of immunity and endocrinology. He was a co-founder of Opotherapy (treatment with oral administration of thyroid): 'Essais de philosophie et d'histoire de la biologie' (in: *Traité Pathol. Gén.* **3;** Paris, 1900). He became a member of the 'Académie de Médecine'.

He did valuable work on the heart muscle (1888). In 1891, he demonstrated the existence of iodine in the blood and the thyroid gland, its internal secretion and pathology ('Sur les fonctions du corps thyroïde': *C.R. Soc. Biol.* (Paris) **43,** 841–847, 1891).

He re-discovered the parathyroids, but later came across Sandstroem's description and acknowledged his priority. He seems, however, to have been the first to understand their real significance and their necessity for the maintenance of life.

His role during the crisis of endocrinology in Spain and antagonism to Marañon, has already been discussed in Chapter 18. Similiarly, the extraordinary affair in connection with the discovery of insulin and Gley's role in it, was discussed in Chapter 19.

GOLTZ, Friedrich Leopold   1834–1902

Friedrich Leopold Goltz was born in 1834 in Posen (Poznan, Poland), at that time in East Prussia. He was one of the pupils of the celebrated Hermann Ludwig Ferdinand von Helmholtz (1821–1894). He became Professor of Physiology at Halle in 1870; he moved to Strasbourg in the same capacity in

1872 and remained there until his death in 1902. His main work was the determination of the functions of the hemispheres of the brain and of the spinal cord. His highly skilled experiments on the decerebrated animal and on that with a severed spinal cord were crucial. He carried out other important studies on the mechanism of shock (1862) and on the semicircular canals (1870).

He and Ernst Julius Richard Ewald (1855–1921) succeeded in impregnating a bitch after her spinal cord had been severed ('Der Hund mit verkuerztem Rueckenmark'. *Pfluegers Arch. Ges. Physiol* **63,** 362–400, 1896) (see also Chapter 15).

De GRAAF, Regnier   1641–1673

Regnier de Graaf was born at Schoonhaven in Holland in 1641, the son of an architect. Regnier became a pupil of Sylvius (1614–72) (= Franciscus de la Boë) in Leyden. Haller related that he had a serious altercation with Jan Swammerdam (1637–80), who contested de Graaf's priority of observations on the gonads. Although de Graaf won his case, the stress of it cost him his life. On the death of Sylvius, de Graaf was offered the chair at Leyden, but he refused to accept it.

Whatever the cause and nature of his death, de Graaf crammed into the short 32 years of his life an amazing number of brilliant experiments and observations, especially on the gonads and on the function of the pancreas. It is, therefore, fitting to count him among the very great scientists of any age. The high reputation he acquired during his life was more than justified. It should be added that his literary style was also of the highest order and his ability to express himself in Latin is still a pleasure to read. Apart from clarity and elegance he was also witty, with a pleasant sense of humour. He died in 1673.

GRAVES, Robert James   1796–1853

Robert James Graves was the son of a Professor of Divinity in the University of Dublin and a descendant of a Colonel in Cromwell's army. He studied medicine in Edinburgh but took his M.B. in Dublin in 1818. He went on a grand tour for three years, where he met J. M. W. Turner in Switzerland and they travelled together for some months. Sailing from Genoa to Sicily, a storm almost wrecked the boat, but Graves saved the ship by repairing the pumps with the leather of his boots.

Graves returned to Dublin in 1821 and was appointed physician to Meath Hospital, where he organized medical education with Stokes. They introduced bedside teaching and encouraged students to take notes and to examine patients. Graves's *Clinical Lectures on the Practice of Medicine* in 1843 was welcomed by Trousseau. Graves was elected a Fellow of the Royal Society in 1849. He was a brilliant student, highly cultured, handsome and charming. He died, probably of congestive heart failure, after a long illness in 1853.

The term Graves' disease is still the one most commonly used in Anglo-Saxon countries for the most important form of hyperfunction of the thyroid gland.

GULL, Sir William Withey, Bart.
1816–1890

William W. Gull was born in Colchester, Essex, in 1816, the youngest son of a barge owner, who died when William was 10 years old. In 1837, Benjamin Harrison, Treasurer of Guy's Hospital, made him an apprentice at Guy's, with residence and fifty pounds a year. In 1841 Gull was medical tutor; for ten years he lived in the hospital, being in turn, assistant to the apothecary, house-physician, superintendent on the lunatic wards and resident physician. In 1849, he became Fullerton Professor of Physiology at the Royal Institution and, in 1851, Assistant Physician to Guy's Hospital. Because of his extensive practice, he resigned from the staff of the hospital in 1865. He was elected F.R.S. in 1869. In 1871 he treated the Prince of Wales for typhoid fever, and was made a baronet in 1872. Although one of the leading London physicians, he never became president of the Royal College of Physicians.

He was a great clinical observer and diagnostician. His description (with H. G. Sutton) of arterio-capillary fibrosis in 1872 was evidence of his wide knowledge of medicine. He showed great interest in J. T. MacLagan's new salicylate treatment of rheumatic fever. He was a versatile man, with a great amount of human understanding, never in a hurry, and known for his aphorisms. He comforted a neurotic: "You are a healthy man out of health". He was religious in the sense of a Christian agnostic and a friend of James Hinton (1822–1875), author of *The Mystery of Pain*. He was an admirer of Sir Thomas Browne's *Religio Medici*. He himself wrote well and in a good style, although he never published a major work. He died at the beginning of 1890 from a third stroke, leaving over £344,000 (much of it "due to well-advised investments").

Gull is, of course, best known for his classical description of myxoedema in 1873.

HABERLANDT, Ludwig   1885–1932

Born in February, 1885, in Graz, Austria, Ludwig Haberlandt was the son of a (non-medical) university professor. He studied medicine in Graz, where he qualified in 1909. He then worked in physiology in Graz, Berlin and in Innsbruck, where he proceeded to Privat-Docent in 1913 and to Professor Extraordinary in 1919. He died of a heart attack in Innsbruck in

July, 1932, aged 47. He was a "thorough research worker, full of new ideas" (obituary by Ernst Theodor von Bruecke, 1880–1941).

Apart from hormonal contraception, Haberlandt made contributions to the physiology of the heart and searched for the so-called 'heart-hormone'. In his research on hormonal contraceptives, he had been stimulated by some of Steinach's experiments. Progesterone was isolated soon after his death, but not then used as a contraceptive. His co-operation and later quarrel with O. O. Fellner was discussed in Chapter 19 (Section I).

HAEN, Anton de   1704–1776

de Haen was born in Holland and was a student with (later Baron) Gerard van Swieten in Leyden, where they were both pupils of Herman Boerhave (1668–1738), the 'Communis Europae . . . magister', as his other pupil, Albrecht von Haller, called him. On van Swieten's (1700–1772) recommendation, he was called to Vienna in 1754, where he was put in charge of six men's and six women's beds at the Buergerspital (= Citizen's Hospital). He was also granted permission to bring patients from other hospitals for teaching purposes. de Haen, like van Swieten, introduced Boerhave's method of teaching at the bedside (i.e. on patients who κλίνειν = are lying in bed), hence the term 'clinical' or bedside teaching. Attempts at bedside teaching were made in Padova in the 16th century, but it did not become established because of student resistance. Like Boerhave, de Haen deprecated rigid systems in the teaching and practice of medicine. His preference was an unbiased approach to the patient at the bedside, meticulous history taking and observation, followed by a thorough clinical examination, on the basis of which one should arrive at the diagnosis and at a plan of rational treatment. This also led to the beginnings of experimental pharmacology under his pupil and assistant Anton von Stoerck (1731–1803), who tried the action of extracts from local plants on animals, nearly a century before Buchheim of Dorpat's (1820–1879) *Textbook of Pharmacology* ('Lehrbuch der Arzneimittellehre', Leipzig, L. Voss, 1856).

De Haen was against direct smallpox inoculation because of its dangers; Jenner's vaccination with cowlymph did not become known until nearly 20 years after de Haen's death. Apart from attempting a diagnosis at the bedside, followed by frequent observation of the course of the disease and of the result of the treatment, de Haen insisted on a post-mortem examination in the case of death. Moreover, he was the originator of the annual publication in book form of the most interesting case histories, the results of examinations and of the treatment given and of post-mortem reports of patients seen during the year, in form of Antonii de Haen's *Ratio Medendi in Nosocomio Practico*. In *Pars Quinta Rationis Medendi* (Viennae, Austriae, 1760), there is on pp. 264–272, the description of a girl of 20, with vomiting, amenorrhoea and loss of vision with severe headache. A trephining operation was carried out, but the patient died five days later.

Post-mortem examination showed inflammation of and pus in the meninges and apparently a tumour in the infundibulum (= pituitary tumour): "Notabile autem maxime infundibulum. 1° Maximum fuit, octo vel novem linearum diametrum habens. 2° Repletum fuit materia grisea, quae partim pultacea, partim calcarea fuit. 3^{tio} Concretum erat cum pia matre Opticos involvente. 4to Insidebat, premebarque ipsum Opticorum coalitum; non quidem ita, ut Optici nervi post coalitum marcescerent, sed saltem sic, ut videretur illorum actio interurbata fuisse, puellaque caeca fuissa mansura, etiam si male haud supcessisset operatio".

From a contemporary report in 1774 on de Haen's method of teaching at the bedside, it is interesting to note how tactful he was in dealing with his students. He himself began work at the hospital at 6 a.m. (winter and summer), and his students assembled at 8 a.m. Leading them to the bedside of a patient, he described the case in great detail as to history, causes and symptomatology. Next, the students examined the patient, and each then whispered his observations into de Haen's ear, who then discussed the correct and incorrect ones without personal reference, thereby saving face for the individual student. At 9 a.m. the consultations for out-patients began. Everyone was carefully questioned and examined by de Haen, in the presence of the students. The history is recorded in a book by an amanuensis, and the condition and the proposed treatment are discussed and written down. If Boerhave had already used the thermometer, de Haen introduced its routine use and, by doing so, he made a number of important observations concerning body temperature.

After de Haen's death in 1776, four years after van Swieten, the method of 'clinical', i.e. bedside, teaching was faithfully continued by all his successors, supported by the use of Leopold von Auenbrugger's (1722–1809) new invention, the percussion of the chest, first published in 1761 ('Inventum novum ex percussione thoracis humani ut signo abstrusos interni pectoris morbos detegendi.' Vindobonae, J. T. Trattner, 1761). (See Wyklicky, H.: Anton de Haen, 1704–1776. *Materia Therapeutica, Dr. Kutiak*; pp. 56–60; Vienna, 1962.)

HALBAN, Josef 1870–1937

Joseph Halban was born in October, 1870 in Vienna, where he also studied. In 1897, he became surgical trainee under the gynaecologist Schauta. Halban was influenced by the work of Alois Lode (1866–1950), later Professor of Hygiene at Innsbruck, who repeated Berthold's testicle transplant experiments in Vienna in 1891, and by Emil Knauer's experiments in 1895 of ovarian transplants in mature castrated female rabbits. In 1897, therefore, he began experimenting with ovarian transplants. In December, 1899, he reported on his experiments. He concluded that the only explanation of Knauer's and his own experiments was an internal secretion of the ovaries, although as recently as 1895, Schaefer in London, had decided against such a possibility. Halban obtained permission to experiment on four female baboons of the Vienna Zoo. He disproved the nervous impulse theory of menstruation in favour of the internal secretion of the ovaries. (To-day, neuroendocrinology seems to favour a combination of nervous and humoral impulses.) Halban also postulated from these experiments that the target organs must respond to the hormones, in order to show an effect. He was then involved in an argument with Ludwig Fränkel (Dec., 1903) on the role of the corpora lutea triggering off menstruation. Contrary to Fränkel's view, Halban could demonstrate in experiments on corpora lutea, with his assistant Koehler, that menstruation starts when the action of the corpus luteum ceases. These experiments were overlooked and forgotten. Halben also observed increased hair-growth in the majority of pregnant women (Halban's pregnancy sign) and amenorrhoea in the case of persistent cystic corpora lutea (Halban's disease). Incidentally Hermann Rubinstein of Dorpat had, in 1899, come to the conclusion of an internal secretion, quite independently of Halban's work.

Halban's most important contribution to endocrinology was perhaps the recognition of an endocrine function of the placenta, mainly by deduction (in 1904–1905) rather than by experiment. The edocrine actions of the placenta were similar to those of the ovaries, but much more marked. That was proved experimentally, about ten years later by O. O. Fellner and Herrmann. Halban was, however, mistaken in his opinion that the secondary sex characteristics are genetically fixed and only influenced by the gonads. He did not know of the isolation and synthesis of pure gonadal hormones. Halban was more a speculative, theoretical researcher than a strictly analytical and experimental one. The experiments he did carry out were, however, carefully thought out and convincing. It must not be overlooked that in addition to his research work, he had an extensive private practice and also carried on busy surgical work as head of a large gynaecological department of a major, though non-teaching, hospital. He proceeded to Private-Docent in 1903 and Professor Extraordinary in 1909.

He was also very interested in the arts, especially in music; his wife was a well known opera singer (Miss Selma Kurz) at the Vienna Opera. He had considerable private means and was used to doing things in style. He died in Vienna in 1937, aged 67.

HALLER, Albrecht von   1708–1777

Albrecht von Haller was born in 1708, scion of an old established bourgeois aristocratic family of Berne, Switzerland. He wrote Latin poetry, when aged 10. At 16, he disproved Professor Coskwitz's theory that the lingual vein was a salivary duct. He graduated at Leyden, his teachers being Boerhave, Albinus, Winslow and John Bernouilli. He soon went to Goettingen, to the newly established university, where he remained for 17 years. There he taught all branches of medicine, founded botanic gardens, wrote about 1300 scientific papers and did a lot of experimental work. In 1753, aged 45, he returned to Berne, where he remained until his death in 1777. There he filled every local post, including that of Public Health Officer.

Von Haller was an eminent botanist, anatomist and physiologist, wrote poetry and historical novels. He had an enormous and international correspondence and became one of the founders of medical and scientific bibliography. He was also a master of anatomical illustration (*Icones anatomicae*, 8 parts, Goettingae, A. Vandenhoek, 1743–1756). The Haller-niaum at Berne represents his work as that of the founder of modern physiology. His main single contribution is his demonstration of Francis Glisson's (1597–1677) hypothesis of irritability (contractility) as a specific, immanent characteristic of all muscular tissue, and sensibility an exclusive property of nervous tissue, thus distinguishing between the two ('De partibus corporis humani sensibilibus et irritabilibus'. *Comment. Soc. Reg. Sci. Goetting.*, **2**, 114–158, 1752/53). This study was based on 567 experiments in Goettingen in 1757, of which 190 were carried out by himself! There he also began his magnum opus *Elementa physiologiae corporis humani* (Lausanne, Berne, 1757–1766). He thus became the greatest systematist since Galen. He also became one of the foremost historians of medicine (*Methodus studii medicinae*, Amsterdam, 1751). Although he also wrote on surgery and compiled an excellent bibliography of the subject (*Bibliotheca chirurgica*. Berne, 1774–1775), he never performed an operation during his life. He was sensitive, humble, charitable and kindly, but not afraid to admit ignorance, but he left no schools of pupils behind. His reputation was enormous.

He also created a niche for himself in German literature and, especially, in alpine and nature poetry, with his long poem '*Die Alpen*' (= the Alps).

He has always been regarded as one of the giants, during his life-time and afterwards.

His grouping of thymus, thyroid and spleen as glands without ducts, was mentioned in the "Introduction" and in Chapter 14.

It was Haller who introduced the term 'Evolution' (evolvere, Latin, = to unroll). As a 'preformationist' (like Spallanzani), he maintained that embryos grew from preformed homunculi in the egg and are 'unfolded'. In contrast, William Harvey (1578–1657) had suggested (in his "De generatione animalium"), his theory of 'epigenesis', i.e. that the organism does not exist preformed in the ovum, but develops from it by gradual building up of its parts. This was long before Caspar Friedrich Wolff (1733–1794) of Berlin and of Wolffian bodies' fame, revived Harvey's ideas in his 'Theoria Generationis' (Halae ad Salam, 1759) and in 'De formatione intestinorum praecipue' (*Novi Comment. Acad. Sci. Petropol.* **12**, 43–47, 1768, etc.), which was translated by Johann Friedrich Meckel the Younger (1781–1833) and popularized in 1812. He was followed by Carl Ernst von Baer (1792–1876), the 'father of new embryology' (Garrison) and of the mammalian ovum fame (see also Chapter 15), and by Johannes Friedrich Blumenbach (1752–1840), who both rejected the preformation theory in favour of epigenesis as the correct explanation of evolution.

HARINGTON, Sir Charles Robert
1897–1972

Charles Robert Harington was born in August, 1897, in North Wales, the son of a clergyman. Harington was a member, by unbroken descent, of the senior surviving branch to Robertus de Hafrinctuna, Lord of the Manor of Flemingby in Cumberland in the 12th century. There had been two peerages in the family, one in the 14th and one in the 17th century, but both became extinct. John Harington of Kelstone, godson of Queen Elizabeth I, was a poet, courtier, soldier and inventor: he invented the water closet.

When Harington was four, his father moved to Herefordshire and from there to Worcestershire in 1912, where he died in 1921. In 1906, Harington was sent to preparatory school at Malvern Wells, where he developed tuberculosis of the hip. He was laid up at home for four years completely immobilized, and for the following two years he could walk only with the help of a stick. It left him with a shortened leg and a permanent limp. Fortunately, he received excellent private tuition at home from a family friend, a retired clergyman and former headmaster of a school. Although excluded from team games and military service, he indulged in long walks over the Pennine moors; in the 1930s, he took up mountaineering in the Alps, and until his mid-sixties he went trout fishing each year, wading in rough upland rivers. In 1912, he won an entrance scholarship to Malvern College, which he took up in 1914. In 1916, he won a mathematical exhibition to Magdalene College, Cambridge, where he went into residence in October, 1916. He had to abandon his planned engineering career for health reasons and took up natural sciences. He obtained a first class in the Natural Sciences Tripos, Part I, in chemistry, physics, physiology and zoology, but he did not stay on to take Part II, perhaps because Cambridge was full of ex-service men. He spent 1919–1920 under George Barger in the Department of Medical Chemistry. Later, he acknowledged a debt of gratitude for Barger's inspiration. Next, he was appointed Research Assistant in the Department of Therapeutics at the Royal Infirmary, Edinburgh under Professor J. C. Meakins, where he remained until 1922, during which time he produced four papers. The fourth paper, on variations in protein metabolism, published in 1924, was co-authored by Dr. J. M. Craig, his future wife. In 1922, he obtained his Ph.D.

On Barger's recommendation, he became Lecturer in Chemical Pathology at University College Hospital Medical School, a newly created post, but was allowed to spend the first year in the United States, mainly at the Hospital of the Rockefeller Institute in New York, under D. D. Van Slyke, but also with H. D. Dakin and Otto Folin. He wrote papers with Van Slyke which were mainly on application of gasometric methods to the analysis of the blood, which Harington later introduced into clinical chemistry in England. He was, however, disappointed by the lack of co-operation between the different departments of the Rockefeller Institute. On his return to England he married Dr. Jessie M. Craig, who was medically qualified.

He returned to the Medical School, and across the road, there were 18 Fellows of the Royal Society, his colleagues. Its reputation was so high that the Rockefeller Foundation of New York had just granted them a considerable donation, part of which enabled Harington to devote himself to the problem of thyroid research. He also developed his talents as a scientific administrator and from 1930 to 1950, he was the editor of the *Biochemical Journal*. In 1938, he was appointed a member of the Medical Research Council for the usual four year term.

On the retirement of Sir Henry Dale as Director of The National Institute for Medical Research in 1942, Harington was elected as his successor as the best candidate, although he himself was not medically qualified. He was admirably suited for the post; moreover, it relieved him from undergraduate teaching, which had never been the favourite part of his duties.

The isolation and synthesis of thyroxine was discussed in Chapter 18. In 1929, Harington and S. S. Randall showed that DL-3:5-diiodotyrosine accounted for 14% of the iodine in the thyroid (*Biochem. J.* **23**, 373, 1929). Harington's book on the thyroid gland, published in 1933, has also been mentioned, It has become a classic, although some of it is now outdated. It is, however, remarkable how superbly he connected the chemistry of the subject with the physiology, history, pathology and the clinical aspects. His scholarship was as evident as his original contributions and his general critical assessment.

Apart from his major research interest, he also made important contributions to the study of antihormones and immunochemistry and to the synthesis of glutathione with T. H. Mead in 1935 (*Biochem. J.* **29**, 1602, 1935). He had become Reader in 1928, Professor in 1931, a Knight Bachelor in 1948. His range of interests in biochemistry was wide; but his particular ability to understand, assess and appreciate the significance of developments outside his own subject, were of particular importance after he had become Director of the National Institute of Medical Research in 1942, which he remained until 1962. Thus it was possible that the progress of the achievements of N.I.M.R. was maintained and enhanced. Although its growth was natural, it was enormous. When Harington started, there was a scientific staff of 45 at Hampstead. At the time of the move to Mill Hill, the staff numbered 80. When he retired in 1962, there were 145 scientists. During his directorship, 14 members of the staff became Fellows of the Royal Society, and five did so shortly after his retirement. Similarly the number of young scientists who came to work at the N.I.M.R. from overseas increased. Obviously, his own time for personal research became more and more restricted, and in 1955 he gave up his appointment as head of the Division of Biochemistry. He gave three important lectures on his views in this direction: in 1957, the Sir David Russell Memorial Lecture on *Leadership in Scientific Research* (Oxford University Press, 1958), in the same year, the Linacre Lecture at St. John's College, Cambridge on 'The place of the research institute in the advance of medicine' (*Lancet;* 1345–1351, 1957); finally, in 1964, the Nuffield Lecture on 'The debt of science to medicine'

(*Proc. R. Soc. Med.* **57,** 1–8, 1964). In his opinion, the director of a large research institute must be a leader of its research campaign. He must be, therefore, a creative scientist himself, and exert understanding, balance, support and – above all – integrity.

From 1962 to 1967, he was consultant adviser to the Secretary of the Medical Research Council at M.R.C. Headquarters and gave unstintingly everything he had, carrying out very important functions, although he had had several coronary heart attacks since 1962, which – like his hip and leg disability – he preferred to ignore. After his final retirement, he reverted to his old love of classic Greek literature, nowadays such a rare accomplishment among the followers of natural science, and biography and history. He also enjoyed the countryside, the love of which he had acquired as a child. Physically he was considerably restrained, and he died in February, 1972.

HARRIS, Geoffrey Wingfield   1913–1972

G. W. Harris was born in Acton, London in June, 1913, the son of Tom Harris, who had studied physics at the Royal College of Science, South Kensington, London and as a research student of J. J. Thompson in Cambridge. For nine years he was a lecturer at the East London College of the University of London, and then obtained a post at the Ballistic Department of Woolwich Arsenal which he kept until his death in 1942.

Geoffrey Harris spent five years at Dulwich College, from where he entered University College London for half a year (early 1932), and Emmanuel College, Cambridge, later in 1932. He won College prizes for three successive years and gained a double first in the Natural Science Tripos. He was much influenced by F. H. A. Marshall of Christ's College, who had shown that the central nervous system played a role in producing ovulation. He was awarded the Marmaduke Shield Scholarship in Anatomy for 1935 to 1936, during which time he produced three important papers, the second of which (with G. T. Popa from Roumania) demonstrated the interaction between brain and pituitary gland in rabbits.

From 1936 to 1940, he studied clinical medicine at St. Mary's Hospital, London, where he won several prizes in ophthalmology, bacteriology and paediatrics. After qualifying in 1939, he did a year in housejobs. His M.D. Thesis in Cambridge was on the activity of the posterior lobe of the pituitary (1944). Harris then returned to Cambridge as demonstrator, later lecturer in anatomy (1940–1948). His brilliance, resourcefulness and technological skill had already emerged by then, tempered by his ability of strictly critical analysis of results. His experiment of avoiding the influence of anaesthesia on vasopressin production in female rabbits by remote control stimulation of the posterior lobe, was a masterpiece, never achieved before. Next followed his studies of the vascular supply of the anterior pituitary with various collaborators (John D. Green), contradicting the previous observations by Popa and Fielding and by Harris and Popa, because in the former observations they had forgotten about the reversal of the visual field by the microscope. With Dr. Dora Jacobsohn from Lund in Sweden, he proved his theory that the blood–borne substances travelled through the portal vessels to the anterior lobe to release (or inhibit the release) of hormones from the anterior lobe. From 1948 to 1952, he became Lecturer in Physiology under E. D. Adrian. Harris showed further that secretion of the pituitary stalk in the rat caused only temporary disturbance unless regeneration of the portal vessels was prevented by the ingenious method of insertion of a small waxed paper plate between the cut ends, in itself a major surgical feat.

In 1952, he accepted the newly created post of Fitzmary Professor of Physiology at the Institute of Psychiatry in London, although the working conditions on his arrival were very primitive indeed. He also taught neuro–physiology to students of psychiatry. His research activities made good progress and in 1953, he was elected Fellow of the Royal Society, aged only 40. During that decade, he was able to prove that the brain is, indeed, "a target organ for ovarian hormones". Harris also became actively interested in the clinical aspects of endocrinology. He travelled a great deal, especially in the United States and, of course, in Sweden. He also became involved with the management of a number of scientific societies, especially those which were connected with his research interests.

In 1962, he was elected Lee's Professor of Anatomy at Oxford, in succession to Sir Wilfrid le Gros Clark. He took over a large department with many researchers and research interests in all sorts of fields, except endocrinology. He was an excellent and enthusiastic teacher of undergraduates and he introduced new ideas and new methods in to the teaching of anatomy, discussing the problems and new methods with the students. He helped to develop the new Physiological Sciences Final Honour School, combining anatomy, biochemistry, pathology, pharmacology and physiology. He also kept up his close contact with clinical medicine, especially with clinical endocrinology. As Fellow of Hertford College which was linked with the Chair of Anatomy, he took part in College Affairs. In order to support his personal research, the Medical Research Council gave him funds for the establishment of a Neuro-endocrinological Research Unit. But the isolation of the LH releasing factor, which he had postulated, could not be achieved in the face of a fierce competition from the United States, which was both determined and well financed as far as the groups of Guillemin and Schally were concerned (see Chapter 22: Interlude: The psychology of teams). In her biographical memoir of Harris, Marthe Vogt said: "A review of Harris's work reads like a chapter in the history of endocrinology. The control of the multiple activities of the pituitary gland, and the study of the reciprocal interactions of brain and endocrine glands are the topics he had made his own. Step by step Harris contributed building stones to our present knowledge, always making sure that his ground was unshakeable before proceeding to the next step. He was one of the founders of the subject of neuroendocrinology." (Biograph. Memoirs of F.R.S. 1972).

Apart from many prizes, many degrees of British and foreign Universities, he was awarded the C.B.E. (Commander of the Order of the British Empire) in 1965, while serving on the Council of the Royal Society. An honour that pleased him particularly was the award of the Dale Medal of the Society of Endocrinology in May, 1971, on which occasion he delivered the memorable Sir Henry Dale Lecture (see Chapters 7 and 18): Humours and hormones (*J. Endocrinol.* **53**, ii–xxiii, 1971). A sudden gastric bleeding which proved uncontrollable caused his death in November, 1971.

Geoffrey Harris was not only an outstanding medical scientist in so many fields, especially in endocrinology, but also a very popular and much loved person, quiet, unobtrusive and generous, His early death was a great loss to modern endocrinology.

HARVEY, William   1578–1657

William Harvey is well-known as the greatest English physician, the discoverer of the circulation of the blood and the personal friend of King Charles I. Extensive and detailed biographies of him have been in existence for three centuries. It may, therefore, suffice to recall that he was born in April, 1578 at Folkestone in Kent, the eldest son of a prosperous business man, who became an alderman and an 'armiger' (bearer of heraldic arms). William went to school in Canterbury and studied medicine at Gonville and Caius College, Cambridge, graduating as a bachelor of arts in 1597. He then went to the University of Padova, where he spent several years; he heard Fabricius, who aroused his interest in blood vessels. Padova, which was a students' university, elected Harvey as the representative of the English students. In 1602 he returned to England as a doctor of medicine of Padova. In 1604, he was admitted to the College of Physicians in London, and married Elizabeth, the daughter of Dr. Lancelot Browne, physician to the court of Elizabeth I and of James I. In 1609, he was appointed physician to St. Bartholomew's Hospital in London, with an annual stipend of £25.00. In 1634, he supervised the examination of four Lancashire women accused of witchcraft.

After being made Fellow of the College of Physicians in 1607, he became its Lumleian Lecturer in 1615 and delivered these lectures on anatomy and surgery twice a week, including dissections of the human body in the winter over a period of five days. His lecture notes (prelectiones) have survived. He described in these lectures his own observations, which differed from those of Aristotle and Galen, but he cautiously added that the shape of the human body must have changed since Aristotle and Galen! Later, he did, however, declare that his teaching of anatomy was not from books, but from his dissections, not from propositions of philosophers, but from "the fabric of nature".

His large private practice among the nobility led to his appointment as Physician Extraordinary to James I, in 1618. He attended him on his deathbed in 1625, and was appointed in the same capacity to Charles I, with whom he became very friendly, presenting to him the more interesting results of his studies. The King permitted him to carry out studies and dissections on the deer of the Royal Game Parks (see Chapter 13); on that occasion, he observed certain changes in their reproductive cycle, especially during 1631. On following a Royal Progress to Edinburgh, he went to look at the multitude of nesting gannets on Bass Rock. Harvey also continued his studies as physician to the special embassy of the Earl of Arundel to Germany and Austria.

The bloody Civil War affected Harvey profoundly and sadly; a violent attack of a hostile mob on his house in London (in his absence) destroyed the fruits of many years of study and observation and other important notes concerning his private patients. He lost his position as physician to St. Bartholomew's Hospital and was even banned from London for a time.

His main work *De Motu Cordis* (= on the movement of the heart) was first published in 1628. It was attacked in Nuremberg, Germany, by one Caspar Hofmann, Professor of Anatomy there, even after Harvey had given a public demonstration by dissection there! The other foolish, but not less unpleasant and dangerous, critic was Jean Riolan of Paris, physician to Maria de Medici, mother-in-law to King Charles I. In fact, the French anatomists persisted for nearly another hundred years in refusing to accept Harvey's findings.

In 1631 Harvey became Physician-in-Ordinary to the King, and in 1639, he became the Senior King's Physician with an annual income of £400 and lodgings in the Palace of Whitehall. In 1641, the King gave him a present of 24 oz. of silver plate. He followed the King during the Civil War, and was at the battle of Edgehill, looking after the Royal children. He was with the King at Oxford, who appointed him Warden of Merton College in 1645. Parliament declared him a 'delinquent', fined him £2000 and banned him from London.

In 1651, his second major work, *De Generatione Animalium,* was published. Failing health prevented him from accepting the presidency of the College of Physicians.

He died in June, 1657, after a stroke. Harvey did not have any children. The last of the male line of his family was Eliab Harvey, born 1758, commanding the *Téméraire* at Trafalgar. He died as Admiral Sir Eliab Harvey., G.C.B.

HELLER, Hans   1905–1974

He was born in Bruenn (Austria, now Czechoslovakia) in 1905, the son of a surgeon. He studied organic chemistry in Prague, where he graduated. He then came under the influence of the pharmacologist E. P. Pick in Vienna, where he began his lifelong study of the control of water metabolism and the influence of neurohypophysial hormones. He was also stimulated by Otto Loewi to consider the problem of neuro-endocrinology. In 1930 he

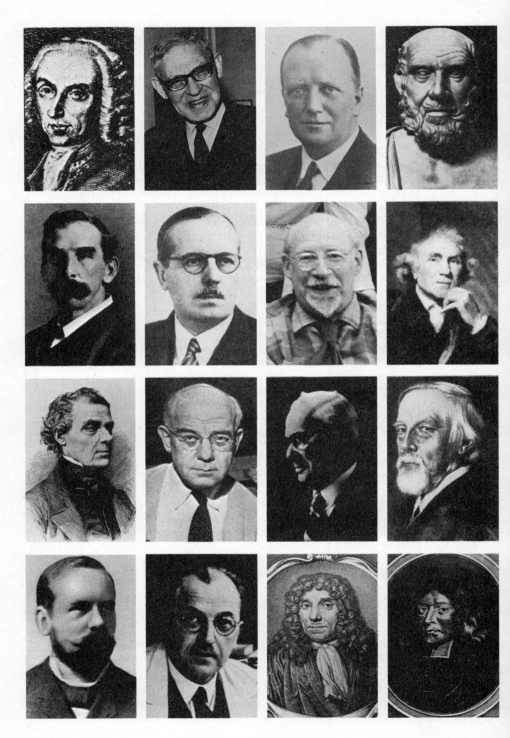

became a medical student at Emmanuel College, Cambridge, where he also worked under W. E. Dixon in the Pharmacology Laboratory. After Dixon's death in 1931, he returned to Vienna, but took up his medical studies again in 1934 at Cambridge and at University College Hospital in London, proceeding M.B., B.Ch. in 1938 and to M.D. Cantab. in 1948. In 1969 he was elected a Fellow of the Royal College of Physicians of London.

He was appointed Lecturer-in-Charge of the newly created Department of Pharmacology in the University of Bristol in 1942 and became Professor of Pharmacology there in 1949

Heller achieved international reputation for his fundamental research on the neurohypophysis and its hormones and his Institute became a centre of such studies. Between 1940 and 1948 a number of classic publications revealed the magnitude of his achievements. In 1949 he spent a fruitful year as Visiting Professor in Homer Smith's laboratory in New York. He also worked at the National Institutes of Health in Washington, D.C., Makerere College, Uganda, the University of Western Australia and other places.

Heller was a great comparative anatomist and his studies covered frogs, fishes and a variety of non-mammalian vertebrates. He was also a pioneer in the use of multiple bioassays. The search for obscure animals made him travel widely. Eventually, he discovered 'the water-balance principle', which he showed to be arginine vasotocin.

He was one of the founders of the journal for *General and Comparative Endocrinology* (with U.S. von Euler) and also of the European Society for Comparative Endocrinology in 1965, of which he became the first president. He became editor of the *Journal of Endocrinology* which he remained until seven months before his death. He was also one of the founder members of the Society for Endocrinology, of which he became a Committee member in 1962 and Chairman in 1971.

Professor Heller was immensely popular with his students, research team, academic colleagues and world wide associates. He was a convivial man and – in the best tradition of his generation – he had many interests. He was an expert in archaeology, on Greek coins from Asia Minor (and became a Fellow of the Royal Numismatic Society) and very interested in literature, music and the arts. He was genuinely interested in people, especially young people and their problems. This was proved to be of great importance when he was Dean of the Faculty of Medicine in Bristol from 1966 to 1969.

Figure 78 (left to right) Top row: Lorenz Heister*; Hans Heller; Thomas Albert Hindmarsh†; Hippocrates. 2nd row: Sir Victor Horsley*; Bernardo Alberto Houssay‡; Arthur Frederick William Hughes; John Hunter. 3rd row: Joseph Hyrtl°; Edward Calvin Kendall; Hans Walter Kosterlitz; Adolf Kussmaul‡. Bottom row: Paul Langerhans; Ernst Laqueur‡; Antony van Leeuwenhoek; Richard Lower[1]. (*by kind permission of Royal Society of Medicine, London; †by kind permission of the University of Newcastle-upon-Tyne (Dr. C. N. Armstrong); ‡from Ciba Monograph No. 10, by kindness of Ciba-Geigy Ltd.; °by kind permission of the Institute for the History of Medicine, University of Vienna, Austria; [1]by kind permission of Department of Medical Illustration, St. Bartholomew's Hospital, London EC1)

HENCH, Philip Showalter   1896–1965

Philip S. Hench was born in 1896 in Pittsburg, where he became M.D. in 1920. In 1921, he went to the Mayo Clinic. In 1929, his studies of rheumatic fever "revealed the profound effect of certain physical states on the course of the disease". In his Heberden Oration in 1948, he said that the remissions associated with them were more satisfactory and common than those with any known treatment. He based 20 years' research on these observations. When his friend Kendall isolated compound E (cortisone), Hench applied it to clinical medicine. "Hench's discovery of (the effect of) cortisone was not a flash in the pan; it was the fruit of a life time's use of experimental method in the treatment of rheumatoid arthritis" (G.W. Pickering, *Lancet* **II**, 81, 1960). Many people were disappointed when, after a year or so, cortisone was found not to be quite the panacea they had thought it might be. Hench was not one of them; in the excitement that attended his success, his was almost a lone voice, preaching restraint. At the International Congress on Rheumatic Diseases in New York in 1949, presenting the results of his work, he insisted that he was not even describing a new treatment, but a study of the effects of a hormone on the mechanism of rheumatoid arthritis (*Lancet* **II**, 24, 1949). His example of patient determination in research, and calm judgement in the moment of discovery may, in the long run, be even more precious than the discovery itself.

He shared the Nobel Prize for medicine with E. C. Kendall and T. Reichstein in 1950.

He died at Rochester, Minnesota, on 31 March, 1965.

HENLE, Friedrich Gustav Jacob   1809–1885

Friedrich G. J. Henle was born in Fuerth in Franken in July, 1809. He studied at the universities of Bonn (under Johannes Mueller) and Heidelberg from 1827 to 1832, and became Mueller's favourite pupil. He proceeded M.D. in 1832 with a dissertation (= thesis) on 'De membrana pupillari . . .' and took his final state exam in Berlin. When Mueller went to Berlin, Henle became his Prosector in 1834. His political activity in 1835 prevented his habilitation as Privat-Docent until 1837. In 1840 he was called to Zurich as Professor of Anatomy (and later of Physiology as well). His main work in Zurich was the *Allgemeine Anatomie* (1841) (= General Anatomy). In 1844, he moved to Heidelberg as Second Professor of Anatomy and Physiology and Anthropology, and after 1849 as 'Director of Anatomy'. In 1852, he succeed Langenbeck in Goettingen as Professor of Anatomy and Director of the Institute of Anatomy; there he remained until his death in 1885. When called to Berlin in 1858 to succeed Mueller, he declined. He received many honours for research and teaching.

His numerous scientific publications comprise, among others: *Handbook of Rational Pathology* (2 vols, Brunswick, 1846–53); *Systematic Anatomy* (3 vols, Brunswick, F. Vieweg, 1855–71). Of his many original papers, several had an endocrine connection, e.g. 'Ueber die Gattung Branchiobdella und ueber die Deutung der inneren Geschlechtsteile bei den Anneliden und hermaphroditischen Schnecken' (= on the internal sex organs of the annelides and hermaphroditic snails) in *Mueller's Archiv*, 1835. 'Ueber die Gewebe der Nebennieren und Hypophysis' (= on the textures of the suprarenals and the pituitary) in *Z. rationelle Medizin*, **24,** (which journal was founded by him and his friends Pfeifer in Zurich in 1844). 'Ueber den Mechanismus der Erection' (= on the mechanism of erection) (ibid., 3.R., **18,** 1863). 'Ueber den Bau und die Funktionen des menschlichen Oviducts' (= on the structure and the functions of the human oviduct) (ibid., 1863).

One of the most unusual and original papers was 'Versuche und Beobachtungen an einem Enthaupteten' (experiments and observations on a beheaded person) (ibid., Neue Folge, 1852).

The looped portion of the tubules of the kidney, the cell layer in the sheath of the root of a hair and other structures are named after Henle.

HOCHENEGG, Julius von   1859–1940

Born as the son of a well-to-do lawyer in Vienna, Julius von Hochenegg had a happy childhood. At the age of 16 a chest complaint compelled him to finish his humanistic education in Bozen (Bolzano) in the South Tyrol. After a short interval as a law student, he changed to medicine and qualified in Vienna in 1884, having worked as demonstrator in anatomy in 1882–1883 under Carl Langer, and as a clerk in medicine under Bamberger. Next, he spent a year working at the Institute of Morbid Anatomy under Kundrat and six months as a surgical trainee under the gynaecologist Gustav A. Braun (1829–1911). Eventually, he became surgical trainee to Eduard Albert; becoming second in 1886, and only a month later first assistant to Albert. In 1891, he became head of the surgical department of the Policlinic and administration director of the whole institution. In 1904, Hochenegg succeeded Billroth's pupil Gussenberger and became a colleague of von Eiselsberg. He had become Privat-Docent in 1889, Professor Extraordinary in 1894 and received the title of an ordinary Professor in 1901. He continued the tradition of his teacher Albert in spreading the practical knowledge of surgery not only among surgeons. but also for the need of the general practitioner. A brilliant speaker and instructor, averse to speculation, he became a most popular and successful surgeon, with an enormous private practice, although he was a somewhat cantankerous character. In 1908, he started an urological unit within his clinic. In 1909 he founded, with von Eiselsberg and Ernst Fuchs, the accident units, but an attempt to achieve the same for orthopaedic surgery did not meet with the same success. Alas, after the war, in 1918, he fell out with Lorenz Boehler (1885–1975), his former pupil and assistant, who became the founder of modern fracture surgery.

Hochenegg was an excellent administrator and designer of modern surgical units. His manifold scientific interests began in 1885, with a study of surgery of the testicle and epididymis. Although he eventually became known for his special interest in major abdominal surgery, he had developed an interest in the surgery of pituitary tumours (3 case histories, published in 1909). He recorded surgical cure of acromegaly due to pituitary tumours in 1923. Of his pupils, Felix Mandl became known as the first who successfully treated generalized osteitis fibrosa by removal of a parathyroid adenoma (1925). During the 1914–18 war, he organized, like von Eiselsberg, mobile surgical groups, which he supervised personally. After the war, he sponsored the idea of a compulsory practical year for doctors after qualifying. His other main interest was the study and treatment of carcinoma, especially of the abdominal organs; he founded the 'Austrian Society for the Study and Treatment of Carcinoma' in 1910. The war prevented the building of a modern cancer hospital, for which he had collected funds.

His relations with his pupils and assistants were, unfortunately, not always happy, mainly due to his autocratic and somewhat suspicious character, especially in the case of the more eminent and successful ones. He was, however, much loved by his patients as a kind, humane and understanding healer. His passion, apart from medicine, was hunting; he was an excellent shot. His only son died, to his grief, in 1914, but he enjoyed the company of his daughter and his grandchildren. He retired in 1930 and died in May, 1940.

HORSLEY, Sir Victor Alexander Haden
1857–1916

Born in Kensington (London) in 1857, Victor Horsley was the son of John Callcott Horsley, R.A. He was educated at Cranbrook School, University College and University College Hospital, qualifying in 1880. He was house surgeon and surgical registrar at University College Hospital, where he made a great number of observations on the action of anaesthetics on his own brain. From 1884 to 1890 he was Professor Superintendent to the Brown Institution of the University of London, in those days of great importance as the main centre of advanced research in pathology and physiology. His three main interests of study were: (1) the action of the thyroid gland; (2) the preventive treatment of rabies, and (3) the localization of function in the brain.

Horsley was a member of the committee set up by the Clinical Society to study myxoedema and cretinism in 1883, after the publication in 1873 of the description by Sir William Withey Gull. Horsley did the experimental work. He proved beyond doubt the action of the thyroid. The committee's report also gave a very good summary of myxoedema. In 1890, Horsley advised transplanting a sheep's thyroid under the patient's skin, as Schiff had suggested. Later came the work of George Murray, whom Horsley strongly encouraged, and others on the administration of thyroid extract. Horsley was the initiator in this country of the modern study of the thyroid gland and postulated the rational treatment of myxoedema and sporadic cretinism.

With others, he went to Paris to study and report back home on Pasteur's preventive treatment against rabies in 1886.

He began his main work on the brain, its physiology and localization of function at about that time. He became Assistant Surgeon at University College Hospital in 1885, Surgeon to the National Hospital for Nervous Diseases in Queen Square in 1886 and was elected F.R.S. in the same year. Having done much experimental work on monkeys, he was well qualified to carry out brain surgery. In one year he carried out ten operations at Queen's Square, nine of them successful. In 1887, he removed a tumour from the spinal cord. He made a long series of experiments on the effect of bullet wounds in the brain. He gave an address at a British Medical Association Meeting in Toronto, which became one of his most significant writings. Horsley took great interest in medical politics and was president of the Medical Defence Union and a leading member of the British Medical Association. He also published a book with Dr. Mary Sturge on *Alcohol and the Human Body* (in 1907). He was noted for his opposition to alcohol and tobacco. Coming from a family of artists, he was temperamental, yet charming and chivalrous. Although dogmatic in politics, he supported woman suffrage. Although in his fifties at the outbreak of the 1914–18 war, he worked in the British Military Hospital in Wimereux in France and, later, in Egypt and Mesopotamia, where he died at Asmara in 1916, of a heat stroke. His brain operations (1886–1890) and the removal of the tumour from the spinal cord (diagnosed by Gowers: Gowers, W. R. and Horsley, V. A. H.: *Med. Chir. Trans.* **71,** 377–430, 1887–88) were pioneering in the field, so that Cushing remarked that after that "certain neurologists began to do their own surgery".

HOUSSAY, Bernardo Alberto   1887–1971

Bernardo A. Houssay was born in April 1887, the son of Alberto Houssay and his wife Clara (née Laffont), both born in the South of France, the father in Bayonne and his mother in the Haut Pyrenées. Houssay's parents returned to France, because Alberto's (senior) baccalaureat was not recognized in Argentina. His father became a doctor of law in France. In 1886, The President of Argentina invited Alberto (senior) to return to Argentina as teacher in the high school 'Colegio Nacional Central' in Buenos-Aires.

Bernardo Alberto was born there in 1887, the fourth child of eight. Bilingual in Spanish and French, he was educated privately from the age of

5 to 8, then went to the State Elementary school to the age of 9. He took his baccalaureat at 13 'Maxima cum laude', being a precocious child, conversant with classical writers and with a passion for reading, especially history, literature and natural sciences. From 1901 to 1904 he studied pharmacy, graduating at 17, top of his class. In 1904, he began to study medicine. A brilliant student, he became assistant for practical work to the Professor of Physiology, H. G. Pinero. He became interested in the pituitary and his M.D. thesis was on 'Studies on the physiological action of pituitary extracts', for which he received not only his M.D. degree but also the Science Prize of the Faculty of Medical Science. The thesis was published in 1911 and was much acclaimed. In 1907, he became Assistant Pharmacist by competitive selection at the Hospital de Clinicas. In 1909, aged 22, he became Acting Professor of Physiology in the Faculty of Veterinary Science. At the beginning, some of the veterinary students boycotted his lecture, because of his age, and because he did not have a veterinary degree. However, he succeeded in converting them, and in 1912, he became Full Professor (aged 25). After medical qualification Houssay started private practice and also served as a house-physician at the hospital. He was soon appointed Chief of the Unit of Clinical Medicine of the Alvear Hospital, where endocrine patients were of special interest to him. As, however, his research work became more absorbing, he gave up both private practice and clinical hospital work.

His Laboratory of Physiology at the Faculty of Veterinary Medicine was not very satisfactory. There was no artificial light, and after dark experiments had to be pursued by candlelight. In winter, it was exceedingly cold in the laboratory. In 1910, Houssay devised a method of removal of the pituitary gland in the frog, later also from dogs, and both enabled him to study the action of pituitary extracts. In cats and cows he studied the action of the posterior pituitary on the secretion of milk; he also received thyroids from horses, cows, goats and sheep. He studied the action of anaesthetics on horses. He was also greatly interested in the venous pulse and in arrhythmias in man (1915).

In 1915, he became Chief of the Section of Experimental Pathology in the Institute of Bacteriology, concerned with the preparations of sera and vaccines; the Director of the Institute was Rudolph Kraus. Houssay held this post until 1919. His studies on snake-, spider-, and scorpion-venoms enhanced his reputation. His biochemist assistant María Angélica Catán, became his wife. Their three sons, Alberto, Héctor and Raúl all became doctors of medicine and worked in research. María Angélica was a great support until her death in 1962, after a long and distressing illness, which left a sad mark on him.

In 1919, aged 32, Houssay was appointed Professor of Physiology in the Faculty of Medicine of the University of Buenos Aires. He became a full-time professor and Director of the Institute, but his financial situation became much more strained. His ideas on teaching were expressed in many articles. He was keen on a careful selection of students and on full-time teaching, but he incurred much opposition. His sphere of interest expanded: endocrinology, neurophysiology, renal function, etc.

In 1943, Argentina went through a crisis. The constitutional government was toppled; the new military government was especially opposed by the universities. With another 150 people Houssay signed a manifesto that constitutional government should be restored. With many others, he was dismissed from his post. Ultimately, the universities were closed. Although an amnesty re-instated him in 1945, he was retired on 'age grounds' in September, 1946, aged 59. He was invited abroad, but he decided to remain at home. An 'Institute of Biology and Experimental Medicine' was created for him by Argentine business men and university graduates, who set up a fund to finance such a venture, and Houssay became its director. The Institute began its work in March, 1944, and has flourished to this day. Houssay was joined later by Juan T. Lewis, formerly Professor in Rosario, Oscar Orrías (Cordoba), Eduardo Brown Menendez and Virgilio G. Foglia (Buenos Aires). Houssay maintained the Institute, when he was re-instated professor after the 'Revolución Libertadora' in 1955. In 1956, he finally resigned from his chair, aged 69, and devoted himself entirely to his work at the Institute, where he carried on until his death in 1971.

HUGHES, Arthur Frederick William 1908–1975

Arthur F. W. Hughes was born in August, 1908 in Cheltenham, England. He studied zoology at Cambridge, obtaining his B.A. in 1930, proceeding M.A. in 1933 and Ph.D. in 1934. The Sc.D. was conferred on him in 1953. From 1933 to 1951 he was Sir Halley Stewart Research Fellow at the Strangeways Research Laboratory at Cambridge University (England). He became a member of the Anatomical Society in 1952, having taken up anatomy after the war (1939–1946) without previous medical qualification. From 1951 to 1953, he was Demonstrator in Zoology at Cambridge, from 1953 to 1964 Lecturer, and in 1964 he was elected a Fellow of Selwyn. In that year he also became Lecturer and Reader in Zoology at the University of Bristol, until he suddenly accepted an invitation to become Professor of Anatomy and Reproductive Biology at the Case Western Reserve University at Cleveland, Ohio, U.S.A., in 1967, where he remained until he became Professor Emeritus in 1975. He carried on work there and was looking forward "to getting ready to teach Human Embryology in 1977" as he said in a letter, received after his sudden death in August, 1975.

His main interests were in developmental biology. After 1957 he made several forays into the Blue Mountains in Jamaica to study the regeneration in lower vertebrates and became known locally as the 'Bearded Doc'. His early work concerned the development of the peripheral nerve fibre (*Biol. Review*, 1960), later he studied the degeneration of neurons in embryos and relations between limbs and the spinal cord. His books *The Mitotic Cycle* (1951) and *Aspects of Neural Ontogeny* (1968) represent his main later work. He also showed great interest in the history of microscopy and published *A*

History of Cytology in 1959. His short, but excellent paper 'A history of endocrinology' was published posthumously and reflected his work on neuro-secretions (see Section I, Preface). He was a likeable, friendly and modest person, shy and a diffident lecturer, but a highly skilled experimenter, a good and honest scientist and a scholarly writer, much loved by his collaborators and students.

HUNTER, John   1728–1793

John Hunter was born in Scotland in 1728 and was a brother of the equally celebrated William. There are many biographies and books about his life; he not only became the most famous anatomist and surgeon of his times, but also had a lasting influence on British anatomy and medical science. He was a pupil of William Cheselden, of Percival Pott at St. Bartholomew's, House Surgeon at St. George's in 1756 and student at St. Mary's Hall, Oxford in 1755–1756. He took part in the Belleisle expedition in 1761 and was with the army in Portugal in 1762. He was, of course, a pupil and associate of his brother William. He began to practise at Golden Square in London in 1763, but kept a dissecting house and a collection of wild animals at Earls Court. He was elected F.R.S. in 1767 and became surgeon to St. George's Hospital in London in 1768. Jenner was his house pupil in Jermyn Street in London. Having lectured in anatomy and physiology for many years, he began lectures in surgery in 1773, having Astley Cooper and Abernethy in his class. He became Surgeon Extraordinary to King George III in 1776. In the same year, he drew up 'Proposals for Recovery of People apparently Drowned'. He was Croonian Lecturer of the Royal College of Physicians in 1776–1782. Hunter bought land in Leicester Square and Castle Street, in London and built a large museum for the incredible number of important specimens and preparations which he had assembled and which later became the Hunterian Collection of the Royal College of Surgeons. He infected himself, experimentally, with *Spirochaeta pallida*, for study purposes, not being able to distinguish *Neisseria* infections from spirochaetal ones, with disastrous late consequences, of which he died miserably in 1793. His outstanding studies, transplant experiments and observations on the freemartin, have been discussed in Chapter 14. The work of this genius certainly deserves study in much greater detail.

HYRTL, Josef   1810–1894

Joseph Hyrtl, the son of a musician, was born in Eisenstadt (then Hungary) where Haydn was director of music to Prince Eszterházy. In 1813 Hyrtl's family moved to Vienna, where he later became a boy-pupil in the choir of the famous Imperial Court Music Orchestra, and where he also received a humanistic education. He studied medicine in Vienna and became prosector (unpaid) as a medical student. Qualifying in 1835, he became Professor of Anatomy and Surgery in Prague only two years later! His main interest was comparative anatomy in continuation of the ideas of Cuvier, John Hunter and Vicq d'Azyr, but regarded obsolete at that time when microscopy and experimental physiology were in the ascendance. On his return to Vienna in 1845 as Professor of Anatomy, he created a museum of comparative anatomy of 5000 specimens (destroyed in 1945 during the war).

An excellent speaker and writer with solid linguistic basis of Latin, Greek and even ancient Hebrew, Hyrtl wrote a celebrated *Textbook of Human Anatomy*, which went into 20 editions, and a *Handbook of Topographic Anatomy* (1847). Empiric in his methods, he was romantic in presentation. His textbook of human anatomy had the subtitle connecting anatomy with physiology and practical clinical application. Unfortunately, the temperamental anatomist had a bitter and unjustified quarrel with his equally celebrated colleague Ernst von Bruecke, Professor of Physiology, and – later in life – with his former pupil and new colleague as second professor of anatomy, Carl Langer. Although he had been Rector (= Vice-chancellor) of the University of Vienna in 1864, Hyrtl suddenly resigned from the Chair in 1874 and withdrew from the academic stage. In his retirement he wrote extensively on the development of anatomic terminology, preparing the ground for reforms, which were to materialize later at the Conferences at Basle and Jena.

In his last years, he founded a scholarship for poor students and an orphanage at Moedling, near Vienna. He died in July 1894, but not before he had witnessed the placement of his bust in the main arcade of the University of Vienna in 1889.

KING, Thomas Wilkinson   1809–1847

Born at Dover in 1809, the son of a doctor, Thomas W. King entered Guy's Hospital in 1824. He became curator of the Museum and lecturer in morbid anatomy in 1837. In 1840 he was lecturer in comparative anatomy and physiology, as well as pathology. He was one of the (300) original fellows of the Royal College of Surgeons of England. He also had private practice in Bedford Square. He wrote two papers on the safety-valve action of the right ventricle of the heart in *Guy's Hospital Reports* 1837 and 1841. His most important paper was 'On the structure and function of the thyroid gland' in 1836, for which many named him a Father of Endocrinology. He was closely associated with Sir Astley Cooper.

He died of pulmonary tuberculosis in March 1847.

KLEBS, Theodor Albrecht Edwin
1834–1913

Klebs of Koenigsberg, East Prussia, was one of the pupils and assistants of Virchow in Berlin from 1861 to 1866. He became Professor of Pathology in Bern in 1866, in Wurzburg in 1871, in Prague in 1873, in Zurich in 1882 and at the Rush Medical College in Chicago in 1886.

He was an outstanding pathologist and bacteriologist who contributed studies and observations of fundamental importance in many fields, but as Garrison puts it (in his 'Introduction to the History of Medicine', p. 581): "A man of irascible, precipitate disposition, Klebs was unfortunate in not following up his discoveries with good generalship", and thus missed much deserved recognition.

His main contributions to endocrinology were his observations, with Christian Friedrich Fritsche (1851–1938), on gigantism and acromegaly: *Ein Beitrag zur Pathologie des Riesenwuchses* (Leipzig, 1884). In the case studied, they thought that the thymus was the primary factor responsible for the condition, as they found it large, persistent and vascular. They noted the enlargement of the pituitary, but they regarded it secondary, like the other changes.

KNAUER, Emil   1867–1935

Emil Knauer was born in February, 1867 in Pressburg (then Hungary, now Bratislava, Czechoslovakia), where he attended grammar school. He studied medicine in Vienna, where he qualified and then became surgical trainee under Billroth. After several years, the gynaecologist Chrobak took him under his wing and he became his assistant. It was then that, following a suggestion of Chrobak, he began his experimental ovarian transplants in rabbits in 1895, which proved that the ovaries possess internal secretion. In recognition of this work and his general ability, his chief recommended him for the Chair of Gynaecology and Obstetrics in Graz (Styria, Austria), in 1903, where he remained for the rest of his life, in spite of invitations to return to Vienna. He was a popular and beloved gynaecologist and teacher. A new clinic was built for him in 1912. He died in May, 1935.

KOCHER, Emil Theodor   1841–1917

Emil Theodor Kocher was a native of Bern, Switzerland, and became a pupil of Langenbeck and Billroth. He was one of the group of modern surgeons like Horsley, Halstead, Crile, Cushing and von Eiselsberg, who revived the traditions of John Hunter and Sir Astley Cooper, and put surgery on a sound anatomical and physiological basis.

Kocher became Professor of Surgery in Bern in 1872 and remained so until his death in 1917, 45 years later. Apart from many innovations of technique in the surgery of hernia (1892), osteomyelitis, dislocations, etc. his study of the thyroid gland and his expertise acquired in over 2000 thyroidectomies (with only 4.5% mortality) after 1878, made him one of the leaders of thyroid surgery. After the first 100 thyroidectomies, he found that in 30 of them 'cachexia strumipriva' occurred, which he described in 1883. This work, together with Moritz Schiff's studies on dogs (1859), and Horley's and Reverdin's observations, laid the foundation of scientific thyroid surgery on a physiological and anatomical basis.

Kocher represented the type of modern surgeon who eschewed the virtuoso technique. He planned each operation carefully and carried it through with slow, meticulous precision and great skill; he knew the clinical history of every patient and based his surgical procedures on the most careful previous examination of the patient. He took great care to maintain absolute asepsis and his method of dissection was of the highest standard. His textbook of operative surgery (1894) bore witness of his methodical, painstaking and safe approach, devoid of all ostentation. His introduction of silk sutures in 1888, was a major step towards improved asepsis. In 1909, he received the Nobel Prize.

KOSTERLITZ, Hans Walter *ca.* 1908–

Hans Walter Kosterlitz was born in Germany, *ca.* 1908, the son of a medical practitioner. He attended school in Germany and studied first law and later medicine in Berlin, where he became M.D. in 1929. He was early attracted to research and worked as a student under Rona, and after qualifying worked for W. His. He became interested in carbohydrate metabolism in relation to liver disease and diabetes mellitus. Under His, he became an assistant diagnostic radiologist, where he studied the radiology of the gastro–intestinal tract.

Kosterlitz left Germany in 1934 and came to work at Aberdeen under J. J. R. Macleod (of insulin fame), who was then professor of physiology. He took his British medical qualification in 1936 and obtained his Ph.D. Aberdeen in the same year. Apart from teaching biochemistry and biology, he continued his research on the problem of conversion of galactose to glucose. In 1944, he obtained a D.Sc. from Aberdeen. Apart from more intensive teaching, he engaged in research on the more fundamental aspects of nutrition, and in the course of this work was elected F.R.S. of Edinburgh. In the early 1950s he became involved in research on the physiology and pharmacology of the peripheral autonomic nervous system, with which he is still concerned. Kosterlitz then spent five months with Dr O. Krayer at Harvard, lecturing, and studying the action of veratramine.

He and his co-workers thought they had made a new discovery, only to find that Luciani, working in Ludwig's laboratory in 1873, had preceded them.

Back in Aberdeen, Kosterlitz became interested in the physiological rôle of the myenteric plexus and, subsequently, in the understanding of the action of morphine. This led to research in the narcotic analgesic field, and on drug dependence. Although there was some interference when he was made professor of pharmacology and director of the new Institute of Pharmacology in Aberdeen from 1968 until his retirement in 1973, he was put in charge of the newly created 'Unit for Research on Addictive Drugs' in Aberdeen after 1973, where he is still working. It was there that he and John Hughes carried out their exciting and fundamental work on the opioid peptides of the brain (the two pentapetides, β-lipotropin and β-endorphin). This was the beginning of the latest phase of development in endocrine history in Britain and in the United States.

Kosterlitz was presented the Baly Medal of the Royal College of Physicians in London at the Harveian Oration on 18th October, 1979.

KUSSMAUL, Adolf   1822–1902

Adolf Kussmaul was born in February 1822 in Graben, near Karlsruhe. He studied at Heidelberg and later served as an army-surgeon of the army of Baden in the campaign of 1864 (Schleswig-Holstein). In 1850–1853, he was in practice in Kanden, carried on post-graduate studies in Wurzburg, becoming Privat-Docent in Heidelberg in 1855, proceeding to Professor Extraordinary two years later in 1857. In 1859, he moved as Professor of Medicine to Erlangen, and in 1863, to Freiburg i.Br. In 1876 he became Professor in Strasbourg, from where he retired in 1886 and returned to Heidelberg, where he died in 1902.

Kussmaul wrote many original papers, including a study on speech disturbances (in von Ziemssen's *Handbook of Pathology*, 1877). He first described periarteritis nodosa, with Adolf Maier (1824–1888) (*Dtsch. Arch. Klin. Med.*, **1**, 484–518, 1866) and the 'paradoxical pulse' in mediastino-pericarditis (1873). From the study of diabetes mellitus, he made the important observation of diabetic coma being due to acetonaemia and the abnormal respiration in this condition ('Kussmaul's respiration') due to air-hunger (*Dtsch. Arch. Klin Med.*, **14**, 1–46; 1874) (see also Chapter 19).

He was the first to attempt oesophagoscopy and gastroscopy in 1869, and to treat gastric ulcer with bismuth. His *Jugenderrinerungen* (= memories of my youth), published in 1899, were widely read, "containing interesting sidelights on the palmy days of the New Vienna School" (Garrison: 'Introduction to the History of Medicine', p. 622). Kussmaul also wrote poetry.

LAMARCK, Jean-Baptiste Pierre Antoine de Monet de la Marck   1744–1829

Lamarck was born at Bazentine-le-Petit, Picardy, France in August, 1744, the youngest of 11 children. His parents were members of the impoverished lesser nobility of Northern France. His father was, traditionally, an army officer. For economic reasons, Jean-Baptiste was destined for the priesthood and sent to a Jesuit seminary in Amiens. After his father's death, at fifteen, he joined the army and fought in the seven years' war (1756–1763). From 1763 to 1768, he served at various French forts along the Mediterranean and on the Eastern borders. During that time he began his botanic studies of the flora of France. Ill health forced him to leave the army in 1768, and he went to Paris; after a while, he studied medicine for four years and also became interested in shell collecting, chemistry and meteorology.

His personal life was one of catastrophe and poverty. He was married three times; all three wives died; perhaps he married a fourth time. Of his eight children (six by his first, two by his second wife) five survived. One son was deaf and one insane. A third did well as an engineer, got married and had children. Two daughters were unmarried in 1829, when he died in Paris, in such poverty that they had to petition the Academy of Sciences to pay for his funeral. His personal belongings, including his books and scientific collections, had to be sold by public auction. Failing health dogged him from 1809 onwards and by 1818 he was completely blind, but carried on work by dictating to one of his daughters (like Milton).

His first recognition stemmed from the publication, in 1779 (not in 1778 as stated on the title page) of his *Flore française*, in which he criticized Linnaeus and introduced a new method of analysis by dichotomous keys. Buffon was impressed (he had arranged that the Government should publish it); it was sold out in a year and reprinted in 1780 (3rd edition in 1805 by de Candelle). Buffon also arranged Lamarck's election to the Académie des Sciences as an adjoint botanist in 1779. He was promoted to Associate Botanist in 1783 and became a pensioner in 1790. The Académie was suppressed in 1793 during the Terror as "a privileged institution of the old order", but resuscitated in 1795 as part of the Institut National des Sciences et des Arts. From that time until his death, Lamarck was a resident member of the botanical section and until his health failed, he attended meetings regularly. The 'Jardin du Roi' became the 'Musée National d'Histoire Naturelle' and Lamarck was made Professor of Zoology for the study of 'insects and worms' ('invertebrates'). He had to give courses and classify the large collection of invertebrates in the museum. He also participated in the administration.

He began to study chemistry in the 1770s, his ideas being based on the four elements (earth, air, water and fire theory); but although his ideas and publications on this subject were ignored, he held on to them, almost paranoically, to the end. He believed that only living beings could produce chemical compounds. The natural tendency of all compounds was to decompose, until they returned to their natural state, in the process producing all organic substances. His theory of evolution from 1800 onwards showed a similar consequential chain: degradation and irrelevance of the species and distinction between the living and non-living.

The third part of his studies became meteorology, having been interested in the effects of climate on living organisms as early as 1776. As always, he emphasized the general principles and not "the little facts". In 1800, he began the publication of his *Annuaire météorologique*, in search for the laws of nature which regulate the changes in the climate (? the moon). He successfully persuaded Chaptal in the Ministry of Interior to establish in 1800 a central meteorological data station, co-ordinating the conditions in the whole of France. This ended in 1810, when Napoleon (foolishly) ridiculed Lamarck's *Annuaire*, which also ceased to exist. (The Emperor would have been better advised to carry out a careful meteorological survey of the climate of Russia before his campaign in 1812.)

His studies of the invertebrates were summed up in his *Histoire naturelle des animaux sans vertèbres* (7 vols, Paris, Verdière, 1815–1822), an extension of his *Philosophie Zoologique* (2 vols, Paris, J. B. Baillière, 1809). All this was leading to his theory of evolution, although he never used that term, but spoke of the order of nature, which it had followed in producing all living organisms. Lamarck was 55, when in 1800 he first made public his new ideas. Until 1790, he had accepted the idea of the fixity of species (see the entry on Albrecht von Haller). His own studies and the influence of men like Cabanis, Cuvier, Buffon, Diderot and others led him to develop his new ideas, although he still believed in the possibility of spontaneous generation after 1800.

In brief, evolution has occurred by the inheritance of acquired characteristics (in animals), due to the use or disuse of organs, responding to external stimuli.

At his death, in 1829, Lamarck and his ideas were ignored. Cuvier, in the official eulogy of the Académie, condemned his theories in all fields as being unacceptable. It was much later, in England, that Darwin was influenced by him and it was Darwin's theory of evolution which ensured Lamarck's fame. In Germany, it was especially August Friedrich Leopold Weismann (1834–1914), of Frankfurt am Main, who opposed Lamarck's ideas. Between 1892 and 1904 he produced some experimental evidence that acquired characteristics are not directly transmitted and presented the theory of the immortality of the germ-plasm. It is mainly 'amphixis', the union of the two parent germs, which is responsible for evolution. ('Aufsaetze ueber Vererbung und verwandte biologische Fragen' Jena, G. Fischer, 1892). Lamarck's ideas were eventually vindicated to some extent, when neo-Lamarckism had a strong following in France, Germany, Austria, Britain and America, and, recently, even in the Soviet Union. Lamarck is now accepted as one of the greatest representatives of biological philosophers.

The latest support to his ideas appears to be given by the work of Sir Cyril Clarke and his team in England, which led Clarke to introduce into biology the term 'The Uncertainty Principle' (*Lancet,* **II,** 784, 1980).

LANDOUZY, Louis Théophile Joseph
1845–1917

Louis T. J. Landouzy was born in Rheims in 1845, the son and grandson of doctors. He studied in Rheims and went to Paris in 1867. There he became a hospital resident in 1870 and physician to the Hôpital Laennec in 1890. In 1893, he obtained the Chair of Therapeutics at the Faculty of Medicine in Paris and also became a Member of the Academy of Medicine. In 1907, he was elected Dean of the Faculty of Medicine in Paris, and in 1912, Member of the Institute. He received the Gold Medal from the Ministry of Interior for his work on infectious diseases and gained an international reputation.

With Déjérine, he described facio-scapulo-humeral myopathy (Déjérine–Landouzy). He also carried out important studies on primary tuberculosis of the pleura. In 1883, he described a type of acute tuberculosis, a typho-bacillose, in which the ordinary morbid lesions of tuberculosis failed to make their appearance. In 1906, he described 'campto-dactylie', the flexure of the little finger in tuberculous subjects: "The little finger of a patient tells his past, shows his temperament, and foretells his future", was Landouzy's dictum. He was in the forefront of the battle against tuberculosis as a social disease; his last work concerned a large scale campaign against tuberculosis in the army. He had a great facility in physical examination of patients and was a great clinical teacher with a clarity of verbal expression.

Landouzy coined the expression 'Opotherapy' ($o\pi\delta\varsigma$ = juice; $\theta\varepsilon\rho\alpha\pi\varepsilon\iota\alpha$ = treatment) in 1898 for the administration of organ-extracts (see also Chapter 1).

LANGDON-BROWN, Sir Walter
1870–1946

Walter Langdon-Brown was born at Bedford (England) on 13 August 1870, the eldest son of the Rev. Dr John Bedford, who was a biographer of Bunyan, and one of whose sisters was the mother of Lord Keynes. He was educated at Bedford School and at University College in London; he then spent two terms at Owens College in Manchester under Arthur M. Marshall, before going to St. John's College, Cambridge, where he was influenced by (Sir) Michael Foster and W. H. Gaskell. He came to St. Bartholomew's Hospital, London, with a scholarship in science in 1894. He qualified in 1897 and became a house physician to Samuel Gee. At the end of 1900, he became casualty physician at Bart's and gained the Raymond Horton-Smith prize for his Cambridge M.D. thesis (on pylephlebitis) the next year. In 1900, he went to Pretoria as Senior Physician in charge of the Imperial Yeomanry Hospital. In 1906 he became Medical Registrar to Bart's; in 1908, he was elected F.R.C.P.; in 1913, he became Assistant Physician and, in 1924, Full Physician to Bart's.

In 1908, Langdon-Brown published *Physiological Principles in Treatment*, a landmark, since it was the first textbook of applied physiology. He became the first English physician to relate the work of Freud and Jung to clinical medicine. This was also expressed in his Croonian Lectures at the Royal College of Physicians in 1918 on 'The Sympathetic Nervous System in Disease', in which he demonstrated the psychosomatic factor, that emotional disturbance may create disorders of bodily function. He began to develop his medical philosophy of scientific humanism.

In 1934 he was Senior Censor to the Royal College of Physicians and gave there the Harveian Oration in 1936: 'The Background to Harvey'. In 1930, Langdon-Brown had retired from Bart's, where he had been a popular teacher and guide to the young. In 1932 he was appointed Regius Professor of Physic at Cambridge and elected professorial Fellow of Corpus Christi. He relinquished the chair in 1935, on reaching the age limit. In the same year he was knighted. He was a big man with bushy eyebrows and of impressive personality, scholarly and widely read in the classics, literature and poetry, who coined many popular phrases. In his later years, he became interested in endocrinology and it was he who introduced the phrase 'the pituitary is the conductor of the endocrine orchestra'. Among his many honorary degrees, he also had a D.Sc. Oxford (1936), but he also became, characteristically, President of the Society of Individual Psychologists and chairman of the Langdon-Brown Committee on postgraduate training in psychological medicine, which reported in 1943.

At the outbreak of the war, he returned to Cambridge, where he delivered the Linacre Lecture in 1941. In 1946, he was elected the first president of the newly formed Section of Endocrinology of the Royal Society of Medicine, but he was too ill and had to have his Presidential Address read for him.

In 1902 Langdon-Brown married Eileen Presland, a Sister at the Metropolitan Hospital in London, where he had been Assistant Physician since 1900 and a Physician from 1906 to 1922. She suffered from a mental disorder for many years, which caused them both much unhappiness. She died in 1931, and he married his secretary, Winifred Marion Hurry (who died in 1953), and there followed 15 happy years. In the year of his death was published *Some Chapters in Cambridge Medical History*, which he had dictated to his wife. He died on 8 October 1946, after a long and difficult illness. His widow founded a lectureship in his memory at the Royal College of Physicians in 1951. At her death, she left £2500 to Corpus Christi College, Cambridge, to endow a Langdon-Brown Scholarship, and £1000 for the formation of a hospitality fund at the Royal College of Physicians.

LAQUEUR, Ernst   1880–1947

Laqueur was professor of pharmacology in Amsterdam. He was the leader of an excellent research team, one of the discoverers of testosterone, which they isolated in 1935. His team was also responsible for research on the standardization of insulin and of the oestrogen (he was a member of the standards committee of the League of Nations). Laqueur was also the discoverer of the oestrogenic activity of male urine (*Klin. Wschr.*, **6,** 1859, 1927). In 1937, he isolated corticosterone, together with T. Reichstein, P. Fremery, et al. (*Nature, London,* **139,** 925–926, 1937). In 1946, he was awarded the Berzelius Medal of the Swedish Medical Society. Laqueur had also been Dean of the Medical Faculty of the University of Amsterdam. He died in August 1947 on a holiday in Switzerland. S. E. de Jongh gave a lively account of the exhilarating atmosphere in the heyday of experimental endocrinology under Laqueur at the Amsterdam Polderweg (*Acta Endocrinol.* **57,** 1–15, 1968).

LEEUWENHOEK, Antony van   1632–1723

Antony van Leeuwenhoek was born in Delft, Holland, in 1632, the son of a basketmaker; his mother was the daughter of a Delft brewer. He went to a rural primary school near Leyden. At the age of 16, he was apprenticed for six years to an Amsterdam linen-draper. When he was 22, he married, bought a house in Delft, the type of which we seem to know so well from Jan Vermeer's paintings, and started in business there as a draper. At the age of 28, he became involved in the local politics of his native town and was appointed Chamberlain of Delft's Worshipful Sheriffs.

Leeuwenhoek devoted all his leisure time to the study of natural science. His long life of over 90 years gave him plenty of scope. His main instrument was the microscope, the accidental discovery of his fellow-countryman Zacharias Jansen, a spectacle-maker of Middleburg. In about 1609, Jansen placed two lenses in a tube (see Chas. Singer: 'Notes on the history of early microscopy', *Proc. R. Soc. Med.* (Sect. History) **7,** 247, 1914). Galileo Galilei put that discovery to practical use, although his name is mainly connected with the use of the other instrument derived from that idea, the telescope. The first to use the primitive microscope for the study of disease was Athanasius Kircher (1602–1680), Professor of Physiology at Wuerzburg in Germany, who examined the blood of patients suffering from the plague.

Leeuwenhoek ground his own lenses and built his own microscopes, of which he had eventually 247 with 419 lenses! On one occasion he sent 26 microscopes as a present to the Royal Society of London, of which he had become a corresponding Fellow in 1680. Although he used a simple lens and did not achieve a magnification beyond 160 at the most, he made important observations and discoveries. It was in 1673, that Leeuwenhoek wrote the first of 308 letters to the Royal Society of London, describing his discoveries. The Royal Society had them translated from Dutch, the only language Leeuwenhoek spoke, and most of them were published in English. All of them have been preserved in the Society's archives (see Clifford Dobell:

Antony van Leeuwenhoek and his Little Animals. London, John Bale, Sons & Danielson, Ltd, 1932).

Leeuwenhoek extended the knowledge of the capillary circulation, which Malpighi had discovered. He described the red blood corpuscles (1674), the spermatozoa (1674), the muscle fibres, and even bacteria (1683), using lenses of very short focal length. He was a hard working, persistent observer, with a truly scientific mind, although he had no university education nor any professional medical training. During his life, he sent 375 scientific papers to the Royal Society in London and 27 to the French Academy of Science.

LINACRE, Thomas   1460–1524

Born in 1460, Thomas Linacre became one of the best known English physicians and scholars of his time. Educated at Oxford, he became Fellow of All Souls College at Oxford in 1484. He went to Italy *ca*. 1485–1486, where he became an M.D. of Padova. He returned to England in 1492, becoming one of Henry VIII's physicians in 1509. He lectured at Oxford in 1510, and was instrumental in founding and is, indeed, regarded as the Founder of the College of Physicians of London in 1518. He became Latin tutor to Princess Mary in 1523, for whom he composed a Latin grammar *Rudimenta Grammaticis*. He also founded lectureships in medicine in Oxford and Cambridge. His writings include works on grammar and on medicine and a number of translations from the Greek, especially from Galen. He died in 1524, aged 64.

LOEWI, Otto   1873–1961

Otto Loewi was born in Frankfurt-am-Main in 1873, the first child and only son of Jakob Loewi, a wealthy wine merchant. At school at the Frankfurt City Gymnasium (= humanistic grammar school) he made good progress in the humanities, hoping for a career in the history of art. In 1891, following the wish of his father, he became a medical student in Strasbourg, but was more interested in lectures at the philosophical faculty. He barely passed his 'Physikum' (= second M.B.), following which he spent two semesters in Munich before returning to Strasbourg. He became interested in Naunyn's (see Section II) lectures. After reading Walter Holbrook Gasken's Croonian Lecture on the isolated frog heart, he wrote his doctor's 'Dissertation' (= thesis) on the effects of various drugs on the isolated frog heart under Oswald Schmiedeberg, and proceeded M.D. Strasbourg in 1896. He attended a course in analytical inorganic chemistry under Martin Freund in Frankfurt and studied physiological chemistry in Franz Hofmeister's Laboratory in Strasbourg. From 1897 to 1898, he was Carl von

Noorden's assistant at the City Hospital in Frankfurt. Discouraged by the lack of effective treatment for tuberculosis, he chose basic research in medicine. From 1898 to 1904 he became assistant to Hans Horst Meyer (1853–1939) at the Pharmacological Institute at Marburg, proceeding to 'Privat-Docent' in 1900 on nuclein metabolism in man. In 1902–1903, he spent several months in England, at Ernest H. Starling's laboratory in London and also paid a brief visit to Cambridge to see the work of Gaskell, Langley, Elliott and Dale. In 1904, he became Assistant Professor at Marburg and, for a brief period, he succeeded Meyer as director there. In 1905, he followed Meyer to Vienna as his assistant and became Professor Extraordinary there in 1907. In 1909, he became Ordinary Professor and Head of Pharmacology at the University of Graz (Austria), where he remained, in spite of various invitations (including to Vienna) until his expulsion by the Nazis in 1938, when he and two of his children were imprisoned in March, 1938. In 1936, he had shared the Nobel Prize in Physiology (Medicine) with Henry H. Dale. In September, 1938, he left for London, after being forced by the Gestapo to transfer his Nobel Prize money from Stockholm to a bank under Nazi control. They retained his wife, Guida Goldschmidt, whom he had married in 1908, while dispossessing her of some property in Italy. He received invitations to the Franqui Foundation in Brussels and to the Nuffield Institute at Oxford. From 1940 to his death in 1961, he was Research Professor of Pharmacology at the College of Medicine, New York University. In 1941, his wife was able to rejoin him. After 1946, he became a naturalized citizen of the United States. He spent his summers at the Marine Biological Laboratory in Woods Hole (where he was buried).

His research interests were wide, but two main categories were outstanding. (1) His studies on protein and carbohydrate metabolism; (2) his work on the autonomic nervous system, especially on the innervation of the heart. Other work concerned the physiology and pharmacology of the kidneys and the physiological role of cations. While working in Schmideberg's laboratory, he was introduced to Johann Friedrich Miescher's classic papers on the metabolism of the Rhine salmon during its freshwater phase (to which he later referred as his 'scientific bible'). He also published studies on Phlorizin-induced glycosuria. In his opinion, fat could not be converted into sugar in dogs. In 1902, he published a paper suggesting that protein synthesis might be possible in animals if their diet consisted of the degradation products of a whole organ rather than of an isolated protein. Between 1902 and 1905, he published a series of five papers on the function of the kidney and of the action of diuretics (later utilized by Arthur Cushny in London, 1917). From 1907 to 1918, there followed six additional studies on metabolism, especially on the function of the pancreas and glucose metabolism in diabetes. After Banting and Best (1921), there were studies on the mode of the action of insulin (with H. F. Haeusler).

His interest in the vegetative or autonomous nervous system was 'imported' from England. His early work on vasomotor action, salivary secretion and the action of adrenalin had all been topics of investigation in Cambridge during his visit there. In 1910 he demonstrated, with Alfred

Froehlich, that cocaine increases the sensitivity of autonomically innervated organs to adrenaline. In 1912 three papers on the vagus action on the heart appeared. Between 1913 and 1921, there were three papers on the role of cations (especially calcium) on the heart action, and six on the physiological relationship between calcium ions and the series of digitalis drugs, especially on the frog's heart. The hypothesis of chemical transmission of nervous impulses is usually credited to Thomas Renton Elliott (1877–1961), who published it in 1904 ('On the action of adrenalin', *J. Physiol. Lond.*, **31**, xx–xxi, 1904), but Walter Fletcher (Sir Walter Morley F., 1873–1933) of Cambridge recalled that Loewi proposed it in 1903. In 1920, it had fallen into discredit, because no experimental evidence had been produced, but in 1921, Loewi revived it by a rather elegant experiment which, eventually, brought him the share in the Nobel Prize. It proved, on the frog's heart, unequivocally, "that the nerves do not influence the heart directly, but liberate from their terminals specific chemical substances which, in their turn, cause the well-known modifications of the function of the heart characteristic of the stimulation of its nerves" (Loewi, O.: An autobiographical sketch, p. 17 in *Perspectives of Biology and Medicine*, vol. **4**, pp. 1–25, 1960). In 1926, Loewi and E. Navratil identified the 'Vagusstoff' as a cholinesther, which is abolished by atropine. Loewi was able to demonstrate the experiment before the 12th International Congress of Physiology in Stockholm. It was confirmed by W. B. Cannon in 1934. It was not until 1936, that Loewi definitely identified the 'Sympathicusstoff' with adrenaline (epinephrine). Finally, in the 10th and the 11th papers of the famous series, Loewi and Navratil could show that the effect of the 'Vagusstoff' faded rapidly because it was speedily metabolized by an enzyme, unless protected by the alkaloid physostigmin (eserine). This ability of eserine, even in small doses, helped to detect transmitters in tissues, where the low concentration or rapid destruction previously kept it undetected (see also Sir Henry H. Dale's work).

LOMBROSO, Cesare   1836–1909

Born in November, 1836 in Verona, Cesare Lombroso studied at Turin, Pavia and Vienna, being a pupil of Panizza and of Skoda. He qualified in 1856 and completed his military service as a surgeon in the war of 1859. In 1862, he was appointed Professor of Psychiatry in Pavia and later, Director of the Lunatic Asylum in Pesaro. Finally, he became Professor of Forensic Medicine in Turin, where he died in 1909.

He achieved international fame for his crimino-pathological studies. He formed the view that the causes of crime were somatic conditions combined with heredity and atavismus. He also wrote on genius and madness (*Genio e follia*, Milano, 1864), and published an important study on cretinism in Lombardy (*Ricerche sull cretinismo in Lombardia*, 1895), and studies on pellagra.

LOWER, Richard   1631–1691

Richard Lower was born in 1631 in Tremeere, Cornwall. He was educated at Westminster, and Christ Church, Oxford, and proceeded D.M. in 1665. He worked in Oxford with Thomas Willis on anatomy, physiology and transfusion of the blood. In 1669 his work, *Tractatus de Corde. Item de Motu et Colore Sanguinis, et chyli in eam Transitu* was published, followed by *De Origine Catarrhi* in 1672.

In 1666, after marrying Elizabeth Trelawney, he came to London where he became a popular physician and had a very good practice. However, his practice suffered in 1678 when he protested to the proposed succession of the Duke of York, brother of Charles II. He attended Charles during his last illness and at the post-mortem examination, and lost his Court appointment on James II's accession. He died in King Street and is buried in St. Tudy, Cornwall.

Lower was an outstanding experimental physiologist and an ideal collaborator of his friend, teacher and protector, Thomas Willis. The latter produced the ideas which Lower skilfully translated into experimental proof. Willis gracefully acknowledged Lower's invaluable contribution and help.

MALPIGHI, Marcello   1628–1694

Marcello Malpighi was born in Bologna; he entered the University there in 1646, proceeding to study medicine in 1649. He attended the dissections and vivisections which Bartolomeo Massari conducted in his own house. He qualified as doctor of medicine and philosophy in 1653. Within a year he was called to Pisa as Professor of Theoretical Medicine. There he spent three important years as a colleague of Giovanni Alfonso Borelli, Professor of Mathematics, who also carried out animal dissections in his home-based laboratory. Malpighi returned to Bologna from 1659 to 1662 to teach medicine, from 1662 to 1666 was Professor of Medicine in Messina, but returned again to Bologna. Invited in December, 1667, to undertake scientific correspondence with the Royal Society in London, that Society subsequently printed all his works. In 1691, he became chief physician to Pope Innocent XII in Rome, where he died in his apartments in the Quirinal Palace in November, 1694. His first and main work was *De pulmonibus* (= about the lungs), which contained fundamental microscopical discoveries about the lungs and which was published in Bologna in 1661. He not only described the structure of the lungs, but also the capillaries within them and the arterio-venous connections. His choice of examination of the frog enabled him to study the capillary network with relatively small magnification. During his four years in Messina he managed to study marine animals from the Straits of Messina, making important contributions to neurology, adenology and haematology. Two short works, *De lingua* (= on the tongue), Bologna 1665, and *De externo tactus organo* (= on the external organ of touch), Naples 1665, are closely linked to each other.

His ideas on the mechanism of taste were strongly influenced by Galileo. He thus became the discoverer of sensory receptors, which was only part of his wider research of the anatomy of the nervous system. In the same year, 1665, was published his treatise *De cerebro* (= on the brain), and in 1666: *De cerebri cortice* (= on the cortex of the brain), but his description of the nerve fluid secreted by the 'cortical glands' was due to an artefact. In spite of this, he succeeded in constructing a system from the brain to the peripheral nerve endings, the neuron, in which the transmission of the nervous impulse was compared with that of a mechanical impulse through a liquid mass.

In Messina, Malpighi also studied the structure of the gland, a 'secretion machine', acting like a sieve. His glandular studies were stimulated by the discovery of the pancreatic duct by Wirsung in 1642, the testicular duct by Highmore in 1651, the submandibular duct by Wharton in 1656 and the parotid duct by Steno in 1660.

Next, he turned his attention to the study of the blood, *De polypo cordis,* his main treatise on the subject, being published in 1668. He regarded these 'Heart polyps', found during autopsy in patients who had died of cardio-respiratory failure, as a process of coagulation during life. In it, he also gave a description of the red 'atoms', which were, in fact, the red blood corpuscles. He also studied simpler organisms of insects and fish, to discover more about the more complex ones. Thus, he reported his observations on the silkworm (*De bombyce*), published in London in 1669. He next described his embryological studies in *De formatione pulli in ovo* (= on the formation of the chicken in the egg), in 1673, on the principle that the artisan "in building machines must first manufacture the individual parts, so that the pieces are seen separately, which must then be fitted together".

His main embryological discoveries were the aortic arches, the neural folds and the neural tube, the cerebral and the optic vesicles, the proto-liver, the feather follicles and other items.

Figure 79 (left to right) Top row: Marcello Malpighi; Pierre Marie*; David Marine†; Leonard Mark‡. 2nd row: Gregor Mendel°; Oskar Minkowski*; Paul J. Moebius*; Giovanni Battista Morgagni†. 3rd row: Robert Tuttle Morris; Johannes Müller; George R. Murray[1]; Bernhard Naunyn*. Bottom row: Paracelsus; Caleb Hillier Parry*; N. C. Paulesco; Felix Platter†. (*from Ciba Monograph No. 10, by kind permission of Ciba-Geigy Ltd.; *by kind permission of Royal Society of Medicine, London; ‡by kind permission of Department of Medical Illustration, St. Bartholomew's Hospital, London EC1; °by kind permission of Institute for the History of Medicine, University of Vienna, Austria; [1]by kind permission of the University of Newcastle-upon-Tyne (Dr. C. N. Armstrong))

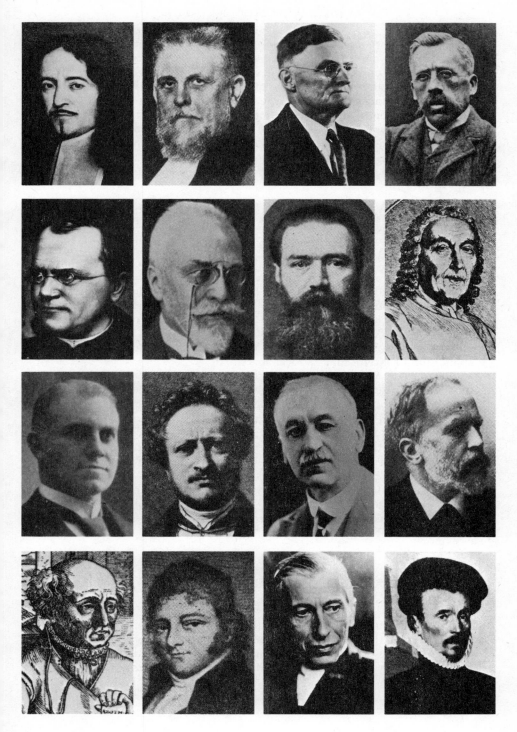

He stressed the importance of his comparative study method again in the introduction to his *Anatomes plantarum idea* (1675): "The nature of things . . . is revealed only by the method of analogy". This work brought him credit as one of the founders of the microscopical study of plant anatomy.

In one of his final works, *De recentiorum medicorum studiio* (= on the study of recent physicians), supported rational medicine against the mere empiricists. This theme was also the basis of his published 'Consultationes', which reflected his ideas in the practice of clinical medicine, which he carried on at the same time as his biological researches.

MANDL, Felix   1892–1957

Felix Mandl was born in Bruenn in Moravia (then Austria) in 1892, son of an industrialist, and attended the local grammar school. He studied medicine in Vienna, his studies being interrupted by the First World War, where he served at the front, the last year as an ambulance man. He continued his studies, qualifying in 1919. He became a surgical trainee under von Hochenegg and his assistant in 1923. He proceeded Private-Docent in 1928, having published 52 original papers. His references mentioned his outstanding work in gastric and rectal surgery and in the application of Novocain as a local anaesthetic.

One of his most outstanding contributions was the study and successful treatment of osteitis fibrosa by removal of a parathyroid adenoma in 1925.

In 1932, he became director of the surgical unit of the newly founded Canning-Child Hospital and Research Institute (for the study of cancer). In 1938, he had to leave Vienna. He went to Jerusalem to chair the surgical department of the Hadassah University Hospital, where he was made Professor of Surgery in 1939. In 1947, the City of Vienna invited him to take charge of the newly re-built surgical department of the Emperor Francis Joseph Hospital, and the University of Vienna granted him the title Professor Extraordinary. In 1953 his monograph was published: *Blockade and Surgery of the Sympathetic*. He died suddenly of heart-failure in 1957 in Vienna. in his 65th year.

MARAÑON, Gregorio   1887–1960

Gregorio Marañon was born in Madrid in May, 1887 and educated at the College San Carlos and at the University of Madrid, where he qualified in medicine in 1911. Just before he graduated, he was awarded the Martinez de Molina Prize by the Academy of Madrid, previously won by Ramon y Cajal. He did some postgraduate study under Ehrlich in Frankfurt/Main. Following his return to Madrid he held many appointments, which culminated, eventually, in the directorship of the Institute for Experimental

Pathology at the General Hospital. At the University of Madrid, he first held the Chair of Pathology and, finally, the Chair for Endocrinology, specially created for him. In the 1920s he was involved in the crisis of endocrinology, as discussed in Chapter 18. He was elected President of the Spanish Academy of Medicine and acquired an international reputation as an endocrinologist, especially in Latin America.

His main scientific interest concerned the sex hormones. He visited Britain under the auspices of the British Council and became foreign corresponding Member of the British Medical Association in 1936 and an Honorary Fellow of the Royal Society of Medicine in London.

He was a Liberal of great influence. Although a personal friend of King Alfonso XIII, it was in his home in 1931 that the monarchist leaders arranged for the transfer of power to the Republic; he thus became the 'Midwife of the Spanish Republic'. During the Civil War, he first lived in the Republican Zone. He then went to the Argentine and later to Paris. In 1942, he returned to Spain and abandoned politics, except for asking clemency for political prisoners. Re-instated as Professor of Endocrinology, he died in Madrid in March, 1960, much mourned by the students and the university.

He was also an essayist of distinction, using the method of 'psychobiographies' of Henry IV of Castile, Tiberius (also translated into English), Antonio Pérez, and others.

After Marañon's death, the doors of the Faculty of Medicine in Madrid were closed for a day in mourning.

MARIE, Pierre   1853–1940

Pierre Marie was born in Paris and first studied law. After completing his medical studies, he became an 'interne des hôpitaux' in 1878 and worked in neurology at the Salpêtrière and Bicêtre under Charcot, becoming Charcot's chief of laboratory and clinic. He became 'médecin des hôpitaux' in 1888 and 'agrégé' at the Faculty of Medicine in Paris a year later. His lectures to the faculty, to achieve that position, were on the diseases of the spinal cord, and were later published (in 1892). From 1897 to 1907, he created at the Bicêtre a neurological service of international reputation. From 1907 to 1917, he was Professor of Pathological Anatomy at the Faculty of Medicine. Supported by Gustave Roussy, his successor, he completely modernized the teaching of pathological anatomy. In 1918, at the age of 65, he succeeded Déjérine to the chair of Clinical Neurology at the Salpêtrière.

A brilliant diagnostician, in the Charcot tradition, he was an equally brilliant teacher. Between 1885 and 1915 he had many outstanding pupils trained at his famed neurological unit.

His literary output was as outstanding as it was enormous. A number of new diseases were described by him and are linked with his name.

Acromegaly (1886–1891) is perhaps the best known; he also defined the Charcot-Marie type of muscular atrophy (1886), pulmonary hypertrophic osteo-arthropathy (1890) cerebellar heredoataxia (1893), cleido-cranial dysostosis (1897) and rhizomelic spondylosis (1898). His opinions on disorders of speech and aphasia were controversial. With E. Brissaud (1852–1909) he founded *Revue Neurologique* in 1893.

He retired from the chair at the age of 72, in 1925, first to the South of France and then to Normandy, where he died in his 87th year.

MARSHALL, Francis Hugh Adam
1878–1949

Francis H. A. Marshall was born in High Wycombe, Buckinghamshire, England, in July, 1878, the fifth son of Thomas Marshall, J.P. His male ancestors were all lawyers, except for a Major Marshall, who was a soldier at the Court of William IIIm Several paternal cousins were distinguished in academic life, e.g. Sir Oliver Lodge and Professor Percy Heawood, the historian. His mother's family, Lucas, were landowners in Warwickshire and could be traced back to Elizabeth I. After school in Southborough he went to University College, London, where he studied Greek with Professor Platt, who encouraged him to go to Cambridge, where he obtained a Natural Science Tripos in 1900, from Christ College. From there he went to Edinburgh where he stayed for eight years, the last four as university lecturer on the Physiology of Reproduction and Assistant to the Professor of Physiology (Schaefer). In 1908, he returned to Cambridge as Lecturer in Agricultural Physiology, and helped to build up the international reputation of the School of Agriculture. In 1919, he became Reader in Agricultural Physiology, which he remained until his retirement in 1943. Although he was for a time Director of the Institute of Animal Nutrition, and had been elected to the Fellowship of Christ College in 1909 and a tutor from 1912 to 1923, Dean in 1926 and Vice-Master in 1939, and served on the Council of the University-Senate, his post was never raised to the status of professor. In 1912, he went to Michigan to deliver a course of lectures on the physiology of reproduction. In 1927, the Ministry of Agriculture sent him as a member of a committee to Algiers, to study Voronoff's methods of the rejuvenation of cattle and sheep. He was elected to the Royal Society in 1920, and became a member of the Council 1933–1935, Croonian Lecturer in 1936 and Royal Medallist in 1940. He also became a D.Sc. Edinburgh and Sc.D. Cantab., and a C.B.E. in 1933 and he received the Baly Medal of the Royal College of Physicians in 1935. He became the principal editor of the *Journal of Agricultural Science* and member of the Council of Management of the *Journal of Endocrinology*, and one of the four honorary members of the Society of Endocrinology.

Marshall's name will always be remembered as one of the foremost pioneers in the physiology of reproduction. His most brilliant research was carried out during his eight years in Edinburgh. Apart from his investigations in the alleged telegony in horses (the Penicuik experiments), he began to study the oestrous cycle in sheep. After making contact with Schaefer, he studied the oestrous cycle in the ferret, and, later, together with W. A. Jolly (1878–1939), that of the dog. For Part II of the paper on the last subject, they chose the title: 'The ovary as an organ of internal secretion'. Strongly encouraged by Schaefer, which fact he freely acknowledged, he published the first edition of his main work: *The Physiology of Reproduction*, in 1910. It became a standard classic. As Sir Alan S. Parkes put it in Marshall's obituary notice: "The appearance of this book, immediately hailed as a masterpiece, was an event in the history of biological literature, and it placed Marshall in the front rank of British biologists and gave him world-wide reputation at the age of 32."

Marshall was a shy, kind person, of simple tastes and addicted to hard work. He died a bachelor in Cambridge in February, 1949 after an emergency operation for acute appendicitis.

MENDEL, Johann Gregor   1822–1884

Johann Gregor Mendel was born in 1822 in Heinzendorf in Austria, the son of a peasant; his mother was the daughter of a gardener, and some of his ancestors were gardeners. Because of his abilities, he was sent to the humanistic grammar school at Troppau. His father's illness forced him to give private tuition. His own health was affected twice, but in 1840 he finished school and began reading philosophy at the University of Olmuetz. With interruptions due to ill health, he completed his course.

In 1843, he entered the Augustinian monastery in Bruenn, assuming the name of Gregor. The monastery was a centre of scientific interest and learning. Many of its members were teaching at the philosophical institute, and the abbot, F. C. Knapp (1792–1867) was an agricultural scientist. He established the tradition of experimenting with plants in the monastery garden. The monastery was well supported by the income from its estates. At the time of Mendel's entry, Matthew Klácel (1808–1882), a teacher of philosophy, was the leader of the experimental garden, investigating variation, heredity and evolution of plants. During his theological studies, Mendel also studied agriculture, pomology and viniculture under F. Diehl (1770–1859). Later, he was sent for further studies to the University of Vienna, where he read physics, botany, zoology and plant physiology under Franz Unger, who also talked on organizing botanical experiments. Mendel read Gaertner's *Experiments and observations on the hybrid procreation among plants* (1849), in which nearly 10 000 experiments of hybridization were described in 700 plant species; he marked the notes on 'pisum' (pea) characteristics specially. He became a member of the Zoological and Botanical Society of Vienna, where he published two short papers in 1853 and 1854. On his return, Mendel became teacher of physics and natural history at the Technical School in Bruenn, where A. Zawadski was his superior. He nominated Mendel a member of the Agricultural Society in Bruenn. He became a popular teacher of large classes of students. It was at that time that he began his experiments with peas and artificial pollination (in 1856). His health broke down again, during a university examination, and he remained a substitute teacher until 1868, when he gave up teaching, because he was elected Abbot of the monastery with many official duties.

In February and March, 1865, Mendel presented to the Natural Sciences Society in Bruenn an account of his experiments on artificial plant hybridization, which was published in the Society's proceedings in 1866, to be completely overlooked and forgotten. In 1900, Hugo de Vries of Amsterdam, Carl Correns of Tuebingen and Erich von Tschermak of Vienna reported on their experiments, carried out independently, in which they obtained the same results. Each of them discovered, towards the end of their studies, that Gregor Mendel's experiments, recorded 35 years before, carefully planned, painstakingly carried out on a large scale, brilliantly analysed, interpreted and clearly presented, formed the real essential basis of the science of genetics. The *Proceedings*, published in 1886, had been distributed to 134 institutions in many countries, including some in New York, Chicago and Washington! Mendel seemed to have sent out 40 reprints personally. Two of them were found in Bruenn, five others elsewhere. One had been sent to Naegeli and another to Anton Kerner, both authorities on hybridization. Mendel wrote up the main results of the experiments and his interpretation in a treatise entitled: 'Versuche ueber Pflanzenhybriden' (1866). He made further experiments to confirm his original findings, and had an extensive correspondence with Naegeli from 1864 to 1873 (published in 1905 by Naegeli's pupil Correns), who remained, however, cautiously sceptical and suspicious, in spite of Mendel's sober, honest, objective and scientific presentation of his case. Naegeli's objections to Mendel's experiments were, later, found to be irrelevant and the rejection of Mendel's conclusions, irrational. Apart from the local gardeners, who used the practical applications for the breeding of new varieties of fruit trees, no one grasped the fundamental significance of Mendel's discoveries. Mendel did not pursue the publication of his further experiments, which proved his theories. He died on 6 January, 1884, a disappointed man.

MINKOWSKI, Oscar   1858–1931

Oscar Minkowski and his brother Hermann were descendants of a German-Latvian family. Hermann, the younger, also became a famous scientist and, in 1896, a teacher of Einstein at the Swiss Technical College in Zurich. At 18, he had been awarded the Gold Medal for Mathematics in Paris and, eventually, became Professor of Mathematics in Goettingen (1901–1909).

Until his death, in 1909, Hermann was interested in the problem of space and time; he died, aged 45.

Oscar was born in June, 1858, near Kovno in Latvia (then Russia). He went to School in Koenigsberg and studied medicine in Strasbourg and Freiburg. He qualified, however, under Naunyn in Koenigsberg. He accompanied Naunyn to Strasbourg, where Naunyn succeeded Kussmaul in 1888. It took, however, another twelve years, before Minkowski got his own department in 1900, first at Cologne, later in Greifswald (in 1905) and, finally, in Breslau (1909).

His scientific work of 14 monographs and over 170 papers covers almost every field of clinical and experimental medicine. He discovered the clinical picture of haemolytic icterus, studied the physio-pathology of purine metabolism and, especially, the role of β-oxybutyric acid in metabolism and diabetic coma, and wrote on biliary acid synthesis in hepatic cells. In 1889, he discovered with J. von Mehring, that pancreatectomy causes diabetes mellitus. Von Mehring originally wanted to demonstrate that rancid fat, containing fatty acids, is absorbed better than ordinary fat. A lucky chance and astute observation changed all that, as has been discussed in Section I.

Minkowski possessed outstanding intelligence and quick perception, which was extended to many other, non-medical fields of life, including art, culture and politics. Although he had an understanding of human weakness, he disliked obscure speculation and incompetence. He possessed the humanity of a great man, with friendliness and nobility of character. He died in Wiesbaden in June, 1931, aged 74.

MOEBIUS, Paul Julius   1854–1907

Paul J. Moebius was born in January 1854 in Leipzig, of a scientific family. He studied theology and philosophy in Leipzig, Jena and Marburg and obtained a Ph.D. He then took up the study of medicine and became M.D. in 1877. He enlisted as an army surgeon and reached the rank of an 'Oberstabsarzt' (= senior staff surgeon or *ca.* surgeon-lieutenant-colonel). In 1878, he published his *Grundriss des deutschen Militaer-Sanitaetswesens* (= Fundamentals of German Military Hygiene). After leaving the army he settled in practice in Leipzig as a neurologist. He became an Assistant at the Neurological Department of the University Policlinic under Ernst Adolf Gustav Gottfried Struempell (1853–1925), and Privat-Docent in Neurology in 1883. After 10 years as Privat-Docent, having achieved no promotion to Professor Extraordinary, he resigned from academic life and retired into private practice and devoted himself mainly to writing.

In endocrinology, he was best known for his description of Moebius' sign, the name being given by Charcot of Paris; it denotes the incomplete convergence of the eyes in toxic goitre, when a finger approaches (*Centralbl. Nervenheilkd. Psychiat.*, **9**, 356, 1886).

Later Moebius became internationally known because of his controversial and polemic writings on the characteristics of the sexes, e.g. *Geschlecht und Krankheit* (= sex and disease), in which he maintained that expectation of life in men is shorter because of alcohol abuse and venereal disease and not because of greater physiological resistance of woman. His main work became his monograph *On the Physiologic Mental Deficiency of Woman* (Ueber den physiologischen Schwachsinn des Weibes), which achieved 7 editions by 1905! On more orthodox lines was his description of 'Moebius Disease', i.e. ophthalmoplegic migraine (Ueber periodisch wiederkehrende Oculomotoriuslaehmung, *Berlin. Klin. Wochenschr.*, **21,** 604–608, 1884), which was later followed by a treatise on headache (Ueber Kopfschmerz. Halle an der Saale, C. Marhold, 1905).

MORGAGNI, Giovanni Battista   1682–1771

Giovanni Battista Morgagni was born in Forli in February 1682. In 1698, he went to the University of Bologna, obtaining a degree in philosophy and medicine in 1701, having studied under Antonio Maria Valsalva and Ippolito Francesco Albertini, both pupils of Malpighi. Morgagni entered the Accademia degli Inquieti in 1699, and became its head in 1704. He reformed the Accademia and modelled it on the Académie Royale des Sciences, incorporating Luigi Marsi's Istituto delle Scienze in 1714. In 1706 his *Adversaria anatomica prima* (= Notes on Anatomy) were published in Bologna.

From 1707 to 1709, he worked in Venice, carrying out research on the anatomy of large fishes and also studying chemistry with Gian Zanichelli. With Gian Santorini, dissector at the medical college in Venice, he carried out dissections on the human body. From 1709 to 1711, he had a successful medical practice in his native city. In 1711, he moved to Padova as second professor of theoretical medicine. His inaugural lecture in 1712 was on: 'Nova institutionum medicarum idea'. He was appointed to the first chair in 1715, on the death of Domenico Gulielmini, and remained in that position until his death in 1771, aged 89!

His *Notes on Anatomy* contain quite a few minor discoveries: the glands of the trachea, of the male urethra, of the female genitalia, etc. His most important work was, however: *De sedibus et causis morborum per anatomen indagatis* (= on the sites and causes of diseases discovered by the (morbid) anatomist), published in 1761, when he was 79 years old! In it he discussed carefully collected case-histories with the clinical signs and manifestations and, eventually, adding the morbid anatomical findings, superbly analysed and interpreted. The collection included observations of Malpighi and Valsalva. Morgagni can thus be regarded the Founder of modern pathological anatomy.

MUELLER, Johannes   1801–1858

Johannes Mueller was born in Coblenz, in July, 1801. He replaced the philosophical speculative methods in German academic medicine by the experimental method of observation and analysis. His empirical research was carried out "with seriousness of purpose and thoughtfulness with incorruptible love of truth and perseverance". He made important contributions to anatomy, histology, embryology and physiology, human as well as animal; and he was regarded by many of his equally famous pupils as a "man of first rank".

The son of a bootmaker who became well-to-do in Coblenz, Mueller was a brilliant student, with great ambition and a vast general knowledge. He became a medical student in 1819 at the newly founded University of Bonn, where he qualified in 1822. He continued his studies in Berlin under the anatomist Carl A. Rudolphi (1771–1832), who attempted to put research on a scientific basis. In 1824, he passed the state medical examination in Berlin and returned to Bonn, where he qualified as lecturer in physiology and comparative anatomy. In 1825, he also became a lecturer in general pathology. In 1826, at barely 25 years of age, he proceeded Professor Extraordinary and in 1830 full Professor, having married a girl from Coblenz in 1827. In 1832, he turned down an invitation from the University of Freiburg but in 1833, he succeeded Rudolphi as Professor of Anatomy and Physiology in Berlin, having outlined the tasks of the holder of that post in a letter to the Minister of Education. In 1834, he became a member of the Prussian Academy of Sciences. He was elected Rector (= Vice-chancellor) of the University in 1838–1839 and in 1848–1849. This position became very invidious during the revolutionary movement of 1848, when he stood between the rebellious student body, who wanted reforms in the university and in government, and between the established authority. He did not favour changes by revolutionary fervour; moreover, he was concerned for the safety of his famous anatomical collections, which might be destroyed. In 1857, he complained of severe insomnia and had symptoms of depression, which he had displayed before. On 28 April, 1858, he was found dead in his bed. As he had forbidden a post-mortem examination, the cause of death was unknown, although suicide was suspected.

With the publication of the final volume of his *Handbook of Human Physiology* in 1840, he seemed to have shifted his interest from experimental physiology to comparative anatomy and zoology, especially of marine animals including protozoa, for the study of which he undertook numerous expeditions in the North Sea and the Mediterranean.

The achievements of Mueller in all the fields he studied are too numerous to discuss in such a thumbnail sketch biography. One of the most important was the law of specific nerve energies, "that is to say, that man does not perceive the changes in the external world, but only the altercations they produce in his sensory systems". In 1830, he published his studies on the development and structure of the glands and also his research on the embryonic development of the genital organs and discovered 'Mueller's duct', which forms the tubes uterus and vagina. His researches in neuro-physiology advanced the knowledge of that field by leaps and bounds. He believed in a combination of experiment and philosophy, which could solve the problems of physiology: "denkende Erfahrung" = critically evaluated experience was the key to most problems.

MURRAY, George Redmayne   1865–1939

George Redmayne Murray was born in Newcastle-upon-Tyne in 1865, son of a physician. He was educated at Eton and Trinity College, Cambridge, then at University College Hospital. In 1886 he was attracted by the teaching of Sydney Ringer and (Sir) Victor Horsley. He won the Fellows and Senior gold medals, and qualified in 1888. He visited Berlin and Paris and returned to Newcastle as pathologist to the Hospital for Sick Children and lecturer at Durham University College in Medicine and Bacteriology. Horsley, who had befriended him, suggested that myxoedema might be improved by grafts of animal thyroid. Murray used extracts of sheep's thyroid by subcutaneous injection, which resulted not only in short-term but also in long-term cure, as his follow-up of a woman patient proved on whom he reported again in 1920. This addition to the knowledge of the role of the endocrine glands was so important that Sir Walter Langdon-Brown termed it the "Birth of Endocrinology", in his inaugural address as the first President of the Endocrine Section of the Royal Society of Medicine in 1946. Alas, Murray's contemporaries in Newcastle were less flattering. He had been appointed Heath Professor of Comparative Pathology at Durham University and physician to the Royal Victoria Infirmary in Newcastle, in 1893, but he decided to accept the chair of medicine at Manchester University in 1908, where his teaching responsibilities deflected him from the pursuit of experimental medicine.

He received many honours subsequently. He became President of the Association of Physicians, member of the Medical Research Committee (later: Council), Bradshaw Lecturer of the Royal College of Physicians in 1905, having been their Goulstonian Lecturer in 1899. He received honorary degrees from Durham and Dublin. As a member of the Departmental Committee of the Home Office, he studied dust diseases in card room workers. During the First World War, he was consulting physician to the British Forces in Italy. He died in Cheshire in September, 1939, in retirement at the age of 74.

NAUNYN, Bernhard   1839–1925

Bernhard Naunyn was the son of a Burgomaster (Lord-Mayor) of Berlin. For seven years he was Friedrich Theodor von Frehrich's assistant in Berlin, but in 1869, he became Professor of Medicine in Dorpat, in 1872 in Bern, and in the same year in Koenigsberg. In 1888, he succeeded Kussmaul in Strasbourg. Following Frehrich's footsteps, his main interest became experimental pathology and pathological chemistry. This soon led him to the study of metabolic diseases and diabetes mellitus. He was co-founder of the *Archiv für experimentelle Pathologie und Pharmakologie* in 1872, and of the *Mitteilungen aus den Grenzgebieten der Medizin und Chirurgie* (= Reports from the borders of medicine and surgery).

His most important work, however, was his monograph on diabetes mellitus (*Der Diabetes mellitus*, Vienna, 1898) and his *Klinik der Cholelithiasis* (Leipzig; 1892). Ernst Stadelmann (b. 1853), of Insterburg was his pupil; he studied the pathological excretion of ammonia in the urine of diabetics and observed an acid substance, which Oscar Minkowski (1858–1931), another of Naunyn's assistants, showed to be betaoxybutyric acid, a year later (*Arch. Exp. Pathol. Pharmakol*, **18**, 35–48, 1884).

Naunyn was a stern taskmaster, but he succeeded in having a splendid new conversion of the old city hospital in 1901. He refused a call to Vienna and eventually gained international reputation. He was a man of culture with a love for music. His *Memoirs* (1925) were widely read and much acclaimed. Many of his pupils (Sadelmann, Minkowski, Magnus-Levy) made names for themselves in the field of diabetes.

NEEDHAM, John Turberville   1713–1781

John T. Needham was born in London in 1713, the son of recusants, and was educated in French Flanders. He was ordained a secular priest in 1738, teaching and accompanying English Catholic noblemen on the Grand Tour. In 1768 he settled in Brussels as director of what later became the Royal Academy of Belgium. His scientific interests were motivated by his desire to defend religion in a scientific age. He became well known for his argument with Voltaire over miracles.

In 1748, at Buffon's invitation, he examined fluids from the reproductive organs of animals under the (weak) microscopes then available. The globules Buffon and he observed were named Buffon's 'organic molecules'. The alleged proof of these 'organic molecules' was based mainly on Needham's experiments, who thus became embroiled in the controversy on generation. Needham's own theory made him a vitalist. In contrast to Buffon's theory, it denied the chance combinations of mathematically countable inherited traits. Needham's theory of spontaneous generation and epigenesis was refuted by Spallanzani's experiment in 1765. Needham's other claims to scientific fame were his observations on plant pollen and on the milt vessels of the squid. He was elected a Fellow of the Royal Society in 1747, of the Society of Antiquaries in London in 1761, as correspondent for the Académie des Sciences in 1768, and a member of the Royal Basque

Société des Amis de la Patrie and first director of the Royal Academy of Belgium in 1773. He died in Brussels on 30 December 1781.

NEEDHAM, Joseph   1900–

Joseph Needham was born in London in 1900, son of the late Joseph Needham, M.D. He was educated at Oundle School and at Gonville and Caius College, Cambridge, where he first read medicine, but later changed to biochemistry, physiology and embryology. Joseph Needham has been appointed to many important positions and has received many honours, some of which are listed here. He was a Fellow of Gonville and Caius College from 1924 to 1966 and Master from 1966 to 1976. He was a University Demonstrator in Biochemistry between 1928 and 1933, and Sir William Dunn Reader in Biochemistry 1933–1966; now he is Emeritus. He was Head of the British Scientific Mission in China and Counsellor and the British Embassy in Chungking and Advisor to the Chinese Natural Resources Commission, the Chinese Army Medical Administration and the Chinese Air Force Research Bureau 1942–1946. From 1946 to 1948 he was Director of the Department of Natural Sciences, UNESCO. He has had visiting professorships to many universities; in 1925 he was visiting Professor of Biochemistry at Stanford University in California. He had given lectures to many universities and societies around the world, and has received honorary degrees from many universities and prizes and medals from many learned societies.

Publications of particuliar importance were: *Science, Religion and Reality* (editor), 1925. *Man and Machine*, 1927. *The Sceptical Biologist*, 1929. *Chemical Embryology*, 1931. *The Great Amphibium*, 1932. *A History of Embryology*, 1934. *Order and Life*, 1935. *Adventures before Birth* (tr.), 1936. *Perspectives in Biochemistry* (Hopkins Presentation Volume; ed.), 1937. *Background to Modern Science* (ed.), 1938. *Biochemistry and Morphogenesis*, 1942. *Chinese Science*, 1946.

In the last 25 years, Needham and his colleagues have undertaken the monumental task of giving the fundamental account of *Science and Civilisation in China*, of which the first eight volumes are now available. This work alone should secure Professor Needham a lasting memorial in the history of science and learning.

OLIVER, George   1841–1915

George Oliver was born in April, 1841, son of Mr. W. Oliver, a surgeon in County Durham. He was educated at Gainford School and at University College Hospital Medical School. After a brilliant career as a medical student, when he was particularly influenced by William Sharpey, then

Professor of Physiology, he won the Gold Medal on obtaining his M.D. London. For a short time he practised in Redcar, but moved in 1875 to Harrogate, where he remained for 33 years, first in general practice, later as a consultant. After the first 12 years or so, he spent the quieter winter months in London or Sidmouth, where he had ready access to medical societies and hospitals to keep him up-to-date. He was, however, especially interested in physiological and experimental problems, and carried on experimental work in his private laboratory and later at University College. After 1901, he bought a house in Farnham, Surrey, where he died in December, 1915. Among his numerous papers, some were on the action of Harrogate waters. He was also very keen on urine testing and developed special methods, using 'Oliver's test papers'. He was an inventor of all sorts of gadgets: of a 'haematocytometer', a 'haemoglobinometer', an 'arterio-meter' and a 'sphygmometer'; the arteriometer played a part in his later major work with Schaefer. He published a book *Studies on Blood Pressure*, which went through three editions and he wrote papers on the suprarenal, thyroid, thymus and pituitary glands. His most important work on the blood pressure raising substance of the suprarenal medulla with Schaefer, was discussed in Chapter 16. Oliver was elected to the Fellowship of the Royal College of Physicians in 1887. He founded, in memory of Sharpey, the Oliver–Sharpey Lectureship, of which he became the first holder in 1904, talking on 'Studies on Tissue Lymph'.

Oliver was a perfectionist and very skilled, not only in his physiological experiments. One of his hobbies was photography, in which he also achieved great perfection; another was cycling in the countryside. His two outstanding characteristics were the clarity of his thought and expression and his perseverance, once he had decided that a certain line of investigation, study or experiment was justified.

In 1910 he had a haematemesis, from which he recovered.

PARACELSUS, Aureolus Theophrastus, Philippus, Bombastus von Hohenheim 1493–1541

von Hohenheim was born in Einsiedeln in Switzerland, *ca.* 1493. The adopted name 'Paracelsus', the meaning of which is not quite clear, dates from *ca.* 1529. His father William was a member of the Banbast family of Swabia, who practised medicine at Villach in Carinthia (Austria). Educated by his father in mineralogy, botany and natural philosophy, and later by the abbot of Sponheim, he worked in the Fugger mines near Villach. Later he studied at various Italian universities. His claim to the title 'Doctor of Medicine' has never been proved.

In 1536, Paracelsus published his book *Grosse Wundartzney* (= great book of the treatment of wounds). He had been a military surgeon in the service of Venice and elsewhere (in the Middle East and Rhodes). He said of himself, he was "In judicando, a physician; in curando, a surgeon". In 1525, he was in Salzburg, but had to leave, as he showed sympathy for the peasants' revolt. He then set up practice in Strasbourg. In Basle, he saved the life of the Humanist Johannes Froben and gave medical advice to Erasmus. He was then appointed Municipal Physician and Professor of Medicine in Basle in 1527. The academic authorities refused permission, however, as he refused to take the oath, did not submit his doctor's diploma and published an anticlerical document. He refuted Galenic medicine and burnt Ibn Sinā's *Canon* at a students' rag on St. John's day. He also lectured in German instead of Latin and offended by admitting barber surgeons to his courses. After Froben's death, his opponents succeeded in forcing him to leave after a year.

After further wanderings, he finished his main medical work: *Opus paramirum* at St. Gall, which he dedicated to Joachim de Watt (Vadianus), humanist and acting mayor. In his further wanderings as a lay preacher in Switzerland and the Tyrol, he studied miners' diseases. In Austria, he was received by Ferdinand of Bohemia, brother of Charles V. In 1538, he returned to Villach where he completed a number of other books. He again practised medicine and was called to Salzburg by Ernest of Wittelsbach; there he died in 1541, aged 48.

His wholesale rejection of traditional medicine and his rough manners made him many enemies. His knowledge of chemistry, pharmacology, his observations on many diseases, including goitre and cretinism, which he recognized as endemic, and his studies of syphilis and its treatment, finally his new concept of disease secure him a permanent place in the history of medicine.

PARÉ, Ambroise   1510–1590

Ambroise Paré was born in 1510 at Laval, Mayenne in France, the son of an artisan. He served an apprenticeship as a barber surgeon in the provinces, then went to Paris to study surgery at the Hôtel-Dieu. About 1536, he became a master barber-surgeon, taking up military service. He served in Italy, returning to Paris in 1539, but took part in military expeditions for the next thirty years. Henry II appointed him one of his surgeons-in-ordinary in 1552. In 1562, he became *premier chirurgien* to Charles IX and, later, to Henry III. He had a large practice at court and as a military surgeon.

He revolutionized the treatment of gunshot wounds after the siege of Turin in 1536, where he ran out of the traditional boiling oil, by abandoning the use of boiling oil for good. He reported his discovery in 1545, in a treatise, published in the vernacular, because he knew no Latin. It brought him immediate fame. He also rejected cautery in favour of the ligature of blood-vessels during amputation.

The invention of printing helped to spread his writings, although the

Royal Faculty of Paris spurned him. He died at the age of 80, in Paris, respected for his honesty, hard work and his concern for the poor and needy.

PARRY, Caleb Hillier (Ap-Harry)
1755–1822

Born at Cirencester, Gloucestershire in 1755, Caleb Parry was the son of a Welsh Nonconformist Minister. He was a school-, and lifelong friend, of Edward Jenner. He went to Edinburgh as a medical student in 1773. After marriage and a tour abroad of about a year, he settled in Bath, and became a member of the Gloucestershire Medical Society with Jenner.

In 1788 he read a paper to the Society entitled 'An inquiry into the symptoms and causes of the syncope anginosa, commonly angina pectoris, illustrated by dissections'. It was not published until 1799. His description of eight cases of 'Enlargement of the thyroid gland in connexion with enlargement or palpitation of the heart' was not published until 1825, three years after his death. The syndrome of hyperthyroidism, commonly known as Graves' or Basedow's disease, should, according to some authorities, really be called Parry's disease.

He was elected fellow of the Royal Society in 1800. He suffered hemiplegia and aphasia in 1816 and died in 1822. He is buried in Bath Abbey Church.

PAULESCO, Nicolas Constantin 1869–1931

Nicolas C. Paulesco was born in Bucharest in 1869 and received his medical education in Paris. He became an intern to Étienne Lancereaux (1829–1910). He wrote his M.D. thesis on the structure and function of the spleen, which was marked 'extrêmement bien'. At the Sorbonne he also obtained diplomas in biochemistry and physiology and later became doctor of science. After qualifying he became assistant physician at Lancereaux's hospital and did clinical and laboratory research. He presented a number of papers to medical societies and journals and acquired the reputation of a careful experimenter and critical observer, and a man of original thought. A collection of his work in Paris indicated his early interest in endocrine research, on the effects of the removal of the thyroid and on the results of injection of suprarenal gland extracts. With Lancereaux, he began to write a major work, *Traité de Médecine*, the first volume of which appeared in 1903. After Lancereaux's death, Paulesco undertook to complete the remaining four volumes. He also wrote another major work on medical physiology in three volumes, published between 1920 and 1922.

In 1900 he returned to Bucharest as Assistant Professor of Physiology. In 1904, at the age of 35, he succeeded to the chair of physiology which he held until he died in 1931 from cancer of the bladder, at the age of 62. In order to keep in touch with clinical medicine he accepted the part-time post of visiting physician to the Hospital St. Vincent de Paul, where he was esteemed as a good clinical teacher. His research work, extending over a wide field and presented in numerous papers and lectures, brought him much credit. There were two main contributions: the study of the result of hypophysectomy and his isolation of pancréine (identical with Banting and Best's 'isletin'), both of which were discussed in detail in section I. He became the forgotten man.

PENDE, Nicola   1880–1970

Nicola Pende was born in Noicattaro, Bari, in April, 1880. He studied medicine and qualified in Rome in 1903. He became an assistant and aiuto, and in 1907, Libero Docente in medical pathology. Later, he obtained the Chair for Medicine in Genoa. He died in Rome in June 1970. His main work was on the vegetative nervous system, on endocrinology and on constitution. He founded the 'Istituto biotipologico-ortogenetico' in Genoa. His book, *Endocrinologia,* was published in 1916. In 1962, at the age of 82, he published a major treatise, "Neuroendocrinología correlativa", proof that he had kept very much up-to-date with modern developments of which he had been the initiator in his own country.

PFLUEGER, Eduard Friedrich Wilhelm 1829–1910

Eduard F. W. Pflueger was born in 1829 in Hanau. His father was a businessman and later, a passionate liberal politician. His mother was of Huguenot descent. He was educated at the humanistic grammar school in Hanau. He studied law in Heidelberg, where he was involved in the politics of 1848 and was arrested in 1849. In 1850, he became a medical student at Marburg and in 1851 in Berlin. There he became a pupil of Johannes Mueller, in whose laboratory he worked. He proved vagus-inhibition on the intestine and proceeded M.D. under Mueller in 1855. His work on electrotonus brought him the title Privat-Docent under Emil du Bois-Reymond in 1858. Pflueger's 'Law of convulsion' became an essential part of physiological teaching in Germany.

In 1859, Pflueger succeeded Helmholtz as Professor of Physiology in

Bonn. Pflueger's resources and space were much reduced to begin with. He introduced research in histology, studying the embryonal development of the ovary (1861–1863) and the nerve endings in the salivary glands (1866). He described 'Pflueger's tubes', the hollow tubes from which the embryonal ovary operates. In their lumina he thought to see closely packed vesicles, probably cells.

He was also concerned with the study of the gas exchange in the blood and in the cells. His idea that the endings of secretory nerves entered directly onto the secreting cells of the ovaries, led him to postulate the reflex theory of menstruation.

Among the many lines of research during his lifetime were the concept of the 'respiratory quotient', studies on protein, carbohydrate and fat metabolism and of glucagon, over which he became involved in controversies. He died of a carcinoma at the age of 81.

Pflueger's Archiv for physiology is still a going concern.

PLATTER, Felix   1536–1614

Felix Platter was born in Bâle, Switzerland, in 1536, son of the headmaster of the gymnasium (= humanistic grammar) school. He became a doctor in Montpellier in 1556. In 1560, he returned to Bâle as Professor of Practical Medicine. His excellent reputation resulted in the University becoming a popular centre for pupils from other countries.

He mentioned cretins in connection with mental deficiency, in his *Praxeos Medicae* in 1602, and his description of thymic death is well known.

He died in Bâle in 1614.

PLINY the Elder (Caius Plinius Secundus)
AD 23–79

Pliny was the scion of a noble family from Como or Verona. In his youth he fought in campaigns in Germany; he was later proconsul in Spain and eventually commanded the Roman fleet at the battle of Misenum.

Of his main works, which were discussed In Chapter 7 of Section I only the *Historia naturalis* remains, in 37 books. It is known that he died during the volcanic eruption of Vesuvius in AD 79, when he was in command of a small squadron in the Bay of Naples and brought his ship into the danger zone, partly to help, partly out of curiosity of the natural scientist, to observe the event at a close range.

PROCHASKA, George P.   1749–1820

Born in April, 1749 at Lipsitz in Moravia (then Austria), George Prochaska first studied philosophy, becoming a Ph.D. at 18. He then took up the study of medicine, first at Prague and later in Vienna, where he proceeded M.D. in 1776. Two years before that, he had become clinical assistant to de Haën. Next, Joseph Barth, professor of Anatomy and Ophthalmology – an unusual combination – made him his assistant and collaborator both of his anatomical studies and in his extensive practice. Prochaska wrote several treatises in Latin on the physiology of the heart and the circulation of the blood (1778) and became Professor Extraordinary of Anatomy, to be invited to the Chair of Anatomy and Ophthalmology in Prague. During the eleven years he worked there, he organized a large anatomical and morbid anatomical collection, and published important studies on the anatomy and physiology of the nervous system (1779), and on general anatomy. In 1791, he was invited to the Chair of Anatomy, Physiology and Ophthalmology in Vienna, in succession to Barth, which post he held until his retirement in 1819. Because of his extensive private practice (he was alleged to have carried out 3000 cataract operations) he left the teaching of anatomy to his prosector Dr. M. Mayer, keeping only the teaching of physiology. His numerous writings of that period concerned mainly physiological problems, which resulted eventually in a textbook of human physiology (1805/1806 and 1820). It was in this that he proposed his general theory of a sympathetic mechanism of the function of the gonads. He was also the first person to describe the reflex mechanism of the nervous system as paramount in the control of many co-ordinated actions.

Prochaska had artistic talents in the field of painting and music. He died in 1820, leaving a profound impression on the development of anatomy and physiology before Hyrtl and Ernst von Bruecke.

REICHSTEIN, Tadeus   1897–

Tadeus Reichstein was born in July, 1897 at Wloclawek, Poland, son of an engineer. His early childhood was passed in Kiev. He was at a boarding school in Jena (Germany) and later in Zürich, where he also attended the State Technical University (Eidgenoessische Technische Hochschule), where he studied chemistry, receiving his diploma in 1920, proceeding to his doctorate in 1922. In 1921, he became a lecturer at the Technical University for organic and physiological chemistry. His early researches were on the composition of the flavouring substances in roasted coffee, which went on for nearly ten years until 1931, when he became assistant to Professor Leopold Ruzicka (b. 1887), of the synthesis of androsterone fame (1934), who was Nobel Prize winner with Butenandt in 1939. In 1934, he was granted the title of Professor in 1937, he became Professor Extraordinary in Zürich, and proceeded in 1938, to Ordinary Professor of Pharmacology and Director of the Pharmaceutical Institute at the University in Basle. From 1946 to 1950, he also held the Chair of Organic Chemistry in Basle. In 1950, a new Director of the Pharmacological Institute was appointed. Between 1948 and 1952, a new Institute of Organic Chemistry was built and equipped in Basle under his supervision: he became its Director in 1960.

In 1933, Reichstein succeeded in synthesizing ascorbic acid, independently of Sir Norman Haworth in Birmingham. He also co-operated with E. C. Kendall and P. S. Hench on the work on the adrenal cortex leading to the isolation of cortisone and its use in rheumatoid arthritis, and shared the Nobel Prize with them in 1950. Between 1953 and 1954 he collaborated with S. A. Simpson and J. F. Tait in London, and A. Wettstein and R. Neher (of CIBA Laboratories, Basle) in isolating aldosterone.

In 1947, he became an honorary doctor of the Sorbonne (Paris), and in 1952, he was elected a Foreign Member of the Royal Society of London.

ROLLESTON, Sir Humphry Davy, Bart.
1862–1944

Humphry Davy Rolleston was born in Oxford in 1862, son of G. Rolleston, M.D., F.R.S., Linacre Professor of Anatomy and Physiology at the University of Oxford. He was educated at Marlborough and St. John's College, Cambridge. There, he worked with C. S. Roy on the mechanics of the heart action. He was elected to a Fellowship at St. John's in 1889, having qualified in 1888, and proceeded M.D. in 1891. In 1893, he became an examiner for the Cambridge M.B. He was elected a Fellow of the Royal College of Physicians in London in 1894. Before qualifying, his clinical medicine was carried out at St. Bartholomew's Hospital in London. He was Goulstonian Lecturer to the Royal College of Physicians on the suprarenal glands in 1895. He was elected Assistant Physician to St. George's Hospital in London and was Physician there from 1898 to 1919. He developed some lung trouble and in 1901 went to South Africa as Consultant Physician to the Imperial Yeomanry Hospital in Pretoria for a year. During the First World War he was a consulting Surgeon Rear-Admiral in the Royal Navy. From 1922 to 1926 was President of the Royal College of Physicians of London, and their Harveian Orator in 1928. In 1925, he succeeded Sir Clifford Allbutt as Regius Professor of Physic at the University of Cambridge. Only Francis Glisson before him held the two offices of P.R.C.P. and Regius Professor at Cambridge. From 1932 to 1936 he was Physician Extraordinary to King George V. He was President of the Royal Society of Medicine 1918–1920, and had many honorary appointments, degrees and decorations. He was also Editor of the *Practitioner* in 1928, Editor of the *British Encyclopaedia of Medical Practice*, and Joint Editor (with Allbutt) of the 2nd edition of *A System of Medicine* (in 11 volumes).

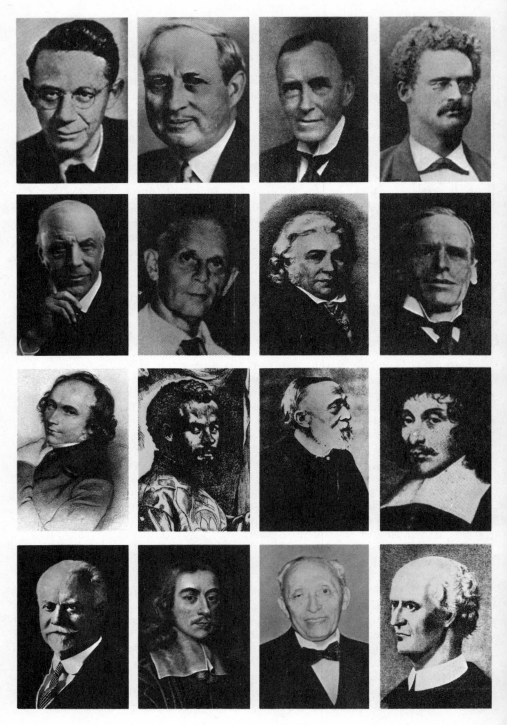

His main interests were, however, the history of medicine and the newly emerging field of endocrinology. In 1932, he published his important *Cambridge Medical History*. In 1936, the celebrated book *The Endocrine Organs in Health and Disease with an Historical Review*, his magnum opus, appeared. It revealed not only his profound knowledge of the subject, but his enormous general knowledge of medical literature, old and new, his only contemporary competitor being Frederick Parkes Weber (1863–1962). It was based on his Fitzpatrick Lectures to the Royal College of Physicians in London on the 'History of the Endocrine Organs', delivered in 1933 and 1934. It has never been surpassed.

RUFUS of Ephesos
[lived in the reign of Trajan   AD 98–117]

Rufus of Ephesos' anatomical writings concerned the eye: he described the membranes, the lens and the chiasma opticum. His (wrong) description of a five lobed liver was carried on in medical literature until Vesalius. He was the first to describe the thymus, and he wrote a good treatise on the pulse, the heart-beat and the systole, which three he declared to be synchronous. Of diseases we have his descriptions of erysipelas and bubonic plague, which latter he perhaps obtained from Alexandria. His major essay on gout was translated into Latin. He introduced an effective purgative, with colocynth, called 'hiera', which became very popular. He was also a successful surgeon, who knew and used digital compression, cautery, torsion and ligature and styptics to stop bleeding.

He belonged to the school of eclectics.

[For a biography of Sajous see Postscript]

SANDSTRÖM, Ivar V.   1852–1889

Ivar Sandström was born in March, 1852, in Stockholm, the son of the Secretary for Agriculture. His brother became a Latin scholar. He himself went to the University of Uppsala in 1871 and a year later, began his

---

Figure 80   (left to right) Top row: Tadeus Reichstein*; Oscar Riddle†; Sir Humphry Davy Rolleston, Bart.†; Ivar Sandström. 2nd row: Sir Edward Sharpey-Schafer†; Hans Selye; Samuel Thomas von Soemmering; Ernest Henry Starling‡. 3rd row: William Stokes‡; Andreas Vesalius; Rulolf Ludwig Vorchow†; Thomas Wharton*; Bottom row: Charles Euchariste de Medici Sajous; Thomas Willis‡; Bernhard Zondek; Abbate Lazzaro Spallanzani†. (*from Ciba Monograph No. 10, by kind permission of Ciba-Geigy Ltd.; †by kind permission of Royal Society of Medicine, London; ‡by kind permission of Department of Medical Illustration, St. Bartholomew's Hospital, London EC1)

medical studies. In 1875–1876, he was a demonstrator in Anatomy. In accordance with the long drawn out plan of medical education in Sweden, he became 'candidate of medicine' (i.e. began his clinical studies after passing the equivalent of the 2nd M.B. in England) in 1878. In 1879/80, he was 'Prosector' in the Department of Anatomy, and in 1881, he became a teacher in histology, which he remained until 1886, while continuing his own studies. In 1887, he finished his medical studies and obtained his diploma as a physician (aged 35, not uncommon in Sweden). Before that time, he fell ill, suffering from a familial mental disorder (from his mother's family) and had to stay in hospital for a short time. The progress of that disease dogged him throughout his life, leading to his early death in 1889, at the age of 37.

His major and almost singular contribution to medical science was the publication in 1880 of 'On a new gland in man and several mammals' (*Upsala Läkareförenings Förhandlinger*, **15**, 441–471, 1880), describing the discovery of the parathyroids. He made it originally during macroscopical dissection in a dog in 1877, while still a medical student. When he examined the structure microscopically, he found that it was an entirely new organ of quite different formation from the underlying thyroid. He continued and completed his investigation in the winter of 1879–1880, when he confirmed the existence of the newly discovered gland in the cat, rabbit, ox, horse and man. In the human species, he investigated 50 individuals and found two such glands on each side in most cases, i.e. four in all. Later studies could not improve on "the admirable precision and accuracy" of his observations (D. A. Welsh: 'Concerning the parathyroid glands: a critical anatomical and experimental study'. In: A critical historical digest of the literature concerning the parathyroid glands. *J. Anat. Physiol.*, **32**, 292–307, 1898). R. L. Thompson added in 1906: "This paper of Sandström is so thorough, that little has been added to our knowledge since their discovery and it is so complete as to leave no doubt that he well deserved all credit for the discovery of these organs." ('A study on parathyroid glands in paralysis agitans', *J. Med. Res.*, **15**, 399–423, 1906). A complete translation (into German) was not accepted by a German scientific journal and the only available information outside Sweden was the report by Magnus Gustav Retzius (1842–1919, Professor of Histology at the Karolinska Institute, Stockholm) in the *Jahresbericht of Hoffmann-Schwalbe*, **9**, 224–226, 1880. This was the one which Gley discovered and duly and fairly acknowledged in 1892.

Sandström was a tall, well built man, with impressive features and a gift for lucid discussion and an analytic mind. He was an excellent teacher whose method of teaching histology "with the microscope at hand" has remained traditional at Uppsala.

An English translation of Sandström's 'Glandulae Parathyroideae' was made by Carl M. Seipel, when he worked at Yale University as a Dental Study Unit Fellow (*Bull. Inst. Hist. Med. Baltimore*, **6**, 192–222, 1938).

SCHÄFER
(after 1918: SHARPEY-SCHAFER),
Sir Edward Albert 1850–1935

Edward Albert Schäfer was born in June, 1850 in London, the son of a merchant of Hamburg and London. He was educated at University College, where he came under the influence of William Sharpey (1802–1880), qualifying M.R.C.S. in 1874. His first paper was published in 1872. He first specialized in histology, and in 1885 the first edition of his *Essentials of Histology* was published (to see another 13 editions during the next 50 years). He became Jodrell Professor of Physiology at University College in 1883, a post he held until 1899. He then moved to Edinburgh accepting the Chair of Physiology which he held for 34 years!

He edited an *Advanced Textbook of Physiology* (1898–1900) and wrote a handbook of *Experimental Physiology, The History of the Physiological Society* (1876–1926). In 1908, he started the *Quarterly Journal of Experimental Physiology*, which he edited until his retirement, when a volume was dedicated to him. He was President of the British Association in 1912, knighted in 1913 and made President of the International Congress of Physiology in 1923.

He became best known, however, for his pioneering work in the endocrine field, first with George Oliver on isolating the blood pressure-raising hormone of the adrenal medulla in 1894–1895, which was discussed in some detail in Section I. This he followed by a lecture on 'Internal Secretions' and, a monograph on the 'Endocrine Organs' in 1916. When he died in 1935, at the age of 85, Sharpey-Schafer had obtained a world-wide reputation, enhanced by his many famous pupils. He had been a Fellow of the Royal Society for many years.

SCHIFF, Moritz 1823–1896

Moritz Schiff was born at Frankfurt-am Main in Germany. He trained originally as a zoologist, with special interest in ornithology. Francis Magendie (1783–1855), the founder in 1821 of the *Journal de Physiologie Expérimentale*, was one of his teachers. Magendie regarded pathology as "the physiology of the sick man". Little wonder that Schiff became an extremely skilled experimental physiologist (see Section I, Chapter 15) and Professor of Comparative Anatomy in Berne, Switzerland, from 1845 to 1863, Professor of Physiology in Florence, Italy, from 1863 to 1876, and in Geneva (1876–1896). His experimental methods were of great ingenuity and carefully designed, far ahead of his time. He investigated many physiological problems, such as the action of the vagus nerve on the heart and the behaviour of the muscle fibres before rigor mortis sets in; he was one of the first to remove the cerebellum and study its effect, and also of the hemisection of the cord. His work of the greatest interest in this book was the investigation of the result of the complete removal of the thyroid gland in dogs; he could show that its effects could be prevented by thyroid grafts and/or by injection of thyroid juice (see Section I, Chapter 15). He also produced experimental diabetes mellitus (in 1856) and demonstrated the role of the nervous system in its production. His original ideas and the influence of his experimental work is not well remembered or appreciated today.

SCHROEDINGER, Erwin   1887–1961

Erwin Schroedinger was born in August, 1887, in Vienna. His father, who had inherited an old established oil-cloth factory, was comfortably off. He (the father) had studied chemistry in Vienna, then turned to painting and later to botany (in which subject he published scientific papers). His mother was the daughter of Alexander Bauer, Professor of Chemistry at the Technische Hochschule (= Technical University) in Vienna. Erwin was educated by a tutor at home and mainly by his father for whom he retained a lifelong affection and admiration. In 1898 he entered the Akademisches Gymnasium, one of the best-known humanistic grammar schools in Vienna. He was a promising student, fond of literature, the theatre and especially of the dramatist Grillparzer. He studied at the University of Vienna and in 1907 he attended lectures on theoretical physics by Friedrich Hasenoehrl, which he continued for eight terms! He also attended the mathematical lectures of Wilhelm Wirtinger and those on experimental physics of Franz Exner, whose assistant he became from 1911 to 1914, having obtained his Ph.D. in 1910. During that time he came under the influence of Egon von Schweidler, who was a Privat-Docent at the Institute. During World War I, he served as an officer in the Fortress Artillery. It was during that time, in 1916, that he learned the fundamentals of Einstein's General Theory of Relativity. He returned to Vienna at the end of the war, but went in 1920 to Jena as assistant to Max Wien, in the experimental physics laboratory. Only four months later he went as Professor Extraordinary to the Technische Hochschule in Stuttgart, and another six months later as Ordinary Professor to Breslau, where he remained, however, for only a few weeks, before being appointed Ordinary Professor in Zürich. His main work there concerned the development of the statistical theory of heat. In 1924, Louis de Broglie defended his doctoral thesis in Paris on his researches into the quantum theory. Only Einstein believed him. Schroedinger was confronted with it in 1925, when reading Einstein's 'Quantumtheorie des einatomigen idealen Gases' (= quantum theory of the single-atom ideal gas). This led eventually to Schroedinger's 'Quantisierung als Eigenwertsproblem' in 1926, containing the first appeearence of his famous wave equation, which forms the basis for the description of the propagation of light. Since then 'Schroedinger's Equation' has been used extensively, concerning various atomic processes (e.g. applied to the exchange of energy between electrons and light rays). In 1927, he succeeded to Max Planck's Chair of Theoretical Physics in Berlin, at Max Planck's personal invitation. In 1933, his dislike of Hitler's régime made him accept a Fellowship at Magdalen College, Oxford (in November). At that time, he shared the Nobel Prize in Physics with P. A. M. Dirac. Homesick for the Alps (he was a keen mountaineer), he accepted a call to Graz in Austria, where he was in 1936–1937. After the 'Anschluss' (the takeover of Austria by Hitler) he was exposed to great pressure. Hitler had not forgotten that Schroedinger had gone to England in 1933. He was dismissed from his post in Graz on 1 September, 1938. Meantime, Eamon de Valera in Eire, who had taught mathematics at the University of Dublin, passed a law establishing the Dublin Institute for Advanced Studies and offering the Department for theoretical physics to Schroedinger. Fortunately, the Germans had left him in possession of his passport, so that he could slip out of the country clandestinely. While waiting for the Institute in Dublin to be opened, Schroedinger was a guest lecturer in Ghent. There he was caught as an 'enemy alien' when war was declared, but de Valera managed to get him a safe conduct via England to Dublin, where he arrived on 5 October 1939. He spent 17 'happy years' there, where he also turned to the study of the foundations of physics and their implications for biology and philosophy. In his lectures *What is Life*, which were published in 1945 (Cambridge University Press), he encouraged the study of molecular biology and examined the application of mathematics and of the laws of physics on heredity and biology. Although his views appear to-day slightly out of date, the ideas represented a great innovation at the time.

Schroedinger spoke four modern languages fluently, was a Greek and Latin scholar; he also published a volume of poetry. He refused to return to Austria while there was a Soviet presence. He eventually returned in 1956 and was given his own Chair in Theoretical Physics. He died in 1961 in Alpbach, in his beloved mountains.

SELYE, Hans   1907–

Hans Selye was born in Vienna in January, 1907, the son of a Hungarian medical officer to an Austro-Hungarian regiment of hussars, stationed at that time in Vienna, and of an Austrian mother. He studied medicine in Prague, Paris and Rome, qualifying in Prague in 1929 and obtaining a diploma in chemistry in 1931. In Prague, he worked under Biedl. A Rockefeller Foundation Scholarship enabled him to spend a year at Johns Hopkins University in Baltimore. From there he went to McGill in Montreal as lecturer in biochemistry and later, in histology. In 1945, he became Professor and Director of the Institute for Experimental Medicine and Surgery at the French University in Montreal, a post specially created for him.

His name is particularly linked to the concept of the 'Stress–General Adaptation Syndrome' which he first presented in a paper in *Nature (London)* in 1936; but he also made extensive studies in the endocrine field and published a *Textbook of Endocrinology*. His international reputation is reflected in the possession of 18 honorary doctor titles from many universities. A popular teacher and writer, his knowledge of nine languages is of great advantage. Although in his 73rd year, he is still carrying on with his research work and with his teaching. As principle for a healthy living, he suggested: 'Find your own stress level, be an altruistic egoist and earn thy neighbours' love'.

SORANOS of Ephesos   AD 98–138

Soranos of Ephesos studied in Alexandria and, later, practised in Rome. He was the leading authority on gynaecology, obstetrics and paediatrics of antiquity. His interests included the study of contraception (N. E. Himes dedicated his book *Medical History of Contraception*, 1936, to Soranos). His treatises on midwifery and diseases of women were translated into Latin, German and French from the original Greek text (edited by Dietz in Koenigsberg, East Prussia, in 1838). On it was based Roeslin's *Rosengarten* (1513) (see also Section I, Chapter 13), and its English translation by Richard Jonas: *The byrth of mankynde*, printed by Thomas Raynalde (London, 1540).

Soranos described the podalic version, which was revived by Ambroise Paré (1510–1590) in 1549. He also described the atresia of the vagina. He packed the severely bleeding uterus to stop haemorrhage, and he performed hysterectomy for the treatment of marked prolapse. Equally outstanding is his chapter on paediatrics with its contribution to infant nutrition and hygiene, and diseases of infants, with a good description of rickets.

His observations with a possible endocrine background were discussed in Chapters 6 and 7. His use of a vaginal speculum has also been mentioned.

SPALLANZANI, Lazzaro (Abbate)
1729–1799

Lazzaro Spallanzani was born the son of a lawyer in Scandiano, Modena (Italy), in 1729. Educated at Reggio, he studied law in Bologna. Apparently influenced by the example of Antonio Vallisnieri (1661–1730) and his zoological studies (1715), he took holy orders to pursue the study of natural science. His appointment in the University of Reggio in 1754 was remarkable as he became Professor of Logic, Metaphysics and Greek Literature. In 1760, he moved to Modena, where he investigated the regeneration of the polyp *Hydra* and the physiology of circulation. He was then invited to the Chair of Natural History at Pisa, where his translation of Charles Bonnet's (1720–1793) *Contemplation de la nature* into Italian evoked his interest in Bonnet's ideas (Bonnet was an 'organistic preformationist') and inspired him to carry out his studies on infusoria. For teaching purposes (in order to explain the mechanism of digestion) he began to study the action of saliva and confirmed Réaumur's findings on the digestive powers of gastric juice in animals. He also showed that it prevented putrefaction and inhibited it once begun, although he did not recognize its acid nature. He demonstrated that gastric juice was produced by the stomach itself and not introduced into it from outside. Some of the decisive and even daring experiments he carried out on himself (English translation: *Dissertations relative to the natural history of animals and vegetables, translated from the Italian of the Abbé Spallanzani*. London, J. Murray, 1784, 2 Vols.) In 1768, he established the doctrine of the regeneration of the spinal cord (*Prodromi sulla riproduzione animale Riproduzione della coda del girino* Modena; 1768). He further demonstrated that the sexual posture in the frog is maintained as a spinal reflex after decapitation or after section of the two brachial nerves (1768; ibidem). His study of respiratory exchanges in warm- and cold-blooded animals demonstrated that hibernating animals can live comfortably in carbon dioxide for a time, whereas warm-blooded animals die immediately. Cold-blooded animals can live in hydrogen and continue to give off carbon dioxide; living tissue, removed from a freshly killed animal, will take up oxygen in an atmosphere not only of air, but also hydrogen and nitrogen. His specially important and ingenious researches were on the doctrine of spontaneous generation, as already discussed in Section I, Chapter 14. Finally, he produced regenerations of the heads, limbs and tentacles of earth worms, tadpoles, salamanders and snails (in 1768: See *Prodromo di un'opera sopra le riproduzioni animali*. Milan, 1829). He was thus, with René Antoine de Réaumur, 1683–1757, Abraham Trembley, 1710–1784, Charles Bonnet, 1720–1793, and Henry Baker, 1698–1774, one of the early experimental morphologists. He was an incredibly brilliant experimenter, not only with an incisive mind and highly skilled technically, but apparently with a puckish sense of humour. His merits are perhaps not sufficiently appreciated outside Italy.

STARLING, Ernest Henry   1866–1927

Ernest Henry Starling was born in London in 1866 and educated at King's College School and Guy's Hospital. A distinguished student, he became demonstrator of physiology and then head of the physiology department of that hospital. He made his laboratory the best equipped in London. At the age of 33, in 1899, he was elected to the Chair of Physiology as Jodrell

Professor at University College, a post which he held until 1922. He was elected a Fellow of the Royal Society in 1899 and awarded the Society's Royal Medal in 1913, having received the Baly Medal of the Royal College of Physicians in 1907. He was also the recipient of many honorary doctorates. In 1922, he was appointed the first Foulerton Research Professor of the Royal Society. He wrote a number of books, one of the most outstanding being the *Principles of Human Physiology* in 1912, the classical textbook of its time.

At University College, he had a longstanding collaboration with (Sir) Edward Sharpey-Schafer, but especially with (Sir) William Maddock Bayliss (1860–1924). Theirs was a really remarkable co-operation. Bayliss, who was six years older than Starling, had switched from the study of medicine to physiology (not unlike Joseph Needham, much later); qualifying as a physiologist in Oxford in 1888, he became assistant at the Institute of Physiology at University College in London in the same year. Although he became eventually Professor of General Physiology in University College, Starling became his chief in 1899, on his appointment to Jodrell Professor, in succession to Schaefer. Bayliss was not young (40) when he began to make a name for himself; he was financially comfortably off and independent, a short, plumpish, kind, reticent and shy person, a dedicated, methodical, skilled, even-tempered experimenter, who loved his work; although a good teacher, he was only a moderate orator. Starling, in contrast, was a romantic personality, in appearance, attitude and behaviour. Generous, but quick on the uptake, in his reactions, repartee, a brilliant speaker, restless, energetic, driven by enthusiasm, a systematic man, whereas Bayliss was the more methodical (it was he who received the Copley Medal of the Royal Society). The two not only complemented one another, but they were also brothers-in-law. This is not the place to discuss in detail their co-operation which culminated in the discovery of secretin, and the effect it had on the development of endocrinology. H. H. Simmer has written a beautiful little study not only on the discovery of secretin, with all the controversies and arguments it produced, but also on the personalities of Bayliss and Starling, representing two important types of research workers, as the Inaugural Address on his (Simmer's) appointment as Professor of the History of Medicine at the University Erlangen-Nurenberg (*Med. Welt.*, **29,** 1991–1996, 1978).

The other subjects Starling studied were the secretion of lymph and other body fluids, and the laws which govern the activity of the heart.

In 1892 he went to Breslau to work with Rudolf Peter Heinrich Heidenhain (1834–1897) on the subject of lymph formation. It is said that Starling verified Heidenhain's experiments, but disproved all his conclusions. He carried out many crucial experiments of his own. Starling showed in fact that most of the phenomena which govern the flow of lymph could be explained, if proper account was taken of the factors which govern the hydrostatic processes of blood in the capillaries together with the osmotic properties of the fluids concerned. In this connection, special stress was laid on the osmotic pressure of the colloid constituents of those fluids. The work, although undertaken with special reference to lymph flow, soon extended to the secretion and absorption of other fluids, such as urine and serous fluids generally. This work put Starling in the first rank of experimental physiologists.

Before the First World War, he devoted time to the study of the action of the heart. He also worked on other subjects, such as the movement of the gut, and on renal secretion. During the war, he joined the Royal Army Medical Corps. He worked at Woolwich and then with the Italian Army. He perfected a respirator which was effective against a gas attack by the Austrians.

He was described as having a magnetic personality, inexhaustible energy and a generous heart.

STEINACH, Eugen   1861–1944

Eugen Steinach was born in January, 1861 in Hohenems (Vorarlberg, Austria). He studied medicine in Vienna, where he qualified in 1886. He then worked as assistant at the Institute of Physiology at Innsbruck for two years. He moved to Prague to work under the celebrated physiologist Ewald Hering. In 1902, he founded a 'Laboratory for General and Comparative Physiology', the first of its kind in the German academic orbit. In 1912, he moved to Vienna as head of the Biological Experiment Station, which two years later was linked to the Academy of Sciences. In 1894, he began systematic experimental work on the physiology of the gonads. The experiments were well planned and continuous, but unfortunately, they were taken up by the press, popularized and distorted. Steinach attempted to verify the hypothesis of the French scientists Ancel and Bovin, that hormonal action of the gonads, which controls the secondary sex characteristics, is a function of the interstitial (Leydig) cells, which Steinach named the 'puberty gland'. His great skill in gonadal transplant experiments produced masculinized female and feminized male animals. Testicular transplants into senile male rats had a rejuvenating effect. On his suggestion, the urologist Robert Lichtenstern carried out the first ligation of the vas deferens in man, a method which had stimulated the puberty gland and had a rejuvenating effect in old male rats, according to Steinach's observation. The human experiment had a spectacular, though transient, result and many similar operations were carried out. With the isolation and synthesis of gonadal hormones, Steinach's method became obsolete. Hitler's occupation of Austria ended his scientific work, and he emigrated to Switzerland. His wife's death and his enforced inactivity depressed him, and he died in May, 1944, a disappointed man.

STOKES, William 1804–1878

William Stokes was born in Dublin in 1804, son of Regius Professor of Medicine at the University of Dublin. He was trained in classics and mathematics by a Fellow of Trinity College, and in science by his father. He took his M.D. degree in Edinburgh in 1825, and in 1826 was elected physician to the Meath hospital in the place of his father. He became a colleague and friend of Graves. He founded the Dublin Pathological Society in 1838, was President of the Royal Irish Academy and elected F.R.S. in 1861, and became Regius Professor of Medicine in 1845. He published work on diseases of the chest, heart and aorta in 1854 and 1874. In his *Diseases of the Heart* (1854), the account of the 'increased action of the heart and of the arteries of the neck followed by enlargement of the thyroid gland and eyeballs', was much fuller than Graves's earlier account. Stokes was regarded as a great clinician by his colleagues. He died in January 1878.

STOPES, Marie Carmichael 1880–1958

Marie Carmichael Stopes is a good example of the influence of innate temperament, family background, emotional conflicts and personal relations with the opposite sex, on the development of her career, her ideas and the movement, which she created and represented and which cannot be understood without her personal history.

She was born in October, 1880, in Edinburgh, daughter of Mary Charlotte Carmichael Stopes, the first woman in Scotland to take a University Certificate, and a Shakespearean scholar. Her father, Henry Stopes, was the son of a Colchester brewer, who became an engineer and architect specializing in the building of breweries. His real interest in life was, however, archaeology. Charlotte fought for women's Reform. Henry was a passionate and loyal man. At the time of his marriage, he was 28 and Charlotte 39! Ruth Hall, who published an excellent biography of Marie Stopes (1978) (characteristically by a publishing company called 'Virago') describes Charlotte from photographs as "a thin-lipped, rather hard-eyed woman, secure in her rectitude".

For the first twelve years Marie was taught by her mother. She took great interest in the archaeological work of her father, whom she adored. She and her younger sister were then sent to St. George's High School, Edinburgh. Two years later, they returned to London, to attend the North London Collegiate School, near home, where the teaching standards were high. Marie received a leaving scholarship in science and enrolled as a student at University College. After the first year, she won a gold medal; after two years she obtained first class honours in botany and third class honours in geology and her B.Sc. degree. Unfortunately, her father died at that very time. She was also awarded the University's (of London) Gilchrist Scholarship for a year's postgraduate work abroad. In October, 1903, she went to Munich, to take up her scholarship and work in palaeobotany, "a chapter in the Book of Life". In Munich, she worked well under Professor K. Goebel and not only learned German, but also obtained a doctorate (based on her thesis on cycads), the first woman there to do so, 'magna cum laude'. She also participated in the gay cultural life of Munich, with all the reservations of a well brought up young English girl. She became friendly with Kenjiro Fujii, a Japanese botanist on study leave in Europe, 14 years her senior and married (with his wife in Japan). German men did not seem to attract her. She discovered music, the opera and especially Wagner.

At the end of June, 1904 Marie returned to England. She applied for a post as junior lecturer in botany at Manchester University. Surprisingly, she was appointed, the first woman to be so. She remained there for three years, during which time she became the youngest doctor of Science (D.Sc.) (London) in Britain (in 1905). Manchester's proximity to the coalfields made her take up the study of coal, an interest she never lost. Her (platonic) love affair with Kenjiro Fujii deepened when he came to work in London and also visited her in Manchester. She published their (edited) correspondence in 1911 under the title *Love letters of a Japanese* under the pseudonym 'G. N. Mortlake'. At 24, she was kissed for the first time by a man whose race disdained the Western habit of kissing. Although his marriage was not yet dissolved, they agreed on a secret betrothal. Addressing one another as husband and wife in their letters, their affair remained platonic. In January, 1906 Fujii's marriage ended in divorce. His feelings for her cooled, however, and in August, 1907, when Marie arrived in Yokohama on a grant of the Royal Society, they were nearly at an end. Marie spent 18 months in Japan, going on a fossil-hunting expedition to Hokkaido. She disliked the inferior status Japanese women had. Professor Fujii became ill, "in danger of losing his sight", she wrote home. It is possible, however, that Fujii exaggerated his ill health in order to extricate himself from the situation, without hurting Marie's pride, Yet he lived to be 86, and had – after Marie's departure from Japan – two common law wives, the last one of whom he eventually married when he was 82! After a period of depression because of the failed love affair, Marie returned to work. In January, 1909, she sailed for England, via Vancouver. Back home, there were more emotional involvements, but her scientific career proceeded. For the next year she lectured in Manchester and published seven major papers.

At 31, Marie's book knowledge of sex was merely from poetry (Browning, Swinburne, Shakespeare) and from Edward Carpenter's *Love's Coming of Age*. It was a presentation of a romantic view on sex, being transformed into a spiritual and emotional experience; but Carpenter himself was a homosexual. In this frame of mind, with two other emotional upsets behind her, Marie met Dr. Reginald Ruggles Gates, a geneticist, at a meeting in St. Louis. He was 29, and they were married within two months. At the same time, Marie was appointed Lecturer in Palaeobotany at University College, the first such post in Britain. Gates was merely teaching biology to medical students at St. Thomas's Hospital. He was also impotent. To complicate things, there was Aylmer Maude, 22 years older than Marie, handsome, separated from his wife, who became a lodger and admirer of Marie. Although their relationship remained platonic, it became a 'ménage à trois'.

In 1914, Marie had read (1) all the books on sex in the British Museum, in English, French and German; (2) as much on English law as possible; (3) Marshall and Starling's papers on the physiology or reproduction and on the hormones; (4) the complete works of Professor August Forel, especially his *Sexual Ethics* and *The Sexual Question*; (5) Havelock Ellis's *Man and Woman* and his *Studies in the Psychology of Sex*. She also openly supported the suffragettes. In 1916, her nullity petition, also proving her virginity, succeeded; but her wish to live with Aylmer Maude was not fulfilled. This experience of her first marriage became Marie Stopes' justification for sexual reform. Her book: *Married Love*, published in 1918, centred on sexual education. In July, 1915, she had met Mrs. Margaret Sanger, the American pioneer of birth control and struck up a friendship and collaboration, which later ended, however, in enmity. Financially, Marie got into difficulties.

When *Married Love* was published, it became a great success. Marie was 38 and had just married for the second time, to Humphrey Verdon Roe, who was then 39. This time, she achieved her desire.

Within a short time, in November 1918, the second book on her new subject was published: *Wise Parenthood*; this she considered a necessary sequel, by public demand, to *Married Love*, being a concise guide to birth control. The suggestion in the book for the necessity of the "sacramental rhythmic performance of the marriage rite of physical union throughout the whole of married life . . . separate and distinct from its value as a basis for the procreation of children" (*Wise Parenthood*, p. 21, London, Fifield, 1918), was too much for the public of the day, for many publishers and, especially, for the Protestant Church. Her medical recommendations were also incorrectly conceived, especially her advice on handling the cap.

At 38, Marie Stopes was pregnant at last. She hoped for a girl, 'Margaret'. At the same time, she developed a urinary infection, and she refused to stop work. On 17 July, 1919, she gave birth to a stillborn boy.

Marie, however, had become a national figure. Whether the Church (and others) protested, criticized, or just disapproved silently, members of the public, including vicars, curates and their wives, wrote to her and asked her advice on their sexual problems. If the bishops followed St. Paul and advocated celibacy or, at least, continence and self-denial, the public, including the lower clergy, became interested in birth control and the enjoyment of sexual relations in marriage by both husband and wife. Needless to say, the Catholic Church was harsher in the condemnation of birth control. The medical profession were split in their attitude. There were supporters of birth control like Dr. C. Killick Millard, Medical Officer of Health for Leicester and also a member of the Birth Rate Commission. Others did not go beyond accepting the 'safe period' in the middle of the cycle. Dr. George Jones, of the West End Hospital for Women (London), was even more liberal, by demanding – logically – birth control even more importantly in the case of unmarried women; but the majority of doctors were antagonistic.

Marie sent out questionnaires to the clergy and to doctors on their married sexual habits, and received a sufficient number of replies to be able to form a picture of the existing position. She also tackled the public and the politicians (MPs). She wrote to Queen Mary and Queen Alexandra, though without much success. The great number of men who had acquired venereal disease while in the forces during the war, was another point that needed consideration. The working classes came in for criticism for thoughtlessly 'destroying the race' (letter to the *Daily Mail*, 12 June, 1919).

Her next book, *Radiant Motherhood*, was published in 1920 and, on the whole, well received, but also criticized that it catered mainly for families with an income of £1000 a year! Marie was annoyed. Following the publication of *Married Love*, she had been, since 1919, a member of the National Birth Rate Commission by invitation and thought she had broadened her knowledge of the general situation. Moreover, she had, in 1919, written a pamphlet: 'A Letter to Working Mothers; on how to keep healthy children and avoid weakening pregnancies' (published by M. C. Stopes), which had been, however, coldly received; "the poor just would not bother", her friend, Mrs. E. B. Mayne, concluded. So Marie decided to set up her own birth-control clinic. There is no room here to discuss in detail the further developments which followed the setting up of the Mothers' Clinic; they were briefly mentioned in Section I.

In 1921, was published *The Truth about Venereal Diseases* (by Putnam & Sons), and in 1922, *A New Gospel to All Peoples: A revelation of God uniting the physiology and the religions of man* (A. L. Humphreys).

Lord Dawson of Penn spoke up for birth control at the Church Congress in Birmingham in 1921. In November, 1921, eight months after Dr. Stopes' clinic came into being, the Malthusian League opened their clinic in South London's slum area (Walworth), run by Dr. Norman Haire, an Australian Jew, favouring the Dutch cap. Marie added her own disapproval, to the general abuse they were exposed to. In August, 1921, she founded the 'Society for Constructive Birth Control and Racial Progress (CBC)', to which she added a newspaper in May, 1922: *Birth Control News*. There was also disagreement with Mrs. Sanger in the U.S.A.; but the main event to follow was Marie Stopes' court case for libel against Dr. Halliday Sutherland, Secretary of the 'League of National Life', an anti-contraception (mainly Catholic) organization. He published a book against birth control, and also argued that it was a class conspiracy against the poor. The trial opened in the High Court on 21 February 1923, before Lord Chief Justice Hewart. Marie's sister Winnie was dying at the age of 38, of heart disease. Marie did not have time to visit her before her death on 28 February. The case was fought in all three instances, before the Lord Chief Justice, before the Appeal Court and before the House of Lords. The final decision, in November, 1924, went against Dr. Stopes, but a moral victory, a tremendous increase in popularity and in the sale of her books, was hers. In 1922, she had also published: *Early days of Birth Control* (Putnam's Sons), to which she added in 1923: *Contraception, its Theory, History and Practice* (Bale, Sons and Danielson), and in 1925, *The First Five Thousand* (first report of the Mothers' Clinic for Constructive Birth Control), John Bale & Co. She also wrote a filmscript: 'Maisie's Marriage', which was eventually filmed, in spite of objections by the British Board of Film Censors, and proved a success outside London. Her greatest achievement at that time, was, however, that she became pregnant again and, at the age of 43, her son was born by Caesarean section on 17 March, 1944; but *The Times* refused to print the announcement of the birth of Harry Verdon Stopes-Roe. Her possessiveness and vanity, concerning the child, strained her relations with her husband. Her possessiveness as a mother, strained, later, her relations with her son.

Of her many subsequent publications, *Enduring Passion* should be mentioned, published in 1928 (Putnam & Sons). She was then 48. It was to be a sequel to *Married Love*, to re-assure the middle-aged that monogamous marriage could survive to ripe old age. Her own marriage proved, however, far from successful, but her personal success had increased beyond any expectation. In the special issue of *The Practitioner* of July, 1923, devoted to Birth Control, the medical profession retained their opinion that the subject should remain in their control. More court cases followed (in June, 1924, to her disgust as against "Mrs. Humphrey Roe"), occasionally Dr. Stopes winning them, but always with the benefit of achieving greater popular acclaim. She was invited to become a member of the National Birth Control Council (later the Family Planning Association), founded in 1930. The ensuing years were of less importance to the now almost independent movement on birth control.

Her husband suffered bankruptcy in the wake of the Wall Street disaster of 1929. He became more and more depressed and subdued. From July, 1938, they began to live apart and after 1940, they never lived together again. Marie refused to let him come home, soon after the beginning of the war, when he had rejoined the Royal Air Force. In 1942, he was 65 and she was 63, but she still felt a young woman. In 1938, she had met Keith Briant, a young man, just down from Oxford, aged 25. She developed a romantic attachment ('erogamic love'). She also struck up a close friendship with Lord Alfred Douglas (Oscar Wilde's 'Bosie'), then sixty-eight. Always interested in poetry, and writing and publishing poems for many years, Marie now began to write erotic poetry, which she then read to her guests, often to their embarrassment. Her *Love Songs for Young Lovers* had been published in 1938; it was believed that they referred to Keith Briant. Her husbend died in 1949, aged 70. She visited him a few weeks before, and on his death, she wrote a sonnet of somewhat doubtful taste.

She tried to interfere with her son's marriage plans, unsuccessfully. Harry's marriage turned out to be a happy one, but nevertheless, she cut him out of her will. By 1950, Ruth Hall, remarks, "Marie Stopes was a figure from the past" (p. 304). The Family Planning Association had overtaken her efforts, with its hundreds of clinics. Her own five clinics were taken over by the National Health Service in 1948. She did not participate in the international organizations of birth control, nor in new ideas.

At the age of 73, she fell in love again, this time with Baron Avro Manhattan, aged 38, a writer and painter. She had originally met him in 1938, but her interest in him really began in 1952. She was convinced that he was her true soul-mate, but the age difference was too great to let the affair go beyond platonic limits, although she seriously contemplated marrying him.

In 1957, she began to feel ill; cancer was diagnosed too late. In November, she went to Bavaria for unorthodox treatment at a much publicized private clinic. There she underwent very painful therapy for six weeks, returning home to Norbury Park, where she still remained active. She died on 2 October 1958, nearly 78 years of age.

According to her will, she was cremated and her son scattered her ashes into the sea from Portland Bill, in the presence of his wife Mary, and of Avro Manhattan.

SUDHOFF, Karl Friedrich Jakob   1853–1938

Karl F. J. Sudhoff was born in November, 1853 in Frankfurt am Main, the son of a Protestant minister. He attended humanistic grammar school (Gymnasium) in Frankfurt, Zweibruecken and Kreuznach. He studied medicine at the universities of Erlangen, Tuebingen and Berlin, and proceeded M.D. in 1875. He did postgraduate hospital studies in Augsburg and Vienna. In 1878, he settled in general practice in Bergen near Frankfurt, moving to Hochdahl near Dusseldorf in 1883, where he practised until 1905 (a total of 27 years in practice). All his spare time was dedicated to the study of the history of medicine. His first major contribution was the *Bibliographia Paracelsica* (2 vols, 1884–1899). He studied not only the life of Paracelsus in detail, but also Paracelsus' manuscripts. In 1901, he founded the German Society for the History of Medicine and Science. In 1905, this entirely self-taught man in the subject, was offered and accepted the chair for the History of Medicine in Leipzig, the first in Germany. It was endowed with 500 000 marks (= £25 000) by the widow of Theodor Puschmann of Vienna, and helped to develop the Institute for the History of Medicine. He developed an incredibly busy programme of meticulous, painstaking research, during the course of which he travelled tirelessly all over Europe, to study important manuscripts first hand, and made a number of important discoveries. He retired in 1925, but when his successor, Henry Ernest Sigerist (1891–1957) accepted a call to the Johns Hopkins University in 1932, Sudhoff returned as acting director until 1934.

Sudhoff's main fields of interest were medicine in ancient times, mediaeval and Renaissance medicine. He had a particular interest in epidemiology and hygiene and in the history of syphilis, to all of which he made important contributions. He also wrote a detailed monograph on the iatro-mathematicians of the 15th and 16th centuries (1902), on German medical incunabula (1908), an early history of anatomical illustrations (1908), on Greek papyrus documents (1909), an early history of syphilis (1912). In 1921, he published a history of dentistry and in the same year, with Theodor Meyer-Steineg (1873–1936), a survey of the history of medicine (5th edition in 1965). In 1925, he published facsimile reproductions of the three earliest printed works on paediatrics. In addition, he founded in 1908 the *Archiv fuer die Geschichte der Medizin,* to which he contributed numerous papers. He also published a number of rare medical texts in the form of inexpensive reprints: *Klassiker der Medizin.* Of his discoveries perhaps the most interesting was Gutenberg's purgation calendar of 1457, which he found in the Bibliothèque Nationale in Paris. His superb catalogue of the Dresden Historical Exhibition in 1911 opened up a survey of the History of Hygiene.

He was a great scholar and, although intolerant of sloppy work, a modest, kindly and generous man. The only person who can be regarded as approaching his standards was Max Neuburger (1868–1955) in Vienna. He was 15 years his junior and had succeeded Theodor Puschmann (1844–1899), whose widow had endowed the chair of medical history in Leipzig.

Sudhoff died at Salzwedel, Germany, in October, 1938.

TANDLER, Julius   1869–1936

Julius Tandler was born in February, 1869 at Iglau in Moravia (then Austria), but moved with his parents to Vienna when he was very small. There they lived in difficult and poor circumstances. However, he managed to enter grammar school and later to study medicine, when he worked under the anatomist Emil Zuckerkandl. He became his assistant after qualifying in 1895, and proceeded to Privat-Docent in 1899 and to Professor Extraordinary in 1903. He succeeded Zuckerkandl in 1910 and gave his celebrated inaugural address on 'Anatomy and the Clinic', stressing his idea that anatomy must be studied and taught in relation to the needs of clinical medicine and of the sick patient. In 1916, he gave a lecture on the effects of war on the population, and he became increasingly interested in social problems. In 1919, the Social Democratic Government made him an Under-Secretary at the Ministry of Health, but he relinquished the post in October, 1920. He then became the City Councillor of Vienna in charge of the Health Department, which he remained for almost 14 years. In this capacity he planned and carried out far-reaching social medical reforms, including re-organization of the City of Vienna's (non-university) hospitals, adding new buildings, tuberculosis out-patient clinics, and ante-natal clinics. The crematorium was built at that time. He was also concerned with social care for the young, opening new Kindergartens, organizing presents of baby linen to the mothers of all children born in Vienna, etc. He was also interested in the treatment of malignant disease and brought the first radium for treatment to Vienna. He also founded marriage guidance clinics, VD clinics and clinics for the treatment of alcoholics.

All that time, he carried out his normal duties as Professor of Anatomy. He published a much appreciated textbook of anatomy in 4 volumes in

1928. His other scientific work was carried out mainly before 1914, of which his research into eunuchoidism with S. Grosz became best known.

He was interested in sport and the Sport Stadium in Vienna was built in his time of office.

After the Social Democratic rising in 1934, he was in prison for a short time; he then was compulsorily retired from his post as Professor of Anatomy. He began his travels to the U.S.A. and to China, advising the Chinese government (of Chiang-kai-shek) on hospital planning and building and administration. In 1936, he was invited to Moscow, to advise on hospital administration. He died there in August, 1936; his body was brought home and cremated and his ashes rest in the crematorium he helped to build.

As already mentioned (see Chapter 14), he and K. Keller were, in 1911, the first to appreciate that in freemartins the twins of opposite-sex shared a common placental circulation.

He was a lively, controversial figure, a brilliant teacher and speaker, often very sarcastic, much admired and, at the same time, much criticized, with a passionate nature and high ideals. He appreciated people who stood up to him, provided that they had a good case and could present it adequately.

TIGERSTEDT, Robert Adolf Armand
1853–1923

Robert A. A. Tigerstedt was born in February, 1853, in Helsinki, son of a Lecturer in History, of Swedish ancestry. Robert matriculated at 16, and passed his examination as a candidate of philosophy at the age of 20. He then studied medicine, proceeding to Licenciate after seven years in 1880 and to Dr. med. et chir. in 1881. Even before passing his 2nd M.B. (to become candidate of Medicine) he was 'Laborator' in Physiology, a post which he gave up after 2 years. In 1877, he worked as an 'assistant in medicine'. Following an invitation by Christian Lovén, the first holder of the the Chair of Physiology at the Karolinska Institute, he moved to Stockholm in 1881, first as locum and later as Laborator in Physiology. In 1883, he published a *Guide for Practical Exercises in Physiology*, mainly on optics and nerve- and muscle-physiology.

He had spent the summer of 1881 with Carl Friedrich Wilhelm Ludwig (1816–1895) in Leipzig. Ludwig was one of the pioneers of modern scientific and experimental physiology, with a wide range of subjects; he made important contributions to the study of renal secretions, blood pressure, innervation of the heart, innervation of the salivary glands and invented the perfusion technique to keep excised parts of organs alive. Tigerstedt repeated his visit to Ludwig's Institute in 1883, when he also visited a number of other European centres. In 1885, Tigerstedt was granted an addition to his official salary through the intervention of Lovén, his chief. Lovén took a long leave in the autumn 1884, because of ill health, and Tigerstedt deputized for him. Two years later, Lovén retired and Tigerstedt succeeded him as Professor of Physiology. He remained there for another 14 years, until he was invited to succeed Hällstén in Helsinki, on his retirement in 1899. Tigerstedt carried on there until he retired in 1919, aged 66. He died suddenly, in his sleep, in December, 1923, aged 70.

His many outstanding contributions to modern physiology can not be discussed in such a brief sketch. In this place, the most important studies concerned those carried out in collaboration with P.G. Bergman on the kidney and the circulation ('Niere und Kreislauf'; *Skand. Arch. Physiol.*, **8**, 223–271, 1898), in which the discovery of a kidney hormone is described, of the pressor substance 'renin', which enters the circulation via the renal veins. Six years before, in 1892, Brown-Séquard is believed to have demonstrated, together with D'Arsonval, that injections of a renal extract improved the condition of nephrectomized animals. Tigerstedt and Bergman also assumed that renin may play a role in the causation of cardiac hypertrophy in renal disease. The value of these classic experiments was not fully recognized until Henry Goldblatt's (b. 1891) studies on the connection between hypertension and kidney damage. In 1921 to 1923 the 2nd edition of his magnum opus (in 4 volumes) on the *Physiology of the Circulation* was published, a worthy sequel to William Harvey's work.

Tigerstedt inherited from his father a definite interest in history. He wrote a number of biographical sketches of famous medical and non-medical people: Vesalius, William Harvey, Du Bois-Reymond, Ludwig and Helmholtz, both in form of obituaries and as *Documents from the History of Medicine* (1921), an excellent work which is hardly known. He was also interested in intelligent dissemination of scientific achievements in popular form, and in problems of school hygiene and of alcoholism.

He acquired an international reputation and was due to preside over the 9th International Congress of Physiology in Paris in 1916, but the war intervened.

TROUSSEAU, Armand   1801–1867

Armand Trousseau was born in Tours in 1801. He studied medicine in Paris and became a pupil of Pierre Bretonneau (1778–1862) of diphtheria fame. In 1837 he received the prize of the Academy of Medicine for his monograph on tuberculosis of the larynx. In 1850, he became Professor of the Medical Faculty in Paris and physician at the Hôtel Dieu.

He described gastric vertigo, and Trousseau's sign of infantile tetany; he was one of the first (after Bretonneau) to perform tracheotomy in croup and intubation. His *Clinique médicale de l'Hôtel Dieu* (1861) became a standard text. He was of generous nature, popularizing Addison's and other contemporary achievements.

VERZÁR, Friedrich   1886–1779

Friedrich Verzár was born in September, 1886 in Budapest where he studied medicine, in addition to studying in Tuebingen and Cambridge. He qualified in Budapest in 1909 and entered there Tangl's Institute for General Pathology and Physiology. Later he worked at Halle/Saale in Germany under Bernstein. He became Privat-Docent in Budapest in 1913, obtained the Chair of Physiology in Debrecen (Hungary) in 1918, from where he moved as Professor of Physiology to Basle in Switzerland in 1930, where he remained.

His scientific work covered nerve–muscle physiology, metabolism, vitamins, blood gas exchange, resorption studies from the intestine and endocrine problems, especially concerning the adrenals.

He died in 1779.

VESALIUS, Andreas   1514–1564

Andreas Vesalius was Flemish by birth, of German extraction. His family name was Witing, later changed to Wesel, where they had once lived. His coat of arms displayed three weasels (wesel). He became a pupil of Jacobus Sylvius (Jacques Dubois, 1478–1555) of Paris, a stern and bigoted Galenist. Although in his graduating thesis, Vesalius appeared to be a strict adherent of Galen, he soon developed a new, superior technique of dissection from which he was able to construct a new live view of anatomy, which found its crowning result in the outstanding work *De Humani Corporis Fabrica libri septem* (Basileae, ex off. Ioannis Oporini) in 1543. It departed from the book-ridden Galenic tradition and put the basis of anatomy on the observation of nature. He had five years' intensive work as public prosector in Padova behind him. The antagonism and the furious attacks upon him, especially by Sylvius and his former pupil Columbus (= Matteo Realdo Colombo, 1516–1559) made him burn his manuscripts in despair, leave Padova and accept service as court physician to the Emperor Charles V in Madrid.

He married, had a family, built up a large private practice and gave up anatomy completely. His favourite pupil Fallopio had become his successor in Padova and his own name seemed to be forgotten. On reading Fallopio's *Observationes anatomicae* in 1561, Vesalius' aspirations were revived. In 1563, he went on a pilgrimage to Jerusalem. On his way back, he received an invitation to resume his post in Padova, following Fallopio's (1523–1562) death. However, he died suddenly of an unknown disease, on the island of Zanthe, a lonely death.

VILLANOVA, Arnold of *ca.* 1235–1311

Arnold of Villanova was born near Valencia *ca.* 1235–50. After studying medicine in Naples he travelled extensively, practising in Paris, Montpellier, Barcelona and Rome. This Catalan physician was an alchemist, astrologer, diplomat, social reformer and visionary. Approximately 123 treatises, most of them short, have been attributed to him, but many are apocryphal.

He was a doctor of theology, law, philosophy and medicine, and counsellor or consultant to Peter III of Aragon. A follower of the Arabian chemists, he also sought a universal elixir of life, and was one of the earliest European writers on alchemy. These tendencies, along with his theological heresies, caused him to be anathematized after his death. He is credited with the introduction of tinctures and of brandy (aurum potabile) into the pharmacopoeia. He translated Avicenna on the heart and probably Avenzoar on diet. He was a pioneer of the classification of diseases and opposed the abuse of dialectics, the tendency of Parisian scholastics to lose themselves in universal theories and ignore particulars, as well as their footless therapeutic empiricism. He was a copious, elegant, uncritical writer, who declined to revise any copy once he had penned it; and his *Breviary of Practice* (Milan, 1483), one of the best of the medical handbooks, contains many independent observations, and many citations from now unknown physicians. His greatest work was the *Parabolae*, a set of 345 pithy aphorisms, dedicated to Philip the Fair (1300), and containing much original thought.

VINCENT, T. Swale   1868–1933

T. Swale Vincent was educated at Birmingham, later studying at the universities of London, Edinburgh, and Heidelberg, and becoming an M.D. London. He was a demonstrator in Physiology in Birmingham, a British Medical Association Research Scholar. He worked with Schaefer at University College in London, becoming Assistant Professor of Physiology. He was a Mason Scholar and Research Fellow at the University of Edinburgh. From 1904 to 1920, he was Professor of Physiology in Manitoba, Canada. From 1920 to 1930 he was Professor of Physiology at the Middlesex Hospital (University of London), examiner in Physiology in London, Leeds and for the Royal College of Physicians in London. He was a member of many medical societies in England, Scotland and overseas.

Although he published *An Introduction to Mammalian Physiology* in 1929, his main interest over many years was in the field of the endocrine glands, on which he published many papers, but his books are especially notable: *Internal Secretion and the Ductless Glands* published in 1912, and in 1924 *An Introduction to the Study of Secretion* (with S. Wright).

As we discussed (see Chapter 18), Vincent, who was a man "with a highly critical mind", attempted "to clear the new science of endocrinology from many pseudo-scientific weeds". He was a man "of firm principles and ideals", and quite "uncompromising". He was strongly supported by A. J. Clark, Professor of Pharmacology at University College and by Schaefer. In France, Eugène Gley was another of the puritans of endocrine physiology. The 'crisis' in the 1920s centred around their figures, contrasting people like Starling and Gregorio Marañon. This should not mean that the many outstanding contributions of these scholars to endocrinology should be belittled, because their general attitude appeared somewhat narrowminded. They resented any appearance of romanticism in science, of which Starling and Marañon were good examples. For the progress of science both types of research workers are necessary.

VIRCHOW, Ludwig Karl   1821–1902

Ludwig Karl Virchow was born at Schievelbein in the Province of Pommern, Prussia. He studied in Berlin, where he qualified. He was a pupil of Johannes Mueller and became Assistant to Robert Froriep at the Charité, when aged 24. Only a year later he became Prosector and in 1847 he founded *Virchow's Archiv fuer Pathologische Anatomie*. In 1848, the government gave him the task of investigating an epidemic of typhus among the weavers of Upper Silesia (also called 'famine fever'). His report revealed the misery of the conditions, which were later so effectively highlighted in Gerhart Hauptmann's social tragedy *The Weavers*. Virchow's liberal political views were also expressed in his medico-political periodical *Die Medizinische Reform* (1848–1849), which got him into difficulties with the authorities. In 1849, he was removed from his post, but obtained the Chair of Pathological Anatomy at Wuerzburg. He made a great success of his new job, and in 1856, he was invited to return to Berlin as Professor of Pathology and Director of a newly built Institute for Pathological Anatomy. With incredible energy he developed new lines of research in the fields of anatomy, pathology, epidemiology, hygiene, anthropology, archaeology and social medicine. This activity was broadened by his election to the Prussian Parliament in 1862. After the creation of the German Empire (1871), he was member of the Reichstag from 1880 to 1893. During the Franco-Prussian War of 1870–1871, he organized the Prussian Ambulance Corps and supervised an army hospital on the Tempelhof.

Garrison described him as "a small, elastic, professorial figure, with snappy black eyes, quick in mind and body, with a touch of the Slav, something of a martinet in the morgue or lecture room, often transfixing inattention and incompetence with a flash of sarcasm. Yet he was generous, whole-souled, and broad-minded withal, and none who 'made good' was ever lost from sight or memory" (Garrison). He was an opponent of Darwin's theories, and of the views of Koch and Behring on toxins and antitoxins. He stood up with great courage for the care and protection of the industrial worker, in spite of the hostility of the Prussian military régime in Berlin. His contribution to pathology and pathological histology was enormous. His interest in anthropology was well known and so was his activity in the field of mediaeval history. He wrote biographical studies on Morgagni and Johannes Mueller, and papers on mediaeval hospitals including leper-hospitals. He was also interested in the relations of medicine to the fine arts; he was altogether a very great man. He was also influential in the creation of an efficient sewage system for Berlin. Scientifically, his outstanding merit was the creation of cellular pathology (1858). He declared that the body was a "cell state, in which every cell was a citizen" and disease "merely a conflict of citizens in this state, brought about by the action of external forces". Cell development is continuous and every cell is begotten by another one ("Omnis cellula e cellula"); accordingly, "A new growth of cells presupposes already existing cells". (*Die krankhaften Geschwuelste* = the diseased tumours; Vols. 1–3, Heft 1, Berlin, A. Hirschwald, 1863–1867 (this work was not completed).)

WEISMAN, August Friedrich Leopold
1834–1914

August Friedrich Leopold Weisman was born at Frankfurt/Main (Germany) on 17 January 1834, the son of Johann Konrad August Weisman, a classics master at the humanistic grammar school ('Gymnasium') in Frankfurt. His mother was a talented musician and painter. At an early age he collected butterflies and beetles, bred caterpillars and started a herbarium; but he was also interested in music. He was educated at the Gymnasium at Frankfurt and studied medicine at Goettingen where he came under the influence of Henle. In 1856, he presented his M.D. thesis on the formation of hippuric acid in the organism. In 1861, he read enthusiastically Darwin's *Origin of Species* in one sitting and became a converted Darwinist. Weisman became an assistant at a (clinical) hospital at Rostock, then a private assistant to Schulze, and carried out a chemical investigation of the salt content of the Baltic Sea. Late in 1858, he passed his state examination and entered a practice of medicine at Frankfurt, while at the same time, occupied with studies on the muscle fibres of the heart. During 1859, he acted as a doctor in the field (of war) in Italy. In 1860, he visited the Jardin des Plantes in Paris and attended lectures of Geoffroy Saint-Hilaire. In 1861, he worked for two months under Leuchart in Giessen, who aroused his interest in developmental studies of insects, especially Diptera. He then took up practising medicine again in Frankfurt. From 1861 to 1863, he was private medical attendant to the Archduke Stephan of Austria at Schaumburg Castle, studying insect development in his spare time.

Weisman then turned to zoology, proceeding to Privat-Dozent in

Zoology and Comparative Anatomy in Freiburg in 1863, extraordinary professor in 1866 and full professor ('ordinarius') in 1874, the first to hold the chair of Zoology in Freiburg, where he remained for the rest of his life. In 1864, he suffered for the first time from a serious eye infection, which made microscopy impossible for the time being, but he continued with his work, assisted by his wife, Dorothy Gruber of Genoa. It was ten years before Weisman could use his eyes and a microscope again. From insects, he turned to the study of small crustaceans, daphnoids and ostracoids. Next came the examination of the hydrozoa, followed by the study of the sexual cells through generations of Hydro-medusae, the results of which he published in 1883: *Die Entstehung der Sexualzellen bei den Hydromedusen* (Jena). He concluded that there was strong evidence for a continuity of the germ plasm. He further decided that acquired characteristics can *not* be inherited, for to become inheritable, changes would have to affect the germ plasm itself.

Weisman was not the first to conceive of a continuity of the substance of heredity. In 1872, Galton had outlined it; and Gustav Jaeger had actually written of a 'continuity of the germ-protoplasm' in 1875, although this was, at the time, unknown to Weisman. Moritz Nussbaum and August A. Rauber later claimed to have originated the theory, but it was Weisman who first developed it into a coherent explanation of inheritance and brought it into agreement with the new understanding of the cell. He later modified his theory and it became a presupposition of his views on the sources of evolution. In 1881 he gave his lecture on 'The Duration of Life', in which he contrasted the 'immortality' of one-celled organisms, which reproduce by division to form two organisms of the same age; this potential immortality was, of course, abrogated by accidents and other vicissitudes – he contrasted them with the division of labour that natural selection had brought about in the more complex forms of life. In the latter, there was an early separation of the elements that were to form the 'immortal' reproductive cells from the elements that were to form the body cells, which perished in each succeeding generation. In 1883, in his book *On Heredity*, he still conceived the germ cells as containing configurations of molecules which led to the reproductive cells as well as other configurations for the somatic cells. The germ cells contained the 'Anlagen': these were the hereditary tendencies or predispositions for certain characteristics to develop. They were not affected by outer conditions which affected the organism, but they were subject to natural selection.

Later Weisman's concept of germ plasm changed again. He borrowed from the botanist Naegeli (see also under Gregor Mendel), the term 'idioplasm' (i.e. the protoplasm concerned with inheritance as distinguished from the rest of the protoplasm). Following the observation and description of 'mitosis' from 1873 onwards (Oscar Hertwig, Walther Flemming, Wilhelm Roux), Weisman now attributed the main rôle in heredity to the nucleus (as Haeckel did in 1886). Germ cells did not necessarily lead directly to other germ cells, for germ plasm might be transmitted through a series of cells – its particles remaining discrete – before reproductive cells were again formed.

In 1885, his new views on 'The Continuity of Germ Plasm', now located it in the nucleus and contained in the 'idioplasm' of Naegeli. Germ cells did not necessarily lead directly to other germ cells, for germ plasm might be transmitted through a series of cells, its particles remaining discrete, before reproductive cells were again formed. In 1887, he postulated that sexual reproduction must lead to variation through the ever new combination of Anlagen (see his thesis *On the number of Polar Bodies*). In 1892, he summmed up in: *Das Keimplasma: Eine Theorie der Vererbung* (Jena). Stressing the new chromosome theory, he regarded it as proof for the repudiation of the inheritance of acquired characteristics, although Oscar Hertwig declared that Weisman's theory 'smacked of preformation'.

Thus Weisman became the most notable of the Neo-Darwinists, in contrast to the Neo-Lamarckians, like Herbert Spencer, with whom he developed a controversy in 1893–1894.

The outbreak of the 1914 war brought Weisman a great deal of worry and heartache, not only because of the many friends he had in England, but because one of his daughters was married to the English zoologist W. Newton Parker. Weisman was given many honours, among others that of 'Wirklicher Geheimer Rat' (Real Privy Councillor) and Foreign Member of the Royal Society. He died on 5 November 1914, in Freiburg/Breisgau, a worried and unhappy man.

WHARTON, Thomas   1614–1673

Thomas Wharton studied at Cambridge in 1638 and at Oxford, where he proceeded M.D. in 1674. He was elected a Fellow of the College of Physicians in London in 1650 and became a Censor in 1658, 1661, 1666, 1667, 1668 and 1673. He was a physician to St. Thomas's Hospital from 1659 to 1673. With great courage and devotion to his patients, he remained in London throughout the plague epidemic in 1665–1666.

He was the discoverer of the duct of the submaxillary salivary gland (Wharton's duct). He also described the thyroid more accurately than had been done before, and named it 'thyreoidea' (from the Greek=oblong shield). We have already referred to Wharton's work: *Adenographia: sive glandularum totius corporis descriptio* (= adenographia: description of the glands of the whole body), published in London in 1656.

WILKS, Sir Samuel, Bart.   1824–1911

Samuel Wilks was born in London in 1824, the son of a cashier at the East India House. He was apprenticed to Dr. Prior, his family doctor, in 1840 and entered Guy's in 1842, qualifying in 1847. He was elected Fellow of the

Royal College of Physicians in 1856 and consulting physician to Guy's Hospital in 1885, after being physician there since 1866. He lectured in pathology, medicine and morbid anatomy and was curator of the museum. He was made a Fellow of the Royal Society in 1870 for his work in establishing the visceral lesions due to syphilis, published in *Guy's Hospital Reports* (1863).

He played a great part in establishing the authenticity of Addison's disease. When his paper, an account of 'a peculiar enlargement of the lymphatic glands', was finished in 1856 he discovered Hodgkin's paper written in 1832 and added a paragraph giving Hodgkin priority.

He was President of the Royal College of Physicians from 1896 to 1898. He died in 1911 in Hampstead in London.

His lectures on *Pathological Anatomy* published in 1859, became the standard textbook for three decades. His second important book, *Lectures on Diseases of the Nervous System* appeared nearly 20 years later, (1878), but from the endocrine point of view, his most important contribution was his staunch support of Addison.

WILLIS, Thomas   1621–1675

Thomas Willis, the son of a farmer, was born in Great Bedwin, Wiltshire, in 1621. He went to school in Oxford where he became a retainer of Canon Iles of Christ Church and matriculated from there. He took the B.A. degree in 1637 and B.M. in 1646. He also served in the Royal Garrison at Oxford. He was in Oxford when it was in the hands of Cromwell but after the Restoration he was made Sedleian Professor of Natural Philosophy. His great work *Cerebri Anatome* was published in 1664.

He moved to London in 1666 and became very busy and made a lot of money. He was spoken of as 'The first inventor of the nervous system'. He also played a part in introducing what is now called biochemistry. He described the sweet taste of urine in diabetes mellitus in 1674, although Avicenna is reputed to have done so before him.

Willis is best remembered from the description of the circulus arteriosus Willisii of the brain, but he also gave a good description of such clinical conditions as myasthenia gravis, epilepsy, whooping cough and of the paracusis Willisii. In Oxford, he was a contemporary of Robert Boyle, John Locke and other future members of the Royal Society. John Oldham expressed the high esteem in which he was held in the lines: "I've known physicians, who respect might claim Tho' they ne'er rose to Willis his great fame". With Richard Lower he formed one of the first research 'teams', which proved to be so fruitful, Willis providing the ideas and Lower the experimental proof.

He died in St. Martin's Lane, London, in November 1675.

ZONDEK, Bernhard 1891–1967

Bernhard Zondek was born in July, 1891 in Wronke, Germany, into a professional family. He was educated at the Gymnasium (= humanistic grammar school) in Rogasen, and entered the medical Faculty of the University of Berlin in 1911, proceeding M.D. in 1918. In 1919, he became assistant to Professor K. Franz, at the University Department of Obstetrics and Gynaecology in Berlin. In 1923, he became Lecturer (Privat-Docent) in Obstetrics and Gynaecology, in 1926 Associate-Professor and in 1929, Director of the Department of Obstetrics and Gynaecology at the Municipal Hospital of Berlin-Spandau. He was a Jew and left Hitler's Germany in 1933. From 1934 to 1961, he was Professor of Obstetrics and Gynaecology and Head of the Hormone Research Laboratory, Hebrew University, Hadassah Medical School, Jerusalem, Israel. In 1961, he became Emeritus, but carried on working. From September to December 1953 he was visiting professor at the Temple University School of Medicine in Philadelphia, PA, U.S.A. In 1966, on the occasion of his 75th birthday, the CIBA Foundation Study Group No. 26 in London, organized a Symposium in honour of Bernhard Zondek on 'The Effects of External Stimuli on Reproduction', which he opened with a paper on 'The Effects of Auditory Stimuli on Reproduction'. Professor (Sir) Alan S. Parkes was in the chair and presented Professor Zondek with the Francis H. A. Marshall medal of the Society for the Study of Fertility, as the Second Medallist. The papers of the symposium were published in a special volume in 1967 (London, Churchill). An interview with Zondek (by Michael Finkelstein) was also published in Volume 12 of the *Journal for Reproduction and Fertility*, in May 1966 (pp. 3–19), explaining the development of his research interests. Although he looked fit, alert and well during the CIBA Symposium, he died in 1967, while the book was in press.

Bernhard Zondek was honoured by many universities and learned societies all over the world. His real merit can be gauged from his scientific achievements, which will be enumerated briefly. Even his early publications bore witness to his permanent interest in endocrinology; his first paper, in 1914, was on the influence of thyroid extracts on lung function. Once he had decided to specialize in gynaecology, the ovaries and their hormones became his main interest. It must not be forgotten, however, that his elder brother, Professor Hermann Zondek (1887–1979) was a pioneer of modern endocrinology. Bernhard pursued experimental research on the ovaries, but also on the effectiveness of organotherapy (1923), the knowledge of the Allen-Doisy test being of great help. On Franz's suggestion, he got in touch with Selmar Aschheim, who was in charge of the gynaeco-pathological laboratory of the hospital. This was the beginning of the celebrated collaboration. The search for an active oestrogenic hormone led to the discovery of hormones in the placenta, and to the conclusion that the anterior pituitary and the placenta produced a 'hormonotrophin', which induced the ovaries to secrete oestrogenic hormone. This conclusion was reached at the same time, but independently, by P. E. Smith in the United

States. Aschheim and Zondek were soon led to believe that "more than one factor was essential for the effect seen with the pituitary tissue" (Finkelstein's Interview, p. 9). This led, eventually, to the development of the pregnancy test, as they did not think that the placental hormone was different from the gonadotrophin of pituitary origin. In the same interview (with Finkelstein) there occurred the following question and answer: ". . . Was the idea of a master gland and of a master hormone yours?" – "Actually, similar ideas were expressed long ago. As far as I can remember, as early as 1905, Heape and then Sand in 1919, and Hammond and Marshall in 1923, and then Lipschütz in 1925, suggested the presence of a 'generative ferment' of a 'substance X'" (Interview, p. 8). The pregnancy diagnosis with Selmar Aschheim was published in 1928 (*Klin. Wochenschr.*, **7,** 8, 1928 and 1404, 1928). In 1930, there followed a number of important papers on the hormones of the anterior pituitary, especially the two prolans, which were first ridiculed by others (see also Section I, Chapter 18). In 1932 appeared 'The relation of the anterior lobe of the hypophysis to genital function' (*Am. J. Obstet. Gynecol.*, **24,** 836, 1932); in 1934 his important observations 'Mass excretion of oestrogenic hormone in the urine of the stallion' (*Nature, London*, **133,** 209 and 494, 1934). After 1935, his publications were all in English. From 1937 onward, he was much concerned with the antigonadotrophic factor (Antiprolan); after 1945, he drew attention to endocrine allergy (I. Allergic sensitivity to endogenous hormones, with Y. M. Bromberg; *J. Allergy*, **16,** 1, 1945). From 1958 onwards, he studied 'Stimulation of the anterior pituitary function with pronounced decrease in fertility by stimulation of the auditory organs' (with I. Tamari: *Bull. Res. Commun. Israel*, **7E,** 155, 1958), which was also the subject of his contribution to the CIBA Symposium in his honour in 1966.

ZONDEK, Hermann 1887–1979

Hermann Zondek was a member of a distinguished medical family in pre-Hitler Germany. His brother was Professor Bernhard Zondek, the gynaecologist, of Aschheim–Zondek's early pregnancy test fame. Another brother was also professor at the University of Berlin. Hermann studied in Goettingen, and Berlin. His early interests were in the fields of renal and heart diseases; in 1920 he carried out extensive investigations into hunger oedema in Germany. He then turned to the study of endocrinology. In this field he not only discovered syndromes and treatments, but also elucidated endocrine function and regulation. He studied the mechanisms of hormone action and the inter-relationships of the endocrine glands with one another and with organ systems. His assertion of the leading role of the pituitary gland and of the existence of two ovarian hormones were received with incredulity and ridicule, until, eventually, they were proved to be correct.

His main book, *Diseases of the Endocrine Glands,* was first published in German in 1923. Thirty-five years later, there were many enlarged and revised editions in English, French, Russian and Italian. It contained a fresh outlook and many new ideas on the subject. Zondek had a particular interest in the thyroid gland and the effect of iodine on it.

The present writer last talked to him in 1960, on the occasion of the Fourth International Goitre Conference in London, when Zondek, at the age of 73, showed the liveliest interest in the proceedings. After he had to leave Germany, he worked in Manchester for a year, and afterwards in Jerusalem. His wife was also a doctor. His many contributions to clinical endocrinology have been discussed in the first section of this book.

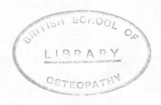

CHRONOLOGICAL TABLES

in alphabetical order

THE ADRENAL CORTEX

1563 AD	Eustachius described the adrenals: De glandulis quae renibus incumbunt. (His *Tabulae anatomicae* published by Lancisi in 1714.) .
1586–1588	Piccolomineus (Ferrara) and Bauhin (Bale) mentioned the suprarenal glands.
1627	Spigelius talked of the capsulae renales.
1651	Highmore suggested that the suprarenals have an absorbent function of exudates from the large vessels.
1716	Montesquieu judged the result of the competition of the Académie des Sciences de Bordeaux: "Quel est l'usage des glands surrénales?" No award was given.
1855	Addison talked "On the constitutional and local effects of disease of the suprarenal capsules".
1856	Brown-Séquard proved in animal experiments that the adrenals are essential for the maintenance of life.
1896	Osler found orally given adrenal extract temporarily effective in a case of Addison's disease.
1905	Bulloch and Sequeira described patients with adrenogenital syndrome.
1926	P. E. Smith showed that hypophysectomy caused atrophy of the adrenals, which Evans prevented by administration of pituitary extracts.
1927	Hartmann and colleagues confirmed this in adrenalectomized cats; so did Rogoff and Stewart in 1928.

1929–1930	Liquid extracts of cortical tissue maintained adrenalecto-mized cats indefinitely (Hartmann and Brownell; Swingle and Pfiffner).
1930	Rowntree and Greene successfully treated a patient with Addison's disease with Swingle and Pfiffner's extract.
1932	Cushing connected the "polyglandular syndrome" of pituitary basophilism, first described by him in 1912, with pituitary–adrenal hyperactivity.
1933	Loeb treated the abnormal serum electrolytes in Addison's disease with sodium chloride.
1936	The concept of stress introduced by Selye.
1937–1952	Steroid hormones of the adrenal cortex isolated, their structure determined and synthesized (Kendall, Reichstein; Wintersteiner and Pfiffner, *et al.*)
1942	Isolation of ACTH by Li and Sayers (see also *Pituitary Tables*)
1946	The general adaptation syndrome described by Selye.
1948	Hench and his colleagues discovered the anti-inflammatory effect of cortisone (Kendall's compound-E).
1949	Hench, Kendall and Slocumb described the effect of Compound E and of ACTH on rheumatoid arthritis.
1953–1955	Isolation and analysis of the structure of aldosterone achieved (Simpson and Tait, Wettstein and Neher, Reichstein and van Euw). Aldosterone synthesized by Wettstein and Schmidlin.
1956	Conn described primary aldosteronism.
1958	Angiotensin suggested by Gross to control aldosterone secretion.
1966	Synthesis of β-corticotrophin by Schwyzer and Sieber.

THE ADRENAL MEDULLA

1805 AD	Cuvier defined medulla and cortex of the adrenal gland.
1856	Vulpian's staining method specific for adrenaline.
1886	Felix Fraenkel described a patient with an adrenal tumour and pressor attacks.
1892	Chromaffine cell tumour of the adrenal described by Berdez of Lausanne.

1894	Pressor substances in adrenal extract discovered by Oliver and Schaefer in London and, independently, by Szymonowicz and Cybulski in Cracow.
1898–1904	Adrenaline isolated, its structure determined and synthesized (Fuerth and Abel; Takamine and Aldrich; Stolz and Dakin).
1922	Labbë, Tinel and Doumer connected paroxysmal attacks of hypertension with chromaffinomas of the adrenal.
1927	Successful removal of a phaeochromocytoma by C. H. Mayo.
1945	Discovery of noradrenaline (Holtz, Credner and Kronenberg).
1957	Vanilmandelic acid (VMA) found to be a metabolite of catecholamines (Armstrong).

ANOREXIA NERVOSA

98–138 AD	Soranos described amenorrhoea and anorexia in women.
ca. 155 AD	Galen described an emaciated condition where a patient could not eat.
1689	Richard Morton gave the first description of anorexia nervosa.
1873	Lasègue described 'l'anorexie hystérique.
1873	Gull described anorexia nervosa and gave its name.
1874	Déjérine described "anoréxie mentale".
1934 1935	von Bergmann } claimed successful treatment with anterior Kylin } pituitary gland
1937	Schur and Medvei called it pituitary insufficiency due to disturbance of "correlation".
1948	E. C. Jacobs studied the effect of starvation on sex hormones in the male.
1954	Perloff and colleagues described hypopituitarism caused by starvation.
1962	Srebnik and Nelson observed reduced pituitary LH concentrations in malnutrition.
1969	Dally (London) suggested a three-scale classification: Obsessional (O), hysterical (H) and mixed (M).

1973	Besser believed to have shown that the endocrine dysfunction of AN originates in the hypothalamus.
1976	Beumont and his group found reduced circulating LH levels in AN and reduced response to gonadotrophin-releasing hormone.
1978	Davies and Lewis showed that male rats and guineapigs lost half of their LE receptors after dietary deprivation; their response to hCG stimulation was also reduced. Functional hypopituitarism may be explained by changes of oestrogen metabolism due to loss of body fat, resulting in excessive LE suppression. This would explain the association between menarche and body weight.

THE ANTERIOR PITUITARY (ADENOHYPOPHYSIS)

ca. 1365 BC	Portrait head of Akhenaten (Pharaoh of Egypt, 18th Dynasty) shows acromegalic features.
BC	Giants were repeatedly mentioned in the Old Testament. Dwarfs were regarded as misfits.
129–201 AD	Galen thought that the pituitary drains the phlegm from the brain to the nasopharynx (refuted in 1660 by Schneider in Wittenberg).
1543	Vesalius described the "glandula pituitaria cerebri excipiens".
1660	Schneider refuted Galen's theory.
1670	Lower (Oxford) confirmed Schneider's view experimentally.
1742	Lieutaud described the pituitary stalk ("tige").
1760	de Haën mentioned amenorrhoea in a patient with pituitary tumour.
1772	Saucerotte described Sieur Mirbeck (acromegaly).
1778	Soemmering (Goettingen) called gland the "hypophysis cerebri".
1786	John Hunter described "pigeon's milk".
1822	Alibert described a "géant scrofuleux" (acromegalic).
1838	Rathke described the formation of the pituitary gland.

1840	Mohr described a patient with Froehlich's syndrome.
1851	Nièpce (France) noted enlargement of the pituitary in connection with parenchymatous goitre.
1857	Chalk described "partial dislocation of the lower jaw" from an enlarged tongue (acromegaly).
1864	Verga published the first post-mortem report in a case of acromegaly ("prosopectasy").
1869	Lombroso described "macrosomia" (acromegaly).
1877	Brigidi published the autopsy on Ghirlenzoni, an acromegalic actor, including the histology of a pituitary tumour.
1884	Fritzsche and Klebs (Switzerland) reported on the clinical and post-mortem findings of a patient with "giantism" (acromegaly).
1886	Pierre Marie called the disease "acromegaly".
1887	Minkowski connected acromegaly with a pituitary tumour.
1892	Vassale and Sacchi showed that hypophysectomy affected water and mineral metabolism.
1892	Massalongo (Padova) attributed acromegaly to hyperfunction of the pituitary.
1893	Caton and Paul (Liverpool) attempted surgical treatment of acromegaly to relieve pressure due to a tumour.
1900–1901	Benda demonstrated the connection between acromegaly and eosinophil adenoma of the anterior pituitary.

1900	Babinski (France)	
1901	Froehlich (Vienna)	described dystrophia adiposo-genitalis.
1906	Cushing	

1906–1907	Schloffer (Vienna) operated on a pituitary tumour by the nasal route.
1908	Paulesco (Paris and Bucarest) succeeded in removing experimentally the anterior lobe of the pituitary, but with fatal results.
1909	B. Aschner showed that hypophysectomy in a growing animal caused dwarfism.
1910	Cushing and his team presented the first experimental evidence of the link between the anterior pituitary and the reproductive organs.

1911	Hirsch (Vienna) developed the endonasal surgical approach to the pituitary.
1912	B. Aschner observed atrophy of the thyroid in hypophysectomized puppies and genital hypoplasia.
1913	Glinski (Poland) described post-partum necrosis of the anterior pituitary.
1914	Simmonds described pituitary cachexia (Simmonds' disease).
1915	Gaines demonstrated pituitary function in lactation.
1916	Erdheim described pituitary dwarfism ("Nanosomia pituitaria").
1921	Evans and Long showed the effect of anterior lobe extract on the growth rate of rats.
1926	Foster and P. E. Smith found that atrophy of the thyroid and lowered BMR in hypophysectomized animals could be restored by using pituitary homoplastic implants.
1927	P. E. Smith and Engle demonstrated that gonadal activity is maintained by the anterior lobe of the pituitary.
1928	Bernhard Zondek and Aschheim isolated the gonadotrophic hormones (Prolan A and B) of the anterior pituitary.
1929	Putnam, Benedict and Teel produced experimental acromegaly in dogs by anterior lobe extract injection.
1929	Stricker and Grueter discovered prolactin.
1929	Aron (Strasbourg) and, independently, Loeb and Bassett described the action of TSH of the anterior pituitary.
1930	Houssay and Biasotti succeeded in removing the pancreas in the hypophysectomized dog.
1932	Cushing described pituitary basophilism.
1932	Anderson and Collip described the thyrotrophic hormone (TSH) of the anterior pituitary.
1933	Collip and his team isolated an impure "adrenotropic hormone".
1933	Ridde and colleagues identified and assayed prolactin.
1936	Evans and his group isolated the interstitial cell stimulating hormone (ICSH).
1937	F. G. Young described the diabetogenic hormone.

1937	Lambie and Trikojus obtained purified TSH.
1939	Sheehan (Liverpool) described panhypopituitarism caused by pituitary necrosis after post-partum haemorrhage.
1940	Choh Hao Li isolated luteinizing hormone (LH).
1943	Choh Hao Li and Evans isolated pure adreno-corticotrophic hormone (ACTH) from sheep pituitaries.
1943	Sayers isolated ACTH from swine pituitaries.
1945	Choh Hao Li and Evans isolated anterior pituitary growth hormone (GH).
1948	Wilhelmi, Fishman and Russel obtained almost pure crystalline bovine growth hormone.
1949	Choh Hao Li and Evans isolated follicle stimulating hormone (FSH).
1955	Knobil and Greep showed that GH extracts from monkeys were active in man and were species-specific.
1957	Raben developed a method for the extraction of human GH from the pituitaries of cadavers.
1959	Liddle and his group developed the metyrapone test for pituitary reserve.
1961	The amino acid sequence of bovine adrenocorticotropin described by Choh Hao Li, Dixon and Chung.
1963	Glick, Roth, Berson and Yallow described a radioimmunological assay (RIA) method for the measurement of human GH.
1965	Choh Hao Li and his group isolated beta-lipotrophin (β-LPH) which is manufactured and released together with ACTH.
1966–71	Choh Hao Li described the structure of human GH and synthesized it.
1970	Mitchell and colleagues introduced the glucagon stimulation test to detect GH deficiency.
1971–79	Formulation of present day ideas on the mechanism of hormonal action.
1971–75	Hughes, Kosterlitz and colleagues identified the pentapeptides from the brain to possess potent opiate agonist activity.
1971	Pierce, Liao and colleagues determined the structure of TSH.

| 1973 | Solomon Snyder and his group (Johns Hopkins) Eric Simon and his group (New York) Lars Terenius and his group (Upsala) | demonstrated that opiates attached themselves to receptor sites in the brain as their target cells (see also The Brain). |

1975   Bradbury, Smyth and Snell isolated beta-endorphin and described its structure.

1978   Feldberg reported on the pharmacology of the central actions of endorphins.

1978   Wm. Jeffcoate, L. Rees, G. M. Besser and colleagues designed a RIA for human β-LPH.

1975–1979   Hyperprolactinaemia, the "galactorrhoea-amenorrhoea syndrome" described and studied. Pituitary prolactinomas recognized by various groups. Treatment with long-acting oral dopamine agonists introduced ("bromocriptine"). The same preparation has been used, in a different dosage, for an attempted longterm medical treatment of acromegaly. Medical management of Cushing's disease has been attempted with metyrapone. New methods of microsurgery have been developed for the transphenoidal approach to small pituitary tumours, e.g. prolactinomas.

THE BRAIN

129–201 AD   Galen thought that the pituitary drains the phlegm from the brain to the nasopharynx (refuted in 1660 by Schneider in Wittenberg).

1543 AD   Vesalius wrote in "De fabrica . . ." that waste material excreted by the brain, "a glandular organ", passes through the infundibulum into the pituitary and from there to the nasopharynx.

1637   Descartes considered the brain as the organ integrating the functions of mind and body.

1664   Willis argued that "some humour out of the ventricles of the cerebrum is carried into the pituitary gland".

1733	Morgagni	
1792	Soemmering	observed absence of the adrenal cortex in anencephaly.
1802	Meckel	

| 1849–1850 | Bernard demonstrated that "piqûre diabétique" of the floor of the posterior part of the 4th ventricle in the dog causes temporary glycosuria. Piqûre a little anterior to the glycosuric centre causes polyuria. |

| 1870 | Eckhard (Giessen) observed that injury to the vermiform process of the cerebellum and to other parts of the brain may also cause polyuria. |

| 1951 | L'Hermite published "Le Cerveau et la Pensée" stressing the regulation of mental life by the hormones. |

| 1971–1975 | Hughes, Kosterlitz and colleagues identified the pentapeptides from the brain to posses potent opiate agonist activity. |

| 1973 | Snyder and his group (Johns Hopkins)
 Eric Simon and colleagues (New York)
 Lars Terenius and his group (Uppsala) } demonstrated that opiates attached themselves to receptor sites in the brain as their target cells. |

| 1975 | Bradbury, Smyth and Snell isolated beta-endorphin and described its structure. |

| 1978 | Feldberg reported on the pharmacology of the central actions of endorphins. |

| 1979 | Kosterlitz believed that the discovery of the enkephalins was one of the most important in British pharmacology. |

| 1979 | Besser, Rees and their group (London) and Wen (Hong Kong) found that, during withdrawal effects of heroin addicts treated with acupuncture, the CSF met-enkephalin levels showed a clear rise. |

| 1980 | The same investigators demonstrated increased levels of β-endorphin, but not of met-enkephalin in human CSF after acupuncture for the treatment of recurrent pain. They concluded that β-endorphin may be released from the pituitary or from the brain. |

| 1979 | The International Health Foundation organized a workshop on "The brain as an endocrine target organ in health and disease", held in Bordeaux. |

GUT HORMONES

| 1902 | Bayliss and Starling reported on their discovery of "secretin" in the duodenum. |

829

1905–1906	Edkin described gastric secretin ("gastrin").
1915	Keeton and Koch confirmed the specific nature of gastrin.
1935–1953	Feyrter (Danzig) described the peripheral paracrine endocrine glands in man.
1955	Zollinger and Ellison described the Z–E syndrome.
1958	Verner-Morrison described the watery diarrhoea hypokalaemic achlorhydric syndrome.
1966	Gregory isolated gastrin and defined its structure.
1969	Pearse introduced the APUD concept.
1975–1980	Numerous peptides have been described, located in the islet organ, the stomach, the duodenum, jejunum, ileum and colon. Some peptides are common to the brain and the gastrointestinal tract. The diagnostic methods used for their detection are:

    RIA (blood and tissues).
    Immunohistochemistry
    Gel filtration
    Bioassay
    Electron microscopy.

THE HYPOTHALAMUS

1742	Joseph Lieutaud discovered the pituitary–portal system as the hypothalamo-hypophysial connection (in the pituitary stalk).
1860	von Luschka (Germany) described the primary capillary loops of the pituitary portal vessels.
1865	Luys (France) described the hypothalamus ("nucleus of Luys").
1909	Karplus and Kreidl (Vienna) reported on the first experimental studies on the hypothalamus.
1913	Camus and Roussy produced experimental diabetes insipidus (DI) in dogs by injury to the hypothalamus.
1930	Popa and Fielding described the vascular link between the pituitary and the hypothalamic region as a portal circulation.
1936	Selye described the stress syndrome.

1944	Berta and E. Scharrer compared the intercerebral cardiacum-allatum system of the insects with the hypothalamo-hypophysial system of the vertebrates.
1947	Verney postulated osmoreceptors in the anterior hypothalamus for the release of ADH.
1948	G. W. Harris published his paper on "Neural control of the pituitary".
1948–1951	Harris carried out intensive experimental studies on the hypothalamic control of the pituitary.
1951	Bergmann and Scharrer described the sites of origin of the hormones of the posterior pituitary in the hypothalamic nuclei.

First reported evidence for the presence of hypothalamic releasing or inhibiting factors (hormones):

1955	CRF	Saffran and Schally; Guillemin and Rosenberg
1960	LRF	McCann et al.; Harris et al.
1960	PRF	Meites et al.
1965–1966	Avian PRF	Kragt and Meites; Nicoll.
1961–1963	PIF	Talwalker, Ratner and Meites; Pasteels.
1961–1962	TRF	Schreiber and Kmentova.
1963–1964	GRF	Deuben and Meites.
1964	FRF	Igarasei and McCann; Mittler and Meites.
1965	MIF	Kastin et al.
1968	GIF	Krulich and McCann.

1966	Greenwood, Landon and Stamp introduced the insulin-induced hypoglycaemia to investigate adrenal insufficiency due to hypothalamic or pituitary disease.
1969	Jacobs and Nabarro (London) found the insulin test clinically most useful in a large series of hypothalamic-pituitary disease.
1966	Price and Lauener used the assessment of serum and urine osmolalities in the differential diagnosis of polyuric states.
1971	James and Landon (London) reviewed the hypothalamic-pituitary–adrenal function tests.
1971	Schally, Arimura and colleagues isolated LH/FSH–RH.
1972	Luizzi and colleagues described the inhibitory effect of L-dopa on GH release in acromegalics.

1973	Brazeau, Guillemin and colleagues defined GH–RIH.
1974	Macleod and Lehmeyer studied the dopamine-mediated inhibition of prolactin secretion.
1974	Rosalyn Yalow described the heterogeneity of peptide hormones.
1975	Introduction of cytohistochemical bioassays for the measurement of polypeptide hormones.
1975	Daniel and Marjorie Prichard published the results of 25 years of studies of the hypothalamus and the pituitary gland.
1976	G. M. Besser summarized the theoretical and clinical application of GH-Dopamine Agonists and Antagonists.
1977	Daniel and Treip published their study of the pathology of the hypothalamus.
1977	Rees, Stuart Mason and Besser *et al.* described longterm treatment of acromegaly with bromocriptin.
1978	Henderson and Daniel discussed portal circulations and their relations to countercurrent systems.
1978	Dorothy Krieger (New York) reported on the factors influencing the circadian periodicity of ACTH and the corticosteroids and on 'free-running periodicity' in some of the blind.

NEURO-ENDOCRINOLOGY

See also the Chronological Tables on The Brain, The Hypothalamus and The Pituitaries

1818	Gall	reported that unilateral castration causes atrophy of the contralateral hemisphere of the cerebellum in the animal experiment.
1835	Vimont	
1849		Berthold in his experiment of testicular transplant implicated the nervous system (NS) as target organ.
1856		Maestre de San Juan (Spain) observed gonadal hypoplasia in men with agenesis of the olfactory lobes.
1914	Weidenreich	
1929	Mirsalis	
1940	Kanai	confirmed the above observation.
1960	Gauthier	
1963	E. and B. Scharrer (experimentally)	

1877	Du Bois Reymond (Germany) suggested a chemical transmission from motor nerve-endings to striated muscle.
1905	Schiefferdecker (Bonn) described the secretion of endocrine substances by neurons as a means of communication between neurons or between a neuron and an effector cell in muscle or gland. This was based on some ideas of Tigerstedt ("automatic" irritation by metabolic products) and on Schiefferdecker's own observations.
1908	Laignel-Lavastine discussed the connection between psychiatry and internal secretions.
1913	Camus and Roussy stressed the predominance of the hypothalamus.
1914	Dale published "The action of certain esters and ethers of acetylcholine".
1914	T. R. Elliott conceived the idea of chemical transmission in the autonomic NS.
1915	Cannon published *Bodily Changes in Pain, Hunger, Fear and Rage*.
1923	Starling's lecture on "The wisdom of the body".
1921–1924	Loewi (Graz, Austria) proved the theory of chemical intermediaries in nervous stimulation.
1928	Berta and Ernest Scharrer reported on the function of the hypothalamus in teleost fishes.
1929	F. H. Lewy declared that the vegetative nuclei of the CNS form with the posterior pituitary one single consecutive system.
1931	Cannon and Bacq described "sympathin", a hormone produced by sympathetic action on smooth muscle.
1933	Feldberg and Sir John Gaddum (London) produced evidence that acetylcholine acts in the transfer of nerve impulses from neuron to neuron in sympathetic ganglia. (J. Physiol., **80**, 12p–13p, London)
1934	Cannon discussed the chemical mediation of nerve impulses.
1936	F. H. A. Marshall referred in his Croonian Lectures to the higher animals in whom "the internal rhythm is brought

into relation with . . . other external phenomena . . . in part . . . through the NS and probably through the hypothalamus upon the anterior pituitary and thence upon the testis and the ovary . . .".

1942	Feldberg and Fessard reported on the cholinergic nature of the nerves of the electric organ of the Torpedo.
1946	Roussy and Mosinger published *Traité de Neuro-Endocrinologie*.
1949	Hoskins introduced Wiener's idea (1948) of the (servo-) feedback mechanism into the field of endocrinology.
1951	Max Reiss discussed the application of endocrine research methods in psychiatry.
1954	Bleuler published his book *Endocrine Psychiatry*.
1955	Harris discussed the relationship between endocrine activity and the development of the NS.
1956	Conference at Columbia University on "Hormones, Brain Function and Behaviour" (Proceedings edited by Hoagland).
1963	Berta and E. Scharrer summarized their work and views in their book *Neuro-Endocrinology*.
1968	Butler and Besser reported on pituitary–adrenal function in severe depressive illness.
1971	Harris' Dale Lecture on "Humours and Hormones".
1974	Bacq (Liège) published "Les transmissions chimiques de l'influx nerveux".
1975	Weitzman and colleagues demonstrated the relationship of sleep and sleep states to neuro-endocrine secretions and biological rhythms in man.

THE OVARIES

BC	In Ancient Egypt ovariotomy was performed on humans. The Ancient Jews knew that hysterectomy in cows and sows caused fattening and prevented breeding.
700–500BC	In the Old Testament (and in Ancient Rome) women were regarded unclean during the menstrual period.
384–322 BC	Aristotle described ovariotomy in sows and camels for increased growth and strength.

4th cent. BC	Herophilos described the ovaries ('female testicles').
1555 AD	Vesalius described the "female testicles".
1561	Fallopio described the tubes, ovaries, corpus luteum, hymen, clitoris and round ligaments.
1573	Coiter discussed the corpus luteum.
1621	The term "ovarium" used by Fabricius.
1651	Harvey published *De Generatione Animalium*.
1667	Stensen suggested that the female testes contained ova and should be called ovaries.
1668	Malpighi coined the term "corpus luteum".
1672	de Graaf published his studies on the female reproductive organs, described the Graafian vesicles and demonstrated ovulation.
17th and 18th cent.	Chinese iatro-chemists produced preparations of oestrogens from urine.
1775	Pott recorded cessation of menstruation after removal of two herniated ovaries in a woman of 23.
1778	von Haller described the conversion of the follicle into the corpus luteum. He coined the term "ova Graafiana".
1786	John Hunter reported on the effect on fertility after removing one ovary in a sow.
1797	Haighton described induced ovulation in rabbits.
1814	Davidge attributed menstruation "to a peculiar condition of the ovaries".
1824	Prévost and Dumas described ovulation and the formation of corpus luteum in the bitch.
1827	von Baer discovered the human ovum.
1842	Bischoff called Graafian vesicles "Graafian follicles".
1843	Martin Barry observed the spermatozoon inside the ovum.
1876	O. Hertwig demonstrated the union of sperm and ovum.
1896	Sobotta described the formation of the corpus luteum in the mouse.
1896	Knauer (Vienna) and Halban (Vienna) proved the existence of ovarian hormones (independently) by implanting ovarian tissue into castrated rabbits.
1898	Prenant and Born suspected a connection between corpus luteum and pregnancy.

1900	Heape (Cambridge) published "The 'sexual season' of mammals and the relation of the 'Pro-estrum' to menstruation".
1901	Fraenkel and Cohn studied the corpus luteum.
1905	Marshall and Jolly (England) showed that ovarian extracts produced oestrus in castrated animals.
1908	Hitschmann and Ludwig Adler (Vienna) described the cyclical changes in the endometrium as a normal physiological process.
1917	Stockard and Papanicolau introduced the vaginal smear test for oestrus.
1923	Allen and Doisy isolated oestrin.
1926	Parkes and Bellerby extracted oestrin.
1927	Allen and Doisy described withdrawal bleeding in *Macacus rhesus*.
1927	Laqueur and his team discovered female hormone (menformon) in male urine.
1928	Aschheim and B. Zondek published their pregnancy test from the female urine.
1929	Corner discovered progesterone.
1929	Marrian isolated pregnanediol.
1930	Marrian obtained crystalline oestriol.
1930	Doisy isolated crystalline oestrone from the urine of pregnant women.
1930	Collip demonstrated an anterior pituitary-like factor in the placenta.
1933	Browne obtained oestriol from the placenta.
1933	Kaufmann (Germany) used oestrogenic hormone in ovariectomized women.
1934	Butenandt obtained crystalline progesterone.
1936	MacCorquodale, Thayer and Doisy isolated oestradiol.
1938	Dodds and colleagues (London) described the first synthetic oestrogen (stilboestrol).

THE PANCREAS

1550 BC	Papyrus Ebers (discovered in 1862 AD in Thebes, Egypt) described polyuria and its treatment.

4th cent. BC	The Ayur Veda of Suśruta (India) described "sugarcream" urine which attracted ants.
3rd cent. BC	Demetrius of Apameiz described a condition resulting in diabetes.
30 BC–50 AD	Celsus described polyuria.
131–201 AD	Galen regarded diabetes as due to weakness of the kidneys (diarrhoea urinosa). The "kallikreas" (pancreas) was a protective organ guarding the great veins.
5th cent. AD	Furunculosis and TB noted as complications of diabetes mellitus (DM).
7th cent. AD	In China, Chen Chuan recorded "sweet urine" in DM. Li Hsuan wrote a monograph on DM.
860–932	Rhazes introduced a regime of treatment in DM.
1020	Avicenna mentioned a multitude of urine and noted the occurrence of impotence and furunculosis in DM.
ca. 1530	Paracelsus regarded DM as a generalized disease.
1621–1675	Willis observed the sweetness of diabetic urine which has a honied taste.
1624–1689	Sydenham regarded DM a general disease with its main site in the blood.
1642	Wirsung (Padova) discovered the pancreatic duct in the human body, shortly after Hoffmann had discovered it in a turkey.
1614–1672	Franciscus de le Boe (Sylvius) suspected that a juice was discharged from the pancreas into the intestine.
1664	Regnier de Graaf published his experiments on obtaining pancreatic juice which he found similar to salivary gland secretion.
1650	Sganarelle in Molière's Le médecin volant tasted the urine for sweetness.
1689	Morton mentioned an hereditary factor in DM.
1765	Morgagni said that DM is a disease of unknown location (morbus in sede incerta locatus).
1774	Wyatt demonstrated the presence of a substance similar to sugar in the urine as well as in the blood of diabetics.
1776	Dobson (Liverpool) published his "Experiments and observations on the urine in diabetes". He proved that the sweetness was caused by sugar which was present in the urine and in the blood (hyperglycaemia).

1788	Cawley observed that diabetes may follow injury (e.g. calculi) to the pancreas.
1797	Rollo, Surgeon-General to the British Army, described a successful meat diet in the treatment of DM.
1785–1830	Prout described diabetic coma.
1815	Chevreul proved that the sugar in DM is glucose.
1841	Trommer (Heidelberg) published his test for glucose in the urine.
1848	von Fehling described his test for sugar in the urine.
1849	Discovery of glycogen in the liver and of the "piqure diabétique" in the dog's brain by Claude Bernard. He also estimated quantitatively sugar in the blood.
1857	Petters (Berlin) isolated acetone from diabetic urine.
1869	Langerhans described the islet cells of the pancreas.
1871	Troisier described "diabète bronzé".
1874	Kussmaul explained diabetic coma to be due to aceto-naemia and described "Kussmaul's respiration".
1875	Bouchardat used the fermentation test, polariscope and copper solutions to detect DM. He invented gluten bread and used it in his "traitement hygiénique".
1876	Ebstein reported on the treatment of DM with sodium salicylate.
1877	Lancereaux connected two cases of DM causally with pancreatic calculi.
1886	von Mering produced experimental diabetes by means of phloridzin.
1889	von Recklinghausen named bronze diabetes "haemochromatosis".
1890	von Mering and Minkowski produced experimental diabetes by successful surgical removal of the pancreas of a dog.
1891	Vassale experimentally destroyed the pancreatic acini by ligation of the excretory duct without destruction of the islet cells (which was confirmed by Ssobolew in 1902).
1892	Minkowski succeeded in obtaining temporary cure of diabetes in pancreatectomized dog by subcutaneous re-implantation of the excised organ (confirmed, independently, by Hédon in Montpellier).
1893	Laguesse suggested that the islet cells produce a hormone.

1895	von Noorden presented his diet therapy of DM, using oats as part of the treatment.
1900–1901	Opie proved the association of DM with failure of the islets of Langerhans.
1902	Bayliss and Starling published the discovery of secretin.
1906	Bang described his method for the estimation of sugar in the blood.
ca. 1906	Joslin (USA) and Naunyn (Germany) improved the treatment of DM and studied diabetic acidosis.
1906	Lydia de Witt (USA) ligated the duct in cats and found that the surviving islet tissue had glycolytic properties.
1909	Jean de Meyer (Brussels) suggested the name "insuline" for the hormone of the islet cells.
1913	F. M. Allen introduced prolonged fasting for the treatment of DM.
1918	Watanabe (Japan) achieved hypoglycaemia in rabbits after injecting guanidine.
1919	Folin and Hsien Wu presented their test for blood sugar estimation.
1920	Moses Barron confirmed the experimental work of Ssobolew.
1920	Foetal hyperinsulinism was recorded in the offspring of diabetic mothers by Dubreuil and Anderodias.
1921	Paulesco reported on "pancréine", a bloodsugar lowering extract from the pancreas of animals, in June, 1921, discovered by him between 1914 and 1916.
November 1921	Banting and Best reported on the discovery of "insulin".
1922	First clinical application of insulin in the treatment of diabetes by Banting, Best, Collip, *et al.*
1923	Collip purified insulin.
1923	Murlin and his colleagues discovered pancreatic glucagon.
1924	Houssay and Magenta recorded that hypophysectomy increased sensitivity to insulin.
1926	Crystallization of insulin by J. J. Abel.
1926	Frank, Nothmann and Wagner introduced biguanides into the treatment of diabetes (abandoned 1940)
1927	Wilder, Allan, Power and Robertson reported the first case of hyperinsulinism due to carcinoma of the islands of the pancreas.

1929	Howland, Campbell, Maltby and Robinson removed an isletcell tumour achieving the first cure of hyperinsulinism.
1930	Ruiz and colleagues (Argentine) described the hypoglycaemic effect of certain sulphonamide derivatives.
1936	Hagedorn, Jensen and their colleagues introduced the first insulin with protamine to delay the absorption rate.
1937	F. G. Young discovered the anterior pituitary diabetogenic hormone (see also pituitary gland).
1937	Alloxan hyperglycaemia described by Jacobs.
1942	Janbon (Montpellier) noticed the hypoglycaemic action of a sulphonamide product.
1943	Dunn, Sheehan and MacLetchie discovered alloxan diabetes.
1944	Loubatières (Montpellier) described the mode of action of some oral hypoglycaemic agents.
1951	Hallas-Møller and his group described the first clinical trials of lente, ultralente and semilente zinc–insulin suspensions.
1953	Staub and colleagues achieved isolation of glucagon and obtained it in crystalline form.
1954	McQuarrie described idopathic hypoglycaemia in infants.
1955	Franke and Fuchs (Berlin) described the hypoglycaemic effect of the sulphonylureas.
1955	Sanger (Cambridge) published the structure formula of the bovine insulin molecule.
1955	Zollinger and Ellison described islet-cell tumour of the pancreas with peptic ulceration of the jejunum.
1956	Structure of glucagon discovered by Bromer and his colleagues.
1957	G. Ungar introduced phenetyl biguanide into the treatment of diabetes.
1957	Berson and Miss Yallow described their radioimmunological method for the measurement of plasma insulin.
1957–1958	Re-appraisal of salicylates in the treatment of diabetes by Reid and colleagues, and Hecht and Goldner.
1961–1968	Glucagon synthesized by Wunsch and his team (Munich).
1964–1966	Insulin synthesized independently by Katsoyannis (USA), Zahn (Germany) and Niu Ching-I (China).

1966	First description of pancreatic glucagonomas by McGauran, R. H. Unger and their colleagues.
1967	Steiner and Oyer isolated pro-insulin.
1969	The three-dimensional structure of pig-insulin determined by Mrs Hodgkin.
1969	Mssrs. Boehringer introduced glibencamide for the oral treatment of diabetes.
1973	Stress-release of glucagon reported by Daniel, Bloom and colleagues.
1979	Deborah Doniach and Bottazzo reported on auto-immunity in diabetes.

THE PARATHYROIDS

1852	One of the first descriptions of the parathyroids in the rhinoceros by Sir Richard Owen (London).
1880	The parathyroids in man first described by Sandström (Upsala).
1891	Gley demonstrated that the parathyroids are essential for life.
1895	Independence of the parathyroids from the thyroid stated by Kohn.
1896	Vassale and Generali (Italy) showed experimentally that tetany follows removal of the parathyroids.
1904	Askanazy (Tuebingen) connected osteitis fibrosa cystica with a parathyroid adenoma found at post-mortem.
1906	Erdheim (Vienna) described hyperplasia of parathyroids in osteomalacia in man.
1909	MacCallum and Voegtlin showed that post-parathyroidectomy tetany and hypocalcaemia can be controlled by calcium administration.
1909	Auto- and iso-transplantation of parathyroid glands in dogs by Halsted.
1914	Erdheim described compensatory parathyroid hyperplasia in spontaneous rickets in rats (secondary hyperparathyroidism).
1923	Hanson obtained the first really effective parathyroid extract from cattle.

1925	Collip isolated parathormone and with Leitch used it in the treatment of tetany.
1926	Mandl (Vienna) achieved the first cure of primary hyperparathyroidism (osteitis fibrosa) by surgical removal of a parathyroid adenoma.
1934–1948	Fuller Albright (Boston, Mass.) described the biochemistry of primary hyperparathyroidism and kidney stones as one of the important diagnostic features.
1959	Isolation of parathyroid hormone and definition of its structure as a polypeptide hormone by Rasmussen and Craig.
1962	Isolation of a hormone (Calcitonin) from the parathyroids with hypocalcaemic action by Copp and his group.
1963	Hirsch found calcitonin in the mammal thyroid.
1963	Berson introduced a radio-immunological method for estimation of parathyroid hormone in serum.
1965	The hypocalcaemic factor (calcitonin) was found to be a polypeptide hormone (Tenenhouse).
1967	Immunological methods introduced for the estimation of serum calcitonin.

THE POSTERIOR PITUITARY (NEUROHYPOPHYSIS)

1794	Johann Peter Frank distinguished diabetes insipidus (DI) from diabetes mellitus (DM).
1838	Robert Willis described several forms of DI ("hydruria", "anazoturia" and "azoturia") according to the associated excretion of urea.
1877	Samuel Gee (London) observed (?) nephrogenic diabetes insipidus.
1895	Oliver and Schaefer described the bloodpressure-raising effect (vasopressor effect) of pituitary gland extract.
1901–1908	Schaefer and his team studied the action of pituitary extract on the kidneys.
1906	Dale described the oxytocic action of posterior pituitary extract.

1908	Schaefer and Herring demonstrated a diuretic principle in the posterior pituitary. "Herring bodies" discovered.
1909	Blair Bell used posterior pituitary extract in shock, uterine atony and intestinal paresis.
1910	Foges and Hofstaetter (Vienna) used pituitrin in the treatment of post-partum haemorrhage.
1911	Ott and Scott (Philadelphia) described the milk-ejection action of infundibulin in mammals.
1912	Alfred Eric Frank connected the posterior lobe with DI.
1913	Herring confirmed the milk-ejection activity of the posterior pituitary in teleosts and amphibia.
1913	Farini (Venice) and von den Velden (Duesseldorf) reported on the antidiuretic effect of pituitary extracts.
1913	von den Velden also reported on the treatment of a patient with DI with posterior pituitary extract.
1921	Brunn (Vienna) discovered a hydrosmotic action of posterior pituitary extract in the frog.
1924	Starling and Verney demonstrated the antidiuretic effect of posterior pituitary extracts on the isolated kidney.
1925	Hogben observed the avian depressor activity of posterior pituitary extract.
1928	Kamm and his team isolated vasopressin and oxytocin.
1940–1947	Heller's studies of the antidiuretic (AD) principle in numerous non-mammalian species (elasmobranch, teleost, amphibian, reptile).
1947	Verney postulated osmoreceptors in the anterior hypothalamus for the release of ADH.
1947	Richardson (London) confirmed Ott's and Scott's results in the goat.
1951	Bergmann and Scharrer described the site of origin of the posterior pituitary hormones in the nuclei of the hypothalamus.
1953	du Vigneaud and his group synthesized oxytocin.
1954	du Vigneaud and his group synthesized vasopressin.
1963	Dashe, Cramm, Crist, Habener and Solomon described the water deprivation test for the diagnosis of polyuria.
1966	Klein, Roth and Petersen described a radioimmunoassay (RIA) for arginin vasopressin (ADH).

THE TESTICLES

Pre-historic times	Castration (human and animal) known.
ca. 2737–1600 BC	The *Pen Tsao* (Great Herbal) recommended the use of semen of young men for treatment of sexual weakness in men.
1600 BC	Important role of eunuchs in ancient China at Court and in the Civil Service.
5th cent. BC	Taoism believed that the brain was the source of sperm.
ca. 1300–650 BC	In the Old Testament the human and animal testicle had different names.
	In the Bible, castrates and eunuchs were known. Eunuchoids were called "Sun castrates"; (also by the Egyptians).
	In the Old Testament (and in Egypt) married eunuchs were known (e.g. the husband of Potiphar).
	Stress, distress, disease, fatigue and starvation diminished the amount of sperm according to the Bible.
	The Talmud used the same name for testicle and ovary. Hermaphrodites were known and described.
ca. 460–400 BC	Hippocrates wrote "On the Seed". He also knew that mumps can be followed by orchitis and sterility.
384–322 BC	Aristotle wrote on the sperm. He said that the semen was the formative, activating agent or "soul", the female element being the passive soil to be fertilized. The right testicle produced male offspring, the left, female. He knew the effects of castration and its use in husbandry.
23–79 AD	Pliny recommended eating of animal testicles to improve sexual function in men.
2nd cent. AD	Aretaeus taught that it is the semen which turns youths into men.
777–837 AD	Mesuë the Elder prescribed testicles as an aphrodisiac and in the treatment of pulmonary tuberculosis.
1132 AD	Hsu Shu-Wei (China) used desiccated pig testicles for the treatment of spermatorrhoea, hypogonadism and impotence.
ca. 1250 AD	Albertus Magnus recommended the powdered testicles of a hog in wine for men of poor sexual power.
1626	Jean Riolan the Younger described the seminiferous tubules.

1651	Highmore described the mediastinum testis.
1668	de Graaf gave an accurate account of testicular structure and of the seminiferous tubes. He also practised ligation of the vas deferens.
1677	Leeuwenhoek and Ham discovered the spermatozoa.
17th and 18th cent.	Chinese iatro-chemists produced preparations of androgens from urine.
1745–50	von Haller described the rete testis.
1771	John Hunter mentioned his testicular transplant experiments.
1775	de Bordeu stated that the male gonad formed an internal secretion which he regarded identical with the semen.
1780	Spallanzani carried out artificial insemination in various animals.
1786	Accurate description of the testis by J. Hunter.
1790	John Hunter suggested artificial insemination in man.
1830	Astley Cooper published his *Observations on the Structure and Diseases of the Testis.*
1841	Koelliker demonstrated the cellular origin of the spermatozoa.
1849	Berthold showed that transplant of a cock's testis prevented atrophy of the comb after castration.
1850	Leydig described the interstitial cells (in animal testes).
1854	Koelliker demonstrated the Leydig cells in man.
1865	Schweigger-Seidl proved that the spermatozoon possessed a nucleus and cytoplasm.
1889	Brown-Séquard reported on the effect of testicular extract injections on himself.
1891	Poehl (Russia) isolated "spermin" from the testis.
1911	Pézard produced an effective testicular extract.
1920	Steinach ligated the vas deferens to rejuvenate the ageing "puberty gland".
1923	Voronoff (Algiers) reported on his rejuvenation experiments by means of testicular implants of monkey glands.
1927	McGee obtained an active extract of male hormone from bull testicles.

1929	Moore, Gallagher and Koch described the capon–comb test for the assay of male hormone.
1929	Funk and Harrow obtained active male hormone from male urine.
1931	Butenandt isolated androsterone in crystalline form.
1933	Hodgson Boggon (England) described true polyorchidism.
1934	Ruzicka and his team synthesized androsterone.
1935	Laqueur and colleagues isolated testosterone from the testis.
1942	Klinefelter's syndrome described by Klinefelter, Reifenstein and Albright.
1973	Lazerda and colleagues studied circadian variations of plasma testosterone in normal men.
1979	Male infertility due to auto-immunity to sperm discussed by Hendry (London).

THE THYROID

1600 BC	The Chinese used burnt sponge and seaweed for the treatment of goitre.
4th cent. BC	The Ayur Veda (India) discussed goitre.
ca. 50 BC	Caesar spoke of big neck among the Gauls as one of their characteristics.
30 BC to 50 AD	Egyptian relief of Cleopatra showing goitre.
30 BC to 50 AD	Celsus defined bronchocoele (a tumour of the neck) and described cystic goitre and its surgery.
30 BC to 50 AD	Catullus referred to the woman's honeymoon enlargement of the neck.
30 BC to 50 AD	Pliny, Vitruvius and Juvenal referred to epidemics of goitre in the Alps and mentioned burnt seaweed.
98–138 AD	Soranus noted swelling of the neck after pregnancy.
130–200 AD	Galen also mentioned spongia usta for treatment of goitre. He regarded the thyroid as a lubricant for the larynx.
340 AD	Ko Hung (China) recommended seaweed for goitre.
625–690 AD	Paul of Aegina discussed two varieties of bronchocoele and recommended surgical treatment for one of them.
ca. 650 AD	Sun Ssu-Mo used combined seaweed, dried powdered mollusc shells and thyroid gland (organotherapy) for goitre.

ca. 990 AD	Ali–ibn–Abbas discussed surgery of goitre.
ca. 1050 AD	Albucasis mentioned operation for "elephantiasis" of the throat.
1110 AD	Jurjani's "Treasure of Medicine" connected exophthalmos with goitre.
12th cent.	The Bamberg Surgery described removal of goitre by surgery.
1235–1311	Arnold of Villanova recommended burnt sponge and seaweed for the treatment of goitre.
1271	Marco Polo reported on goitre in the Province of Karkan.
1330	Hu Ssu-Hui wrote that seaweed will cure goitre.
ca. 1345	Guy de Chauliac considered goitre a local and hereditary disease.
1475	Wang Hei described the thyroid gland and recommended treatment for goitre by taking dried thyroid.
ca. 1530	Paracelsus attributed goitre to mineral impurities in drinking water. He also realised the connection between cretinism, endemic goitre and congenital idiocy.
1543	Vesalius described the "Glandes laryngis radici adnatae".
1562	Realdus Columbus noted that women's thyroids are larger than men's.
ca. 1560	Josias Simmler ⎫
ca. 1560	Johannes Stumpf ⎬ described cretins in Swiss cantons.
ca. 1560	Ambroise Paré regarded exophthalmic goitre as examples of aneurysm.
1563	Eustachius used the term "isthmus" for the part connecting the two thyroid lobes.
1602	Platter described cretinism in his native Canton.
ca. 1606	Shakespeare mentioned goitre in *The Tempest*.
1656	Wharton's description of the thyroid.
1657	Hoefer (Vienna) discussed the cause of goitre by air, water and food.
1657	First reference to bronchocoele in English by Tomlinson.
1659	Wharton used the term "thyroid" in his "Adenographia".
ca. 1730	Ruysch (Leyden) thought that produce of the thyroid poured into the veins.
1742	Heister described surgical removal of goitre.

1752	de Bordeu's observations on goitre in the Pyrenees.
1761	Morgagni described the two glands in the neck connected by an isthmus.
1769	Prosser described treatment and cure of Derby Neck with a powder of calcined sponge.
1776	von Haller grouped thyroid, thymus and spleen as glands without ducts pouring their fluid into the circulation. He also used the word struma in its modern (German) sense.
1779	Bate and later Wilmer used the "Coventry treatment" to cure bronchocoele by means of burnt sponge.

1722	de Saint-Yves	described patients with exophthalmos and palpitations without realizing the connection.
1800	Testa	
1802	Flajani	

1786–1820	(published posthumously in 1825) Parry (Bath) observed and first described correctly exophthalmic goitre (Parry's disease).
1786	de Saussure described goitrous cretinism in the Alps.
1789	Malacarne reported on endemic goitre in the Aosta valley.
1792	Desault (Paris) described successful surgical removal of part of the thyroid.
1792	Fodéré's "Essai sur le goître et le crétinage" published.
ca. 1800	Dupuytren (Paris) described effect of pressure of goitre on the windpipe.
ca. 1800	Benjamin Smith Barton's "Memoir concerning the disease of goiter as it prevails in different parts of North America".
1802	The brothers Wenzel classified cretinism.
1802	Flajani (Rome) reported on successful treatment of two patients with exophthalmic goitre (without realizing the connection).
1811	Courtois (Paris) discovered iodine in ashes of seaweed.
1812	Coates successfully ligated the superior thyroid arteries.
1819	Prout claimed (in 1834) that he first recommended iodine for the treatment of goitre at St. Thomas's Hospital.
1820	Coindet (Geneva) first used iodine in the treatment of goitre.

1822	Hedenus reported on six successful excisions of goitre since 1800.
1829	Lugol recommended the use of Lugol's solution.
1833	Boussingault (Paris) suggested iodized salt for goitre prevention.
1835	Graves published his account of exophthalmic goitre.
1840	von Basedow described the "Merseburg triad".
1844	Johannes Mueller called the thyroid a "bloodgland".
1848	Morris described the only instance of endemic cretinism in England, in Chiselborough (Somerset).
1849	Dalrymple's eye sign reported by White Cooper.
1850	Curling (London) described defective cerebral development due to absence of thyroid body.
1850	Chatin (France) showed that endemic goitre and cretinism could be prevented by the iodine content of plants.
1859	Rilliet (Geneva) described toxic effects of the use of iodine.
1860	Boussingault's experiment in France to use iodized salt for the prevention of goitre failed because high dosage given caused toxic effects.
1864	von Graefe described "Graefe's sign" in exophthalmic goitre.
1871	Fagge (London) described sporadic cretinism.
1873	Gull gave a classical account of myxoedema in women.
1878	Ord coined the term "myxoedema".
1880	Rehn carried out the first thyroidectomy in exophthalmic goitre.
1884–1886	Horsley confirmed Semon's postulates and so did a committee of which he was a member.
1886	Moebius postulated that exophthalmic goitre is due to hyperfunction of the thyroid.
1891	Murray reported on his successful treatment of myxoedema with thyroid extract.
1895–1896	Baumann (Germany) isolated "thyrojodin" (later called "iodothyrin") from the thyroid.
1896	Pendred described the association of goitre with deaf-mutism.
1896	Description of Riedel's thyroiditis.

1896	Charcot described exophthalmic goitre as "cachexia exophthalmica" and stressed tremor as one of the signs.
1897–1925	Oswald's studies of the iodine content of the thyroid.
1907	Charles Mayo first used the term "hyperthyroidism".
1907	Brissaud described thyroid infantilism.
1909	Marine proved that iodine is necessary for thyroid function.
1910	Kocher coined the term "Jod-Basedow".
1910	Marine and Lenhart prevented goitre formation in animal experiments by using iodine.
1911	Marine proposed treatment of Graves' disease with iodine.
1912	Hashimoto's disease (struma lymphomatosa) described.
1912	Gudernatsch observed the acceleration of metamorphosis in tadpoles by feeding thyroid.
1914	Kendall isolated thyroxine in crystalline form.
1915	Cannon produced exophthalmic goitre experimentally.
1917	Marine and Kimball reported on their successful revival of iodide prophylaxis of goitre in Akron, Ohio, USA.
1918	Hermann Zondek published his studies of the heart in myoedema.
1924	Plummer and Boothby reported on the pre-operative use of iodine in exophthalmic goitre.
1926	Harington determined the chemical structure of thyroxine.
1927	Harington and Barger synthesized thyroxine.
1928	Webster and Chesney observed endocrine goitre in rabbits.
1931	Naffziger introduced orbital decompression for treatment of exophthalmos.
1932	Marine described cyanide goitre.
1943	Hertz and Roberts ⎫ introduced radioactive iodine for the assessment of Graves'
1943	Leblond (independently) ⎬ disease and, later, for its treatment.
1943	Astwood used thiourea and thiouracil in the medical treatment of Graves' disease.
1949	Jones, Kornfeld, McLaughlin and Anderson synthesized methimazole.

1949	Commercial synthesis of laevo-thyroxine was achieved.
1951	Lawson, Rimington and Searle synthesized carbimazole.
1953	Gross and Rosalind Pitt-Rivers isolated tri-iodothyronine from the thyroid gland and synthesized it (lio-thyronine).
1956	Roitt, Deborah Doniach *et al.* demonstrated auto-antibodies in Hashimoto's disease.
1956	Adams, Purves and McKenzie discovered LATS in the serum of thyrotoxic patients.
1965	Mass neonatal screening programme was started in Switzerland for metabolic disorders.
1974	Thomas and Hart introduced retrobulbar repository corticosteroid therapy in thyroid ophthalmopathy.
1972–1978	Screening begun for neonatal (congenital) hypothyroidism in USA, Canada, England, Japan and some other countries.

POSTSCRIPT

Several items of information obtained during the course of production of the book are given below.

ENDOCRINE HORMONE PRODUCTION BY NON-ENDOCRINE TUMOURS
(see also p. 548)

Hormones secreted by tumours of tissues other than those normally responsible for their synthesis are called 'ectopic', which term was coined by G. W. Liddle and his colleagues[1], during their studies between 1962 and 1965. Their existence may indicate the neoplasm long before other manifestations. The tumour may not necessarily be malignant, such as a bronchial carcinoid. Removal of the tumour may mean disappearance of the ectopic hormone production; recurrence may cause return of such secretion. The cause and mechanism of this phenomenon has not been finally established yet.

There are, at present, nearly twenty such ectopically produced hormones known, some identical with the natural hormones in a wide variety of biological and immunological procedures. The most important is perhaps the ectopic ACTH syndrome. W. H. Brown described in 1928 a patient with Cushing's syndrome and bilateral adrenal cortical hyperplasia[2]; after his death an oat cell carcinoma of the bronchus was found in the post-mortem examination. Usually, β-Melanocyte-stimulating-hormone is also secreted in excess with excessive ACTH production causing the pigmentation.

Apart from the oat cell carcinomas, bronchial adenomas (carcinoid tumours) and tumours of the thymus and pancreas and, rarely, others may cause the ectopic ACTH syndrome. Bronchial carcinomas can also produce excessive vasopressin, such inappropriate secretion causing excretion of hypertonic urine (high rate of sodium excretion), in spite of hypotonic plasma and expanded extracellular fluid volume, and water retention[3].

853

Finally, tumours have been described which secreted two or more hormones. They were mainly oat cell carcinomas and bronchial carcinoids.

References

1. Liddle, G. W., Givens, J. R., Nicholson, W. E., Island, D. P.: Cancer Res., **25,** 1057; 1965
2. Brown, W. H.: Lancet, **2,** 1022; 1928
3. Bartter, F. C., Schwartz, W. B.: Am. J. Med., **42,** 790; 1967

THE PANCREAS AS A SINGLE ORGAN

The present trend of endocrine research points towards integration in medicine rather than towards segregation into subspecialities. The recognition of the brain as 'master gland' is just one indicator.

Recently, evidence has been accumulating that the endocrine and exocrine parts of the pancreas are not independent of each other, but are, in fact, functionally related. Microsphere injections in the living rabbit's pancreas proved that blood flows from the islets to the exocrine gland[1]. Insulin increased the flow of pancreatic juice and amylase release in the isolated, perfused rat pancreas[2]. In insulin-requiring diabetics, the plasma concentration of trypsin was found to be about one quarter of that in normal subjects[3]. J. R. Henderson, P. M. Daniel and P. A. Fraser (London) summed up the results of the studies on the vascular anatomy of the pancreas, on the effect of insulin and of glucagon on exocrine function, on the effect of pancreatic polypeptide (PP) as an inhibitor of the exocrine gland and, finally, the 'Halo' phenomenon around islets (which could be abolished by alloxan), in the following table:

Islet hormone	Effect on function of exocrine pancreas
Insulin	Increases uptake of amino acids Increases synthesis of amylase (independently from effect on amino acids) Increases cell division Is necessary for normal release of bicarbonate
Glucagon	Inhibits synthesis of enzymes Inhibits release of enzymes Stimulates release of bicarbonate
Somatostatin	Inhibits the production of pancreatic juice
Pancreatic polypeptide	Inhibits release of enzymes

References

1. Lipson, N., Kramlinger, K. G., Mayrand, R. R., Lender, E. Jane: Blood flow to the rabbit pancreas with special reference to the islets of Langerhans. Gastroenterology: **79,** 466–73; 1980
2. Saito, A., Williams, J. A., Kanno, T.: Potentiation of cholecystokinin-induced exocrine secretion by both exogenous and endogenous insulin in isolated and perfused rat pancreata. J. Clin. Invest.: **65,** 777–82; 1980.
3. Adrian, T. E., Barnes, A. J., Bloom, S.R.: Hypotrypsinaemia in diabetes mellitus. Clin Chim. Acta: **97,** 213–16; 1979
4. Henderson, J. R., Daniel, P. M., Fraser, F. A.: The pancreas as a single organ: the influence of the endocrine upon the exocrine part of the gland. Gut: **22,** 158–67; 1981.

HASHIMOTO, HAKARU 1881–1934

Hashimoto was born in the village of Midau, Nishi-tsuge, in the Mie prefecture in Japan, on 5th May, 1881. He was the fifth generation of medical practitioners and his grandfather was a well known physician. After attending his village school and other schools for higher education, he entered the newly established medical school of Kyushu University in 1903. As a student he was reputed to be diligent and had an unassuming manner. He was also one of the founders of a student's cultural society; he was a religious Buddhist. He graduated in 1907 as one of the first medical graduates of his university. From 1908 to 1912 he worked in Kyushu in the surgical department of Professor H. Miyake on his MD thesis on a hitherto unknown condition: 'Struma lymphomatosa (see Chap, 21, p. 571). He published it in Germany, which caused it to go unnoticed in Japan.

Next, Hashimoto spent two years on a European tour, in Germany and London, but returned home at the outbreak of World War I. The death of his father made him take up practice and he became a much thought after surgeon with an interest in major abdominal surgery. He published another two papers, on erysipelas and one on penetrating wounds. He died of typhoid fever in January, 1934. He was buried in his home county. In 1937, the local Physicians' Association placed a bronze bust of him in front of the town hall of the village where he is buried.

MARRIAN, GUY FREDERIC 1904–1981

Guy Frederic Marrian was born on 3rd March, 1904 and educated at Tollington School and University College, London (England), where he became BSc with honours in 1925. In 1930 he proceeded to DSc and in the same year he became lecturer in the Department of Biochemistry at University College under Sir Jack Drummond. At University College, he had begun his work on oestrin, which subtance produces oestrus in animals, and in 1929 he obtained the isolation of crystalline oestriol from human pregnancy urine. His work was virtually single-handed (see p. 400), leading in a competitive field of German, Dutch and American research teams. He was disbelieved, but later his results were fully vindicated!

In 1933, Marrian became first Associate then Professor of Biochemistry at the University of Toronto, where he continued work on oestrogens. In 1939, he was appointed Professor of Chemistry in relation to Medicine at the University of Edinburgh as successor to George Barger, himself of thyroxine research fame. He remained there for 20 years and at the beginning of the 1950s established, with Gaddum and Dunlop, the Medical Research Council's Endocrinology Research Unit in Edinburgh, which became a centre for steroid biochemists and endocrinologists. In 1959, he was appointed Director of Research of the Imperial Cancer Research Fund in London, where he remained until he retired in 1968. His profound knowledge of the sex hormones and of steroid biochemistry put the Imperial Cancer Research Laboratories into the lead of fundamental biochemical cancer research.

He had a delightful personality, great charm, good sense of humour and perfect manners. At the same time, he had a clarity of thought and did not tolerate superficial or shoddy work. He himself was a superb and indefatigable bench worker, whose example was both forceful and inspiring. Marrian's hopes for the creation of a multidisciplinary research laboratory were, eventually, fulfilled, alas for the benefit of his successors, not for himself. He was also an excellent teacher, who carried out these duties most conscientiously, even as regards courses for junior medical students. He himself was presentable, well dressed, quietly mannered, popular with colleagues and students. When young, he was a good athlete and would have become a sprinter of international standard, had he turned to sport instead of biochemistry.

Marrian became a Fellow of the Royal Society of London in 1944, an Honorary MD Edinburgh in 1975 and was created CBE (Commander of the Most Excellent Order of the British Empire) in 1969. His name will remain in chemistry in the form of 'marrianolic acid', an oestriol derivative. The Germans marked his 70th birthday by arranging a special meeting in Berlin. The British Society of Endocrinology organized a meeting in London in 1980, to mark the 50th anniversary of his discovery of oestriol. He died on 24th July, 1981.

NEUBURGER, MAX 1868–1955

Max Neuburger was born in Vienna in December, 1868, the son of Ferdinand. His father was a brilliant linguist, a native of Munich, who came to Vienna as a young man and settled there. Max studied medicine in Vienna at the time of Billroth, Nothnagel, Krafft-Ebing, Fuchs and Politzer. He qualified in 1893. In 1896 he became Assistant at the Poliklinik to Mortiz Benedikt, the neurologist, and remained with him until 1908. He practised as a neurologist until 1914. During the war of 1914–1918 he was in charge of several military hospitals; the end of the war marked the end of his active clinical career.

Already as a student, he had published short historical–philosophical articles, encouraged by Theodor Puschmann, who held the chair of History of Medicine. Neuburger published his major thesis for 'Privat-Docent' in 1897, a history of experimental physiology of the brain and the spinal cord from Willis to Fleurens and Magendie. He proceeded to 'Docent' in 1898. The other Privat-Docent was his friend Robert Ritter von Töply, a military surgeon, who eventually became the Austrian equivalent of Director General Medical Services, Army. He wrote the long section on Anatomy in the famous *Handbuch der Geschichte der Medizin*. After Puschmann's death in 1899, Neuburger and Töply carried on the teaching, but Puschmann's wish to found an Institute for the History of Medicine did not come to fruition, especially as his widow left a large sum of money towards the foundation of such an institute in Leipzig, which was achieved in 1905 with Sudhoff as director. Neuburger became professor extraordinary in 1904 and ordinary professor for the history of medicine in 1912. From then on his work has to be considered in two parts:

(1) Writings: He became editor of the monumental *Handbuch* originally planned by Puschmann, jointly with Julius Pagel of Berlin. The first volume, to the Middle Ages, was published in 1902. The second and third volumes, dealing with the histories of individual subjects, appeared in 1903 and 1905. Neuburger's long introduction to the second volume marked an important contribution. His own 'History of Medicine' achieved the publication of the first volume in 1906 and of the second, to the close of the Middle Ages, in 1910. He never finished the work. He was preparing a section on the Renaissance in 1920. An English translation was sponsored by Osler from 1910–1925. It was meant for the general reader and was very thorough, but had only a few references. Other studies concerned the biography of Hermann Nothnagel and many contributions to the history of the Vienna medical school. In 1926 was published his

major book on the 'vis medicatrix naturae'. Having given up clinical medicine, he found himself in poor financial straits, especially after the war ended in 1918.

(2) The long drawn out struggle against great odds to establish an Institute for the History of Medicine made progress when, in 1919, he was given three rooms in the historical building of the 'Josephinum', originally a training school for army surgeons. Töply, although no longer an active participant, gave 1000 books and reprints. Later the Library of the Josephinum and the magnificent collection of 1200 medical wax models were transferred to the Institute, which is still housed in the same building. Needless to say, Neuburger's own library is incorporated.

On his 60th birthday a "Festschrift" was issued in his honour and his portrait medal was struck in Vienna. In 1930, Garrison published 12 of his studies in English.

At the age of 70, he had to leave Vienna, after Hitler's occupation of Austria. On 26th August, 1939, he arrived in London on the last plane, with two suitcases and 5 shillings, to join the scientific staff of the Wellcome Historical Medical Museum. His wife had died in 1930, his elder son had gone to Tasmania, the younger to the United States, where he entered medical practice in Buffalo. Neuburger stayed in London throughout the war, in spite of the bombs and a major operation he had to undergo. He began to write in English, his most important contribution being a book: *British Medicine and the Vienna School: Contrasts and Parallels*. He carried on his studies, although now very deaf and myopic. In 1948, aged 80, he left London for Buffalo, to live with his son. In 1952, he left Buffalo, aged 83, and returned to Vienna to a cordial welcome. At the end of 1953, he fell at home and fractured his femur, which made him an invalid to the end of his life. However, he still carried on some research. Neuburger died in Vienna after a long illness on the 15th March, 1955, in his 87th year.

During his lifetime, Dr. Emanuel Berghoff published a biography of Max Neuburger in Vienna. The Royal Society of Medicine of London made him an honorary Fellow on 1st December, 1943 and arranged an exhibition of his books and papers on the occasion of his 75th birthday. Walter Pagel said about Neuburger that he was the last exponent of the 'heroic' generation of medical historians: Julius Pagel (1851–1912), Karl Sudhoff (1853–1938) and Neuburger. 'Heroic' because of the stupendous achievements against heavy odds, when historical studies were frowned on and the subject was not recognized for university teaching, departments or research grants. As his life's motto may be given 'Primum philosophare, deinde vivere.'

He left behind a flourishing Institute for the History of Medicine of the University of Vienna and his successors gave every help towards the completion of this book. Their names are mentioned in the Acknowledgments.

SAJOUS, CHARLES EUCHARISTE DE MEDICI 1852–1929

Charles Sajous (see photograph p. 792) was born at sea when his family returned from America to France. After early schooling in France, he studied medicine in California and graduated from the Jefferson Medical College of Philadelphia. He first specialized in diseases of the nose and throat and his early papers were on that subject.

At the end of the 1880s he became Editor-in-Chief of the monumental *Annual of the Universal Medical Sciences* of 45 volumes between 1888–1896, followed in 1898 by *Sajous Analytic Cyclopaedia of Practical Medicine* (60 volumes).

In 1892, he suddenly devoted himself to the study of internal secretions, especially in France. This resulted in the publication of *The Internal Secretions and the Principles of Medicine* in 1903 (Philadelphia, F. A. Davis Co.), the first book on the subject in the United States, to which he added a second volume in 1907. The work went into ten editions. He propounded some interesting theories of his own, particularly concerned with the role of the adrenal system and the body's defence (immune) mechanisms including the leukocytes, a very modern idea but not seriously accepted at the time.

He became the first president of the Association for the Study of the Internal Secretions (1916–1917). At the age of almost 70 he became the first professor of endocrinology in the United States: Professor of Applied Endocrinology in the University of Pennsylvania Graduate School of Medicine.

In the 1920s (to 1925) he was also Editor of the *New York Medical Journal* (1865–1925). His son Louis Theo also specialized in endocrinology.

Sajous died in the United States in 1929.

NAME INDEX

B indicates Biography; R indicates a reference

882

SUBJECT INDEX